CHOLESTEATOMA

FIRST INTERNATIONAL CONFERENCE

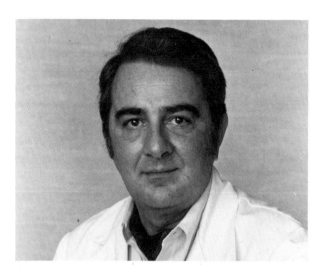

Brian F. McCabe, M. D.

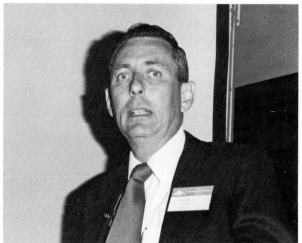

Jacob Sade, M. D.

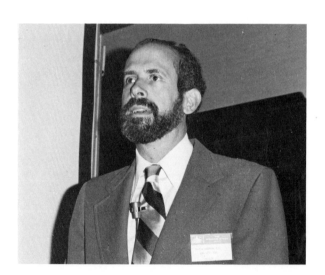

Maxwell Abramson, M. D.

CHOLESTEATOMA

FIRST INTERNATIONAL CONFERENCE

An interdisciplinary consideration of the etiology, basic mechanisms, pathophysiology, and management of aural cholesteatoma.

Brian F. McCabe, M. D.
Professor and Chairman
Department of Otolaryngology and Maxillofacial Surgery
The University of Iowa
Iowa City, Iowa

Jacob Sade, M. D.
Chief, E. N. T. Department, Meir Hospital
Kfar Saba, Israel
Consultant, Polymer Department, Weizmann Institute of Science
Rehovot, Israel

Maxwell Abramson, M. D.
Associate Professor
Department of Otolaryngology and Maxillofacial Surgery
The University of Iowa
Iowa City, Iowa

AESCULAPIUS PUBLISHING COMPANY
Birmingham, Alabama
U. S. A.

Aesculapius Publishing Company
903 South 21st Street
Birmingham, Alabama 35205

Distributors for Europe and Middle East
Shimon Kugler
Medical Publishers b. v.
P. O. Box 516, Amstelveen 1134,
The Netherlands

Copyright 1977, by AESCULAPIUS PUBLISHING COMPANY
Library of Congress Catalog Card Number 76-42368
International Standard Book Number 0-912684-11-9.

Printed in the United States of America

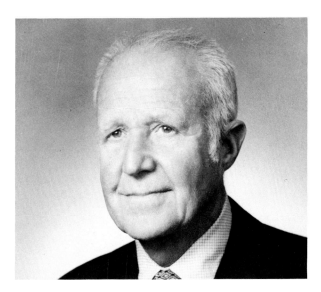

George E. Shambaugh, Jr., M.D.

Dedicated to George E. Shambaugh, Jr., M.D., in recognition of his numerous and valuable contributions to clinical and basic otology, in appreciation of the wisdom and guidance he has provided for hundreds of otolaryngologists, and in recognition of his preeminence in continuing otologic education.

PREFACE

So far as we know, an international conference devoted exclusively to aural cholesteatoma has never before been held. Forty-one speakers from 26 countries participated in this meeting and their contributions have resulted in this book.

That such a conference was held in Iowa City, or indeed held at all, was due to several interesting coincidences. The first: at the Bristol, England meeting of the Collegium ORLAS in 1974, Dr. Jack Duval, a previous Fellow at Iowa, inquired if any visiting professorships were available at Iowa. Since there were, he introduced a man to me that I had never met though whose fine work I knew quite well—Dr. Jacob Sadé. He was planning his sabbatical leave, and he expressed polite interest in coming to Iowa, but obviously was thinking of a larger medical center in a megacity. The second: he was flying to Chicago for a special NIH conference the following month, and could spend a day with us. After visiting our University and Department, he accepted a Visiting Professorship from us. The third: on our staff was Dr. Maxwell Abramson, an authority on the basic mechanisms of cholesteatoma. Since Dr. Sadé had been deeply interested in cholesteatoma during his entire medical career, these two authorities discussed this subject intensively during the next few months. When they presented to me the idea of a conference on cholesteatoma, I pointed out the danger of committing the Department's resources to a meeting of this magnitude, off the beaten path in a discipline already over-rich in meetings and conferences. However, the discussions continued and it became evident that Dr. Sadé had been consciously or subconsciously planning such a meeting for years. The organization, topics and speakers he listed so impressively signalled the ample thought and extensive research already given to this idea. Dr. Abramson, from his knowledge of this field and research associates, ably arranged most of the basic science considerations. I became convinced that this would be a landmark conference on cholesteatoma. The commitment was made and the diligent work began.

Throughout the long planning months, Dr. Sadé was the guiding light. He became involved in all facets of the program—advertising, program balance, proper depth, selecting the proper speaker for the correct subject, program timing, entertainment, special menus—inspiring us all to greater achievement. During this exciting time, and throughout the meeting, there was a marvelous sense of troika: although each of us had certain areas of ultimate responsibility, decisions were made jointly. Yet, the fact stands out quite clearly that without Jacob Sadé, there would not have been a cholesteatoma conference.

Brian F. McCabe, M.D.

FOREWORD

The conference began with the introduction of the guest of honor, George E. Shambaugh, Jr., M.D., the father of aural microsurgery (although he modestly gives this credit to Holmgren), and probably our era's greatest teacher of ear surgery. His job was the hardest of all: to attempt in the final panel to apply what we learned during the conference to cholesteatoma management.

We wanted to have another honor guest, a special one, whose name may not be so familiar to residents and young otologists but which was for decades virtually synonymous with the term cholesteatoma—Mr. Frank McGuckin, F.R.C.S. For medical reasons he could not travel the distance from Newcastle-upon-Tyne to Iowa City, but sent a delightful letter so typifying the spirit of this conference that I insisted on his permission to read parts of it into the minutes of the meeting.

"May an old duffer, now long retired, say how welcome was your almost nostalgic letter? Of course, you must accept my best wishes for the success of the 'First International Conference on Cholesteatoma,' if only because some future conference may herald the final interment of a term bequeathed to us by Virchow, then of Wurtzburg, about 120 years ago. You mention that 'cholesteatoma and the name McGuckin have been virtually synonymous for many decades.' Now it is true, at the Royal Society of Medicine in London, I made a tentative but also serious effort to abolish the traditional terminology, because of my belief that it led to inexact thinking and false logic. The 'cholest' part of the word seemed inacceptable, since cholesterol was no essential element in the entity, if it is an entity. Moreover, it is not an 'oma' in the accepted sense of that suffix from the Greek. Unquestionably, I was on a hiding to nothing, so that my trial balloon, of about 1952 or 53, proved too outrageously unorthodox to stand a chance. My thesis was greeted, not with encouragement and still less with acclamation, but with something close to derision. Today I must admit that one of my objectives was to stir up howls of derision and ever since then, I have found the injection of a liberal dose of poison into any discussion to be a most effective remedy for platitudinous boredom.

"My last performance about this subject on the London platform was perhaps 10 years ago, in discussion of a paper presented by Brian Pickard and the late Sir Terence Cawthorne. These two were very old friends of mine but they were given ample notice that my remarks would be derogatory, not to say hostile (which possibly they were), because they had adopted certain fashionable views about congenital rests here, there and everywhere inside the middle ear, ideas propounded mainly by some of the younger chaps in Chicago.

"Now Hal Schuknecht had discussed the terminological problem with me from time to time over the years and I think with a certain amount of pity for a fellow who must be a crank. It must have been in Edinburgh about 1971 that we had our last contretemps and his change of view, moderate though it was, proved balm to my soul. In the recent edition of his text-book, the term keratoma had been substituted for cholesteatoma. I agreed that the 'kera' was suitable but it was still not an 'oma.'

"There was also the dogma that cholesteatoma destroyed tissues because of its pressure. Here was a notion quite unacceptable to any clinician who listened to the stories told by patients, not all of whom could be dismissed as poor witnesses and even fewer as deliberate liars. For several decades a patient may unwittingly have suffered a slow destruction of the middle ear cleft, and even beyond, to the point that the whole labyrinth may have been eliminated; if pressure be the cause of so much havoc, how can such a person still retain perfect function in the facial nerve?* Furthermore, I see no essential difference between non-malignant destruction of the external auditory canal and similar changes inside the middle ear cleft—and both these insidious lesions may be unappreciated by the subject until some additional pathology causes a crisis. In parenthesis I should add that, in my terminology, keratosis obturans was abandoned many years ago, since keratosis in the auditory canal may be present for months, and indeed for years, before it comes to act as an obturator. For similar reasons, 'external otitis' was dismissed because it was a term covering a multitude of external auditory sins.

"I would be most happy to drink to a toast celebrating the demise of the word cholesteatoma. Moreover, I would love to look down from 'elsewhere' if, after another conference or two, or three, the grand toast could celebrate the final elimination of this pestilential bit of pathology from the ears of the human race.

"Since I cannot take part in your First Conference on Cholesteatoma, I have felt it proper to write about something of the past, of what is for you an age of unreason, as your age will be so judged not so many years ahead. 'Sic transit gloria mundi,' but do not be abashed by the knowledge that it must be so."

His thoughts typify what we have tried to build into this conference: a spirit of critical analysis, of self-criticism, of transition. If Dr. Shambaugh is our guest-of-honor in person, let Mr. McGuckin be our guest-of-honor in spirit.

Brian F. McCabe, M.D.

---

*Editor's Note: A clear example of Mr. McGuckin's prescience. We now know that pressure is not a significant factor in bone destruction in this disease, but that it occurs primarily by enzymatic digestion.

ACKNOWLEDGEMENTS

It is obvious that the organizing co-chairmen could never have mounted a meeting of this complexity without a strong and dedicated staff. They are particularly grateful to Mr. James Good, Administrator of the Department of Otolaryngology and Maxillofacial Surgery, and Mrs. Marie Matthes. Mr. Good quickly realized the importance of the success of the conference to the Department, the Medical Center and the University, and immediately brought his unique abilities to bear on making a smooth flow of every aspect, especially during the four climactic May days. The excellence of the overall coordination of the meeting itself in terms of the scientific sessions and the evening entertainments is a tribute to him and his staff. Especially deserving of citation here is Mrs. Patricia Edberg. Mrs. Matthes bore the great burden of early correspondence among us and the many participants as the idea of the conference crystallized, along with her regular load as chief secretary of a large Department. Also, she bore the responsibility for innumerable organizational details with her usual equanimity and many helpful suggestions.

Our wives deserve our special thanks for helping us with our planning, and when we decided to go forward with our international conference, they had little time to organize the social part of the program. Yet, we are told by most of our registrants, that this was "the best part of the meeting".

We salute them all.

Jacob Sadé, M.D.
Maxwell Abramson, M.D.
Brian F. McCabe, M.D.
Co-chairmen

LIST OF CONTRIBUTORS

Maxwell Abramson, M.D. Associate Professor, Dept. of Otolaryngology, and Maxillofacial Surgery, University of Iowa, Iowa City, Iowa.

Cyrus S. Amiri, M.D. Head of Otolaryngology, Firouzgar Medical Center, Tehran, Iran.

Richard G. Asarch, M.D. Resident, Dept. of Dermatology, University of Colorado, Denver, Colorado.

David F. Austin, M.D. Attending Staff, Grant Hospital and Columbus Hospital. Associate Professor, Dept. of Otolaryngology, College of Medicine, University of Illinois, Chicago, Illinois.

Shirley H. Baron, M.D. Clinical Professor Emeritus, Dept. of Otolaryngology, University of California. Chairman, Dept. of Otolaryngology, French Hospital, San Francisco, California.

Eugene A. Bauer, M.D. Assistant Professor, Division of Dermatology, Washington School of Medicine, St. Louis, Missouri.

Quinter C. Beery, Ph.D. Research Assistant Professor of Otolaryngology, University of Pittsburgh, School of Medicine. Director of Clinical Studies, Dept. of Otolaryngology, Children's Hospital, Pittsburgh, Pennsylvania.

Richard J. Bellucci, M.D. Professor and Chairman, Dept. of Otolaryngology, Flower & Fifth Avenue Hospital, New York Medical College. Chairman, Dept. of Otolaryngology, Manhattan Eye, Ear and Throat Hospital, New York, New York.

E. Berco, M.D. Resident, ENT Department, Meir Hospital, Kfar Saba, Israel.

Joel M. Bernstein, M.D., M.A. Assistant Otolaryngologist, Surgery, Buffalo General Hospital. Consultant, Clinical Staff, Roswell Park Memorial Institute. Medical Staff, Otolaryngology, Sisters of Charity Hospital of Buffalo, New York.

Herbert G. Birck, M.D. Clinical Professor in Otolaryngology, Ohio State University. Chief, Dept. of Otolaryngology, Children's Hospital, Columbus, Ohio.

Charles Bluestone, M.D. Professor of Otolaryngology, University of Pittsburgh School of Medicine. Director of the Dept. of Otolaryngology, Children's Hospital of Pittsburgh, Pennsylvania.

Derald E. Brackmann, M.D. Assistant Clinical Professor of Otorhinolaryngology, University of Southern California, Los Angeles, California.

Wesley H. Bradley, M.D. Associate Director, National Institute of Neurological and Communicative Disorders and Stroke, National Institutes of Health. Director, Communicative Disorders, National Institutes of Health, Bethesda, Maryland.

Edward C. Brandow, Jr., M.D. Clinical Associate Professor, Dept. of Otolaryngology, Albany Medical College, Albany, New York.

Georges A. Bremond, M.D. Professor of Otorhinolaryngology, Marseille, France.

P. Bretlau, M.D. ENT Dept., Righospitalet, Copenhagen, Denmark.

Erdem I. Cantekin, Ph.D. Assistant Professor of Otolaryngology, University of Pittsburgh School of Medicine, Director of Research, Dept. of Otolaryngology, Children's Hospital, Pittsburgh, Pennsylvania.

Constance Clancey, Research Assistant, Dept. of Obstetrics and Gynecology, University of Iowa, Iowa City, Iowa.

D. Thane R. Cody, M.D., Ph.D. Professor of Otolaryngology, Mayo Medical School, Rochester, Minnesota.

William B. Coman, F.R.A.C.S., Otologist, University of Queensland, Brisbane, Australia.

Jean-Michel Dayer, M.D. Research Fellow in Medicine, Harvard Medical School. Clinical and Research Fellow in Medicine, Massachusetts General Hospital, Boston, Massachusetts.

Eugene L. Derlacki, M.D. Otolaryngologist, Otologic Professional Associates, Chicago, Illinois.

Herman Diamant, M.D. University Professor and Head of the ENT-department, University of Umea. Chief Doctor and Head of the Dept. of Otorhinolaryngology, the Regional Hospital of Umea, Umea, Sweden.

Marcus Diamant, M.D. Professor of Otorhinolaryngology, Halmstad, Sweden.

Gavin S. Douglas, M.D. Pediatric Otolaryngology Fellow, Dept. of Otolaryngology, University of Pittsburgh, Pittsburgh, Pennsylvania.

William J. Doyle, M.A. Research Assistant, Dept. of Otolaryngology, Children's Hospital, Pittsburgh, Pennsylvania.

R. Bruce Duncan, F.R.C.S. (Eng.), F.R.A.C.S., F.R.C.S. (Edin). Consultant Otologist, Wellington Hospital, New Zealand.

H. Paul Ehrlich, Ph.D. Assistant Professor of Pathology, Harvard Medical School, Shriners Burns Institute, Boston, Massachusetts.

Arthur Z. Eisen, M.D. Professor of Medicine and Head, Division of Dermatology, Washington School of Medicine. Dermatologist in Chief, Barnes Hospital, St. Louis, Missouri.

Irwin Freedberg, M.D. Professor of Dermatology, Harvard Medical School. Chief of Dermatology, Beth Israel Hospital and Children's Hospital Medical Center, Boston, Massachusetts.

Imrich Friedmann, M.D. Professor of Pathology, University of London, London, England.

J. M. Friot, M.D. Centre Hospitalier Regional de Nancy, Nancy, France.

Bruce J. Gantz, M.D. Resident, Dept. of Otolaryngology and Maxillofacial Surgery, University of Iowa, Iowa City, Iowa.

Michael E. Glasscock, III, M.D. Clinical Assistant Professor of Surgery (Otology and Neurotology), Vanderbilt University, Nashville, Tennessee.

Steven R. Goldring, M.D. Research Fellow in Medicine, Harvard Medical School. Clinical and Research Fellow in Medicine, Massachusetts General Hospital, Boston, Massachusetts.

Victor Goodhill, M.D. Surgeon in Residence, Department of Surgery, Section of Head and Neck, UCLA, Los Angeles, California.

Malcolm D. Graham, M.D. Assistant Clinical Professor of Otolaryngology, University of Southern California, Los Angeles, California.

A. Halevy, M.D. Resident, ENT Department, Meir Hospital, Kfar Saba, Israel.

Lee A. Harker, M.D. Associate Professor, Dept. of Otolaryngology and Maxillofacial Surgery, University of Iowa, Iowa City, Iowa.

Ernest Hausmann, D.M.D., Ph.D. Department of Oral Biology, School of Dentistry, State University of New York at Buffalo, New York.

Ron Hinchcliffe, M.D., Ph.D. Consultant Neuro-Otologist to the Royal National Throat, Nose and Ear Hospital, London, England.

Lewis B. Holmes, M.D. Associate Pediatrician, Massachusetts General Hospital. Assistant Professor of Pediatrics, Harvard Medical School, Boston, Massachusetts.

J. V. D. Hough, M.D. Clinical Professor of Otolaryngology, University of Oklahoma Medical School. Otolaryngologist, Baptist and Presbyterian Hospitals, Oklahoma City, Oklahoma.

Cheng-Chun Huang, Ph.D. Dept. of Otolaryngology and Maxillofacial Surgery, University of Iowa, Iowa City, Iowa.

Claus Jansen, M.D. Head of ORL Department, Gummersbach, West Germany.

John J. Jeffrey, Ph.D. Associate Professor of Biochemistry in Medicine, Washington University School of Medicine, St. Louis, Missouri.

M. B. Jørgensen, M.D. Professor of University, Righospitalet, Copenhagen, Denmark.

P. Karma, M.D. Instructor in Otolaryngology, Helsinki University, Helsinki, Finland.

Thomas J. Koob. Pre-Doctoral Student in Biochemistry, Washington University, St. Louis, Missouri.

Franklin P. Koontz, Ph.D. Associate Professor, Dept. of Pathology, University of Iowa, Iowa City, Iowa.

C.M. Kos, M.D. Clinical Professor of Otolaryngology and Maxillofacial Surgery, University of Iowa, Iowa City, Iowa.

Stephen M. Krane, M.D. Professor of Medicine, Harvard Medical School. Chief, Arthritis Unit and Physician, Massachusetts General Hospital, Boston, Massachusetts.

Charles J. Krause, M.D. Professor and Vice Chairman, Department of Otolaryngology and Maxillofacial Surgery, University of Iowa, Iowa City, Iowa.

H. K. Kristensen, M.D. Professor, Chief of University ENT Dept., Righospitalet, Copenhagen, Denmark.

Bryan Larsen, Ph.D. Dept. of Microbiology, University of Iowa, Iowa City, Iowa.

Edna B. Laurence, Ph.D. Research Associate, Birkbeck College, University of London, London, England.

Neil Lewis, M. A. Senior Lecturer in Audiology AB Original Hearing Conservation and Treatment Program, Faculty of Medicine, Queensland, Brisbane, Australia.

David J. Lim, M.D. Professor, Dept. of Otolaryngology, Ohio State University College of Medicine. Director, Otological Research Laboratories, Dept. of Otolaryngology, Ohio State University College of Medicine, Columbus, Ohio.

John R. Lindsay, M.D. Professor Emeritus, Dept. of Surgery, University of Chicago, Chicago, Illinois.

Ward B. Litton, M.D. Otolaryngologist, private practice, Moline, Illinois.

Ian C. Mackenzie, Ph.D., F.D.S., B.D.S., L.D.S. Associate Dean for Research and Program Development. Professor of Periodontology, Dept. of Periodontology, University of Iowa, Iowa City, Iowa.

J. Magnan, M.D. Otorhinolaryngology, Marseille, France.

Brian F. McCabe, M.D. Professor and Head, Dept. of Otolaryngology and Maxillofacial Surgery, University of Iowa, Iowa City, Iowa.

Gerard McCafferty, F.R.A.C.S. Otologist, University of Queensland, Brisbane, Australia.

Gregory R. Mundy, M.D. Assistant Professor of Medicine, Division of Endocrinology and Metabolism, University of Connecticut Health Center. Consultant Physician, V.A. Hospital, Newington, Connecticut.

George T. Nager, M.D. Professor and Chairman, Dept. of Laryngology and Otology, Johns Hopkins University, School of Medicine, Baltimore, Maryland.

A. Palva, M.D. Professor in Otolaryngology, Helsinki University, Helsinki, Finland.

T. Palva, M.D. Professor of Otolaryngology and Head of Department at Helsinki University. Deputy Medical Director of the University Hospital of Helsinki, Helsinki, Finland.

Michael M. Paparella, M.D. Professor and Chairman, Department of Otolaryngology, University of Minnesota Medical School, Minneapolis, Minnesota.

Gary L. Peck, M.D. Dermatology Branch, National Cancer Institute, National Institutes of Health, Bethesda, Maryland.

Dietrich Plester, M.D. Professor and Head, ENT Department, Tübingen University, Tübingen, West Germany.

Lawrence G. Raisz, M.D. Professor of Medicine, Head of Endocrinology and Metabolism, University of Connecticut Health Center, Farmington, Connecticut.

P. Ratnesar, F.R.C.S. Consultant E.N.T. Surgeon, E.N.T. Unit, Farnborough Hospital, Orpington, Kent, England.

Frank N. Ritter, M.D. Clinical Professor, Dept. of Otorhinolaryngology, University of Michigan Medical Center, Ann Arbor, Michigan.

Stephen Roth, Ph.D. Department of Biology, Johns Hopkins University, Baltimore, Maryland.

Jacob Sade, M.D. Chief of ENT Department, Meir Hospital, Kfar Saba, Israel. Consultant, Polymer Department, Weizmann Institute of Science, Rehovot, Israel.

William H. Saunders, M.D. Chairman, Dept. of Otolaryngology, Ohio State University, College of Medicine, Columbus, Ohio.

H. F. Schuknecht, M.D. Professor and Chairman, Department of Otolaryngology, Massachusetts Eye and Ear Infirmary, Boston, Massachusetts.

Jo L. Seltzer, Ph.D. Research Assistant in Medicine, Washington University School of Medicine, St. Louis, Missouri.

Larry R. Severeid, M.D. Otolaryngologist, Maxillofacial Plastic Surgeon, Gunderson Clinic, La Crosse, Wisconsin.

George E. Shambaugh, Jr., M.D. Attending Staff, Northwestern Memorial Hospital. Consulting Staff, Henrotin Hospital. Chicago Courtesy Staff, Hinsdale Sanitarium and Hospital. Professor Emeritus, Otolaryngology, Northwest University Medical School, Hinsdale, Illinois.

Elizabeth Shaw, B.Sp.Thy. Audiologist, University of Queensland, Brisbane, Australia.

James L. Sheehy, M.D. Clinical Professor of Otolaryngology, University of Southern California, Los Angeles, California.

Gordon D. L. Smyth, M.D. Reader, Department of Otorhinolaryngology, Queens' University. Consultant, Northern Ireland Hospitals Authority in Ear, Nose & Throat Disease, Royal Victoria Hospital, Belfast, North Ireland.

Sylvan E. Stool, M.D. Professor of Otolaryngology and Pediatrics, University of Pittsburgh School of Medicine. Director of Education, Department of Otolaryngology, Children's Hospital, Pittsburgh, Pennsylvania.

George P. Stricklin, Medical Science Training Program Student, Washington University School of Medicine, St. Louis, Missouri.

William F. Taylor, M.D. Otorhinolaryngology, Mayo Clinic, Rochester, Minnesota.

Jens Thomsen, M.D. University ENT Department, Righospitalet, Copenhagen, Denmark.

Paul A. Toller, F.D.S.R.C.S. Consultant Maxillo-Facial Surgeon at Mount Vernon Hospital, Northwood, England. Consulting Oral Surgeon to King Edward VII Hospital for Officers, London, England.

Robert Trelstad, M.D. Chief of Pathology, Shriners Burns Institute. Assistant Pathologist, Massachusetts General Hospital. Assistant Professor of Pathology, Harvard Medical School, Boston, Massachusetts.

Charles F. Tschopp, M.D. Chief, Otolaryngology, Alaska Native Medical Center, Anchorage, Alaska. Chairman, Indian Health Service, Otitis Media Project, Alaska.

Michel R. Wayoff, Professor, M.D. Centre Hospitalier, Regional de Nancy, Nancy, France.

Ziva Weismann, Ph.D. Polymer Department, Weizmann Institute of Science, Rehovot, Israel.

John Wright, M.D. Dept. of Pathology, School of Medicine, State University of New York at Buffalo, New York.

William K. Wright, M.D. Clinical Professor of Otolaryngology, Baylor College of Medicine, Houston, Texas. Attending Otolaryngologist at Methodist Hospital, Hermann Hospital, St. Joseph's Hospital, St. Luke's Hospital, Texas Children's Hospital, and Twelve Oaks Hospital, Texas.

I. Yarowitzkaya, M.D. Resident, ENT Dept., Meir Hospital, Kfar Saba, Israel.

CONTENTS

CHOLESTEATOMA

FIRST INTERNATIONAL CONFERENCE

SECTION I
BASIC PROBLEMS

Chapter 1

Biology and Pathology

of

Keratinizing Epithelium

THE NATURE OF THE INTERDISCIPLINARY PROBLEM IN CHOLESTEATOMA

Maxwell Abramson, M.D.

One of the greatest challenges of otology is that we must be physicians as well as surgeons—scientists as well as practitioners. Urologists have nephrologists to help them and thoracic surgeons may depend upon findings of respiratory physiologists; however, we otologists must be our own physiologists.

What actually happens in the middle ear disease of cholesteatoma? Because of the great technical advances we have made in the last 20 years, we can take the middle ear apart, remove the cholesteatoma and reconstruct the ear again, even with normal hearing in some cases. Yet, many cholesteatomas return. We are not always sure of when and if to operate on a dry cholesteatoma. We do not have the answers for many questions. How do we tell a retraction pocket from a cholesteatoma? Can the disease be prevented? Can we leave the matrix? Should we leave the posterior canal wall intact? Should we return to the ear for a second look?

On the dissection table and in the operating room, many of us try to find the answers to these and other questions. We must know more about the patho-physiology of the ear before we can answer these questions. First we need to find out how cholesteatomas form and understand the mechanism of the associated destructive process.

We have brought together here a very unusual and diverse group—otologists willing to spend four days at a meeting without the expectation of learning a new technique, and clinical and basic scientists willing to discuss their work in the context of a disease that many had previously never heard of or remember dimly from medical school days.

What are the expectations of this meeting? We are not going to solve all the problems of cholesteatoma in the next four days, but we will be greatly influenced here. Our old ideas are going to be subjected to critical review. We are going to see the problems of cholesteatoma in a new context. A 2 sq. meter sac of skin enclosing the body may not be very different than a 2 mm sac of skin in the ear. The factors affecting cell growth and movement in the uterus may apply to the ear as well. Bone resorption at the metacarpophalangeal joint may not be so different than bone resorption at the incudo-stapedial joint. We shall see that the organism responds to injury and inflammation in a rather standard way.

My expectation is that we will leave here with the desire to communicate with scientists in other disciplines; to apply basic principles and biologic models to problem solving in our clinical area.

THE DEFINITION OF CHOLESTEATOMA

D. Thane R. Cody, M.D., Ph.D.

Introduction

A definition of cholesteatoma that describes its histologic features is easy, but such a relatively simple definition is not satisfactory for the otologist. His definition of cholesteatoma must be expanded to include the characteristics of the disease and the associated pathologic alterations in the middle ear cleft. Certain observations that I have made in managing many patients who have had active chronic suppurative otitis media have helped me define cholesteatoma in this expanded sense.

The narrower definition of cholesteatoma is one of stratified squamous epithelium trapped and growing in foreign sites within the temporal bone, resulting in the production of a progressively expanding tumor mass consisting of new growth of epithelium, various stages of degenerating epithelium, abundant keratin, and usually associated with cholesterol and chronic inflammatory cells. This definition probably would satisfy most pathologists, but it is incomplete for otologists.

Cholesteatoma is either congenital or acquired. Congenital cholesteatoma is caused by an embryologic developmental defect that gives rise to a nidus of epithelium in the temporal bone. An acquired cholesteatoma originates after birth as a result of a disorder in the middle ear cleft. In a series of 483 ears with cholesteatoma that underwent mastoidectomy at the Mayo Clinic between January 1, 1963, and December 31, 1969, 473 (98%) were acquired cholesteatomas and 10 (2%) were congenital. Traditionally, the acquired cholesteatomas have been further subdivided into primary acquired and secondary acquired cholesteatomas. The primary type arises through the development of an attic defect and, in our series, accounted for 389 (82%) of the acquired cholesteatomas. The sec-

ondary type develops from marginal or central perforations of the tympanic membrane and accounted for 84 (18%) of the acquired cholesteatomas. Therefore, congenital cholesteatomas are rare, and primary acquired cholesteatomas are far more common than are secondary acquired cholesteatomas.

Our study of patients with cholesteatoma has revealed that cholesteatoma is predominantly a disease of the male. Eighty percent of the congenital cholesteatomas occurred in males and 20% in females. Sixty-three percent of the acquired cholesteatomas occurred in males and 37% in females.

In addition, observations of all patients who underwent mastoid surgery for active chronic suppurative otitis media between January 1, 1963, and December 31, 1969, have indicated that the definition of acquired cholesteatoma should include its association with an attic defect, the presence of a very sclerotic mastoid process, and various degrees of eustachian tube dysfunction. I shall describe some of the observations that have led to this conclusion.

Acquired Cholesteatoma

Between January 1, 1963, and December 31, 1969, 473 mastoidectomies were performed at the Mayo Clinic for acquired cholesteatoma. Of the 473 ears, 389 (82%) had an attic defect, 65 (14%) had a total or marginal perforation of the tympanic membrane, and only 19 (4%) had a central perforation. Evaluation of the mastoid processes revealed that 323 ears (68%) were extremely sclerotic with little or no cellular architecture, 87 (19%) had a postoperative mastoid cavity (revision mastoidectomies), and 63 (13%) had a reasonably well pneumatized mastoid process. In the group with a pneumatized mastoid process, mastoid roentgenograms revealed some sclerosis in all patients, and none of the patients had normal pneumatization of the mastoid process. The processes were judged to be relatively well pneumatized on the basis of the roentgenograms and in particular on the surgeon's findings at operation. If the revision mastoidectomies in which pneumatization of the mastoid process could not be determined are excluded from the series, 84% of the mastoid processes were extremely sclerotic and 16% were reasonably well pneumatized but not normal. Therefore, acquired cholesteatoma is usually associated with an attic defect and an extremely sclerotic mastoid process which is suggestive of inadequate function of the eustachian tube.

If chronic dysfunction of the eustachian tube is a primary cause of acquired cholesteatoma, and more specifically of the primary-acquired cholesteatoma, then the intact canal wall mastoidectomies (simple mastoidectomy and simple mastoidectomy with opening of the facial recess) would not be adequate to manage this disease process. If poor function of the eustachian tube existed after an intact canal wall mastoidectomy for acquired cholesteatoma, an attic retraction pocket or a facial recess retraction pocket, when the recess has been surgically opened, should reform in time, and cholesteatoma should eventually recur. The speed at which these complications would develop would depend on the degree of eustachian tube dysfunction.

Analysis of the results of 171 intact canal wall mastoidectomies performed for acquired cholesteatoma between January 1, 1963, and December 31, 1969, revealed this to be true. The patients with intact canal wall mastoidectomies either were followed for a minimum of four years after the operation or the procedures had failed during the first four postoperative years. The mean postoperative follow-up for the mastoidectomies was 70 months, with a range of seven to 150 months.

Of the 171 intact canal wall mastoidectomies,

60 (35%) failed because of recurrent or residual cholesteatoma; 68% of the cholesteatoma failures were due to recurrent cholesteatoma. Twenty percent of the mastoidectomies (34 ears) failed because of a precholesteatoma, which is defined as the formation of an attic or facial recess retraction pocket. Nineteen of the 34 precholesteatoma failures also were associated with chronic infection. Precholesteatoma for retraction pockets has proved to be an appropriate term because the recurrent cholesteatoma first develops a retraction pocket and then forms a cholesteatoma. Since this analysis was completed, at least one of the precholesteatoma failures has formed a recurrent cholesteatoma. Therefore, during this relatively limited postoperative follow-up period, 55% of the intact canal wall mastoidectomies for acquired cholesteatomas (94 ears) have failed because of either precholesteatoma or cholesteatoma formation. In many of these mastoidectomy failures, the cycle that gave rise to the cholesteatoma in the first place was repeated. The only logical explanation for this is eustachian tube dysfunction.

Chronic Infection

We also observed patients who have had intact canal wall mastoidectomies for chronic infection without cholesteatoma who, after an initial seemingly successful operation, gradually developed a retraction pocket and occasionally after still a longer follow-up period have had a primary acquired-type cholesteatoma. This sequence implies the existence of eustachian tube dysfunction in these ears. To further investigate this problem, the mastoidectomies performed for chronic infection without cholesteatoma formation between January 1, 1963, and December 31, 1969, were analyzed. An important question was why the retraction pockets and cholesteatomas developed only after the infection had been eradicated and the tympanic membrane had been repaired.

Of the 159 mastoidectomies performed for chronic infection during this period, 68 (43%) involved ears that had total or marginal perforation of the tympanic membrane and 60 (38%) involved ears that had central perforation. However, only

10% (16 ears) involved an attic defect, and the remaining 9% (15 ears) had an intact tympanic membrane, the chronic infection being limited to the mastoid cavity. These latter 15 cases involved revision mastoidectomies. Evaluation of the mastoid process in these 159 patients revealed that 43% (68 ears) had a postoperative mastoid cavity (revision mastoidectomies), 41% (65 ears) had an extremely sclerotic mastoid process, and 16% (26 ears) had a relatively well pneumatized mastoid process, but all 159 had some sclerosis. If the revision mastoidectomies are excluded, then 72% of the mastoid processes were extremely sclerotic and 28% were relatively well pneumatized. A comparison of the pathologic alterations that were found in the middle ear cleft of patients undergoing mastoidectomy for acquired cholesteatoma and those undergoing mastoidectomy for chronic infection without cholesteatoma revealed that many in both groups had extremely sclerotic mastoid processes (Table 1). The basic difference in pathologic alterations of the middle ear cleft between these two disease processes was that many of the acquired cholesteatomas had an attic defect, whereas many of the chronically infected ears without cholesteatoma had a total, marginal, or central perforation of the tympanic membrane.

In this group of patients, 52 intact canal wall mastoidectomies were performed for chronic infection. Patients have been followed up for a minimum of four years after operation or the operation failed during the first four postoperative years. The mean postoperative follow-up was 79 months, with a range of four to 159 months. During the postoperative period, three (6%) of the patients developed primary acquired-type cholesteatomas and seven (13%) developed attic or facial recess retraction pockets. Thus, 19% of the patients with intact canal wall mastoidectomies for chronic infection developed retraction pockets or cholesteatoma. The sequence of events through which the cholesteatoma failures passed was identical to that observed in the recurrent cholesteatoma failures among the intact canal wall mastoidectomies for acquired cholesteatoma. A case report of one of these cholesteatoma failures illustrates the iatrogenic development of a primary acquired cholesteatoma.

TABLE 1

Middle Ear Cleft Disease in 632 Mastoid Operations

| Disease | % of patients with | |
	Acquired cholesteatoma	Chronic infection
Attic defect	82	10
Total, marginal, or central tympanic membrane perforation	18	81
Sclerotic mastoid process*	84	72

*Excluding revision mastoidectomies.

Case 1: A 49 year old woman was first seen at the Mayo Clinic in March 1967. She had a life-long history of chronic drainage from her left ear. Examination revealed a purulent discharge in the left ear canal from which Proteus organisms were cultured. A polyp composed of granulation tissue was noted growing from the middle ear through a large, posterior, central perforation in the tympanic membrane. Mastoid roentgenograms revealed a very sclerotic mastoid process. On March 8, 1967, a left simple mastoidectomy with opening of the facial recess revealed hemorrhagic granulation tissue throughout the tympanic cavity, epitympanum, and mastoid antrum. The perforation of the tympanic membrane was repaired with a temporalis fascia graft, but no attempt was made to reconstruct an ossicular chain defect. The ear healed satisfactorily, and on August 18, 1967, a transcanal tympanoplasty was performed to reconstruct the ossicular chain. The ear again healed uneventfully. The patient was not seen again at our clinic until April 21, 1972. She had had no trouble with her left ear, and she returned because of a throat complaint. Examination revealed a large, posterosuperior retraction pocket of the left tympanic membrane extending into the facial recess but no cholesteatoma. In June 1974, the patient began to have postural unsteadiness and developed vertigo when she pressed on her left ear, and one month later, otorrhea developed on the left. When these symptoms persisted, she returned to the Mayo Clinic in October 1974, where examination revealed a purulent discharge in the left ear, and extensive cholesteatoma in the mastoid process, and findings consistent with a fistula of the horizontal semicircular canal. A left modified radical mastoidectomy on October 17, 1974, confirmed the findings. The mastoid process was packed with cholesteatoma, which had obviously arisen from a retraction pocket that had formed through the previously opened facial recess.

In some of the ears that have undergone intact canal wall mastoidectomies for chronic infection, the sequence of events that gave rise to the acquired cholesteatoma could be observed. The only logical explanation for the gradual development of these complications in ears that have undergone what seems to be an initially successful intact canal wall mastoidectomy for chronic infection is eustachian tube dysfunction. The theory that primary acquired cholesteatomas are caused by inadequate eustachian tube function is certainly not a new one. However, the present observations suggest agreement with this theory and that the development early in life of a large perforation of the tympanic membrane which exteriorizes the middle ear cleft is nature's way of protecting most of these ears with eustachian tube dysfunction from developing a cholesteatoma. When these ears with large perforations of the tympanic membrane and chronic infections are operated on and the middle ear cleft is turned back into a closed system, tubal dysfunction causes retraction pockets to develop and acquired cholesteatomas to eventually develop.

Conclusion

Analysis of patients with active chronic suppurative otitis media and of their courses after mastoidectomy has contributed data that help define cholesteatoma in terms that are broader than the histologic characteristics. Besides the histologic definition—that is, stratified squamous epithelium trapped and growing in foreign sites within the temporal bone, resulting in the production of a progressively expanding tumor mass consisting of new growth of epithelium, various stages of degenerating epithelium, and abundant keratin and usually associated with cholesterol and chronic inflammatory cells—the otologist defines the cholesteatoma as usually being associated with an attic defect, an extremely sclerotic mastoid process, and eustachian tube dysfunction. Cholesteatomas may be congenital or acquired, and they predominantly occur in the male.

THE PATHOLOGY OF EPIDERMOID CHOLESTEATOMA: HUMAN AND EXPERIMENTAL

Imrich Friedmann, M.D.

The history of the so-called "aural cholesteatoma" bristles with controversial problems, both real and artificial, and presents a bizarre picture of theories abandoned, revived, and again abandoned. The principal points of contention have changed little and the definition, terminology, and histogenesis have remained focal points of discussion and arguments generating more heat than light.

The histopathologist has the function of both disgnostician and experimental pathologist in trying to answer some of the questions based on clinical observation.

Observation is important: all persons have the innate ability to identify patterns which they have seen before or to agree that two such patterns are essentially equivalent. Knowledge gained in this way is perfectly "scientific", although pattern recognition cannot be reduced to a mathematical formula. This seems to be the "so-called intuitive element in science which is often stressed by biologists but pooh-poohed by the physicists" (Ziman, 1973).

Otologists have been and are in the forefront of the study of the pathology of the ear and, ceteris paribus, of the cholesteatoma problem. Pathologists have largely ignored this field, deceived perhaps by the comparatively simple and straightforward histopathological features contrasting sharply with the often dramatic clinical evidence.

The duty of interpreting the findings should be a joint effort, but pathologists are often busier in other spheres of their work. Often the pathological diagnosis differs considerably from the clinical finding (Table 2). In the majority of the cases, the

TABLE 2

Clinical Diagnosis	Histopathology
Cholesteatoma	Epidermoid cholesteatoma confirmed
Cholesteatoma	Unconfirmed
No clinical evidence	Epidermoid cholesteatoma present
Cholesteatoma	C.O.M. and cholesterol granuloma
C.O.M.	Squamous epithelium present (non-keratinizing)

clinical and histopathological diagnoses would agree but there remains a considerable proportion of cases in which there will be disagreement. Sampling error or loss of relevant tissue may explain why in certain cases histopathological confirmation may be impossible. Pathological definition is essential.

Aural cholesteatoma is a usually cystic structure produced by keratinizing squamous epithelium; the laminated keratin from its inverted surface accumulates in the cyst-like cavity and may contain an admixture of purulent and necrotic matter (Figs. 1 and 2).

If this symposium achieves no more than to clear up some of the confusion surrounding the definition of epidermoid cholesteatoma and cholesterol granuloma, this alone will be important (Friedmann, 1959 and 1974; Dota, et al, 1963).

Goodhill (1960) rightly points out that "cholesteatoma may lurk behind central perforations, behind dry ears and in many rare ear conditions.

Of great interest are some cases where the

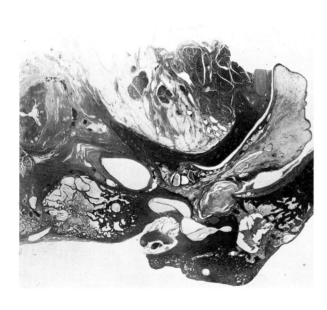

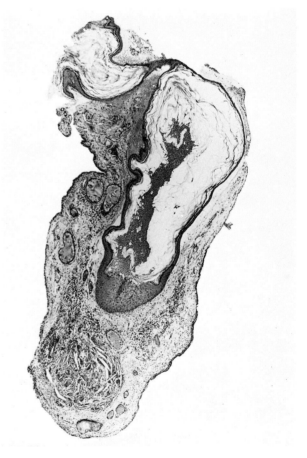

Fig. 1: This is the classical histopathological picture of an epidermoid cholesteatoma presenting as a cystic structure formed by hyperkeratotic squamous epithelium.

Fig. 2: Aural polyp containing both epidermoid cholesteatoma and cholesterol granuloma.

histopathological diagnosis differs from that of the surgeon and, in particular, where in spite of the negative clinical evidence, the specimen obtained at operation or at autopsy furnishes definite histopathological evidence of a latent epidermoid cholesteatoma.

Latent Epidermoid Cholesteatoma

Case 1: A 24 year old male complained of a left earache on and off with discharge for 20 years. Admitted on September 15, 1975, with left earache. He ran a high temperature and the left mastoid process was swollen. The swelling fluctuated and the tympanic membrane was perforated discharging a foul-smelling exudate. Radical mastoidectomy was performed and the mastoid antrum was filled with granulation and purulent exudate surrounded by necrotic bone. There was no clinical evidence of cholesteatoma.

Microscopy confirmed the diagnosis of chronic otitis media (Figs. 3, 4, and 5). There was a good deal of inflammatory granulation tissue, some filling the mastoid air cells, some surrounding a microscopical finding apparently not observed at operation; in one area the bone was covered by keratinizing squamous epithelium forming a cyst-like structure filled with laminated keratin, i.e., epidermoid cholesteatoma.

It is interesting to note that the surrounding bone, which showed signs of reconstruction and irregular cement lines, was absorbed by the inflammatory fibrous perimatrix of the epidermoid lining of the cholesteatoma.

Histogenesis of Epidermoid Cholesteatoma

The structure and cytology of the middle ear mucosa has remained a controversial issue. A thorough understanding of its normal morphology is essential in any consideration of pathological changes (Tos, et al, 1973).

The healthy middle ear lining consists of a thin layer of fibrous tissue covered by flattened endothelium-like cells. There are areas where columnar epithelium normally occurs as on the medial

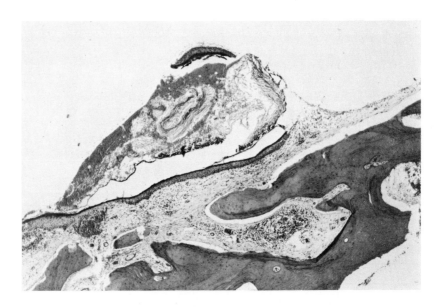

Fig. 3: Mastoid bone fragments from a 24 year old man with a long history of chronic otitis media. There was an apparently latent e.ch. present in the sectioned material not observed at operation.

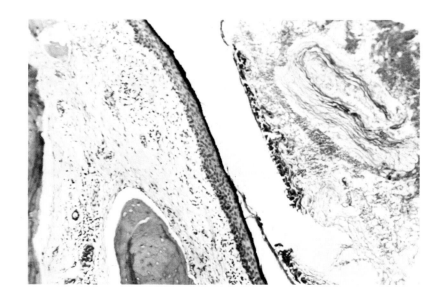

Fig. 4: Detail of Figure 3.

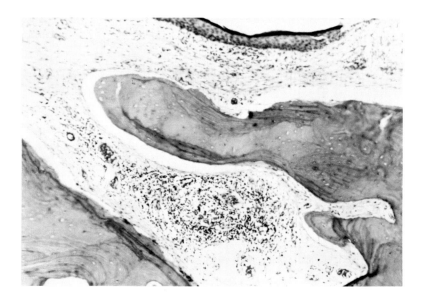

Fig. 5: Detail of Figure 3 to show bone absorption.

wall, near the orifice of the eustachian tube and on the promontory. The entire epithelial lining is, essentially, of respiratory epithelial character and its true nature is revealed in pathological circumstances, as for instance in the experimentally infected tympanic bulla of the guinea pig, in chronic otitis media and in the "glue ear".

The cellular lining of the middle ear cavity may be replaced by stratified keratinizing squamous epithelium. This usually results in the development of an epidermoid cholesteatoma complicating chronic (and acute) infections of the middle ear cleft.

Sadé (1971) believes that it is important to distinguish between simple stratified squamous epithelium (SSE) and cholesteatomatous SSE. It is, however, doubtful that "simple SSE metaplasia is found all over the ear in chronic otitis media" (Sadé and Weinberg, 1969). Local conditions may perhaps be responsible for the different findings in different countries. Vitamin A deficiency and malnutrition are known to be common in the countries of the Middle East. Fell and Mellanby (1953) and Fell and Rinaldini (1965) have shown that vitamin A played an important role in metaplasia. Vitamin A deficient media enhanced the growth of squamous epithelium; hypervitaminosis A produced columnar metaplasia.

The unique relationship between vitamin A deficiency and squamous metaplasia of respiratory epithelia is well established. The association of infection with vitamin A deficiency is also recognized but it has not been known whether viral or bacterial infections precede or follow the keratinizing lesions. Bang, et al, (1974 and 1975) have shown that in the trachea of vitamin A deficient chicks, keratotic changes occurred mainly in areas regenerating following infection with Newcastle virus (not before).

It is noteworthy that recent research workers have found no evidence of metaplastic transformation in the middle ear cleft and in his thesis Karma (1972) has concluded that "cholesteatoma formation cannot be explained on a metaplastic basis". Lim and Saunders (1972) found no evidence of keratinization in metaplastic squamous epithelium, a prerequisite of cholesteatoma formation.

Non-keratinizing squamous epithelium of metaplastic origin is unlikely to produce an epidermoid cholesteatoma and the presence of both keratotic squamous epithelium and of the columnar epithelium of the middle ear mucosa argues against metaplasia (Figs. 6 and 7).

In his comprehensive monograph on cholesteatoma, Schwarz (1966) categorically rejects not only the theory of metaplasia but also the theory of activation of embryonic cell nests as a cause or source of cholesteatoma.

There is general agreement that the congenital origin of aural cholesteatoma is a myth based only on clinical impressions and on the fallacious concept of an "intact" tympanic membrane. It was rejected by Wittmaack (1926) as an "unnecessary theory". Wittmaack, in common with some other authors, failed to find embryonic cell nests as confirmed by Schwarz (1966), Friedmann (1974), and others. The cell nests may be overwhelmed by inflammatory processes.

Activation of epithelial cell nests or cell nests in the gum, described by Malassez as studied by Ten Cate (1922), depends both in vivo and in vitro on a switch in their metabolism consequent to an alteration of the supporting connective tissue. Their potential to dental cyst formation is due to their anatomic location. Intraepithelial cavitation or cell death may be the mechanism initiating cyst formation and local changes in pH, etc., may be responsible. This has not been demonstrated by the proponents of the congenital theory.

Some Experimental Studies

Habermann's immigration theory (1892) remains the most plausible and well founded theory of the origin of cholesteatomatous squamous epithelium (Kern, 1958 and Ruedi, 1959; Friedmann, 1959; Schwarz, 1966; Friedmann, 1974). According to Ordmann and Gillmann (1966) there are two requisites for the immigration and spread of squamous epithelium: (1) Intradermal epithelial

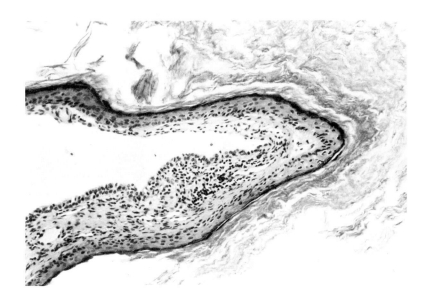

Fig. 6: Epidermoid cholesteatoma in a 12 year old child with C.O.M. Note that there is both the lining of the epidermoid "cyst" present and the mucosal epithelium of the middle ear separated by inflammatory granulation tissue. This not uncommon finding advocates strongly against metaplasia.

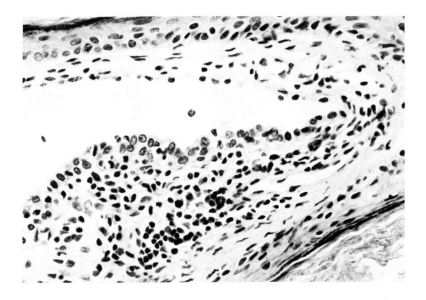

Fig. 7: Detail of Figure 6.

elements must be injured; (2) the injury must be kept patent (as in the tympanic membrane). The maintenance of even a tiny tear in the tympanic membrane for a short period of time—say 24 hours—would suffice to encourage epidermal invasion. Its advancing edge is secreting some proteolytic enzymes capable of degrading both fibrin and denatured collagen (Gillmann and Penn, 1956).

Friedmann (1959 and 1974) described the development of epidermoid cholesteatoma in the bulla of the guinea pig following experimental injection of bacterial cultures, especially pseudomonas pyocyanea and confirmed the earlier work of Hayman (1914) and Ruedi (1959) concluding that migration of the squamous epithelium of the external auditory meatus and/or tympanic membrane leads to the formation of epidermoid cholesteatoma.

I have reported studies of the spontaneous development of epidermoid cholesteatoma in the nude mouse*. Nude mice lack the thymus and are immunodeficient (Flanagan, 1966, Pantelouris, 1968, and Rygaard, 1973). This often leads to spontaneous infection. Figure 8 shows the infected bulla and perforated tympanic membrane with cholesteatomatous material in the tympanic cavity.

Figure 9 shows, in contrast, an intact tympanic membrane and purulent labyrinthitis. There is no evidence of cholesteatoma. This suggests that on

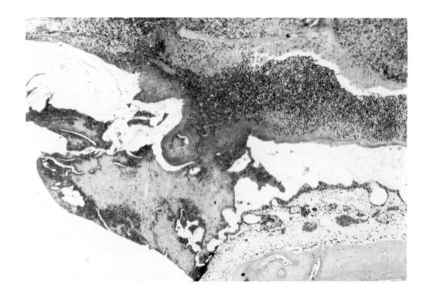

Fig. 8: Infected middle ear of a "nude" mouse with cholesteatoma. Note damaged tympanic membrane.

---

*The mouse mutant "nude" has been described by Flanagan only in 1966 as an autosomal recessive. The homozygotes are hairless and their growth is retarded. Other parts of the syndrome include: sulphydril-group deficiency and abnormal keratinization of hair follicles, necrosis of the liver associated with toxoplasma gondii infection. In 1968, Pantelouris added congenital absence of the thymus in homozygots in both sexes and all ages of the nude mouse. Rygaard in 1973 concluded that the untreated nude mouse has a similar short life expectancy as the neonatally thymectomized mouse and that it is similarly prone to infection not only by pathogens but also by other organisms usually described as commensals. Rygaard points out that the wasting syndrome occurs as a sum-total of various isolated insults to which the animal has no resistance.

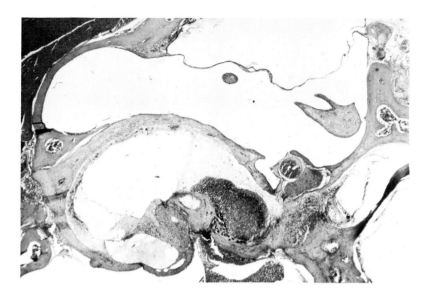

Fig. 9: "Nude" mouse. Note purulent labyrinthitis behind an intact tympanic membrane.

its own the infected middle ear cleft may not provide the histological basis for the formation of an epidermoid cholesteatoma unless "invaded" by migratory squamous epithelium.

Billingham and Silvers (1968) used suspensions of epidermal cells virtually uncontaminated by fibrous elements. When injected into the tongue of rats histological examination (after 30, 70, 90 days) revealed that there were small epidermal cysts present with masses of cellular debris inside and viable Malpighian cells on the outside. Experimentally (trypsinization) disaggregated epidermal cells are thus capable of reassembling and producing a continuous layer of fully stratified epidermis in the form of a cyst on inocultation into various types of mesenchymal tissues unrelated to dermis.

Guggenheim (personal communication) correctly ascribes to the mesenchyme an important role (McLoughlin, 1961 and 1968). But this is an inductive force and the transformation of the mesenchyme, which Hay (1968) calls secondary mesenchyme, into squamous epithelium has not been substantiated. Billingham and Silvers (1968) believe that "there is no predetermined regional specificity in the embryonic ectoderm, both its differentiation and regional differentiation being initiated by morphogenic stimuli from the subjacent mesenchyme". In this respect the mesenchyme may play an important role also in the formation of epidermoid cholesteatoma.

Tissue Culture Studies

Friedmann and Hodges (1975) noted on organ cultures of the primordial submandibular gland that following a soak in trypsin considerable changes occurred in the basal lamina and in the mesenchymatous cells. Variable bullous protrusions containing mitochondria and organelles of the cytoplasm passed through the apparently weakened basal lamina and the mesenchymatous cells were converted into bizarre "ropalocytes" (Ghadially and Skinnider, 1971). The observations support the view that the capacity of the epithelial cells to spread might be due to their ability to produce collagenolytic enzymes. Dresden, et al, (1972) have referred to an "overproduction of normal enzymes in some tumors" and this is the case in the matrix of a cholesteatoma (Abramson, 1969).

Embryonic otocyst cultures have served well as

a model of the study of differentiation of the neuro-epithelial structures of the inner ear and of the effect of ototoxic agents on them. Friedmann has used mainly the chick embryo. Ruben and Van de Water have developed successfully a technique for the organ culture of the mouse embryo otocyst.

The squamous epithelium from the cutaneous areas of the primordial otocyst may migrate into the deeper portion of the developing culture forming either a solid epithelial mass or cystic structures resembling and reproducing the features of an epidermoid cyst of, if the analogy is not too far-fetched, a cholesteatoma. The model can be used for the study of metaplasia (Fig. 10).

Spread

Sadé and Halevy (1972) have concluded that the most important cause of bone destruction or absorption in chronic otitis media with or without cholesteatoma is the inflammatory process itself and, in fact, the granulation tissue. Other processes may be involved (Abramson, 1969). The illustrative case described above shows clearly that the granulation tissue readily absorbs and replaces the bone surrounding an epidermoid cholesteatoma.

It is interesting to note that squamous epithelium resting on bone in the external auditory meatus did not absorb bone but when there was inflammatory granulation tissue present underneath, bone was absorbed (Figs. 11, 12, 13, and 14).

Epilogue

The interpretation of scientific evidence, be it histopathological or clinical and even "intuitive," may have to switch from one way of interpretation to another. When such switching of interpretation occurs past knowledge need be disregarded; we merely restructure the pattern and change the meaning and emphasis of various features (Ziman, 1973). Some of these might be new or may have been obtained by newer techniques but we are not bound to accept an argument just because it is new and exciting. This may serve as the motto of the symposium.

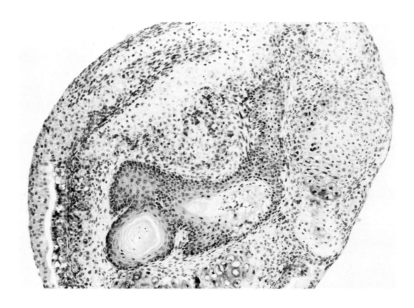

Fig. 10: Organ culture of chick embryo otocyst showing ingrowing keratinizing squamous epithelium forming small keratocyst.

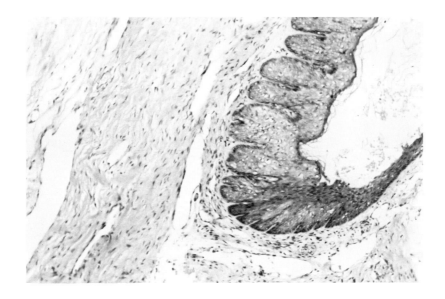

Fig. 11: Human tympanic membrane with acanthotic squamous epithelium.

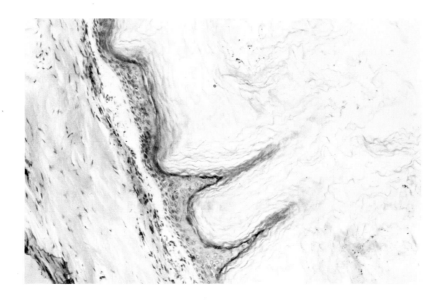

Fig. 12: Hyperkeratotic squamous epithelium of the human external auditory meatus. There is no bone absorption.

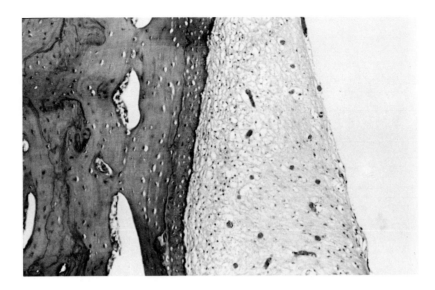

Fig. 13: Non-keratinizing squamous epithelium of the human external auditory meatus. There is direct contact with bone, but there is no evidence of bone absorption.

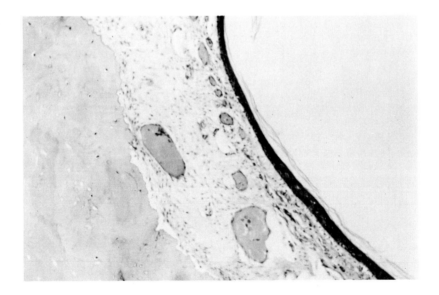

Fig. 14: Epidermis of the human external auditory meatus and underlying vascular granulation tissue causing bone absorption.

References

1. Abramson, M.: Collagenolytic activity in middle ear cholesteatoma. *Ann. Otol. Rhinol. Laryngol.*, 78: 112, 1969.

2. Abramson, M.; Asarch, R. G.; and Litton, W. B.: Experimental aural cholesteatoma causing bone resorption. *Ann. Otol. Rhinol. Laryngol.*, 84: 425, 1975.

3. Bang, F. B.; Bang, B. G.; and Foard, M.: Acute Newcastle virus infection of the upper respiratory tract of the chicken. I. A model for the study of environmental factors on upper respiratory tract infections. *Amer. J. Pathol.*, 76: 333, 1974.

4. Bang, F. B.; Bang, B. G.; and Foard, M.: Acute Newcastle viral infection of the upper respiratory tract of the chicken. II. The effect of diets deficient in vitamin A on the pathogenesis of the infection. *Amer. J. Pathol.*, 78: 417, 1975.

5. Billingham, R. E. and Silvers, W. K.: Dermoepidermal interactions and epithelial specificity. In Fleischmajer, R. and Billingham, R. E.,: (Eds.). *Epithelial-Mesenchymal Interactions. 18th Hahnemann Symposium.* Williams and Wilkins Company, Baltimore, Maryland, 1968, p. 252.

6. Birrell, J. F.: Black cellular cholesteatosis in childhood. *J. Laryngol. Otol.*, 70: 260, 1956.

7. Craigie, David: *Elements of General and Pathological Anatomy.* Ed. 2, Presenting a view of the present state of knowledge in these branches of science. Lindsay and Blakiston, Philadelphia, Pennsylvania, 1851, p. 343.

8. Dota, T.; Nakamura, K.; Saheki, M.; and Sasaki, Y.: Cholesterol granuloma—experimental. *Ann. Otol. Rhinol. Laryngol.*, 72: 346, 1963.

9. Fell, H. B. and Mellanby, E.: Metaplasia produced in cultures of chick by high vitamin A. *J. Physiol.*, 119: 470, 1953.

10. Fell, H. B. and Rinaldini, L. M.: The effects of vitamin A and C on cells and tissues in culture cells. In Wilmer, E. N.: (Ed.). *Tissues in Culture.* Vol. I. Academic Press, New York, New York, 1965, p. 659.

11. Ferlito, A.: Le "cholesteatome" de l'oreille moyenne et le granulome a cholesterol: considerations histopathologiques et cliniques. *Ann. Oto. Laryngol.*, 90: 697, 1973.

12. Fernandez, C. and Lindsay, J. R.: Aural cholesteatoma. Experimental observations. *Laryngoscope*, 70: 1119, 1960.

13. Flanagan, S. P.: "Nude," a new hairless gene with pleiotrophic effects in the mouse. *Genet. Res.*, 8: 295, 1966.

14. Fleischmajer, R. and Billingham, R. E.: *Epithelial-Mesenchymal Interactions. 18th Hahnemann Symposium.* Williams and Wilkins Company, Baltimore, Maryland, 1968.

15. Friedmann, I.: The comparative pathology of otitis media—experimental and human. II. The histopathology of experimental otitis of the guinea pig with particular reference to experimental cholesteatoma. *J. Laryngol. Otol.*, 69: 588, 1955.

16. Friedmann, I.: The pathology of otitis media with particular reference to bone changes. *J. Laryngol. Otol.*, 71: 313, 1957.

17. Friedmann, I.: Epidermoid cholesteatoma and cholesterol granuloma. *Ann. Otol. Rhinol. Laryngol.*, 68: 57, 1959.

18. Friedmann, I.: *The Pathology of the Ear.* Blackwell, Oxford, England, 1974.

19. Friedmann, I. and Hodges, G. M.: Morphogenesis and ultrastructure of the mouse embryonic salivary gland in tissue culture. *Acta Otolar.*, 79: 197, 1975.

20. Ghadially, F. N. and Skinnider, L. F.: Ropalocytosis. A new abnormality of erythrocytes and their precursors. *Experientia*, 27: 1217, 1971.

21. Goodhill, V.: The lurking latent cholesteatoma. *Ann. Otol. Rhinol. Laryngol.*, 69: 1199, 1971.

22. Goodhill, V.: A cholesteatoma chronicle. *Arch. Otol.*, 97: 183, 1973.

23. Guggenheim. Personal Communication.

24. Habermann, J.: Cholesteatomentstehung. In: Schwartze *Textbook of Otology.* Vogel, FCW Leipzig, Germany, 1892.

25. Harris, A. J.: Cholesteatosis and chronic otitis media: The histopathology of osseous and soft tissues. *Laryngoscope*, 72: 954, 1962.

26. Harris, M. and Toller, P.: The pathogenesis of dental cysts. *Brit. Med. Bull.*, 31: 159, 1975.

27. Hay, Elizabeth D.: Organization and fine structure of epithelium and mesenchyme in the developing chick embryo. In Fleischmajer, R. and Billingham, R. E.: (Eds.). *Epithelial-Mesenchymal Interactions. 18th Hahnemann Symposium.* Williams and Wilkins Company, Baltimore, Maryland, 1968, p. 31.

28. Haymann, L.: Experimentelle Studien zur Pathologie der akuten entzundlichen Prozesse im Mittelohr. *Arch. Ohrenheilk.*, 93: 1 and 95: 99, 1913.

29. Karma, P.: Middle ear epithelium and chronic ear disease. *Acta Otolar. (Stockh) Supple.*, 307: 1, 1972.

30. Kern, G.: Zur Entwicklung des Cholesteatoma hinter intaktem Trommelfell. *Schweiz. Med. Wschr.*, 88: 777, 1958.

31. Lim, D. J. and Saunders, W. H.: Acquired choleste-

atoma: light and electron microscopic observations. *Ann. Otol. Rhinol. Laryngol.*, 81:1, 1972.

32. McLoughlin, C. B.: II. The importance of mesenchymal factors in the differentiation of chick epidermis. *J. Embryol. Exp. Morphol.* 9: 385-409, 1961. Also, Part I. The differentiation in culture of the isolated epidermis of the embryonic chick and its response to excess vitamin A. *J. Embryol. Exp. Morphol.*, 9: 370, 1961.

33. McLoughlin, C. B.: Interaction of epidermis with various types of foreign mesenchyme. In Fleischmajer, R. and Billingham, R. E.: (Eds.). *Epithelial-Mesenchymal Interactions. 18th Hahnemann Symposium.* Williams and Wilkins Company, Baltimore, Maryland, 1968, p. 244.

34. Ordmann, L. J. and Gilman, T.: Studies in healing of cutaneous wounds. *Arch. Surg.*, 93: 857, 1966.

35. Pantelouris, E. M.: Absence of thymus in a mouse mutant. *Nature*, 217: 370, 1968.

36. Sadé, J.: Cellular differentiation of the middle ear lining. *Ann. Otol. Rhinol. Laryngol.*, 80: 376, 1971.

37. Sadé, J. and Halevy, A.: The etiology of bone destruction in chronic otitis media. *J. Laryngol. Otol.*, 88: 139, 1974.

38. Sadé, J. and Weinberg, J.: Mucus production in the chronically infected middle ear. A histological and histochemical study. *Ann. Otol. Rhinol. Laryngol.*, 78: 148, 1969.

39. Schuknecht, H. F.: *The Pathology of the Ear.* Harvard University Press, Boston, Massachusetts, 1974.

40. Schwarz, M.: *Das Cholesteatom im Gehörgang und im Mittelohr.* G. Thieme, Stuttgart, Germany, 1966.

41. Ten Cate, A. R.: The epithelial cell nests of Malassez and the genesis of the dental cysts. *Oral Surgery*, 34: 956, 1972.

42. Virchow, R.: Uber Perlgeschwülste (Cholesteatoma Joh. Müllers). *Virchows Arch. Pathol. Anat.*, VIII: 371, 1855.

43. Wagner, B. M.: Collagenase activity. In: Mandl, Ines (Ed.) *Collagenases.* Gordon and Breach, London, England, 1972, p. 77.

44. Wilkes, D. L.: Upper respiratory tract and ear (Chap. 25). In Anderson, W. A. D.: *Pathology.* [Ed. 6] Vol. 2. C. V. Mosby, St. Louis, Missouri, 1971, Figs. 25-29, p. 1063.

45. Wittmaack, K.: Das Gehörorgan. Die Entzündlichen Erkrankungsprozesse des Gehörganges. In Henke, E. and Lubarsch, O.: (Eds.). *Handbuch der Speziellen Patholog. Anatomie und Histologie*, Vol. 12. J. Springer, Berlin, Germany, 1926.

46. Ziman, J.: Is science to be believed? *Proc. R. Inst. of Great Brit.*, 46: 267, 1973.

FACTORS AFFECTING THE ORGANIZATION AND RENEWAL OF EPIDERMIS

Edna B. Laurence, Ph.D.

Introduction

Experimental studies on the regulation of tissue kinetics have suffered in the past years from the emphasis being placed on cell birth without reference to those equally important events which lead to cell maturation and cell death. This has been due mainly to the development of techniques for the visualization and quantitation of cell proliferation (a process common to all tissues) in comparison to the more difficult task of studying the events intrinsic to cell maturation and death; a process which is complicated by superimposition of tissue specific functions. In a normal tissue cell, birth is always balanced by cell death to maintain homeostasis. It is the imbalance of cell birth to cell maturation and to cell death that results in abnormal growth.

During the past few years there has been a shift in emphasis so that attempts now are being made to correlate the well documented happenings at cell birth with the subsequent events during maturation and consequent death of the cell. For the visualization of these processes there is no better model than the epidermis itself where there is histological and horizontal stratification demarcating the regions in the life-cycle of the tissue.

This short review attempts to give a general overall picture. It is in no way comprehensive and contains flagrant generalizations and by necessity it is biased. More detailed knowledge however, may be obtained from the cited literature.

Origin, Function, and Organization of Normal Epidermis

The epidermis is formed from embryonic ectoderm (Holbrook and Odland, 1975). Its function is to form a renewable selectively permeable, protective barrier over the body (the stratum corneum) (Elias and Friend, 1975). This barrier consists of layers of tightly cemented cornified cells (corneocytes) which are shed continuously from the surface (cell death). However, the mechanism underlying this process is little understood. This functioning, cornified layer is the final stage in the differentiation of an epidermal cell and the ultimate fate of a cell which has been produced in the deepest layer of the epidermis (cell birth) (Breathnach, 1975).

Dividing cells (keratoblasts) occur almost exclusively in the basal layer of cells (Christophers and Laurence, 1973) that are attached to the basement membrane which separates the epidermis from the dermis (Briggaman and Wheeler, 1975; and Kefalides, 1975). After division and during the ensuing differentiation process (keratinization) (Lavker, 1975) these cells lose their connections with the basement membrane (Christophers and Wolff, 1975), and move over their neighboring attached basal cells (Christophers, 1971), making connections with neighboring keratocytes to form the stratum spinosum. They are carried passively towards the surface by the continual production of cells below and the loss of cells from the surface (Matoltsy, 1975). As the cells differentiate they lose their reproductive potential and synthesize such specific components as fibrillar and amorphous proteins, keratohyalin (Fukuyama and Epstein, 1975; and Ugal, 1975) and membrane-coating granules. During this maturation process these cells become progressively flattened, their cell membranes and contents become modified (Buxman and Wuepper, 1975) and they resorb their organelles and nuclei. Thus a distinctive layer is formed, the stratum granulosum (Montagna and Parakkel, 1974), where the primary barrier to water loss was found (Elias and Friend, 1975). Very little is known about this layer but the biochemical events (Bernstein and Sibrack, 1972; and Bernstein et al, 1975) and the changes in shape of the cells in this layer determine the final structure and shape of the cornified cells. It is also considered that the loss of cellular turgidity causes a reduction in pressure on the underlying cells, thus giving room for a loosely connected basal cell to move away from the basal layer (Christophers, et al, 1974; and Christophers and Laurence, 1976) probably as a result of the combination of maturation (Christophers and Wolff, 1975) and the pressure of the neighboring cells (Bullough and Deol, 1975; and Bullough and Mitrani, 1976). The stratum granulosum is thus a much neglected focal point in epidermal architecture (Christophers and Laurence, 1976). It is not only the focus for the development of the functional membrane but also it may determine the architecture of the whole epidermis.

Recently, some regions (e.g. mouse ear and back, hamster ear, human scrotum, etc.) of the epidermis have been shown to have distinct vertical architecture so that the cells are arranged in columns or stacks (Christophers, 1971; and Mackenzie, 1972, 1973, and 1975). There has been much conjecture about the organization of these stacks, but it is known that they occur in regions with slow cell proliferation and maturation rates (Christophers, 1972; and Christophers and Laurence, 1973) so that adjacent cells in neighboring stacks have different ages (Christophers, et al, 1974). Proliferative cells are usually located around a central cell at the base of the column (Mackenzie, 1975), a factor which has led Potten and co-workers (Potten, 1974) to refer to a column as an "epidermal proliferative unit" (EPU) since he believes that all the cells on one EPU are a single clone. He also presents the hypothesis that the central basal cell of an EPU is a committed stem cell thus bringing the epidermis into line with the blood system for its pattern of prolifera-

tive activity (Potten, 1976). This central cell he considers to be a Langerhans cell (Allen and Potten, 1975).

The Langerhans cell (Wolff, 1972) is of unknown origin which is found in varying numbers in different layers of most keratinizing epithelia as well as dermis, lymph nodes, and the thymus of some animals. Potten's contention that the Langerhans cell is an epidermal stem cell is based on the fact that in mouse skin one is found at the central position at the base of each EPU. Yet Mackenzie, et al, (1975) have shown mouse is an exception and that stacked epidermis of other animals has a very sparse supply of Langerhans cells. More recently, the Langerhans cells have been considered as playing an immunological role in contact allergy (Silderberg, et al, 1974) but Hunter, et al (1976) found them in athymic hairless mice, thus suggesting that they are not of thymic origin. Thus the origin and function of Langerhans cells is still obscure and there is considerable evidence against their function being the controlling force in the maintenance of the epidermal proliferative unit.

The melanocytes found also in epidermis are of neural crest origin and are a system where the cells interact with the keratinocytes for the distribution of pigment (Montagna and Parakkal, 1974). They are a tissue in themselves (Quivedo, 1972) and apparently have their own cell proliferation regulating mechanism (Thronley and Laurence, 1976).

Merkel cells are the only other cells of unknown origin and function in the epidermis. They may be related in some way to nerve cells. They are attached by numerous desmosomes to their adjacent epidermal cells in the area surrounding certain hair follicles (Montagna and Parakkal, 1974). They have not yet been involved in any hypothesis concerning epidermal architecture or cell proliferation.

Langerhans and Merkel cells and melanocytes make up a very small percentage of the total epithelial cell population.

Regional Variations in Keratinizing Epithelia

The very organized structure of the epidermis is not the only form of architecture that exists. Depending on the region of the body (Christophers and Petzold, 1969) and the species studied, it may vary from this thin, compact, highly organized form of ear and back skin epidermis, e.g., in the mouse, to the thickened, vertically disorganized, highly keratinized epidermis of the sole of foot or palm of hand (Bullough, 1972; and Christophers and Laurence, 1973). In general it may be said that the thicker the epidermis the more cells are in division and the faster the maturation rate. Thus, the transit time through the living epidermis, which is a measure of maturation rate, is faster (Christophers and Laurence, 1976). The number of proliferating cells is greater in the thicker epidermis, but the cell cycle length may not be different (Cameron and Thrasher, 1971; Christophers and Laurence, 1973; Laurence, 1973; and Potten, 1975).

Ectodermally derived keratinizing epithelium extends in the head to line the buccal cavity, so that the mucosae that cover the palate, gingiva, and tongue have highly specialized, regionally defined histological characteristics; each with their own organization proliferative pool size and cell cycle time (Laurence, 1973; and Hansen, 1967). Besides extending into the mouth, it also lines the external nares and most important in the context of this symposium, it extends into the auditory canals.

Evolutionarily and developmentally one of the last organs to be formed in mammals is the hair. This develops from the epidermis late in fetal life or even after birth. This pilary unit develops from an epidermal plaque (Pinkus, 1958) differentiating into the sebaceous glands and the highly keratogenous hair. The follicle itself is lined with keratinizing epithelium which becomes less and less keratinized as the opening into the sebaceous gland is reached. Here the keratinized cells no longer adhere to each other to form a cohesive barrier. This is particularly well demonstrated in the so-called sebaceous follicles found on the human face and shoulders (Kligman, 1974; and Plewig and Kligman, 1975) and in the external auditory canals of other mammals. It is the increased formation of horny cells (corneocytes) and the increase in cohesion of these follicle cells that forms the typical acne comedone (Plewig, et al, 1971; Plewig, 1974; and Plewig and Kligman, 1975).

It is interesting to note that comedones can be produced experimentally in the sebaceous follicles of the external ear canal of rabbits (Mills and Kligman, 1975).

In contrast to this type of cyst formation the reverse may happen and the epidermal cells are shed before they become fully cornified and a cohesive barrier is poorly formed as seen in such diseases as psoriasis. It is not known why there should be these differences in production and cohesiveness of the cornified cells in different regions of the body. This emphasizes the lack of information concerning the maturation processes involved in epithelial cells, Keratinizing epithelium is not all ectodermally derived. It may also be of endodermal origin as in the esophagus and fore stomach or (in a modified form) in the mammalian bladder which has an epithelium that is able to keratinize under certain circumstances (Hicks, 1975).

Epidermal Derivatives

Besides forming stratified, keratinizing epidermis, the embryonic ectoderm may be non-keratinizing as in the cornea and the highly specialized lens epithelium. It may become mucous secreting as in the mucous membrane of the nose. Besides the hair, it forms the sebaceous, mammary, lacrimal, salivary, and sweat glands. It forms part of the teeth.

Metaplasia of one type of epithelium into another occurs in adults in addition to the well-known examples in embryos (McCloughlin, 1963). The mechanism underlying these transformations is still unknown, but factors involving the dermis or mesenchyme itself apparently are involved (McCloughlin, 1961, 1963, and 1968; and Fleischmajor and Billingham, 1968).

Dermal Involvement

There is no doubt that there is ample evidence for the dermis being intimately involved in the architecture of the epidermis. Christophers and Laurence (1976) have shown the influence of the dermal skeleton (papillary body) on the formation of rete pegs and their constancy in number even in hyperplastic conditions. The mere fact that embryos have regional variations in e.g. the thickness of epidermis of the soles of feet indicates that the external environment (in the form of wear and tear) need not be responsible for the epidermal architecture. The role of the dermis forms an extensive study in itself which is beyond the scope of this study, but mention should be made here of the pioneering work of Billingham and coworkers, (1972) who have shown that the epidermis can be structurally remodelled by the underlying dermis. However, very little emphasis has been placed on the fact that normal regional variations are so stable. This is particularly well demonstrated in e.g. the vermillion border of the lip where the abrupt change in form of the papillary layer is reflected in an equally abrupt difference in the overlying epidermis (Christophers and Laurence, 1976).

Wound Healing

The function of the epidermis is to maintain a protective barrier over the body, and in this study to this point, the normal constant replacement of this barrier has been emphasized. However, during the life of the animal the epidermis is constantly subjected to insults from chemical irritants, abrasions, burns, cuts, and extirpation. In these circumstances the demands on the epidermis to renew completely the living layer as well as the cornified barrier are countermanded by an activity which has different requirements from the ordinary tissue turnover.

Removal of the cornified layer by cellotape stripping results in enormously increased cell proliferation rate and shortening of the cell proliferation cycle and maturation rates until the cornified layer is restored and the living epidermis returns to its normal tissue kinetics and thickness (Christophers, 1971 and 1972). However, deeper wounding involves cell migration in order that resurfacing may take place. This is achieved by migration from the cut edges of the epidermis (Bullough and Laurence, 1960; and Winter, 1972) accompanied by a vast increase in cell proliferation at that point. In shallow excised wounds the repopulation of the surface originates from the hair follicles, sebaceous ducts or sweat ducts (Winter, 1972) as well as the wound edges.

Factors affecting epidermal migration have been studied extensively since they are of prime importance medically. Experiments involving re-epithelialization emphasize the need for oxygen, even hyperbaric conditions (Winter, 1972; and Silvers, 1972) and the composition of the substrate (Ryan, 1970; and Ryan, et al, 1971) as well as the cellular components within that substrate (Winter, 1975; and Schellander and Marks, 1973). These conditions are reflected in vitro situations and have caused much confusion since the conditions necessary for epithelial maintenance are different from those required for cellular migration (Karasek, 1975; and Marks, et al, 1972).

Epidermis is invasive unless it either meets itself, as in the opposite edge of a wound or is inhibited or directed by architecture, endothelial-epithelial interactions or mesenchymal-epithelial interaction. Thus in corneal transplants the epithelium may migrate over the inner corneal surface obstructing the aqueous drainage tract. Apparently, in normal circumstances, it is held in check by the interaction with the endothelium (Cameron, et al, 1974). However, in corneal healing the timing of the response is slower in endothelium than in the epithelium and if retarded still further, the epithelium takes over and continues on its suicidal course.

Similar migratory response was particularly well demonstrated when pieces of skin were implanted into the pinna of guinea pigs. The epidermis always migrated round the cut explanted dermis so that a cyst was formed with the cornified cells innermost and basal cells outermost. "It was a constant observation that horny material was shed into the lumen of the cyst and in no instance could different patterns be found. Close contact between the dermis of the implant and the host connective tissue was always established. Heavy inflammatory reaction predominantly consisting of polymorphonuclear leucocytes was seen near or above the stratum corneum" (Christophers, 1972).

This is in marked contrast to the in vitro conditions when migration (epiboly) completely enclosed the dermal explant so that the cornified layer was external. Christophers concludes from these experiments that a suitable microenvironment including nutritional requirements and available space are dominating factors in the orientation of migrating epidermis. This is also emphasized by Winter (1975) who found that cellular migration in burns was impeded not because of changes caused by the heat to the dermis but because granulation tissue was absent from the wound site. This situation was also found in skin wounds in rabbit fetuses where no inflammation occurred nor granulation tissue formed and no epithelialization of the wound resulted (Somasundaram and Prathap, 1970). Winter (1975) also demonstrated that the resulting architecture of the epidermis was directly dependent on the structure of the newly formed dermis.

The Mesenchymal Factor/Antichalones

For many years now the epidermal architecture has been known to be dictated by cells from other tissues, particularly of mesenchymal origin (McCloughlin, 1961; Billingham and Silvers, 1971; and Fleischmajer and Billingham, 1968). Following the work in embryology on induction, it has been shown that the epidermis is under the influence of stimulating substances. From the point of view of a unified concept for all tissues, such considerations as the nature of these substances, where they are synthesized, their specific target sites and biochemical pathways involved are still unresolved. That they exist there is no doubt and Bullough and Mitrani (1976) point out that for every tissue that has been studied for mesenchymal factor effect, evidence has been found for their action.

Direct indications that these substances may act by antagonizing epidermal chalone action was first given by Laurence, et al (1972), since it was impossible to explain site variations in response to epidermal G_2 chalone solely by a negative feedback process (Laurence and Hansen, 1971 and 1972). Argyris (1972) also gave evidence from the effect of tumor implants on overlying epidermis and adjacent hair follicles that the chalone must be inactivated. Since then it has been established that cell proliferation cannot be controlled by negative feedback processes alone (Bullough, 1975; and Bjerknes and Iversen, 1974). Whether the epidermal growth factor (Cohen, 1972 and 1975) acts directly on the epidermal chalones is not known.

Chalones

The high mitotic activity encountered at the edges of wounds was considered for very many years to be a result of stimulants coming from the wound and were termed "wound hormones". It was in the pursuit of these substances that Bullough and Laurence (1960) performed their differential wounding experiments and realized that their results could only be explained in terms of release of an inhibitor produced by the epidermis itself which acted by repressing the normal epidermal cell proliferation. Bullough (1962) recognized that all tissues should be controlled by similar negative feedback process which he called "chalones". Although experiments had previously been performed showing evidence for the existence and effects of substances which act by means of a negative feedback principle (Houck and Attallah, 1975) and theories had been proposed formulating such a feedback mechanism (Iversen, 1961 and 1965; and Weiss and Kavanau, 1957), the implications of the concept as a whole were only realized when extensive experimental evidence was produced using fractionated tissue extracts (Houck and Daugherty, 1974; Houck, 1976; and Rytömaa, 1976). The first chalone (Laurence, 1973) to be prepared in almost pure form was an epidermal chalone extracted from pig skin acting on mitosis (Hondius, Boldingh, and Laurence, 1968). This is now known as the epidermal G_2 chalone (Marks, 1973). Since then Marks has isolated a chalone which acts in G_1 of the epidermal cell cycle; the epidermal G_1 chalone (Marks, 1973, 1975, and 1976). Extensive experiments with these two purified epidermal chalones have shown that each one is specific for its own phase of the cell cycle, it is cell-line (tissue) specific, and it is species unspecific since both were isolated from pig skin and tested on DNA synthesis and mitosis in mouse pinna epidermis and the associated epidermal derivative, the sebaceous gland (Thornley and Laurence, 1975 and 1976; Thornley, et al, 1976, in press; and Laurence and Thornley, 1976). Results of experiments illustrating these properties are shown in Tables 3 and 4. By expressing the results in terms of cell cycle kinetics it was recognized that the epidermal G_1 chalone acted at the G_1/S phase boundary and the G_2 chalone at the G_2/M phase boundary (Fig. 15). The more crude extract (the 72-81% ethanol extract)

TABLE 3

Cell-Cycle and Cell-Line Specificity of Epidermal G_1 Chalone

N = 10= Number of animals	DNA Synthesis 5 h test (16.00-21.00 h)		Mitotic Index 4 h test (11.00-15.00 h)	
	d.p.m. / mg	Labelling Index	Colcemid	
Control	3760 ± 320	26.0 ± 0.95	8.95 ± 0.84	
G_1 chalone	2770 ± 220	20.0 ± 0.76	8.40 ± 0.81	Epidermis
Depression	$-26\%^*$	$-23\%^*$	0%	
		$^*P < 0.01$		
Control	1005 ± 170	81.8 ± 2.12	19.3 ± 1.41	
G_1 chalone	885 ± 70	82.9 ± 2.71	17.8 ± 1.35	Sebaceous glands
Depression	-12%	0%	-8%	

TABLE 4

Cell-Cycle and Cell-Line Specificity of Epidermal G_2 Chalone

N = 15= Number of animals	DNA Synthesis 5 h test (16.00-21.00 h)		Mitotic Index 4 h test (11.00-15.00 h)	
	d.p.m. / mg	Labelling Index	Colcemid	
Control	3380 ± 230	25.8 ± 0.78	10.6 ± 0.36	
G_2 chalone	3700 ± 315	25.6 ± 1.07	5.7 ± 0.26	Epidermis
Depression	0%	0%	47%*	
			*P 0.01	
Control	820 ± 45	90.2 ± 2.16	23.9 ± 1.50	
G_2 chalone	995 ± 90	86.5 ± 2.57	22.2 ± 1.28	Sebaceous glands
Depression	0%	4%"	7%"	
			"P 0.01	

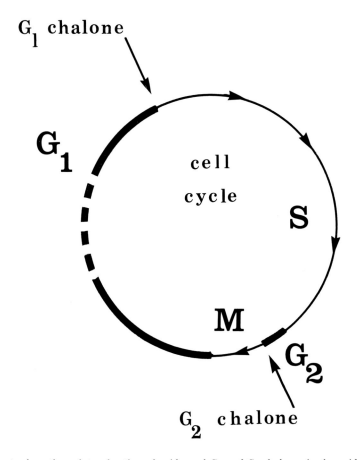

Fig. 15: Diagram to show the points of action of epidermal G_1 and G_2 chalones in the epidermal cell cycle.

affected the cell proliferation of both epidermal and sebaceous gland tissues and both phases of the cell cycle indicating the presence of at least four chalones (Table 5). What is not known is whether these chalones in their pure form act on other keratinizing epithelia of e.g. esophagus of endodermal origin or non-keratinizing epithelia of ectodermal origin (Laurence and Thornley, 1976). They do not affect the cell proliferation in intestine (Thornley and Laurence, 1976).

The mechanism of action of chalones is still unknown (Laurence and Thornley, 1976). Simms and Stillman (1936) considered that these endogenous inhibitors were primarily inhibitors of cell proliferation so that the cell remained in a "dormant state" from where it could be modulated either to differentiation or proliferation. Bullough (1973) regarded chalones as being primary inhibitors of cell proliferation and so promoting maturation and consequently differentiation for function of a cell. Bullough and Rytömaa (1965), and Laurence, et al (1972) considered the inhibition of cell proliferation to be secondary and resulting from the cell's promotion of maturation. Bullough (1975) regarded chalones as being a factor which maintained the balance in the organ of cell gain as well as cell loss. Attallah and Houck (1976) consider that the changes in the chalone concentration regulate the cellular cyclic AMP system.

Unfortunately, chalones in general are very difficult to isolate and the stringent care in assessing the results in terms of DNA synthesis inhibition can lead to the recognition of artefacts rather than chalones (Laurence and Thornley, 1976; Christophers and Laurence, 1976; and Duell, et al, 1975). Only when pure substances are available and stringent experiments performed will the mode of action of chalones be elucidated.

Epidermal Chalones and Cyclic AMP

Since the discriminative test for epidermal G_2 chalone revealed that adrenalin was needed as a co-factor (Bullough and Laurence, 1964; Marrs and Voorhees, 1971; Voorhees, et al, 1973) it was natural that, once the presence of the c-AMP system in skin was established (Sutherland, 1972), chalones should be linked with c-AMP (Voorhees and Mier, 1974). As with all work on the substances of this sytem the interpretations have been complicated by the concentrations of the substances and methods used (Flaxman and Harper, 1975; Halprin, et al, 1975; and Voorhees, et al,

TABLE 5

Cell-Cycle and Cell-Line Non-Specificity of 72-81% Ethanol Extract Pig Skin

N = 10= Number of animals	DNA Synthesis 6.5 h test (07.30-14.30 h)		Mitotic Index 4 h test (11.00-15.00 h)	
	d.p.m. / mg	Labelling Index	Colcemid	
Control	8100 ± 620	42.1 ± 1.60	11.25 ± 0.63	
Ethanol extract	4750 ± 450	26.7 ± 0.90	5.50 ± 0.20	Epidermis
Depression	41%	31%	51%	
Control	1625 ± 185	91.6 ± 2.24	23.9 ± 1.50	
Ethanol extract	985 ± 105	54.7 ± 1.66	13.0 ± 0.41	Sebaceous glands
Depression	39%	40%	46%	
		In all cases P < 0.01		

1975). Thus, although the epidermal G_2 chalone appears to act in relation to the c-AMP system, at present, there is no direct evidence that the epidermal G_1 chalone is operating in a similar manner (Elgjo, 1975; and Grimm and Marks, 1974). In other tissue-chalone-systems a link with c-AMP system has been proposed (Attallah and Houck, 1975). It is known that cellular cyclic-AMP levels fall when the cells are in division but it is not known whether this is a cause or an effect of other c-AMP limiting substances. Thus any interpretation of results using c-AMP as a mediator are subject to scrutiny.

The Diurnal Rhythm and the Stress Hormones

The well-known diurnal rhythm in all phases of the cell proliferation cycle (Izquierdo and Gibbs, 1974; and Grube, et al, 1970) make it necessary to have well conditioned mice in controlled conditions before any experiments are performed (Laurence, 1973). Even so, it has been shown that the degree of response of DNA synthesis to epidermal G_1 chalone is independent of the diurnal variation (Thornley and Laurence, 1976). This does not apply to the epidermal G_2 chalone where certain phases of the diurnal rhythm mask any chalone (G_2) inhibition.

None of the substances so far mentioned have been shown experimentally to affect the maturation or functional processes of the epidermis. The chalones and adrenalin have been shown to affect the cell proliferation cycle but long term administration has never been attempted to discover if the tissue maturation rate or the cellular death rate has been increased or if they affect the functional processes of the cells of the epidermis. However, glucocorticoids are known to reduce the thickness of the epidermis. Wilson and Marks (1976) and Laurence and Christophers (1976) have shown that the effect of long term administration of hydrocortisone affects the rate of maturation of the cells, but not the cell proliferation rate. The highly organized epidermis of the mouse ear shows this dramatically (Fig. 16), although it may be easily seen and quantified in the thicker, ver-

tically organized sole of foot. If this type of study is repeated with such substances as the epidermal chalones, then a more positive approach to chalone action should be established. Whether corticosteroids mediate their action via prostaglandins as they apparently do in other tissues would be interesting to discover (Tashjian, et al, 1975; Kantrowitz, et al, 1975; and Lewis and Piper, 1975).

Vitamin A

The dramatic effects of vitamin A on acne (Plewig and Kligman, 1975) has led to a thorough study of this group of substances on cell proliferation and hyperplasia. Zil (1972) reported an increase in the cell proliferation rate, thickness and cellularity. Christophers and Langner (1974) showed that it stimulated cell proliferation in confluent epidermal cell cultures whereas lymphocytes and fibroblasts showed no response. This indicated a tissue specific effect. In a further study, Christophers and Wolff (in press) showed that the cellular attachments were also increased. Vitamin A acid also affects the maturation or functional differentiation for the cells. Thus, Chopra and Flaxman (1975) reported a decreased number of keratohyalin granules with vitamin A alcohol as well as the increase in cell proliferation and growth of cultures while Christophers and Wolff (in press) not only showed this disappearance of keratohyalin in vivo but a decrease in tonofilaments and desmosomal membrane specifications. The tissue specific nature of the substance and the action on differentiation lead to speculation on the interaction with chalone which, however, would not only be premature at this stage but, without considerable amount of extensive experimentation would be dangerous. It was interesting that none of these experiments reported any signs of mucous metaplasia of the epidermis although this has been reported as a major effect of this substance.

Conclusions

This review has attempted to correlate the evi-

Mouse Pinna Epidermis.

CONTROL

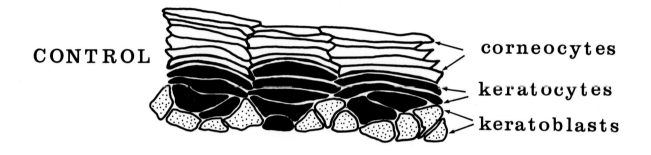

corneocytes

keratocytes

keratoblasts

HYDRO-

CORTISONE

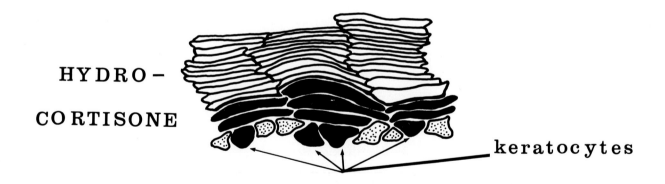

keratocytes

Fig. 16: Diagram to show the effect of three week oral administration of hydrocortisone on mouse pinna epidermis. There is a noticeable reduction in the number of cells in the basal layer and a reduced number of stacked keratocytes in each column. Diagram drawn from fluorescein isothiocyanate stained section prepared by Dr. Enno Christophers.

dence that exists for some of the factors which are involved in the maintenance of site specific structural organization of the epidermis and the effect of endogenous regulators of that system. Gurdon, et al (1975) in a series of dextrous experiments, transplanted the nucleus from an epidermal cell of the web of a frog to the enucleated egg. By further transplantation in a similar way he was able to obtain a tadpole with normal histologically developed tissues which functioned in a normal manner. From this it can be concluded that it is not the genetic composition of the nucleus that dictates the nature of the tissue but the interaction of many factors on that nucleus and cytoplasm. These are intercellular, extracellular, endogenous and exogenous in origin. In the case of epidermis they are also environmental.

With the correct experimental procedures, the architectural anatomy of epidermis is such that it is possible, although laborious, to visualize and quantitate the effects of substances on cell proliferation and maturation/differentiation. Thus a long term study of substances on the tissue life cycle can be pursued. The deviations from the normal that are recorded should help to elucidate some of the many abnormalities that occur in pathological conditions, whether these are organizational, metaplastic or structural defects.

Acknowledgements

I am indebted to my colleagues Professor Enno Christophers, University of Kiel, Dermatology Department and Dr. Alan Thornley, University of Witswatersrand, Zoology Department for their contribution to many of the ideas incorporated here. Whereas they have given so much they are in no way responsible for any inaccuracies and gross generalizations recorded here. I am also indebted to the Wellcome Trust and the Cancer Research Campaign for grants which have made the cooperation possible.

It is my pleasure to express gratitude to Professor Ian Mackenzie and the Staff of the Dental College, The University of Iowa, for their help in the preparation of this manuscript.

Also, my thanks to Professor F. Marks of the Cancer Research Center, Heidelberg and Dr. W. Hondius Boldingh, N. V. Organon, Holland, for the gifts of epidermal G_1 and G_2 chalone respectively.

References

1. Allen, T. D. and Potten, C. S.: Fine-structural identification and organization of the epidermal proliferative unit. *J. Cell Sci.*, 15: 291, 1975.

2. Argyris, T. S.: Chalones and the control of normal, regenerative, and neoplastic growth of skin. *Am. Zoologist.*, 12: 137, 1972.

3. Attallah, A. M. and Houck, J. C.: Lymphocyte chalone. In Houck, J. C.: (Ed.). *Chalones.* Elsevier, Amsterdam, North Holland, Chapter 15, 1976.

4. Beer, A. E. and Billingham, R. E.: In vivo approaches to the analysis of the conservation of epidermal specificities. In Maibach, H. I. and Rovee, D. T.: (Eds.). *Epidermal Wound Healing.* Year Book Medical Pub., Chicago, Illinois, 1972, pp. 187.

5. Bernstein, I. A. and Sibrack, L. A.: Chemical dynamics in epidermal differentiation. *J. Invest. Dermatol.*, 59: 77, 1972.

6. Bernstein, I. A.; Kaman, R. L.; Malinoff, H., et al.: Translation of polysomal messenger RNA during epidermal differentiation. *J. Invest. Dermatol.*, 65: 102, 1975.

7. Billingham, R. E. and Silvers, W. K.: A biologist's reflections on dermatology, *J. Invest. Dermatol.*, 57: 227, 1971.

8. Bjerknes, R. and Iversen, O. H.: "Antichalone". A theoretical treatment of the possible role of antichalone in the growth control system. *Acta Path. Microbiol. Scand. (A)*, Suppl. 248: 33, 1974.

9. Boldingh, W. H. and Laurence, E. B.: Extraction, purification and preliminary characterization of the epidermal chalone. A tissue specific mitotic inhibitor obtained from vertebrate skin. *European J. Biochem.*, 5: 191, 1968.

10. Breathnach, A. S.: Aspects of epidermal ultrastructure. *J. Invest. Dermatol.*, 65: 2, 1975.

11. Briggaman, R.A. and Wheeler, C. E.: The epidermal-dermal junction. *J. Invest. Dermatol.*, 65: 71, 1975.

12. Bullough, W. S.: The control of mitotic activity in adult mammalian tissues. *Biol. Rev.*, 37: 307, 1962.

13. Bullough, W. S.: The control of epidermal thickness. *Brit. J. Dermatol.*, 87: 187, 347, 1972.

14. Bullough, W. S.: The chalones. A review. *Natl. Cancer Inst. Monogr. Suppl.*, 38: 5, 1973.

15. Bullough, W. S.: Mitotic control in adult mammalian tissues. *Biol. Rev.*, 50: 99, 1975.

16. Bullough, W. S. and Laurence, E. B.: The control of epidermal mitotic activity in the mouse. *Proc. Soc. Biol.*, 151: 517, 1960.

17. Bullough, W. S. and Laurence, E. B.: Mitotic control by internal secretion: the role of the chalone-adrenalin complex. *Exp. Cell Res.*, 33: 176, 1964.

18. Bullough, W. S. and Rytömaa, T.: Mitotic Homeostasis. *Nature* (London), 205: 573, 1965.

19. Bullough, W. S. and Deol, J. U.: Dermo-epidermal adhesion and its effect on epidermal structure in the mouse. *Brit. J. Dermatol.*, 93· (4) 417, 1975

20. Bullough, W. S. and Mitrani, E.: An analysis of the epidermal chalone control mechanism. In Houck, J. C.: (Ed.). *Chalones*. Elsevier, Amsterdam, North Holland, 1976.

21. Buxman, M. M. and Wuepper, K. D.: Keratin cross-linking and epidermal transglutaminase. *J. Invest. Dermatol.*, 65: 107, 1975.

22. Cameron, I. L. and Thrasher, J. D.: *Cellular and Molecular Renewal in the Mammalian Body.* Academic Press, New York, New York, 1971.

23. Cameron, J. D.; Flaxman, B. A.; and Yanoff, M.: In vitro studies of corneal wound healing: epithelial-endothelial interactions. *Invest. Ophthalmol.*, 13: 575, 1974.

24. Chopra, D. P. and Flaxman, B. A.: The effect of Vitamin A on growth and differentiation of human keratinocytes in vitro. *J. Invest. Dermatol.*, 64: 19, 1975.

25. Christophers, E.: Die epidermale Columnarstruktur Voraussetzungen und Moglicher Entstehungsmechanismus. *Z. Zellforsch. Mikrosk. Anat.*, 114: 441, 1971.

26. Christophers, E.: Cellular architecture of the stratum corneum. *J. Invest. Dermatol.*, 56: 165, 1971.

27. Christophers, E.: The architecture of stratum corneum after wounding. *J. Invest. Dermatol.*, 57: 241, 1971.

28. Christophers, E.: Correlation between column formation, thickness and rate of new cell production in guinea pig epidermis. *Virchows Arch. (Zellpathol.)*, 10: 286, 1972.

29. Christophers, E.: Kinetic aspects of epidermal wound healing. In Maibach, H. I. and Rovee, D. T.: (Eds). *Epidermal Wound Healing*. Year Book Medical Publishers, Chicago, Illinois, 1972, pp. 53.

30. Christophers, E. and Petzold, V.: Epidermal cell replacement: topographical variations in albino guinea-pig skin. *Brit. J. Dermatol.*, 81: 598, 1969.

31. Christophers, E. and Laurence, E. B.: Regional variations in mouse skin: quantitation of epidermal compartments in two different body sites. *Virchows Archiv (Zellpathol)*, 12: 212, 1973.

32. Christophers, E. and Langner, A.: In vitro effects of Vitamin A acid on cultured fibroblasts, lymphcytes and epidermal cells: a comparative study. *Arch. Dermatol. Forsch.*, 251 (2): 147, 1974.

33. Christophers, E., Wolff, H. H. and Laurence, E. B.: The formation of epidermal cell columns. *J. Invest. Dermatol.*, 62: 555, 1974.

34. Christophers, E. and Wolff, H. H.: Differential formation of desmosomes and hemidesmosomes in epidermal cell cultures treated with retinoic acid. *Nature*, 256: 209, 1975.

35. Christophers, E. and Laurence, E. B.: Kinetics and structural development of the epidermis. In Mali, J. W. H.: (Ed.). *Current Problems in Dermatology.* Karger, Basel, Switzerland, 1976.

36. Cohen, S.: Epidermal growth factor. *J. Invest. Dermatol.*, 59: 13, 1972.

37. Cohen, S. and Carpenter, G.: Human epidermal growth factor: isolation and chemical and biological properties. *Proc. Nat. Acad. Sci.*, 72: 1317, 1975.

38. Duell, E. A., Kelsey, W. H. and Vorhees, J. J.: Epidermal chalone—past and present concept. *J. Invest. Dermatol.*, 65: 67, 1975.

39. Elgjo, K.: Epidermal chalone and cyclic AMP: an in vivo study. *J. Invest. Dermatol.*, 64: 14, 1975.

40. Elias, P. M. and Friend, D. S.: The permeability barrier in mammalian epidermis. *Cell Biol.*, 65: 180, 1975.

41. Flaxman, B. A. and Harper, R. A.: In vitro analysis of the control of keratinocyte proliferation in human epidermis by physiologic and pharmacologic agents. *J. Invest. Dermatol.*, 65: 52, 1975.

42. Fleischmajer, R. and Billingham, R. E.: *Epithelial-Mesenchymal Interactions. 18th Hahneman Symposium.* Williams and Wilkins Company, Baltimore, Maryland, 1968.

43. Fukuyama, K. and Epstein, W. L.: Heterogenous proteins in keratohyaline granules studied by quantitative autoradiography. *J. Invest. Dermatol.*, 65 (1): 113, 1975.

44. Grimm, W. and Marks, F.: Effect of tumor-promoting phorbol esters on the normal and the isoproterenol-elevated level of adenosine 3', 5'-cyclic monophosphate in mouse epidermis in vivo. *Cancer Res.*, 34 (11): 3128, 1974.

45. Grube, D. D.; Auerbach, H.; and Brues, A. M.: Diurnal variation in labeling index of mouse epidermis: a double isotope autoradiographic demonstration of changing flow rates. *Cell Tissue Kinet.*, 3: 363,

1970.

46. Gurdon, J. B.; Laskey, R. A.; and Reeves, O. R.: The developmental capacity of nuclei transplanted from keratinized skin cells of adult frogs. *J. Embryol. Exp. Morphol.*, 34 (1): 93, 1975.

47. Halprin, K. M.; Adachi, K.; Yoshikawa, K., et al.: Cyclic AMP and Psoriasis. *J. Invest. Dermatol.*, 65 (1): 170, 1975.

48. Hansen, E. R.: Mitotic activity and mitotic duration in tongue and gingival epithelium of mice. Effect of chalone. *Odont. T.*, 75: 480, 1967.

49. Hicks, R. M.: The mammalian urinary bladder: an accommodating organ. *Biol. Rev.*, 50 (2): 215, 1975.

50. Holbrook, K. A. and Odland, G. F.: The fine structure of developing human epidermis: light, scanning, and transmission electron microscopy of the periderm. *J. Invest. Dermatol.*, 65 (1): 16, 1975.

51. Houck, J. C.: *Chalones.* Elsevier, Amsterdam, North Holland, 1976.

52. Houck, J. C. and Daugherty, W. F.: *Chalones: A Tissue Specific Approach to Mitotic Control.* Med. Com. Press. Update Series. New York, New York, 1974.

53. Houck, J. C. and Attallah, A. M.: Chalones (specific and endogenous mitotic inhibitors) and cancer. In Becker, F. F.: (Ed). *Cancer. A Comprehensive Treatise.* Plenum Press, New York, New York, 1975, pp. 287.

54. Hunter, J. A.; Fairley, D. J.; Priestley, G. C., et al.: Langerhans cells in the epidermis of athymic mice. *Brit. J. Dermatol.*, 94 (2): 119, 1976.

55. Iversen, O. H.: The regulation of cell numbers in the epidermis. A cybernetic point of view. *Acta Pathol. Microbiol. Scand. Suppl.*, 148: 91, 1961.

56. Iverson, O. H.: Cybernetic aspects of the cancer problem. *Progr. Biocybern.*, 2: 76, 1965.

57. Izquierdo, J. and Gibbs, J. S.: Turnover of cell-renewing populations undergoing circadian rhythms in cell proliferation. *Cell. Tissue Kinet.*, 7: 99, 1976.

58. Kantrowitz, F.; Robinson, D.; McGuire, M. B., et al: Corticosteroids inhibit prostaglandin production by rheumatoid synovia. *Nature*, 258: 737, 1975.

59. Karasek, M. C.: In vitro growth and maturation of epithelial cells from postembryonic skin. *J. Invest. Dermatol.*, 65 (1): 60, 1975.

60. Kefalides, N. A.: Basement membranes: structural and biosynthetic considerations. *J. Invest. Dermatol.*, 65 (1): 85, 1975.

61. Kligman, A. M.: An overview of acne. *J. Invest. Dermatol.*, 62: 268, 1974.

62. Laurence, E. B.: Experimental approach to the epidermal chalone. *Natl. Cancer Inst. Monogr.* 38: 37, 1973.

63. Laurence, E. B.: The epidermal chalone and keratinising epithelium. *Natl. Cancer Inst. Monogr.* 38: 61, 1973.

64. Laurence, E. B. and Hansen, E. R.: An in vivo study of epidermal chalone and stress hormones on mitosis in tongue epithelium and ear epidermis of the mouse. *Virchows Arch. (Zellpathol.)*, 9:271, 1971.

65. Laurence, E. B. and Hansen, E. R.: Regional specificity of the epidermal chalone extracted from two different body sites. *Virchows Arch. (Zellpathol.)*, 11:34, 1972.

66. Laurence, E. B.; Hansen, E. R.; Christophers, E.; and Rytömaa, T.: Systemic factors influencing epidermal mitosis. *Rev. Eur. Etude Clin. Biol.*, 17: 133, 1972.

67. Laurence, E. B. and Christophers, E.: Selective action of cortisol on post mitotic epidermal cells in vivo. *J. Invest. Dermatol.*, 62:222, 1976.

68. Laurence, E. B. and Thornley, A. L.: Chalone tissue specificity and the embryonic derivation of organs. An appraisal of the problems. In Houck, J. C.: (Ed.). *Chalones.* Elsevier, Amsterdam, North Holland, 1976, chapt. 11.

69. Laurence E. B. and Thornley, A. L.: The influence of epidermal chalone on cell proliferation. In Cairnie, A.: (Ed.). *Stem Cells in Various Tissues.* Academic Press, 1976.

70. Lavker, R. M.: Lipid synthesis in chick epidermis. *J. Invest. Dermatol.*, 65 (1): 93, 1975.

71. Lewis, G. P. and Piper, P. J.: Inhibition of release of prostaglandins as an explanation of some of the actions of anti-inflammatory corticosteroids. *Nature*, 254 (5498): 308, 1975.

72. Mackenzie, I. C.: The ordered structure of mammalian epidermis. In Maibach, H. I. and Rovee, D. T.: (Eds.). *Epidermal Wound Healing.* Year Book Medical Publishers, Chicago, Illinois, 1972, pp. 5.

73. Mackenzie, I. C.: Ordered structure of the epidermis. *J. Invest. Dermatol.*, 65 (1): 45, 1975.

74. Mackenzie, I. C.: Spatial distribution of mitosis in mouse epidermis. *Anat. Rec.*, 181 (4): 705, 1975.

75. Mackenzie, I. C. and Linder, J. E.: An examination of cellular organization within the stratum corneum by a silver staining method. *J. Invest. Dermatol.*, 61:245, 1973.

76. Mackenzie, I. C.: Zimmerman, K. L.; and Wheelock, D. A.: Patterns of mitosis in hamster epidermis. *Am. J. Anat.*, 144 (4): 461, 1975.

77. Marks, F.: A tissue-specific factor inhibiting DNA synthesis in mouse epidermis. *Natl. Cancer Inst. Monogr.*, 38: 79, 1973.

78. Marks, F.: Isolation of an endogenous inhibitor of epidermal DNA synthesis (G_1 chalone) from pig skin. *Hoppe Seyler's Z. Physiol. Chem.*, 356 (12): 1989, 1975.

79. Marks, F.: The epidermal chalones. In Houck, J. C.: (Ed.). *Chalones.* Elsevier, Amsterdam, North Holland, 1976.

80. Marks, R.; Bhogal, B.; and Dawber, R. P.: The

migratory property of epidermis in vitro. *Arch. Dermatol. Forsch.*, 243: 209, 1972.

81. Marrs, J. M. and Voorhees, J. J.: Preliminary characterization of an epidermal chalone-like inhibitor. *J. Invest. Dermatol.*, 56: 353, 1971.

82. Matoltsy, A. G.: Desmosomes, filaments, and keratohyaline granules: their role in the stabilization and keratinization of the epidermis. *J. Invest. Dermatol.*, 65 (1): 127, 1975.

83. McCloughlin, C. B.: The importance of mesenchymal factors in the differentiation of chick epidermis. I. The differentiation in culture of the isolated epidermis of the embryonic chick and its response to excess Vitamin A. *J. Embryol. Exp. Morphol.*, 9: 370, 1961.

84. McCloughlin, C. B.: The importance of mesenchymal factors in the differentiation of chick epidermis. II. Modification of epidermal differentiation by contact with different types of mesenchyme. *J. Embryol. Exp. Morphol.*, 9: 385, 1961.

85. McCloughlin, C. B.: Mesenchymal influences on epithelial differentiation. *S. E. B. Symposia XVII Cell Differentiation*, pp. 359, 1963.

86. Mills, O. H. and Kligman, A. M.: Assay of comedolytic agents in the rabbit ear. In Maibach, H.: (Ed.). *Animal Models in Dermatology*. Churchill and Livingstone, Edinburgh, Scotland, 1975, pp. 176.

87. Montagna, W. and Parakkal, P. F.: *The Structure and Function of Skin*. (3rd ed.) Academic Press London, New York, New York, 1974.

88. Pinkus, H.: Embryology of hair. In Montagna, W. and Ellis, R. A.: (Eds.). *Biology of Hair Growth*. Academic Press, New York, New York, 1958, pp. 1.

89. Plewig, G: Follicular keratinization. *J. Invest. Dermatol.*, 62: 308, 1974.

90. Plewig, G. and Kligman, A. M.: *Acne: Morphogenesis and Treatment*. Springer-Verlag, New York, New York, 1975.

91. Plewig, G.; Fulton, J. E.; and Kligman, A. M.: Cellular dynamics of comedo formation in acne vulgaris. *Arch. Dermatol. Forsch.*, 242: 12, 1971.

92. Potten, C. S.: The epidermal proliferative unit: the possible role of the central basal cell. *Cell Tissue Kinet.*, 7: 77, 1974.

93. Potten, C. S.: Epidermal cell production rates. *J. Invest. Dermatol.*, 65: 488, 1975.

94. Potten, C. S.: Identification of clonogenic cells in the epidermis and the structural arrangement of the epidermal proliferation unit. In Cairnie, A.: (Ed.). *Stem Cells in Various Tissues. A symposium in tribute to C. P. Leblond*. Academic Press, New York, New York, 1976.

95. Quivedo, W. C.: Epidermal melanin units: melanocyte-keratinocyte interaction. *Am. Zoologist*, 12: 35, 1972.

96. Ryan, T. J.: Factors influencing the growth of

vascular endothelium in the skin. *Brit. J. Dermatol.*, 82: Supp. 5, 99, 1970.

97. Ryan, T. J.; Nishioka, K.; and Dawber, R. P.: Epithelial-endothelial interaction in the control of inflammation through fibrinolysis. *Brit. J. Dermatol.*, 84: 501, 1971.

98. Rytömaa, T.: The chalone concept. In Richter, G. W. and Epstein, M. A.: (Eds.). *International Review of Experimental Pathology*. Academic Press, New York, New York, 1976, p. 155, vol. 16.

99. Rytömaa, T.; Vilpo, J. A.; Levanto, A.; and Jones, W. A.: Effect of granulocyte chalone on acute and chronic granulocytic leukemia in man. Report of seven cases. *Scand. J. Haematol., Suppl.* 27:1, 1976.

100. Schellander, F. S. and Marks, R.: The epidermal response to subepidermal inflammation. An experimental study. *Brit. J. Dermatol.*, 88: 363, 1973.

101. Silderberg, I.; Baer, R. L.; and Rosenthal, S.A.: Circulating Langerhans cells in a dermal vessel. *Acta Derm. Venereol. (Stockh.)*, 54:81, 1974.

102. Silvers, I. A.: Oxygen tension and epithelialization. In Maibach, H. I. and Rovee, D.T.: (Eds.). *Epidermal Wound Healing*. Year Book Medical Publishers, Chicago, Illinois, 1972, pp. 291, 1972.

103. Simms, H. S. and Stillman, N. P.: Substances affecting adult tissue in vitro; growth inhibitor in adult tissue. *J. Gen. Physiol.*, 20: 621, 1936.

104. Somasundaram, K. and Prathap, K.: Intra-uterine healing of skin wounds in rabbit foetuses. *J. Path.*, 100: 81, 1970.

105. Sutherland, E.W.: Studies on the mechanism of hormone action. *Science*, 177: 401, 1972.

106. Tashjian, A. H.; Voelkel, E. F.; McDonough, J.; and Levine, L.: Hydrocortisone inhibits prostaglandins production by mouse fibrosarcoma cells. *Nature*, 258 (5537): 739, 1975.

107. Thornley, A. L. and Laurence, E. B.: Chalone regulation of the epidermal cell cycle. *Experientia*, 31 (9): 1024, 1975.

108. Thornley, A. L. and Laurence, E. B.: Current status of melanocyte chalones. In Houck, J. C.: (Ed.). *Chalones*. Elsevier, Amsterdam, North Holland, 1976, chapt. 10.

109. Thornley, A. L. and Laurence, E. B.: The specificity of epidermal chalone action: the results of in vivo experimentation with two purified skin entracts. *Developmental Biology*. In press.

110. Thornley, A. L.; Spargo, D.; and Laurence, E. B.: A simple method for measuring DNA synthesis in the epidermis and sebaceous glands. Submitted for publication.

111. Ugel, A. R.: Bovine keratohyalin: anatomical, histochemical, ultrastructural, immunologic and biochemical studies. *J. Invest. Dermatol.*, 65 (1): 118, 1975.

112. Voorhees, J. J.; Duell, E. A.; Bass, L. J.; and Harrell, E. R.: Role of cyclic-AMP in the control of

epidermal cell growth and differentiation. *J. Natl. Cancer Inst. Monogr.* 38:47, 1973.

113. Voorhees, J. J. and Mier, P. D.: The epidermis and cyclic-AMP. *Brit. J. Dermatol.*, 90:223, 1974.

114. Voorhees, J. J.; Marcelo, C. L.; and Duell, E. A.: Cyclic-AMP, Cyclic-GMP, and glucocorticoids as potential metabolic regulators of epidermal proliferation and differentiation. *J. Invest. Dermatol.*, 65 (1): 179, 1975.

115. Weiss, P. and Kavanau, J. L.: A model of growth and growth control in mathematical terms. *J Gen. Physiol.*, 41: 1, 1957.

116. Wilson, I. and Marks, R.: (Eds.). *Mechanisms of Topical Corticosteroid Activity.* Churchill Livingstone, Edinburgh, London, 1976.

117. Winter, G. D.: Epidermal regeneration studied in the domestic pig. In Maibach, H. I. and Rovee, D. T.: (Eds.). *Epidermal Wound Healing.* Year Book Medical Publishers, Chicago, Illinois, 1972, pp. 71.

118. Winter, G. D.: Histological aspects of burn wound healing. *Burns*, 1: 191, 1975.

119. Wolff, K.: The Langerhans cell. In Mali, J. W. H.: (Ed.). *Current Problems in Dermatology.* Karger, Basel, Switzerland, 1972, pp. 79, vol. 4.

120. Zil, J. S.: Vitamin A acid effects on epidermal mitotic activity, thickness and cellularity in the hairless mouse. *J. Invest Dermatol.*, 59: 228, 1972.

EPIDERMAL DIFFERENTIATION AND KERATINIZATION

Irwin M. Freedberg, M.D.

At least three facets of the biological and biochemical aspects of epidermal differentiation and keratinization are relevant to a conference on cholesteatoma. These are the gross and microscopic structure of epidermis, the pathways and controls of protein synthesis in epidermis and the characteristics of the two phenotypic protein products of epidermal differentiation, keratin and keratohyalin. In this paper I shall review each of these topics.

Structure of Epidermis

The skin itself is an organ composed of three distinct tissues—the subcutaneous tissue, the dermis and the epidermis. The subcutaneous tissue is primarily composed of adipose cells, the dermis contains connective tissue cells, blood vessels and nerves and the avascular epidermis consists of two distinct cell lines, the keratinocytes and the melanocytes. Since there is no evidence that melanocytes are in any way involved in the pathophysiology of cholesteatoma, they will not be discussed.

The skin of an embryo contains a germinative layer from which arise the cells of the general epidermis as well as the epithelial components of the cutaneous appendages, the hair follicles, sebaceous glands, eccrine and apocrine sweat glands and the nails. In adult epidermis there is evidence from a variety of sources which indicates that appendageal cells can migrate and become keratinizing cells of the general body epidermis. Each of the epithelial components, hair, nails, sebaceous glands, sweat glands, and the general body epidermis are involved in the major function of the skin which is protected. The contribution of several of the appendages in this area is minor in man, but of major significance in certain animal species.

The epidermis (Freedberg, 1976) is a stratified tissue with a basal layer, several spinous layers, a variable number of granular layers and a superficial stratum corneum. Cell division and much of the protein synthesis in the tissue takes place in the basal cell layers and the cells go through a maturation process which can be considered to be programmed cell death. The end result of the maturation is formation of the stratum corneum which is the major protective barrier in man. During this process of maturation several specific intracellular organelles are formed including the tonofilaments in the basal layer and the keratohyaline granules and membrane-coating granules in the more superficial strata.

The epidermis is not a homogenous tissue throughout the body but is heterogenous on both gross and microscopic levels. The gross difference between the epidermis on the palm and on the volar surface of the forearm is obvious to even the untrained observer. This same heterogeneity is present on a microscopic level with major differences in thickness, organization and number as well as distribution of appendages in the several body areas. The structural differences, in large part, are related to functional specialization and a general description of the structure of the tissue can be drawn in spite of the heterogeneity.

The basal layer cells are the site of cell division in epidermis (Weinstein, 1965). It has recently been shown that after prolonged exposure of epidermal cells to tritiated thymidine essentially all cells in the basal layers become labelled (Duffill, et al, 1976). This means that the percentage of epidermal cells which are in the G_0 portion of the cell cycle is quite small and that all cells participate in the differentiation processes which have been described previously. The length of the cycle in normal epidermal cells has been determined in several laboratories and although there are differences among the results presented by several groups, the cycle length in normal epidermis is somewhat greater than 300 hours.

In pathological conditions such as psoriasis vulgaris, the cell cycle is much shorter and the migration of cells through the epidermis is much faster. Cells do not have time to mature before they reach the superficial layers of the epidermis and the stratum corneum is thus abnormal.

The cells in the basal layer of normal epidermis are metabolically active with prominent nucleoli, many mitochondria, ribosomes and a well developed Golgi region. There are filaments of several different diameters and the cells are attached to each other at the desmosomes which are specialized areas on the cell membranes which also serve as attachment points for the tonofilaments. The filament density is somewhat greater in cells of the spinous layers than it is in the basal layer cells, probably a manifestation of continuing protein synthesis in the cells.

The granular layer is the site of synthesis of one of the major morphological constituents of mammalian epidermis, the keratohyaline granules (Freedberg, 1976). In hematoxylin and eosin stained specimens these are cytoplasmic bodies of irregular size and shape which on electron microscopic evaluation are amorphous, osmiophilic structures without a limiting membrane but surrounded by large numbers of polyribosomal particles. The polyribosomes may be related to the in situ synthesis of polypeptides which make up the keratohyaline granules. Neither the granules nor their constituent proteins can be identified in the stratum corneum.

In the granular layer the intracellular organelles known as membrane-coating granules or keratinosomes (Krawczyk and Wilgram, 1967) are first seen. These granules which are known by a variety of names have a distinctive, lamellated structure and seem to empty their contents into the intracellular space. The role of the membrane-coating granules in formation of the normal stratum corneum has not been elucidated.

The stratum corneum, which has already been pointed out as the major site of the protective function of epidermis, is composed of anucleate, dehydrated cells which are filled with bundles of fibrous protein (Freedberg, 1976). Cells leave the surface of the stratum corneum at a regular rate and are lost to the environment. It should be apparent that, in the usual steady state condition on a statistical basis, for each cell which divides in the basal layer, a cell must be lost from the stratum corneum.

Epidermal Protein Synthesis

Much of the work of my own laboratory during the past few years has been directed at a study of the pathways and controls of protein synthesis in mammalian epidermis and hair root cells (Freedberg, 1970). One of our reasons for working in this area is that we believe we may eventually be able to affect benign and malignant proliferative lesions of the skin by interfering with the processes of epidermal protein synthesis. The processes which result in formation of a cholesteatoma, also a proliferative lesion, may be influenced successfully by interference with protein synthesis in the affected tissue.

In epidermis, as in all other eukaryotic tissues which have been studied, there are three species of ribonucleic acid (RNA) whose synthesis is directed by the desoxyribonucleic acid (DNA) of the tissue (Fig. 17). Ribosomal RNA complexes with a number of proteins (ribosomal proteins) to form the ribosomes which are the structural units upon which protein synthesis takes place. Transfer RNAs, of which there are at least one for each of the natural amino acids which make up the primary structure of proteins, complex with specific amino acids in the cytoplasm of cells. As is shown in Figure 17 this complex formation requires the presence of adenosine triphosphate and a specific enzyme for each transfer RNA-amino acid pair. The enzymes, known as amino acyl-transfer RNA synthetases, lead to the formation of charged

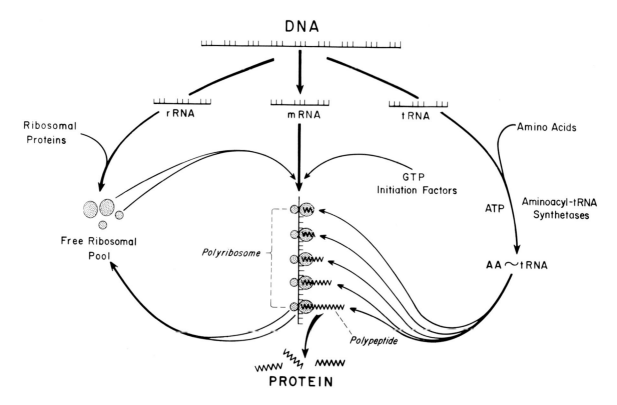

Fig. 17: Summary of the pathways of protein synthesis in eukaryotic cells. *(by permission: The Journal of Investigative Dermatology.)*

transfer RNA species. The charged transfer RNA species reach the surface of ribosomes which, in epidermis as well as all other protein synthesizing tissues studied, are found in polyribosomal configuration. On the surface of the ribosomes the actual processes of protein synthesis take place and an equivalent polypeptide or protein chain is formed on each ribosome of a polyribosome complex. These chains may subsequently be modified by intra- or interchain reactions. Specificity of the synthetic process depends upon the triplet nucleotide sequences of the messenger RNA which is the third species of RNA in the cell.

Figure 18 summarizes the reactions which take place on the surface of the ribosome during the process of protein synthesis. These reactions may be divided into three phases, initiation, elongation and release, and only the first two are detailed in the illustration since no studies of the release

reactions in mammalian epidermis are available. Protein synthesis is initiated by a reaction between the initiator transfer RNA, which is methionine-tRNA, GTP and an initiation factor known as IF MP. A ternary complex is formed which is then bound to a specific site on the 40S ribosomal subunit. A second initiation factor, IF M3, is involved in the subsequent binding of messenger RNA to the 40S subunit in such a way that the methionine codon on the messenger reacts with the anticodon of the methionine transfer RNA. Formation of the initiation complex is completed as the 60S subunit is joined through the reaction with two more initiation factors, IF M2A and IF M2B. The transfer RNA for the next amino acid, specified by the subsequent triplet nucleotide sequence of the messenger RNA, is then bound to the 40S ribosome, the first peptide bond is formed, the methionine transfer RNA returns to the

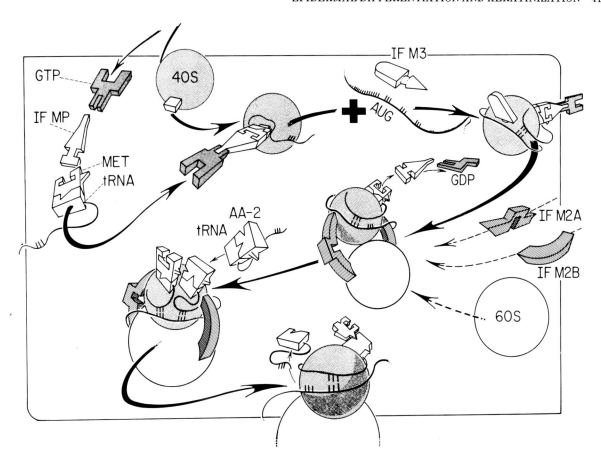

Fig. 18: The initiation and elongation reactions of protein synthesis.

cytoplasm of the cell and translocation occurs so that the entire sequence can be repeated sequentially. The polypeptide grows until a codon signifying a stop signal is reached and at that time, under control of specific release factors which have not been identified in epidermis, the protein is released from the surface of the ribosome. The 80S ribosome then breaks up to its 40 and 60S subunits.

All of these reactions have been shown to occur in epidermis and several points of potential qualitative and quantitative control have been identified (Freedberg, 1972). A protein corresponding to IF MP has been identified and partially purified, and activities corresponding to those of IF M3, IF M2A and IF M2B have been documented. An endogenous inhibitor of the in-

itiation reactions has been identified in the 0.5 M potassium chloride wash of epidermal ribosomes and this inhibitor may be of importance in overall control of protein synthesis in epidermis (Gilmartin and Freedberg, 1976). At the present time its specific site of action has not been determined. A large number of exogenous inhibitors of the initiation reactions, predominantly antibiotic agents, have been identified and these are also potentially valuable substances in control of proliferation in epidermis and other keratinizing tissues.

Keratin and Keratohyalin

Within the past several years much progress has been made in elucidating the biochemical structures of the two specific products of epidermal differentiation, keratin and keratohyalin. In addition to the studies which have been reported from our laboratory (Bhatnagar and Freedberg, 1976) major contributions to this area have come from the work of Baden at Harvard (Lee, et al, 1975), Steinert and Idler (1975) and Ugel (1975) at the National Institutes of Health, Dale and Stern (1976) at the University of Washington, Fukuyama and Epstein (1975) and their coworkers at the University of California in San Francisco, Bernstein (1975) at the University of Michigan and Matoltsy (1975) and his coworkers at Boston University. The studies have been done with a variety of epidermal tissues including newborn rat, guinea pig and human epidermis and bovine snout and hoof.

Solubilized components of keratin have been obtained by extraction of tissue, usually with denaturing solvents such as 8M-urea. The polypeptides obtained have been found to be high in a helical content by x-ray diffraction or circular dichrotic studies. The amino acid content of the polypeptides isolated in our laboratory from newborn rat epidermal tonofilaments are summarized in Table 6. Most investigators have found that there are several polypeptides which can be isolated from the solubilized keratin and their molecular weights vary from 50,000 to 70,000. Using acrylamide gel electrophoresis in the presence of sodium dodecyl sulfate, we have been able to identify two polypeptides whose relative molecular weights are 60,000 and 68,000. The two polypeptides are immunologically identical.

TABLE 6

Amino Acid Analysis

	Urea Extract		Desoxycholate Extract
	68,000	60,000	
LYS	4.9	4.9	5.5
HIS	0.4	0.6	3.3
ARG	3.3	4.7	8.2
ASP	8.7	10.1	7.5
THR	5.2	4.7	5.4
SER	12.3	9.3	9.3
GLU	10.8	11.2	14.5
PRO	5.2	4.7	3.8
GLY	23.5	19.8	10.6
ALA	4.3	3.7	10.1
VAL	4.5	4.5	4.6
MET	1.8	1.9	1.0
ILE	2.9	3.7	3.8
LEU	6.5	8.0	7.5
TYR	2.5	3.7	2.4
PHE	2.7	3.2	2.9
Cysteic Acid	0.4	1.3	1.6

m Moles/100m Moles

Keratohyaline granules have been extracted with detergents such as desoxycholate or with buffers with high salt concentrations. The solubilized proteins are not alpha helical, they do not crossreact with anti-keratin antibodies and, as can be seen in Table 6, their amino acid composition is different from that of the keratin polypeptides. Within the past several years studies in our laboratory have been directed at an analysis of the proteins solubilized from the keratohyalin granules.

The components are heterogeneous and we have focused upon a group of low molecular weight proteins (10,000-18,000 daltons). Among six species in this region we have isolated and partially purified four fractions. Two of these are polypeptides with amino acid compositions resembling that of the histidine rich protein which was first isolated from keratohyalin granules by Hoeber (1966) and his coworkers. One of the "histidine-rich" fractions has ribonuclease activity. The most predominant of these low molecular weight proteins is a species of 12,800 relative molecular weight whose amino acid composition indicates it to be a lysine-rich basic protein which binds to DNA. Such lysine-rich DNA binding proteins are known to occur in the nucleus of many cell types but their presence in a cytoplasmic organelle is unusual. We believe that these data lead to an as yet unproven hypothesis that keratohyaline granules are related to control of the programmed cell death which characterizes epidermis. The components of the granules destroy or bind macromolecules and thus interfere with the anabolic synthetic reactions in the tissue.

Acknowledgements

My gratitude to the National Institute of Arthritis, Metabolic and Digestive Diseases for supporting my laboratory with grant MA 16262.

References

1. Bernstein, I. A.; Kaman, R. L.; Malinoff, H.; Sachs, L.; and Gray, R. H.: Translation of polysomal messenger RNA during epidermal differentiation. *J. Invest. Dermatol.*, 65:102, 1975.
2. Bhatnagar, G. and Freedberg, I. M.: Solubilized protein of mammalian epidermis. *Biochim. Biophys. Acta*, (in press, 1976).
3. Dale, B. A.; Stern, I. B.; Rabin, M.; and Huang, L. Y.: The identification of fibrous proteins in fetal rat epidermis by electrophoretic and immunologic techniques. *J. Invest. Dermatol.*, 66:230, 1976.
4. Duffill, M.; Wright, N. A.; and Shuster, S.: The cell cycle time in psoriasis. *J. Invest. Dermatol.*, 66:259, 1976.
5. Freedberg, I. M.: Rashes and ribosomes. *New Eng. J. Med.*, 276:1135, 1967.
6. Freedberg, I. M.: Mammalian epidermal and hair root protein synthesis: subcellular localization of the synthetic site. *Biochem. Biophys. Acta*, 224:214, 1970.
7. Freedberg, I. M.: Epidermal protein synthesis. *J. Invest. Dermatol.*, 59:56, 1972.
8. Fukuyama, K. and Epstein, W. L.: Heterogenous proteins in keratohyaline granules studied by quantitative autoradiography. *J. Invest. Dermatol.*, 65:113, 1975.
9. Gilmartin, M. E. and Freedberg, I. M.: Epidermal protein synthesis: initiation factors. *J. Invest. Dermatol.*, 67:, 1976.
10. Hoober, J. K. and Bernstein, I. A.: Protein synthesis related to epidermal differentiation. *Proc. Natl. Acad. Sci. USA*, 56:594, 1966.
11. Krawczyk, W. S. and Wilgram, G. F.: The synthesis of keratinosomes during epidermal wound healing. *J. Invest. Dermatol.*, 64:263, 1967.
12. Lee, L. D.; Fleming, B. C.; Waitkus, R. F.; and Baden, H. P.: Isolation of the polypeptide chains of prekeratin. *Biochem. Biophys. Acta*, 412:82, 1975.
13. Matoltsy, A. G.: Desmosomes, filaments and keratohyaline granules: their role in the stabilization and keratinization of the epidermis. *J. Invest. Dermatol.*, 65:127, 1975.
14. Steinert, P. M. and Idler, W. S.: The polypeptide composition of Bovine epidermal α-keratin.

Biochem. J., 151:603, 1975.

15. Ugel, A.: Bovine keratohyaline: anatomic, histochemical, ultrastructural, immunologic and biochemical studies. *J. Invest. Dermatol.*, 65:118, 1975.

16. Weinstein, G. D. and Van Scott, E. J.: Autoradiographic analysis of turnover times of normal and psoriatic epidermis. *J. Invest. Dermatol.*, 45:257, 1965.

DIFFERENTIATION AND METAPLASTIC PROPERTIES OF STRATIFIED SQUAMOUS EPITHELIUM

Gary L. Peck, M.D.

Since one of the theories of histogenesis of the cholestcatoma is squamous metaplasia of the middle ear epithelium, a review of naturally occurring and experimentally induced metaplasias should serve a useful purpose in defining the differentiative potential of epithelia. I would like to structure this report by addressing the following questions: (1) Is the middle ear epithelium capable of squamous metaplasia? (2) What mechanisms could account for the simultaneous production of both mucin and keratin in the middle ear epithelium as described by Sadé? (3) Is the keratinizing epidermis capable of mucous metaplasia? (4) Does this information provide any direction for future laboratory and clinical investigations?

Is the Middle Ear Epithelium Capable of Squamous Metaplasia?

The recent report by Greenberg, Dickey, and Neely (1973) in which crude tobacco tar was installed at weekly intervals into the middle ear bullae of cats clearly demonstrates squamous metaplasia. One week after the second installation of tar, goblet cell metaplasia was seen in association with a chronic inflammatory reaction. Squamous metaplasia without keratin formation was seen elsewhere in the middle ear. Goblet cell metaplasia was present to a lesser degree in the control middle ear in which an indwelling polyethylene tube had been placed. After seven weeks (six installations) the stratified squamous epithelium keratinized and produced abundant keratohyalin. Epidermal cyst formation and bone resorption did not occur; heterotopic bone formation was present in one cat.

What Mechanisms Could Account for the Simultaneous Production of Mucin and Keratin in the Middle Ear Epithelium?

I would like to approach the answer to this complex question by first describing the morphology of epithelia of vertebrates other than man in which mucin and keratin co-exist normally. Then, after describing naturally occurring squamous metaplasias in the vagina and embryonic esophagus, I would like to discuss experimentally induced mucous metaplasias and squamous metaplasias with particular emphasis on the induction of mucous metaplasia by vitamin A acid in embryonic chick skin in organ culture.

The normal human epidermis is characterized by a stratum corneum, keratohyalin granules, tonofilaments, Odland bodies (lamellar granules, keratinosomes, membrane coating granules), thickened plasma membranes in the superficial epidermis, and desmosomes. Although hyaluronic acid may be demonstrated in the interstices between epidermal cells and in the outer root sheath of the hair follicle, mucin granules do not occur (Graham, et al, 1972).

The fish epidermis, in contrast, does not keratinize and does contain unicellular mucous glands which secrete their contents onto the surface of the fish. Keratohyalin granules and Odland bodies are not seen (Parakkal and Alexander, 1972). The frog epidermis does keratinize, but, instead of having a distinct mucus producing cell, cells within the epidermis contain two types of membrane bound mucous granules. The smaller mucous granules are formed first and migrate to the periphery of the cell and are extruded into the intercellular space, a fate similar to that of the Odland body in the human epidermis. The larger mucous granules are located near the nucleus often in association with the Golgi apparatus. As in the fish, keratohyalin and Odland bodies are not seen.

Membrane bound mucous granules occur both in living and horny layers of the turtle epidermis (Matoltsy and Huszar, 1972). Of particular interest is that in the sheep rumen, epithelium both large and small mucous granules are seen in cells that also contain keratohyalin granules.

Naturally occurring metaplasia includes the changes seen in the vaginal epithelium during the menstrual cycle and the ontogenetic squamous metaplasia of the esophagus. When estrogen (particularly 17-Beta estradiol) is administered to spayed animals, and in normal animals during the follicular phase of the cycle, the vaginal epithelium hypertrophies and the epithelial cells synthesize glycogen, keratohyalin, Odland bodies, and thickened plasma membranes. During the luteal phase of the normal cycle, the epithelium forms mucus instead, as a result of the inhibiting action of progesterone or estrogen (Parakkal and Gregoire, 1972). In normal embryological development of the chick esophagus mucin is seen on the tenth day of gestation and squamous metaplasia begins on the fourteenth day and is complete at hatching (day 21). Of particular interest is that at the time collagen first appears in the subjacent lamina propria of the embryonic chick esophagus there is a decrease in the intensity of the mucin stains in the mucosa. A similar squamous metaplasia occurs in human esophageal development (Mottet, 1970).

Mucous Metaplasia (Fell and Mellanby, 1953)

Vitamin A induced mucous metaplasia of embryonic chick skin has served for over 20 years as a well-defined model system for the study of altered epithelial differentiation. Since 1953 when Fell and Mellanby initially observed the inhibition of keratinization in chick embryo skin and its subsequent transformation into a mucous secreting structure by vitamin A, many studies have been concerned with the mode of action of vitamin A on a variety of epithelia. Results from these studies indicate that the response to vitamin A varies with the dose of vitamin A and the species, age, and site of tissue. In addition to chick skin, excess vitamin A inhibits keratinization in the stratified squamous epithelium of the adult hamster cheek pouch, embryo mouse epidermis and lip vibrissae, chick esophagus and cornea, embryonic rat esophagus, tongue, palate, tail and foot pad, rat vagina, adult rabbit keratoacanthoma, mouse, guinea pig, and human epidermal cells, adult guinea pig ear, as well as in embryonic, normal adult, and diseased human skin. Mucin is produced in chick skin, the cheek pouch, mouse vibrissae, cornea, the esophagus, tongue, and keratoacanthoma. In three tissues the chick esophagus, hamster cheek pouch, and embryonic mouse lip vibrissae, vitamin A induced intraepithelial mucous gland formation. The initial effects of excess vitamin A, as well as vitamin A deficiency induced squamous metaplasia, are focal, reversible, and selectively alter the differentiation of germinative layers of epithelia. Hydrocortisone and citral may reverse or inhibit completely the metaplastic effects of excess vitamin A.

The morphological metaplastic events in 14 day embryonic chick skin induced by a three day exposure in organ culture to 20 iu/ml vitamin A acid include a premature loss of periderm and an inhibition of keratinization. Keratohyalin granules and the stratum corneum do not form. Tonofilaments are finer and fewer in number. Desmosomes are disrupted with resulting loss of the usual horizontal stratification of epidermal cells. The surface cells round up and develop a pattern of microvilli and interconnecting surface ridges. Individual cells vary in this metaplastic response. Initially, these changes are more pronounced in focal areas of the explant. Metaplasia is enhanced at the cut edges of the explant and in the folds between the scales of the metatarsal shank skin. These skin scales eventually flatten completely and the entire explant shrinks in size and becomes spherical in shape. Tight junctions and elongated gap junctions increase in number. The adjacent plasma membranes are highly folded and interdigitate across the widened intercellular space. Surface epidermal cells are hypertrophic and contain glycogen. The basal cells are hyperplastic. A selective metaplastic effect on the basal cells was seen in 17 day and older embryos as the more superficial epidermal cells are already committed to keratinize. A cleavage plane develops and separates the responsive and non-responsive layers of the epidermis. Intracellularly, there are increased numbers of polyribosomes, Golgi elements, and rough endoplasmic reticulum. Lipid droplets and secondary lysosomes are also seen. Large gaps in the basal lamina allow direct contact between the downward extending basal cell processes and fibroblasts. Collagen fibers contact the basal cell membrane above the level of the basal lamina.

Later metaplastic events include the formation of an intraepithelial tubulo-alveolar mucous gland with terminal acini and intercellular canaliculi leading to the surface. Mucin granules are located in the apices of the surface epidermal cells and of the cells forming the acini. Microvilli with internal axial filaments and surface glycocalyx are increased in size and number. With higher doses of vitamin A acid, the microvilli in the acini resemble a brush border seen in normally occurring mucous glands.

The mechanism of action of inductive agents in differentiation is thought to involve primarily the germinative cell population which is capable of DNA synthesis. Most of the evidence in the field of vitamin A effects on epithelia tend to support this view. For instance, hyperplasia of the epidermal basal layer after vitamin A exposure has been noted repeatedly, including in this study. Metaplasia secondary to vitamin A deficiency also leads to basal cell hyperplasia. Basal cell effects are most easily observed in organ culture when vitamin A is discontinued and the tissue is exposed to control medium. In the reversal experiment in this study the mucous containing cells were pushed to the surface by a new generation of keratinizing cells. In addition, when older embryos are used metaplasia is limited to the basal epidermis and the superficial epidermis remains keratinized. These data indicate that although the epidermis may modulate between mucin formation and keratin

synthesis depending on the presence or absence of vitamin A acid, the individual epidermal cells, once committed to a specific course of differentiation, cannot reverse themselves. The foci of early mucous metaplasia may also indicate cell cycle specificity. Wong (1975) suggests that the focal mitotic activity seen in the hamster cheek pouch may account for the focal metaplasia induced by vitamin A. The repeatedly observed acceleration of the mitotic rate in skin treated with vitamin A may be a result of lysosomal proliferation with increased release of lysosomal proteinases. Cathepsin D has been found in increased concentration in cultured rabbit skin exposed to vitamin A acid. Proteases in other systems are known to be potent stimulators of mitosis.

Hardy (1974) suggests that the prime effect of vitamin A may be the production of basement membrane gaps which allow extensive dermal-epidermal cell to cell contact. Inappropriate signals from the dermis may then lean to metaplasia, as opposed to a direct action of the vitamin on the epidermis. Additional evidence in favor of a dermal mechanism comes from McLoughlin (1961) who demonstrated that gizzard mesenchyme has the ability to induce mucous metaplasia in overlying isolated chick epidermis. Similarly, Sweeny and coworkers (1975) found that full thickness canine oral mucous membrane when transplanted to the ear began to keratinize. Upon retransplantation to the trachea the graft shed its stratum corneum and underwent a mucous metaplasia with production of a simple tubular mucous gland within its center. Furthermore, in all the studies on isolated epidermal cells, frank mucous metaplasia was not seen indicating that, if there is a direct metaplastic effect of vitamin A on epidermal cells, then a dermal presence is necessary to fully amplify the inductive signal. Whether collagen itself plays a role in determining the direction of epidermal cell differentiation or whether it only serves to amplify the vitamin A metaplastic effect is unclear. Hay and Meier (1975) have demonstrated that collagen-cell surface interactions are necessary for corneal morphogenesis. One possible specific role for collagen in this system could be to participate as a substrate in epidermal cell surface glycosyltransferase reactions, perhaps also involving a retinol glycolipid intermediate (Dorsey and Roth, 1974).

In spite of this preponderence of evidence indicating a vitamin A action on the basal germinative cells, it is clear that there are, in addition, direct effects on the post-mitotic, post-synthetic, superficial epidermal cells. It is conceivable that in this system vitamin A acid may bind to all the epidermal cell membranes with resultant alteration in cell surface morphology. Upon transmission of this surface signal to the genome, perhaps via membrane messengers (Roseman, 1974), new messenger RNA and glycoproteins may be formed only in those cells capable of DNA synthesis.

We cannot as yet determine whether the surface mucin cells seen after three days of incubation are derived from superficial post-synthetic epidermal cells or represent metaplastic basal cells that have migrated to the surface. If the source of the mucin containing cells were indeed the superficial post-synthetic epidermal cells, then this would support the view that the action of vitamin A occurs at the post-translational level as suggested by DeLuca (1972). In this instance vitamin A could serve as a carrier of monosaccharide units and glycosylate pre-existing proteins to form a glycoprotein moiety.

Squamous Metaplasia (Fell and Mellanby, 1953)

Several factors are known to induce squamous metaplasia of epithelia. Among these are carcinogens, such as benzpyrene which induces squamous metaplasia readily when instilled into the trachea. Vitamin A deficiency leads to squamous metaplasia in calf parotid gland, rat bladder, rat trachea, and cornea, hamster trachea, and mouse prostate. Testosterone can inhibit the vitamin A deficiency induced squamous metaplasia of the mouse prostate. Clinically, vitamin A deficiency produces squamous metaplasia of the trachea, urinary tract, salivary gland ducts,

pancreatic ducts, cornification of the vagina, keratinization of the cornea, and hyperkeratosis of the epidermis and hair follicles (Olson, 1972). Citral not only antagonizes the effect of excess vitamin A but also produces squamous metaplasia in chick esophagus and cornea. Estrogen induces squamous metaplasia of the calf prostate and bulbourethral glands (Kroes and Teppema, 1972). Hydrocortisone antagonizes the effects of vitamin A and stimulates the keratinization of the epidermis, but does not lead to squamous metaplasia (Sugimoto and Endo, 1971). Epidermal growth factor stimulates epithelial growth in vivo and in organ culture and is a small polypeptide purified by Cohen and collaborators (1974) from the submaxillary gland of the adult male mouse. Its action appears to be non-specific in that it also enhances fibroblast growth, and enhances vitamin A induced mucous metaplasia of embryonic chick skin (personal communication, S. Cohen, 1976). Of particular interest is Moscona's demonstration (1964) that the gaseous environment may initiate keratinization in the respiratory epithelium of the chick chorioallantoic membrane. At high O_2 and low CO_2 levels the chorionic epithelium thickens and keratinizes. When the CO_2 level is raised to 5%, keratinization is suppressed. Similarly, Hilding (1932) sutured closed one nostril of a rabbit and later found that the increased flow of air in the other nostril led the nasal septal mucosa to develop in the direction of a stratified squamous epithelium. The closed nostril had increased mucin production. These phenomena may help explain the keratinization of the cornea resulting from ectropion (Donaldson, 1968) and the keratinization of the vagina resulting from total prolapse of the uterus. Of interest, when a perineal skin graft is used to reconstruct a vagina in cases of vaginal atresia, the stratum corneum of the graft is shed, the epidermal cells develop glycogen, and eventually the cytological smear becomes similar to the normal smear of the outer third of the vagina (McIndoe, 1959).

What Is The Potential of Adult Human Epidermis To Develop Mucin?

Is there a clinical lesion in the skin similar to the cholesteatoma in which mucin and keratin are simultaneously produced? This question could have added significance if one theorized that the cholesteatoma and the hyperplastic mucous epithelium were both derived from migrating epidermis of the external ear canal. Most cutaneous mucinoses, such as myxedema, consist of accumulations of mucin in the dermis. Very few epidermal diseases contain mucin. The hair follicles in an alopecia mucinose undergo a mucinous degeneration and contain large amounts of hyaluronic acid. The abnormal cells in the epidermis of Paget's disease of the nipple contain mucin, but there is controversy over the origin of these cells (Graham, et al, 1972). They may not be of epidermal origin. There have been reports of variant cutaneous carcinomas which contain mucin (Johnson and Helwig, 1963 and 1966). However, it may be said in summary that adult human epidermis has neither under experimental nor pathological conditions produced goblet cells or mucous glands. In one report, 0.1% vitamin A acid lotion applied for two weeks to normal skin produced electron dense granules, possibly representing mucin, in the intercellular space between basal cells (Plewig, et al, 1971). Mucous cell metaplasia has occured in three-four month old human fetal skin (Lasnitzki, 1958).

Does This Information Provide Any Direction for Future Laboratory and Clinical Investigations?

My recommendations for laboratory research would be to define exactly the morphological sequence of events in the histogenesis of cholesteatoma and then to investigate the factors controlling each event, with particular emphasis on cell surface phenomena and epithelial-mesenchymal interactions.

My concept of cholesteatoma at this point is that the hyperplasia of mucous elements is a nonspecific reaction to inflammation in the middle ear and may be stimulated by the proteases derived from the inflammatory infiltrate seen in chronic otitis media prior to cholesteatoma development. The mitogenic effect of proteases could lead to mucous cell hyperplasia of the middle ear epithelium. Afterwards, possibly as a result of squamous metaplasia, initially focal as in other systems, mucin and keratin containing cells would be observed side by side. Migration of keratinizing cells from foci of squamous metaplasia could complicate the task of attempting to decide between the migration and metaplastic theories of origin of the cholesteatoma. This is particularly true if the focus of squamous metaplasia occurs near the tympanic membrane perforation as a result of a higher O_2 exposure due to a "flow of air". To test these concepts, I would suggest that attempts be made to develop an in vitro system where the various possible contributory factors, such as the effect of proteases and protease inhibitors, excess vitamin A and vitamin A deficiency, and the concentration of O_2 and CO_2 in the gaseous environment, could be tested individually.

The use of the scanning electron microscope may assist in clarifying the metaplasia versus migration controversy. Foci of squamous metaplasia surrounded by mucin should be readily visible in the scanning electron microscope, as should a tongue of epithelium extending through a tympanic membrane perforation. The mechanism of cyst formation in cholesteatoma could likewise be studied, particularly if epithelial fusion, similar to palatal shelf closure (Waterman and Meller, 1974), occurs.

My recommendation for a clinical investigation would be to test the effects of synthetic analogs of vitamin A in the treatment of cholesteatoma. Vitamin A, often in very large doses, has long been used in the treatment of cutaneous disorders of keratinization, such as ichthyosis, Darier's disease, pityriasis rubra pilaris, and psoriasis. Vitamin A acid has in the recent decade been shown to be more potent than vitamin A in this regard. Its topical use in acne is standard practice today. Topical vitamin A acid has also been used with varying results in psoriasis (Peck, et al, 1973). Of particular interest is the development of synthetic analogs which are proving to be more potent and less toxic than the parent compounds (Sporn, et al, 1976). Recent results with the 13-cis analog of retinoic acid in the treatment of these diseases have been encouraging, particularly for pityriasis rubra pilaris (Peck, et al, 1976).

References

1. Cohen, S. and Taylor, J. M.: Part I. Epidermal growth factor: Chemical and biological characterization. In Greep, R. O.: (Ed.). *Recent Progress in Hormone Research.* Vol. 30. Academic Press, New York, New York, 1974, p. 533.

2. DeLuca, L., and Wolf, G.: Mechanism of action of vitamin A in differentiation of mucus-secreting epithelia. *J. Agric. Food. Chem.*, 20: 474, 1972.

3. Donaldson, D. D.: *Atlas of External Diseases of the Eye. Vol. II. Orbit, Lacrimal Apparatus, Eyelids, and Conjunctiva.* C. V. Mosby, St. Louis, Missouri, 1968.

4. Dorsey, J. K. and Roth, S.: The effect of polyprenols on cell surface galactosyltransferase activity. In Clarkson, B. and Baserga, R.: (Eds.). *Control of Proliferation in Animal Cells.* Cold Spring Harbor Laboratory, Cold Spring Harbor, New York, 1974.

5. Fell, H. B. and Mellanby, E.: Metaplasia produced in cultures of chick ectoderm by high vitamin A. *J. Physiol.*, 119: 470, 1953.

6. Graham, J. H.; Johnson, W. C.; and Helwig, E. B.: *Dermal Pathology.* Harper and Row, New York, New York, 1972.

7. Greenberg, S. D.; Dickey, J. R.; and Neely, J. G.: Effects of tobacco on the ear. *Ann. Otol. Rhinol. Laryngol.*, 82: 311, 1973.

8. Hardy, M. H.: Epithelial-mesenchymal interactions in vitro altered by vitamin A, and some implications. *In Vitro*, 10: 338, 1974.

9. Hay, E. D. and Meier, S.: Role of collagen-cell surface interaction in corneal morphogenesis. *J. Cell. Biol.*, 67: 321a, 1975.

10. Hilding, A.: Experimental surgery of the noses and sinuses; change in the morphology of the epithelium following variations in ventilation. *Arch. Otolaryngol.*, 16: 9, 1932.

11. Johnson, W. C. and Helwig, E. B.: Histochemistry of primary and metastatic mucus-secreting tumors. *Ann. N.Y. Acad. Sci.*, 106: 794, 1963.

12. Johnson, W. C. and Helwig, E. B.: Adenoid squamous cell carcinoma (adenoacanthoma). A clinicopathologic study of 155 patients. *Cancer* 19: 1639, 1966.

13. Kroes, R. and Teppema, J. S.: Development and restitution of squamous metaplasia in the calf prostrate after a single estrogen treatment. An electron microscopic study. *Exp. Molec. Pathol.*, 16: 286, 1972.

14. Lasnitzki, I.: The effect of carcinogens, hormones, and vitamins on organ cultures. In Bourne, G. H. and Danielli, J. F.: (Ed.). *International Review of Cytology, Vol. VII.* Academic Press Inc., New York, New York, 1958, p. 79.

15. McIndoe, A.: Discussion on treatment of congenital absence of vagina with emphasis on long-term results. *Proc. R. Soc. Med.*, 52: 952, 1959.

16. McLoughlin, C. B.: The importance of mesenchymal factors in the differentiation of chick epidermis. *J. Embryol. Exp. Morphol.*, 9: 385, 1961.

17. Matoltsy, A. G. and Huszar, T.: Keratinization of the reptilian epidermis: An ultrastructural study of the turtle skin. *J. Ultrastruct. Res.*, 38: 87, 1972.

18. Moscona, A. A.: Studies on stability of phenotypic traits in embryonic integumental tissues and cells. In Montagna, W. and Lobitz, W. C., Jr.: (Eds.). *The Epidermis.* Academic Press, New York, New York, 1964, p. 83.

19. Mottet, N. K.: Mucin biosynthesis by chick and human oesophagus during ontogenetic metaplasia. *J. Anat.* 107: 49, 1970.

20. Olson, J. A.: The biological role of vitamin A in maintaining epithelial tissues. *Israel J. Med. Sci.*, 8: 1170, 1972.

21. Parakkal, P. F. and Alexander, N. J.: *Keratinization. A Survey of Vertebrate Epithelia.* Academic Press, New York, New York, 1972.

22. Parakkal, P. F. and Gregoire, A. T.: Differentiation of vaginal epithelium in the normal and hormone-treated Rhesus monkey. *Biol. Reprod.*, 6: 117, 1972.

23. Peck, G. L.; Key, D. J.; and Guss, S. B.: Topical vitamin A acid in the treatment of psoriasis. *Arch. Dermatol.*, 107: 245, 1973.

24. Peck, G. L.; Elias, P. M.; and Wetzel, B.: Effects of retinoic acid on embryonic chick skin. *J. Invest. Dermatol.*, submitted for publication, 1976.

25. Plewig, G.; Wolff, H. H.; and Braun-Falco, O.: Lokalbehandlung normaler und pathologischer menschlicher Haut mit Vitamin A-Saure. Klinische, histologische elektronenmikroskopische untersuchungen. *Arch. Klin. Exp. Dermatol.*, 239: 390, 1971.

26. Roseman, S.: Complex Carbohydrates and intercellular adhesion. In Moscona, A.A.: (Ed.). *The Cell Surface in Development*. John Wiley and Sons, New York, New York, 1974, p. 255.

27. Sporn, M. B.; Dunlop, N. M.; Newton, D. L. et al: Prevention of chemical carcinogenesis by vitamin A and its synthetic analogs (retinoids). *Fed. Proc.*, 35: 1332, 1976.

28. Sugimoto, M. and Endo, H.: Accelerating effect of hydrocortisone on the keratinization of chick embryonic skin growing in a chemically defined medium. *J. Embryol. Exp. Morphol.*, 25: 365, 1971.

29. Sweeny, P. R.; Farkas, L. G.; Farmer, A. W., et al: Metaplasia of adult oral mucous membrane. *J. Surg. Res.*, 19(5): 303, 1975.

30. Waterman, R. E. and Meller, S. M.: Alterations in the epithelial surface of human palatal shelves prior to and during fusion: a scanning electron microscopic study. *Anat. Rec.*, 180: 111, 1974.

31. Wong, Y. C.: Mucous metaplasia of the hamster cheek pouch epithelium under hypervitaminosis A. *Exp. Molec. Pathol.*, 23 (1): 132, 1975.

THE PHENOTYPIC EXPRESSION OF MIDDLE EAR MUCOSA

Jacob Sadé, M.D.
Ziva Weisman, Ph.D.

Biopsies from the middle ear mucosa in chronic otitis media without cholesteatoma, often show islands of stratified squamous epithelium, with or without keratin (Sadé, 1969). Whole cell populations transformed into goblet cells or glands also appear in the biopsies (Fig. 19). Cholesteatomatous ears, which characteristically show stratified squamous epithelium, are similarly found studded with hyperplastic mucus producing cells and glands (Fig. 20). In both of these situations, the keratin-forming and mucus-forming cells are often intermingled (Fig. 21) and frequently pass abruptly from one type into the other (Figs. 19 and 20). This concomitant presence in the inflamed middle ear mucosa of such different cell types

should not be looked upon as extraordinary, in spite of the traditional acceptance of keratin cells being ectodermal in orgin and mucus cells endodermal in origin. Actually, transformation of a specific cell population (such as mucus cells) into another (such as keratin cells) is a common occurrence under inflammatory conditions and is termed metaplasia (Sadé, 1971). Metaplastic changes in mucosa are seen in chronic bronchitis, sinusitis, rhinitis, cervicitis or urinary tract epithelium. The middle ear mucosa, which was described by Sadé (1966) and later by Lim (1969) and Hentzer (1970) as a respiratory mucosa, is not different in its biologic behavior from other respiratory mucosa. We should therefore, not be

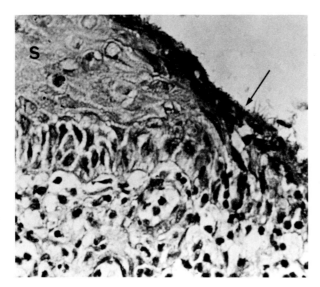

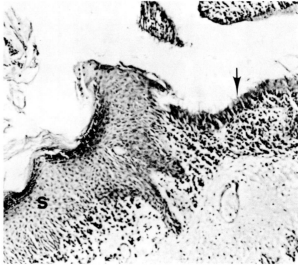

Fig. 19: Biopsy from the middle ear mucosa in case of simple (non-cholesteatomatous) chronic otitis media. Note striated squamous epithelium (s).

Fig. 20: Biopsy from a cholesteatomatous middle ear mucosa—note abrupt transition from keratinizing stratified squamous epithelium (s) into mucus producing respiratory epithelium (arrow).

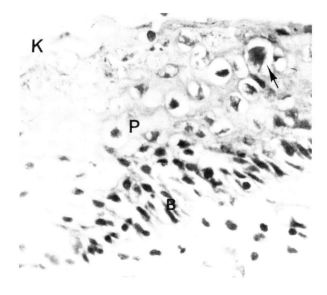

Fig. 21: A lonely mucus producing cell (arrow) in a sea of stratified squamous epithelium (p), keratin (k).

surprised when the middle ear mucosa exhibits metaplastic features in the presence of inflammation.

Theoretically, the transformation of one cell population into another is not astounding, taking into consideration that every cell forming a multicellular organism contains in its chromosomes all the information needed to synthesize any protein in that particular organism and is therefore capable of forming any specific cell in the same animal. The particular path taken by a given stem cell is looked upon as its phenotypic expression. The process through which different morphological cell types result is termed differentiation. Differences in phenotypic (cell type) expression are brought about by selective protein synthesis and are due to activation of some genes (in a given cell) and inhibition of other genes. This will take place whenever cells divide and mature. The above is relevant in the post-embryonic period only in cell populations which divide periodically or cyclically, i.e., exhibiting cellular turnover. It happens to those cells whose life span is relatively short, such as blood cells, mesenchymal cells and mucosa cells. The specific induction of these cells,

i.e., the selective gene activation, is, of course, meticulously programmed in order not to end up in havoc. However, under special circumstances—which can be seen under inflammatory conditions or created in the laboratory—this stability might be lost. Thus, stem cells of each of the "dividing families" (mesenchymal blood, epithelia) have several options open to them after mitosis. Epithelial cells are essentially liable to develop after division into one of the following cells: (a) another stem cell, (b) an intermediate cell, (c) a ciliated cell, (d) a mucus-producing cell, or (e) a keratin-producing cell. A particular epithelial stem cell will "choose" one of these particular paths and will mature into a respective cell type (phenotype) in accordance to a signal from a specific inducer. It is this phenomenon in the middle ear which is the central subject of this study.

In 1922, Wailbach described the transformation of mucosa into keratinizing stratified squamous epithelium in patients suffering from vitamin A deficiency. Thereafter, in vitro experiments by Fell (1957) also showed that maturation of chick embryo skin was really vitamin A dependent. In the presence of vitamin A, mucus-forming cells appeared, while in the absence of vitamin A, keratinizing cells appeared. Later, Moscona (1964) demonstrated that the presence or absence of CO_2 will also bring about similar variations in differentiation of the chorioallantoic membrane which keratinizes in air (containing only 0.03% CO_2), but not in air mixed with 5% CO_2. Clinical observations and in vivo experiments also indicate that ventilation and therefore, composition of the air may affect differentiation of mammalian and human mucosa. Hilding (1932) found that the closure of rabbit nares to the outside atmosphere caused an increase in the number of goblet cells. Similarly, Young (1967) treated ozena in which the mucosa of the nose changes into stratified squamous epithelium by closing the nares for a long period, resulting in retransformation of the epithelium into normal mucosa.

Of special interest are recently reported experiments where tobacco was shown to cause stratified squamous metaplasia in cats' middle ears (Greenberg, et al, 1973). The way vitamin A, CO_2, tobacco, and other agents, such as SO_2 (Reid, 1963), act on the cell is not known. The difference in chemical structures of the various substances which bring about the same phenotypic expression makes it probable that they are unspecific triggers. The action of these triggers may release an "in situ" (possibly from the cell membrane) substance having a specific inductive action on the genes themselves. The various metaplastic changes observed in inflammatory respiratory mucosa are probably the result of such triggering action, by various agents acting solo or possibly even in combination with each other.

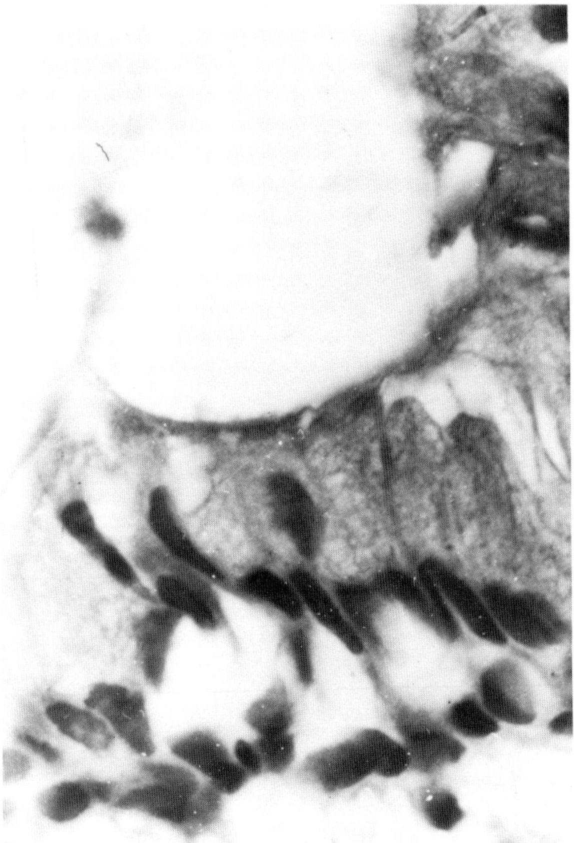

These clinical and experimental observations on mucosa, of which the middle ear is actually only another example, show the diversified differentiating power of its stem cells. Fell actually demonstrated that the very same cell will turn into a mucus cell or keratin cell according to whether vitamin A was present or absent. Mucus forming cells and keratin forming cells should, therefore, be viewed as competitive in nature as they are mutually exclusive as far as the progeny of a certain dividing stem cell is concerned—as a postmitotic cell, with all its potential, will differentiate into one or the other. In other words, agents promoting the emergence of mucus cells can be looked upon as suppressing the formation of keratinizing and cilia producing cells. A simplified example of such cell transformation is seen in secretory otitis media (S.O.M.) where whole areas transform themselves only in mucus processing cells (Sadé, 1971, 1974 and 1976), (Fig. 22). The clinically favorable action of ventilation in cases of S.O.M. is brought about both through the enhancement of clearance (Sadé, et al, 1976) as well as through the probable inhibition of excessive mucus production. The excessive amount of mucus production is at least in part related to the increased number of goblet cells.

Fig. 22: Whole cell population shifting into mucus producing cells—a typical finding in secretory otitis media biopsied—all cells stain intensely PAS positive.

There are theoretical difficulties in accepting the classical ex vacuo theory (Sadé, 1974) since it has lately been demonstrated (Sadé, et al, 1976) that there is only a mild negative pressure (1.7-5 mm) in these ears. Such a mild under-pressure could hardly cause transudation from the capillary bed in the mucosa—although how it may influence cell differentiation is not really known. This might suggest that another factor affects the middle ear secondary to eustachian tube hypoventilating such as differences in the middle ear gas composition. The likelihood that the active variable component in the middle ear gases is CO_2, or possibly oxygen, is supported by the studies of Moscona (1964), Hilding (1932) and Young (1967), which are mentioned above, as well as by measurements of middle ear CO_2 in cases of S.O.M. It was indicated both by Ingelstedt, et al, (1975), and by us*, that CO_2 partial pressure is significantly higher in S.O.M. ears than in normal ears—being 58 mm Hg and 18.2 mm Hg, respectively (Fig. 23).

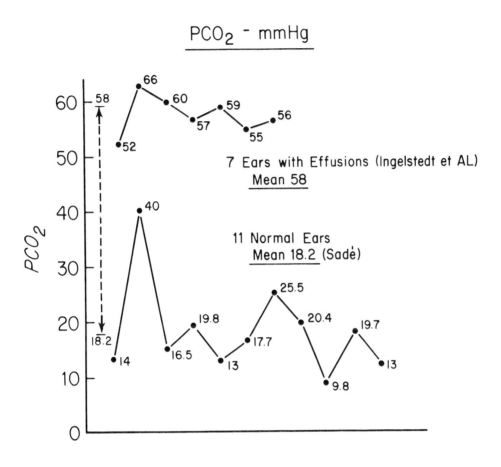

Fig. 23: CO_2 concentrations in normal (lower curve) compared with values from ears with effusions (upper curve). All values are partial pressure in millimeters of mercury. The normal values have been obtained after direct aspiration through gas analysis with Ph blood gas analyzer (313, Instrumentation Laboratory, Inc.). The values for the ears with effusions were measured with a probe (16).

We recently undertook a series of investigations to obtain suitable in vitro models for the study of factors (especially O_2 and CO_2) and mechanisms controlling cell proliferation and differentiation in middle ear respiratory epithelia. Our experimental system included tissue explants and monolayer growths from the following mucosa: the mucociliary membrane of the frog plate (Nevo, et al, 1975), mucosa from the rabbit trachea (Weismal, et al, 1976 and Sáde, et al, 1975),

*The gas analyses were performed with the help of Prof. Y. Bruderman of the Respiratory Unit at Meir Hospital, Kfar Saba, Israel and Prof. A. Boutros, Intensive Care Unit at the University of Iowa Hospitals. I am indebted to both these scientists.

mucosa from human adenoids and a few samples of mucosa from the middle ear (Drucker, et al, 1976). The various tissue explants were cultured for two to three weeks either on the surface of 0.6% agar (semisolid medium) containing the culture medium or on a cover glass in fluid medium. The biological features and the kinetics of cell proliferation and cell differentiation in these systems were characterized under standard culture conditions as reported by us previously. The activity of the cilia at the periphery of the explant and the morphological details of the cells in the monolayer were observed by phase microscopy. For histological observations, the explants and monolayers were fixed in Bouin's fixative and stained by the PAS technique to identify mucus producing cells. Cell nuclei synthesizing DNA (i.e., mitosis) were labeled by a pulse of tritiated thymidine (H-TdR) and autoradiographs were prepared (Fig. 24). The similar patterns of growth, cell division, and differentiation in these various mucociliary epithelia led us to continue the experimentation with rabbit trachea explants as a representative biological model of such epithelia. Medium -199 (semisolid medium) enriched with 10% calf serum was usually used and the explants were incubated at 37°C in an atmosphere of air with 5% CO_2, pH 7.0. In later experiments, the atmospheric composition (CO_2 and O_2) and the pH's were varied as given in Table 7. On the whole, mitosis started to appear at the wounded areas after 24-48 hours following planting (Fig. 25). This was followed by appearance of flat cells covering of the wounded area. Cell

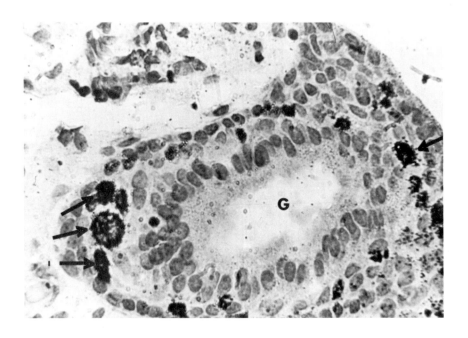

Fig. 24: Tritiated thymidine labeled cells in respiratory mucosa.

TABLE 7

Differentiation into PAS+ and ciliated cells in areas of new growth after 8-12 days in organ culture, expressed in % of explants having 10% or more PAS cells and 20% or more ciliated cells per section. About 100 cells were counted per section.

Group	CO_2 %	O_2 %	pH	Total number of explants examined	No. of explants showing new growth	% explants showing PAS+ cells	% explants showing ciliated cells
A1	0.03	20	6.8-7.0	45	6(12.5%)	17	17
A2	0.03	20	7.2-7.4	30	22(73%)	18	69
B1	5	20	6.8-7.0	52	33(68%)	18	67
B2	5	20	7.2-7.4	136	72(55%)	15	33
B3	5	20	7.6-7.8	41	31(78%)	33	37
C1	16	17	6.8-7.0	76	10(14%)	22	67
C2	16	17	7.2-7.4	84	43(52%)	(46)	42
C3	(16)	17	(7.6-7.8)	41	24(58%)	(90)	26
D	5	50	7.2-7.4	43	20(48%)	10	75
Total:				547	261(48%)		

Table 7: Amino acid analyses of the keratin polypeptides (urea extract) and the proteins solubilized from keratohyalin granules (desoxycholate extract).

Labeled Index (LI) from Rabbits' Trachea

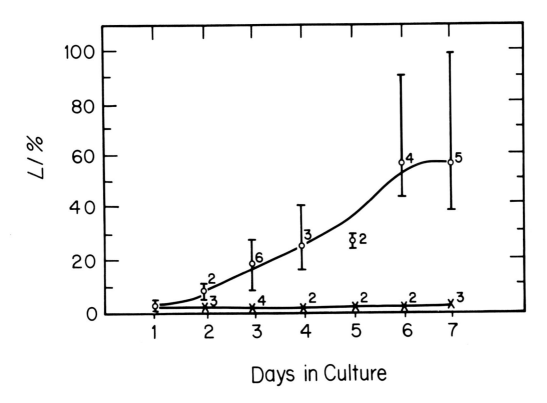

Fig. 25: Labeled index in explants from rabbit trachea during first week of culture on semi-solid medium 199 containing + 10% calf serum. L1 was calculated as % of labeled nuclei per total number of basal cells. (o)—L1 in the epithelium near the wound and in new growth. (x)—L1 in the original epithelium. Two hundred cells counted for each measurement.

maturation started to occur thereafter. This permitted us to consider our experimental system as suitable for inducing and directing cell differentiation by exposing the explants to varying conditions of pH or CO_2 concentrations. Results obtained from tracheal explants grown on agar surface in various gases' composition and pH's can be summarized as follows:

(1) On the average, cilia covered more than 50% of the surface of the original explant in all the different experimental conditions used, with the exception of high oxygen concentrations.

(2) Oxygen concentrations of 80% and 95% appeared to be toxic for the epithelium, causing sloughing of most of the epithelial cells within 8 to 10 days of culture. Oxygen con-

centrations of 50% did not influence the various differentiation patterns.

(3) The new epithelial growth which appeared within 2 to 3 days after planting and covered the denuded connective tissue, developed in many cases into a two to three layered epithelium within eight to 12 days of culture (Figs 26 & 27). The surface layer consisted of many morphological undifferentiated cells but PAS+ cells and ciliated cells also appeared with time.

(4) The percentage of differentiated cells in the surface layer of the new epithelial growth was calculated. The results given in Table 7

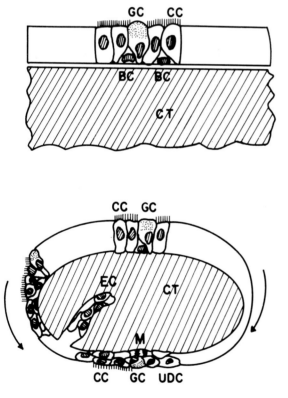

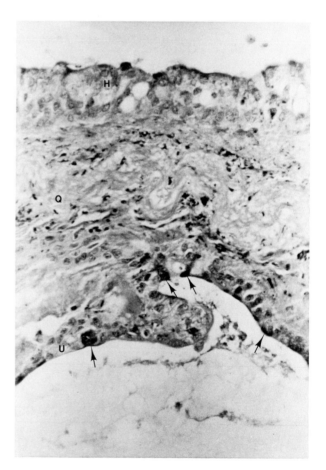

Fig. 26: Schematic representation of a trachea explant before culture (top) and after some days in culture (bottom). Basal cell (BC); ciliated cell (CC); goblet cell (GC); non-differentiated cell (UDC); mitosis (M); connective tissue (CT); epithelial cord (EC); growth direction (arrows).

Fig. 27: An explant of rabbit's respiratory mucosa grown for eight days. (Upper surface) original mucosa (H); connective tissue stroma (Q); new cell growth on (under surface) (U); PAS positive cells differentiated into mucus producing cells in under surface (arrows).

represent the percentage of explants having 10% or more PAS+ cells and 20% or more ciliated cells per section. Each denuded area was composed of 50 to 100 new cells. These results show that increased CO_2 concentration and increased pH enhanced the differentiation of PAS+ cells in the new cell population which developed during the culture period, yet the development of ciliated cells decreased.

Maintenance of precisely controlled environmental conditions in the experiments reported here was met with great technical difficulty, especially that of constant pH. These studies need to be elaborated and the results are, therefore, still preliminary. However, we can summarize that

these experiments indicate that carbon dioxide may be also a non-specific inducer in mucosal cell differentiation (Fig. 28). This might explain the modus operandi of eustachian tube hypoventilation on the middle ear mucosa. It should be emphasized that intracellular pH is affected by the environmental pCO_2 and may be as important as the actual fixation of CO_2 in cell metabolism regulation (McLimas, 1972). The emergence of a greater number of mucus producing cells is by itself an "antikeratinizing" action and vice versa. The microscopic squamous metaplasia found in the presence of central perforations is conceivably related to low pCO_2—which may be responsible for the emergence of fewer mucus secretory cells than when the pCO_2 is higher—therefore of more

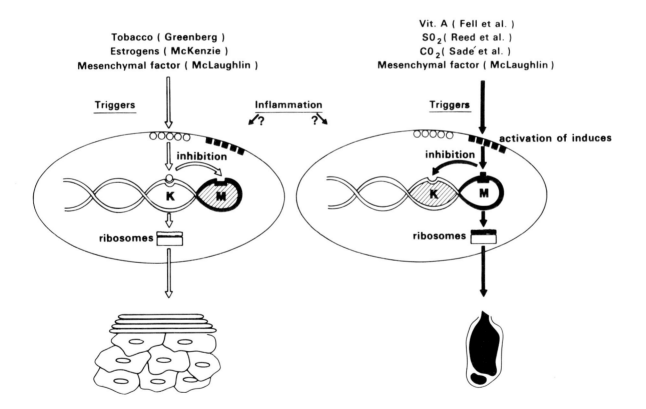

Fig. 28: Diagram of a hypothetical model showing various triggers and their action on the microenvironment of the cell—when a specific inducer will be released. Induction of mucus synthesis inhibiting keratin synthesis—and vice versa.

keratinizing cells. It should be stressed that pCO_2 is by no means the only trigger for mucosal (and probably keratinizing cells) differentiation—and by itself it is not a sufficient mechanism to explain the emergence of epidermoid cysts in the attic.

Finally, an important observation in respect to the metaplastic properties of the middle ear lining comes from yet unpublished data by Gordon Smyth, Michael Glasscock, Blair Simmons, Brian McCabe, and Arnold Shuring, who have deliberately left patches of stratified squamous epithelium in the middle ear (on a fistula or in between the stapedial crura) during conservative surgery for cholesteatoma—only to find some time later (on a "second look") that it disappeared. Thus middle ear mucosa which is seen often to change into stratified squamous epithelium apparently can also occasionally reverse this process, when small patches are involved. The specific conditions which call upon the mucosa to be transformed into S.S.E. or occasionally reverse this process are not known today. Reverse metaplasia is of course expected to occur in ears which produce mucus for a long time (i.e., long standing "glue ears"). The mucus metaplasia apparently returns to normal—especially when ventilating tubes are used. As most S.O.M. ears sooner or later recover, this can't be an exceptional phenomenon.

Summary

The middle ear mucosa is essentially a respiratory mucosa behaving according to the same general biological laws as all mucosae do. As such it is not surprising to find metaplastic changes in the middle ear mucosa either into whole stratified squamous cell populations or into mucus producing cells and glands. There is some clinical evidence that such a process can also reverse itself back to a normal mucosa. Epithelial cells, like other cells, on dividing have the option to mature (i.e., differentiate) into more than one type (phenotype) of cell. Normally, cell maturation is programmed and stable. However, under inflammatory or other abnormal conditions, the dividing cells might mature into "irregular" types. This explains the presence of keratinizing cells in mucosa (chronic bronchitis, ozena, etc.) or the turning of a mucosa into "all" mucus producing cells (S. secretory, O. otitis, M. media). In vitro experiments were performed with tissue explants of adult mucosae from various sources. When tracheal explants were subjected to high CO_2 concentrations, mucus producing cells showed a fourfold increase in new epithelial growths CO_2 concentration is, therefore, viewed as one of the agents which may direct mucosal cell maturation. This conclusion is strengthened by the finding of higher CO_2 levels in secretory otitis media ears than in normal ones. When a given mucosal stem cell divides, it has, however, to "choose" one specific pathway to follow. Therefore, maturation into mucus forming cells, especially in large numbers, is in a sense an "antikeratin" differentiation. The agent or agents which trigger the same mucosa to transform itself under pathological conditions into stratified squamous epithelium is now, however, known.

References

1. Drucker, I.; Weisman, Z.; and Sadé, J.: Tissue culture of human adenoids and middle ear mucosae. *Ann. Otol. Rhinol. Laryngol.* To be published, 1976.

2. Fell, H.: The effect of excess vitamin A on cultures of embryonic chicken skin implanted at different stages of differentiation. *Proc. R. Soc. Med.*, 146:242, 1957.

3. Greenberg, D. S.; Dickey, J. R.; and Neely, J. G.: Effects of tobacco on the ear. *Ann. Otol. Rhinol. Laryngol.*, 82:311, 1973.

4. Hentzer, E.: Histological studies of the normal mucosa in the middle ear, mastoid cavities and eustachian tube. *Ann. Otol. Rhinol. Laryngol.*, 79:825, 1970.

5. Hilding, A. C.: Experimental surgery of the noses' and sinuses' change in the morphology of the epithelium following variations in ventilation. *Arch. Otolaryng.*, 16:9, 1932.

6. Ingelstedt, S.; Jonson, B.; Rundcrantz, H.: Gas tension and pH in middle ear effusion. *Ann. Otol. Rhinol. Laryngol.*, 84:198, 1975.

7. Lim, D. J. and Hussel, B.: Human middle ear epithelium. *Arch. Otolaryngol.*, 89:835, 1969.

8. McLimas, W. F.: The gaseous environment of the mammalian cell in culture. In Rolbact, G. H. and Gristofalo, V.: (Eds). *Growth, Nutrition and Metabolism of Cells in Cultures*. Academic Press, New York, London, Vol. 1, 1972.

9. Moscona, A. A.: Studies on stability of phenotypic traits in embryonic integumental tissues and cells. In Montagna, W. and Lobitz, W. L.: (Eds.). *The Epidermis*. Academic Press, New York, New York, 1964, pp. 83-96.

10. Nevo, A.; Weisman, Z.; and Sadé, J.: Cell proliferation and cell differentiation in tissue cultures of adult mucociliary epithelia. *Differentiation*, 3:79, 1975.

11. Reid, L.: An experimental study of hypersecretion of mucus in bronchial tree. *Brit. J. Exp. Pathol.*, 44:437, 1963.

12. Sadé, J.: Middle ear mucosa. *Arch. Otolaryngol.*, 84:137, 1966.

13. Sadé, J.: Pathology and pathogenesis of the serous otitis media. *Arch. Otolaryngol.*, 84:297, 1966.

14. Sadé, J. and Weinberg, J.: Mucus production in the chronically infected middle ear. *Ann. Otol. Rhinol. Laryngol.*, 78:148, 1969.

15. Sadé, J.: Cellular differentiation of the middle ear lining. *Ann. Otol. Rhinol. Laryngol.*, 80:376, 1971.

16. Sadé, J.: Biopathological aspects of secretory otitis media. *Ann. Otol. Rhinol. Laryngol.*, 83:59, 1974.

17. Sadé, J.; Weisman, Z.; Nevo, A. C.: and Drucker, I.: Effect of environmental factors on respiratory epithelia. Proceedings of the International Symposium on Respiratory Disease and Air Pollution. *OHALO Symposium*, 1975.

18. Sadé, J.; Halevy, A.; and Hadas, E.: Middle ear clearance and middle ear pressures. *Ann. Otol. Rhinol. Laryngol.* (Supplement), 1976.

19. Wallbach, B. S. and Pery, H. R.: Tissue changes following deprivation of vitamin A. *J. Exp. Med.*, 42:753, 1925.

20. Weisman, Z.; Sadé, J.; and Nevo, A. C.: The effect of CO_2 and O_2 concentration on growth and differentiation of cultures of rabbit respiratory epithelium. To be published, 1976.

21. Young, A.: Closure of the nostrils in atrophic rhinitis. *J. Laryng. & Otol.*, 81:515, 1967.

CELLULAR POLARITY AT THE EPITHELIAL-MESENCHYMAL INTERFACE

Robert L. Trelstad, M.D.
Lewis B. Holmes, M.D.

During embryonic development, tissues are basically organized as either epithelial sheets or as relatively free wandering groups of mesenchyme. These two subsets of cells frequently interact with each other during organogenesis, and some of these epithelial-mesenchymal interactions have been studied in detail, including that between somite mesenchyme and notochord; the apical ectodermal ridge and mesenchyme in the limb; the enamel organ and mesenchyme in the tooth; and the mesenchyme and epithelium of a number of exocrine organs such as salivary glands and pancreas. In a number of these systems, attention has recently focused on the possible role of the extracellular matrix as a passive or permissive mediator of the epithelial-mesenchymal interaction. Support for this matrix function stems from studies which suggest that extracellular macromolecules are capable of stabilizing, and perhaps even promoting certain differentiative functions of cells (Slavkin and Greulick, 1975).

We recently have undertaken a series of studies to examine the structure of the cells at the epithelial-mesenchymal interface. In particular, we have directed our attention at the architectural order within the cells in both the epithelia and underlying mesenchyme in respect to the polarity of the individual cells.

Cellular polarity is an old concept derived from morphological studies in which the asymmetry of the cytoplasm of individual cells was noted. Originally, such studies derived from observations on oocytes undergoing various stages of meiotic division (Wilson, 1925). Later studies were directed at the polarity of cells within epithelia, particularly those with an excretory function and the organelle most frequently used as a marker of the polarity has been the Golgi apparatus (Beams and King, 1933). In a recent study of the corneal epithelium in the developing avian embryo, we noted a change in the polarity of the epithelial cells as measured by changes in position of the Golgi apparatus during several distinct stages of development (Trelstad, 1970). These changes in intracellular position of the Golgi apparatus were precisely coordinated temporarily, with the appearance beneath the epithelium of an extracellular matrix (Fig. 29). Subsequent biochemical and ultrastructural studies have confirmed that these epithelial cells in the early avian cornea are producing a substantial amount of highly organized extracellular matrix during the period in which the Golgi apparatus is present in the basal cell pole (Trelstad, et al, 1974 and Meier and Hay, 1974).

The unusual secretory function of these corneal epithelial cells, in which material is moved across the basal cell surface, is integrated into a complex reorientation of the internal architecture of the cell. In addition to Golgi apparatus, the centrioles move to the basal pole of the cell during the period when collagen and glycosaminoglycans are being produced and excreted. This internal arrangement must require a mechanism for reorienting internal organelles. Based on the previously described functions of microtubules, it seems quite likely that this group of internal structures, along with the centrioles, are responsible for the internal translocation of the Golgi apparatus. During the period in which the Golgi apparatus occupies the basal pole of the corneal epithelia, there is relatively little mitotic activity in the epithelium, an observation which is consistent with the possibility that the centrioles, located in the basal

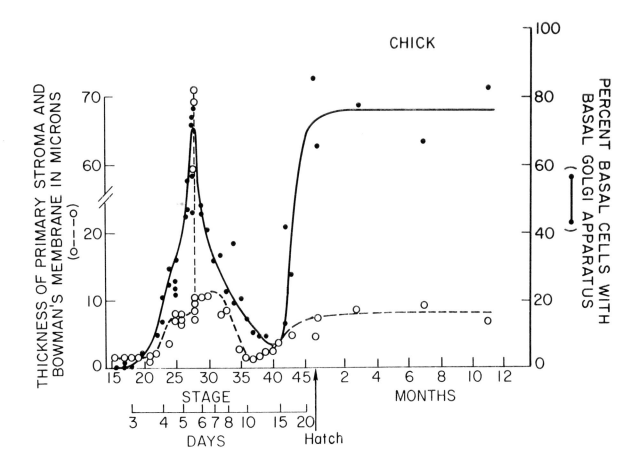

Fig. 29: Percentage of basal cells from the corneal epithelium with basal Golgi apparatuses as a function of time. Corneas at the indicated stages of development were impregnated with silver to stain the Golgi apparatus. Approximately 1000 cells in the basal cell layer of the epithelium were examined at each stage in tissue sections in the light microscope, and the percentage of cells with a Golgi apparatus in the basal cell pole was recorded. The shift of the Golgi apparatuses to the basal cell pole which occurs between day three and day ten correlates with the period when the primary corneal stroma is deposited beneath the corneal epithelium. The second shift of the Golgi apparatus which begins on day 15 correlates with the appearance of Bowman's membrane beneath the corneal epithelium.

position, are unable to act as a normal component of the mitotic apparatus.

In the developing limb, the apical-ectodermal ridge (AER) is a cap of ectoderm which lies at the distal most part of the limb bud and is responsible for its outgrowth (Zwilling, 1961). Removal of the AER results in loss of distal limb development and transplantation to another site on the limb results in limb outgrowth in that region (Saunders, et al, 1976). We examined the organization of the internal organelles in the AER, particularly the

position of the Golgi apparatus, and have found that during the period in which the apical ectodermal ridge is inducing outgrowth of the limb in the mouse, there is no reorientation of the Golgi apparatus to the basal pole of the cell. The epithelium in the AER thus does not manifest the same secretory morphology as seen in the cornea, nor the rearrangement of the internal organelles.

The mesenchyme cells which underlie the apical ectodermal ridge, on the other hand, show a distinct pattern in their orientation, which changes with time. During the early stages of development, the majority of these subectodermal mesenchyme cells are oriented with their Golgi apparatus either laterally or away from the overlying ectoderm. At about the 12th day of development in the forelimb and the 13th day of development in the hind limb, however, there is a remarkable shift in orientation of the cells in the underlying mesenchyme toward the overlying ectoderm (Table 8). At this same time, extracellular matrix accumulates at the interface between the ectoderm and mesenchyme. In addition, a profusion of cellular processes is present at the interface which derives from the mesenchyme, but perhaps also from the epithelium (Fig. 30). Direct cell contact between the epithelium and mesenchyme by such processes has been recently suggested for a number of such interacting tissues (Wartiovaara, et al, 1974; Mathon, et al, 1972; Slavkin, 1974; Meier and Hay, 1975).

TABLE 8

% Cells with Golgi apparatus directed toward the epithelial-mesenchymal interface

Forelimb	Epithelium	Mesenchyme
11 day	0	13
12 day	1	34
13 day	4	47

The internal architecture of both epithelial and mesenchymal cells during organogenesis is thus apparently precisely controlled by the cell. We suggest that the orientation of the internal organelles of the cell is causally related to the development of the final three dimensional structure of the embryo. The order which we readily recognize in a fully formed tissue is thus derived from a succession of ordered morphogenetic subunits which clearly extend to the subcellular level. At

present, we can only crudely measure subcellular structural polarity, by defining the relative positions of organelles, such as the Golgi apparatus and nucleus; we suspect that the centriole is more

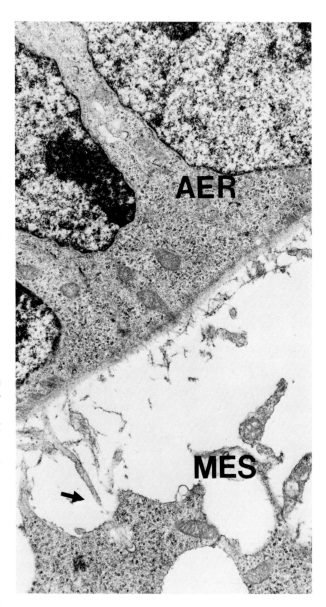

Fig. 30: Electron micrograph of 13 day embryonic mouse limb at the epithelial-mesenchymal interface. The compact epithelial cells in the apical ectodermal ridge (AER) contain numerous free ribosomes, but little endoplasmic reticulum. Unlike the corneal epithelium there are no Golgi apparatuses in the basal pole of the cells. Cellular processes from the mesenchyme (MES) are prominent; interdigitation of such processes with the mesenchymal cell body is common (arrow). Extracellular matrix including collagen fibrils is apparent near the basal surface of the epithelium.

causally related to the positioning of these internal organelles than is either of these other structures. The centrioles, with their associated microtubules, are probably major determinants of the internal architecture of the cell (Porter, 1966).

The epithelial-mesenchymal interaction occurs across an interface bounded by the epithelial cell membrane with its contiguous basement membrane, and the cellular processes of the underlying mesenchyme. This region contains extracellular macromolecules including collagen and the glycosaminoglycans (Toole, 1973 and Bernfield, et al, 1972). In many tissues these extracellular materials are organized in a highly patterned fashion, and it has been suggested that macromolecular self-assembly is responsible in part for the patterns which appear in this region (Trelstad, 1973). The major point to be derived from the present data is that the cells on both sides of this important interface show changing patterns of cellular orientation which presumably influence the geometry and morphogenesis of the matrix materials as they assemble in the extracellular space.

References

1. Beams, H. W. and King, R. L.: The Golgi apparatus in the developing tooth, with special reference to polarity. *Anat. Rec.*, 57:29, 1933.
2. Bernfield, M. R.; Banerjee, S. D.; and Cohn, R. H.: Dependence of salivary epithelial morphology and branching morphogenesis upon acid mucopolysaccharide-protein (proteoglycan) at the epithelial surface. *J. Cell Biol.*, 52:674, 1972.
3. Mathan, M.; Hermos, J. A.; and Trier, J. S.: Structural features of the epithelio-mesenchymal interface of rat duodenal mucosa during development. *J. Cell Biol.*, 52:577, 1972.
4. Meier, S. and Hay, E. D.: Control of corneal differentiation by extracellular materials. Collagen as a promoter and stabilizer of epithelial stroma production. *Dev. Biol.*, 38:249, 1974.
5. Meier, S. and Hay, E. D.: Stimulation of corneal differentiation by interaction between cell surface and extracellular matrix. *J. Cell Biol.*, 66:275, 1975.
6. Porter, K. R.: Cytoplasmic microtubules and their functions. In: *Principles of Biomolecular Organization*. CIBA Foundation Symposium. Churchill, London, 1966, p. 308.
7. Saunders, J. W.; Gasserling, M. T.; and Errick, J. E.: Inductive activity and enduring cellular constitution of a supernumerary apical ectodermal ridge grafted to the limb bud of the chick embryo. *Dev. Biol.*, 50:16, 1976.
8. Slavkin, H. D.: Embryonic tooth formation. *Oral Sciences Reviews*, 4:1, 1974.
9. Salvkin, H. C. and Greulich, R. C.: *Extracellular Matrix Influences on Gene Expression*. Academic Press, New York, New York, 1975.
10. Toole, B. P.: Hyaluronate and hyaluronidase in morphogenesis and differentiation. *Amer. Zool.*, 13:1061, 1973.
11. Trelstad, R. L.: The Golgi apparatus in chick corneal epithelium: changes in intracellular position during development. *J. Cell Biol.*, 45:34, 1970.
12. Trelstad, R. L.: The developmental biology of vertebrate collagens. *J. Histochem. Cytochem.*, 21:521, 1973.
13. Trelstad, R. L.; Hayashi, K.; and Toole, B. P.: Epithelial collagens and glycosaminoglycans in the embryonic cornea. *J. Cell Biol.*, 62:815, 1974.
14. Wartiovaara, J.; Nordling, S.; Lehtonen, E.; and Saxen, L.: Transfilter induction of kidney tubules: correlation with cytoplasmic penetration into nucleopore filters. *J. Embryol. Exptl. Morphol.*, 31:3, 1974.
15. Wilson, E. B.: *The Cell in Development and Heredity*. Macmillan, London, England, 1925, pp. 106-111.
16. Zwilling, E.: Limb morphogenesis. *Advan. Morphogenesis*, 1:301, 1961.

CELL INTERACTIONS AND GROWTH CONTROL

Stephen Roth, Ph.D.

Cholesteatoma is a disease of growth control at some level and the single point to be made by me in this presentation is that growth control is a conceptual phenomenon, but not a phenomenon that can be ascribed to one cell type. It is wrong to make the statement that a particular cell or tissue type is contact inhibited if it shows growth potential or that another cell type does not show growth control if it is not contact inhibited. It is clear from many observations that some cell types may be contact inhibited and may show growth control but, when put in the wrong place, fail to show such behavior.

Table 9 summarizes our laboratory experience in the study of cell surface carbohydrates and cell surface enzymes as mechanisms for recognition and growth control.

TABLE 9

Examples of Biological Specificity
in
The Degree of Growth Control Shown
by
Normal and Malignant Cells in Culture

Labeled, test cells	Percent increase in test cell number when grown (24h) on a lawn of:	
	3T3 cells	3T12 cells
3T3 cells (non-malignant)	0	96
3T12 cells (highly malignant)	−1	54
SV$_{40}$ transformed 3T3 cells (malignant)	105	150

Test cells were prelabeled with ^{3}H-thymidine and seeded, at low concentrations, on confluent lawns of the cells indicated. At various times, the cultures were fixed, developed radioautographically, and the labeled cells were counted directly.

Table 9 shows fibroblasts that are cell lines from newborn mice. These fibroblastic cell lines grow rapidly and show much of the contact inhibition behavior with which we are concerned. Here is shown a growth curve of two different fibroblastic cell lines 3T3 and 3T12. Notice that the non-malignant cell type, when it fills up the available surface area of the culture dish, stops growing. Those cells turn each other off and those cells also happen to be non-malignant in a sense that no number of those cells, when injected back into the syngeneic newborn mice will cause tumors.

Another cell line coming from the same newborn mouse preparation some 10-12 years ago has been transformed and is malignant. A very small number of those cells will kill a mouse in a very short period of time when injected subscapularly. Those cells grow well beyond the monolayer equivalent level. They do level off at a very very high concentration but that leveling is probably due to sloughing of many cells and not due to growth inhibition, even at that level.

Growth curves like this have been done with many cell types and lead to the generalization that non-malignant cells are always contact inhibited and malignant cells are rarely contact inhibited.

Hardly ever in embryology or in pathology is growth control within one cell type a problem. The problem is always when well controlled cells or poorly controlled cells meet other cells. That is where tumors or morphogenetic movements occur.

Some contact inhibited cells are not contact inhibited when grown on some malignant cell types. Similarly, some malignant cell types do show contact inhibition when challenged against a non-malignant cell type.

The contrast in the appearance of a malignant and non-malignant cell type grown together on one plate is striking. The 3T12 cells, malignant, are the same size as the 3T3', non-malignant. The non-malignant cell types are spread out and are flat, and do not tend to overlap one another and are highly contact inhibited. When they contact one another, they stop moving and they stop growing. The 3T12 cells grow rapidly and pile up on top of one another. Sometimes it is impossible to make out even the outlines of single cells in some areas of the slides we study. Yet at the interface between the malignant and non-malignant cell type, the malignant cell type respects the boundaries of this particular non-malignant cell type. The 3T12 cells, although highly malignant and contact inhibited when grown together, do show the ability to receive some sort of a message from the non-malignant, contact inhibited cell type. Even though they are contact inhibited by themselves, 3T3 cells are not contact inhibited by the malignant cell type.

One can quantitate these findings by preparing plates with cells of any type as a lawn and sprinkling on top of that lawn radio-labeled cells of any other cell type. We usually use tritiated thymidine. If for example, 100 cells are placed on the media on day zero, then on day one, day two, or day three, the number of cells that have grown can be determined by radioautographic methods.

3T3 cells, when placed on top of other 3T3 cells, do not grow. So, the non-malignant cell type can turn itself off. However, when a non-malignant cell type is placed on top of a lawn of 3T12 cells, which are themselves highly malignant and non-contact inhibited, there is no apparent message that is sent to these cells to cause them to stop growing. These cells will show growth, even in the presence of large numbers of other cell types, only because those cell types are not their own cell types. The malignant cell type, 3T12, will grow well when placed on their own kind, but not at all when placed on the contact inhibited 3T3 cells.

It is clear that some cells can send messages to other cells and some cells can receive messages from other cells, but not all cells can do both. Every combination seems to exist.

Studies such as I have been describing are related to cholesteatoma because the outer surface of the eardrum is derived from ectodermal epithelium and the inner surface which faces the middle ear is derived from endodermal epithelium. This junction occurs in the mouth as well, at the root of the tongue and in the rectum, and these areas are often the sites of malignant tumors. I had thought previously that tumors occurred in the ear, and a cholesteatoma may fit that category. One epithelial cell type, squamous epithelium, may find itself in a place where it no longer receives the turn-off signal; and it begins to proliferate. Squamous epithelium can turn itself off because that is the basis for wound healing; after a wound is made, the free edges migrate toward each other, and when they meet, mitosis ceases. But it is possible that when the ectodermal epithelium gets in the middle ear, it is not turned off because it is not surrounded by the appropriate cells, and continues to develop. Perhaps this agrees with Dr. Freedberg's informal diagnosis that cholesteatomas in the middle ear are made up of skin.

Additional support is given to this theory from the fact that cholesteatomas rarely form in the outer ear.

Our own work is involved with the kinds of messages cells can send and receive. Our own particular bias is that this occurs by protein-carbohydrate interactions on cell surfaces. One of these proteins is the glycosyltransferases that are usually found in the Golgi and that are often found to a lesser extent on the outsides of cells. It is clear from a number of studies that when two contact inhibited cell types meet in culture one cell can catalyze the transfer of a sugar to the surface of another cell and vice-versa. There may or may not be catalysis but, if there is a reaction, the cells will separate and will be changed by the covalent addition of an additional monosaccharide, or any number of monosaccharides.

This is one way in which two fibroblasts can actually send a message to one another on contact. There is a small number of experiments that causally implicate transferases in the control of cell growth. That is, the addition of monosaccharides to recipient cells can cause them to stop growing for at least one day. In malignant cells, which I did not intend to refer to until I learned of Dr. Peck's work, there are two problems that have turned up with respect to transferases as the recognizing protein. The basic problem is why don't malignant cells catalyze this reaction when contact is made? One possible reason is that the enzyme seems to be taken up with themselves and are not free to react. A second reason comes from the work of several laboratories, indicating that an intermediate product in the transfer reaction on the plasma membrane may be vitamin A. It seems to be a carrier of sugar phosphates across the membrane from the inside to the outside. The vitamin A catalyzed glycosyl transfer reaction is decreased in some transformed cells.

THE ROLE OF EPITHELIAL CELL MIGRATION IN WOUND HEALING

H. Paul Ehrlich, Ph.D.

In response to injury, skin has the ability to repair by regenerating a new epidermis and dermis. In the epidermis, this is accomplished by the migration and proliferation of viable cells which survive the injury. In addition to the migration of sheets of epidermal cells into the wound space, other stationary epidermal cells at the wound margin undergo mitosis, thereby increasing the population of migrating cells. In the underlying dermis repair involves fibroblast proliferation, migration and synthesis of a new connective tissue matrix.

Very small surface wounds can heal entirely by epidermal migration; no granulation tissue synthesis or epithelial cell mitosis appears necessary. In some tissues such as the cornea, cellular migration is the only feature in the repair process and can be observed just one hour after injury (Friedenwald, 1944). In skin, cellular migration takes somewhat longer to initiate, with movement clearly identifiable at 12 hours (Krawczk, 1971). The supply of epidermal cells is from the uninjured edge and from the surviving hair follicles in the injured area. The rate of migration of the skin epidermal cells is 50 to 100μ per hour. Although slow in comparison with white blood cells which can migrate at 500 to 1000μ per hour, this is an adequate rate for wound closure (Abercrombie, 1964).

Epidermal movement continues until the epidermal cells from the edge of the wound meet cells migrating from the opposite edge. The cessation of movement following the collision and adhesion of two cells coming in contact with one another is termed contact inhibition of movement. As long as epidermal cells have a free edge and are in contact with their substratum, they will continue to migrate. Following contact inhibition the newly arrived epidermal cell can round up and take on the appearance of a normal epidermal basal cell.

During epithelization there is progressive extension of a tongue of epidermal cells from the wound edge across the wound space. This sheet of epidermal cells migrates down along the wound edge with the invasive nature of this moving tissue being checked by the underlying connective tissue components of the dermis. The direction and orientation of movement is directed by the substratum which can be fibrin or collagen.

The movement of the epidermal cells is a rolling and sliding one. These cells migrate by moving over the top of fellow epidermal cells which have previously migrated out into the wound space. The moving cells are elongated and flattened as they move over this cellular surface. When they come in contact with the substratum, they acquire a more rounded shape and may cease to move. These epidermal cells attach to their substratum by forming hemidesmosomes which are the same structures responsible for basal cell attachment to basement membrane in uninjured skin. As epidermal cells migrate and cover over the wound area they systematically anchor themselves to their substratum as they move (Krawczyk, 1971).

In response to injury the mitotic rate in the wound edge can be increased as much as 20 times normal. The area for this increase is confined to cells in the edge 0.3 mm from the wound space. Active cells lose their diurnal variation and their cell cycle is reduced from 30 days to only 12 hours. Besides basal cells undergoing mitosis, mature cells in the higher layers of the epidermis can pass back into a basal state and undergo mitosis, which enlarges the mitotically active cell population.

The life expectancy of cells in regeneration is reduced. For example, the half life of a regenerating liver cell is reduced from 450 days to 26 days.

The same is true for epidermal cells; life expectancy drops from 27 days to four. Mitosis is confined to the cells at the wound edge and to a lesser extent to cells actively involved in migration. Migrating cells have a basal cell character and following the cessation of migration they can undergo mitosis. In general a cell in migration does not undergo mitosis until it has stopped moving and comes to rest (Bullough, 1966).

There have been a number of theories put forth to explain the changes in mitotic activity of epithelial cells at the wound margin. Bullough and Laurence (1961) have suggested that chalones, a tissue specific mitosis inhibitor, is responsible for the control of epithelial mitosis. At specific concentrations chalones will inhibit mitosis, following injury with the loss of cells and viable tissue, there is a drop in chalone concentration in the surrounding area. Without sufficient concentration of this inhibitor, cells begin to undergo mitosis and continue to do so until the new cellular population is large enough to produce sufficient quantities of the inhibiting chalone. It is proposed by these authors that chalones will inhibit mitosis by inhibiting DNA synthesis.

Blisters can heal in a single day by epidermal cellular migration, provided the blister is left intact. Blisters made on the backs of mice show epidermal cells migrating from the wound edge and hair follicles. They move over the basement membrane which remains intact and adherent to the dermis (Krawczh, 1971). Healing is rapid in this model because healing involves only epidermal cell migration. There are sufficient epidermal cells migration sites throughout the entire wound area and hence, there is no need for mitosis to increase cell number to cover the defect. In addition, an intact basement membrane is an excellent substratum for epidermal cell migration. Since no injury has been sustained by the dermis, the need for new granulation synthesis is unnecessary. The importance of the substratum for epidermal cell migration is demonstrated in the healing of a perforated tympanic membrane (Johnson, 1966). The epithelial cells on the tympanic membrane surface show an elevated mitotic activity with an increase in cell number but no cellular migration across the perforation. By 36 hours there is a pile up of cells along the margins of the wound but no migration. Not until days three to seven do cells migrate over the defect and this occurs only after the accumulation of new granulation tissue in the wound space.

In recent experimental studies which we have carried out on the effects of topical and systemically administered vitamin A on cortisone-retarded 4 cm^2 open wound in rabbits (Hunt, et al, 1969), we found that vitamin A stimulates the healing of wounds which have been retarded by glucocorticoids (Ehrlich and Hunt, 1968). The end result in animals treated with cortisone and vitamin A showed that the wounds which normally healed largely by contraction healed instead by epithelization, when vitamin A and cortisone were given together. A possible explanation for these results is that vitamin A antagonizes the inhibitory effects of glucocorticoids on fibroplasia and new granulation tissue synthesis. Without a new connective tissue matrix epidermal cells are reluctant to move across the wound space. By the local application of vitamin A, fibroplasia is established in the wound and a new connective tissue matrix is synthesized. The new connective tissue matrix fills in the wound space and forms the substratum necessary for epidermal cell migration.

Wound healing by epithelization requires three components: cellular migration, cell mitosis and substratum. Epidermal cells migration must occur to cover the defect in the epidermis. A rise in the mitotic rate at the wound edge increases the number of epithelial cells involved in migration. Lastly, the substratum which the epithelial cells move over is necessary for both the control of migration and the direction of cell movement. The absence of a substratum will impair the movement of epithelial cells.

References

1. Abercrombie, M.: Behavior of cells toward one another. In Montagna, W. and Billingham, R.: (Eds.). *Advances in the Biology of Skin*, Vol. 5. Pergamon Press, New York, New York, 1964, p. 95.

2. Bullough, W. S.: Cell replacement after tissue damage. In Illingworth, C.: (Ed.). *Wound Healing*. J. and A. Churchill Ltd., London, England, 1966, p. 43.

3. Bullough, W. S. and Laurence, E. B.: The control of mitotic activity in the skin. In Slome, D.: (Ed.). *Wound Healing. Proceedings of a Symposium Held on 12-13 November, 1959 at the Royal College of Surgeons of England*. Pergamon Press, Symposium Publications Division, New York, New York, 1961, p. 1.

4. Ehrlich, H. P. and Hunt, T. K.: Effects of cortisone and vitamin A on wound healing. *Ann. Surg.*, 167: 324, 1968.

5. Friedenwald, J. S. and Buschke, W.: Influence of some experimental variables on epithelial movements in healing of corneal wounds. *J. Cell. Comp. Physiol.*, 23: 95, 1944.

6. Hunt, T. K.; Ehrlich, H. P.; Garcia, J. A. et al: Effect of vitamin A on reversing the inhibitory effect of cortisone on healing of open wounds in animals and man. *Ann. Surg.*, 170: 633, 1969.

7. Johnson, F. R.: Wound epithelialization. In Levenson, S. M.; Stein, J. M.; and Grossblatt, N.: (Eds.). *Wound Healing—Proceedings of a Workshop*. National Academy of Sciences—National Research Council, Washington, D.C., 1966, p. 48.

8. Krawczyk, W. S.: A pattern of epidermal cell migration during wound healing. *J. Cell. Biol.*, 49: 247, 1971.

FACTORS INFLUENCING THE MOVEMENT OF EPITHELIAL CELLS

Ian C. Mackenzie, Ph.D., D.D.S.

An examination of the literature on epidermal cholesteatoma provides no clear consensus of opinion concerning the etiology of this condition (Friedmann, 1974 and Mawson, 1974) and most of the hypotheses proposed were developed many years ago (Goodhill, 1973). Although it appears probable that cells sequestered during embryonic development may proliferate to produce cystic lesions anatomically related to the middle ear (McKenzie, 1931), it is reported that this is a rare occurrence (Friedmann, 1974). Alternative explanations for the presence of keratinizing epithelium in the middle ear have therefore been sought and four general mechanisms have been proposed and are discussed elsewhere in this volume: (1) perforation of the tympanic membrane and subsequent invasion of the middle ear by keratinizing epithelium of the external auditory meatus; (2) proliferation and ingrowth of basal cells of the keratinizing epithelium of an unperforated tympanic membrane under the influence of inflammation; (3) metaplastic change of the cuboidal epithelium of the middle ear to a stratified squamous epithelium; (4) invagination of the pars flaccida of the tympanic membrane as a result of negative pressure within the middle ear.

Given the anatomical relationships of the region and the frequent, possibly invariable, association of inflammation with epidermal cholesteatoma (Friedmann, 1974 and Lim and Saunders, 1972), each of these mechanisms appears feasible. The concept of invagination of the pars flaccida to form a saccule, the occlusion of which produces a cyst, is an attractive one in that the formation of a cyst cavity and the origin and inward polarization of its keratinized lining epithelium are readily explained. Each of the other concepts goes so far as to produce an area of keratinizing epithelium abutting with the epithelial lining of the middle ear but does little to explain the subsequent mechanisms of invasion and replacement of the columnar epithelium. While the mechanism of invasion and replacement of the cuboidal epithelium of the existing epithelial surfaces lining the middle ear appears to be difficult to explain, evidence that such a process actually occurs appears to be available. Hellmann (1925) refers to a "fight for life or death" between stratified squamous and cuboidal epithelia during cholesteatoma formation and Friedmann (1974) has published photographs of histological preparations of cholesteatoma with squamous epithelium poised to burrow beneath the normal epithelium of the malleus. The ultrastructural appearance of the advancing edge of squamous epithelium has been described by Lim and Saunders (1972). If it is accepted that a gradual invasive replacement of the normal cuboidal epithelial lining the middle ear occurs then, irrespective of the origin of the keratinizing epithelium, the question of the stability of a junction which may be formed by two dissimilar epithelia appears to be a central one. The uncertainty about the mechanisms associated with this aspect of the etiology of epidermal cholesteatoma suggests that a general consideration of factors initiating and affecting the direction of epithelial migration and movement could be of interest.

Epithelial Junctions at Various Sites

Junctions between epithelia with dissimilar patterns of differentiation are normally found in many anatomical areas. Several such junctions exist in the oral cavity, for example (Fig. 31) between the keratinizing epithelium of the attached gingiva and the non-keratinizing epithelium of the alveolar mucosa (Lozdan and Squier, 1969 and

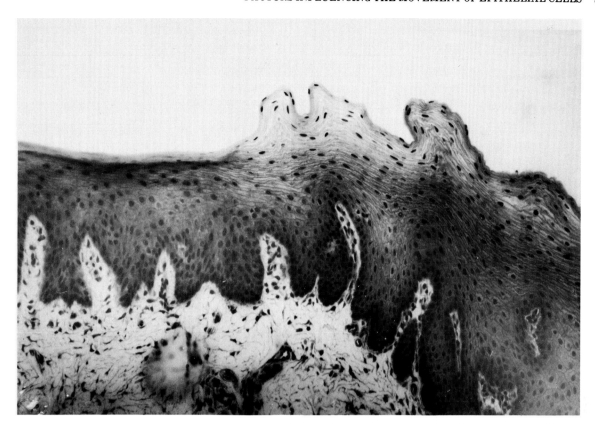

Fig. 31: Photomicrograph of histological section of the region of the mucogingival junction of a rhesus monkey. There is a sharply delined junction between the keratinizing gingival epithelium (left) and the non-keratinizing epithelium of the alveolar mucosa.

Lainson and Mackenzie, 1976), at the vermilion border of the lip (Ham, 1969) and between the "hard" and "soft" keratinizing epithelium in tongue papillae (Cameron, 1966). The mucocutaneous junctions of the eye and various junctions at the orifices of glands (Ham, 1969) provide similar examples. With the possible exception of the cervical junction of the uterus, which has been reported to drift in position with varying hormone levels (Cairns, 1975), it is apparent that the position of such junctions is relatively stable throughout life. Junctions of this type are established during embryonic development and, at that stage, the role of epithelial-mesenchymal interactions appears to be an important one through determination of the local patterns of differentiation and spatial organization of epithelia

(McLoughlin, 1963; Sengel, 1964; and Cohen, 1969). There is evidence from experiments involving transplantation from one site to anther of epithelia with and without their underlying connective tissue, that connective tissue influences may be important in maintaining specific patterns of epithelial differentiation throughout life (Billingham and Silvers, 1967 and 1968).

One of the features of the organization of normal stratified squamous epithelia and of the epithelia on either side of normal anatomical junctions between epithelia is the orderly sequence of maturation of cells as they pass towards the surface from the stratum germinativum. The mechanism of this pattern of cell movement is not well understood but the beautiful patterns of cellular architecture established in the epidermis

(Mackenzie, 1969 and 1975 and Christophers, 1971) and in other epithelial structures such as tongue papillae (Cameron, 1966) and hairs (Mercer, 1961) indicates a close control of cell movement and differentiation during the normal replacement of epithelial structures. Establishment of spatially organized patterns between epithelial cells have been interpreted either in terms of physical packing properties (Christophers, 1972 and Menton, 1975) or cell-surface properties associated with cell adhesion (Mercer, 1961 and Mackenzie, 1972).

Concepts of Epithelial Movement During Wound Healing

Normal patterns of epithelial organization are often disrupted by injury and the ability of epithelial cells to respond to various stimuli by increased proliferation and migration is a basic one. During wound healing the direction of migration of epithelial cells from the wound margin leads to effective re-epithelialization of the wounded surface (Johnson and McMinn, 1960 and Gillman and Penn, 1956). The aphorism that "epithelium will not tolerate a free edge" (Rand, 1915) is now well known but the answers to the questions of what it is that constitutes a "free edge" and what mechanisms are associated with the switching on and switching off of movement are uncertain. Abercrombie (1962 and 1964) from experiments dealing principally with fibroblasts in culture but also from some studies of epithelial cells (Abercrombie and Middleton, 1968), developed the concept of "contact-inhibition of movement" in which contact of one cell with another cell prevents motion in the direction of contact. Some of the problems of interpreting diverse contact-inhibition phenomena in culture and the meaning of "contact" have been discussed by Wallach (1975), but it appears that the direction of migration from a wound margin can be interpreted as a release from inhibition of movement in the direction of the missing tissue. An additional concept of "mobilization" of cells adjacent to a wound has also been proposed in which some change of the

cells of this region releases them from a restraint which normally delays movement (Abercrombie, 1962).

More recently considerable interest has focused on the role of cell-surface glycoproteins and glycolipids in the control of cell movement, cell recognition and cell proliferation (Hakomori, 1973; Edelman, 1976; and Marx, 1976) and the mechanism for the concepts described by Abercrombie has been sought in changes in cell-surface properties. There is a considerable body of biochemical evidence indicating that changes in the cell-surface components of cultured cells occur (a) with the establishment of cell confluence, when cells become contact-inhibited and (b) following cell transformation, after which cell contact inhibition patterns are altered, (Hakomori, 1973; Hynes, 1974; Robbins and Macpherson, 1971 and Gahmberg and Hakomori, 1974). The role of cell-surface changes in the control of the behavior of normal epithelial in vivo has not been studied in depth but there is some histological immunofluorescent evidence for changes in the glycoprotein and glycolipid components which are associated with the expression of blood group antigens on the cell-surfaces of neoplastic and pre-malignant oral mucosal lesions (Prendergast, et al, 1968, Dabelsteen and Pindborg, 1973; Dabelsteen, et al, 1975; Davidsohn, et al, 1969; Cowan, 1962; and Kim and Isaacs, 1975). However, as Dabelsteen and Fejerskov (1974) have shown that there is loss of blood group antigens from the epithelial cells adjacent to healing wounds of human oral mucosa, it appears that such changes are tumor-associated rather than tumor-specific and may be primarily associated with cell movement or cell proliferation.

Epithelial Blood Group Antigens During Wound Healing

Recently, to examine further the relationship between epithelial cell movement and cell-surface antigens, we have examined patterns of cell proliferation and distribution of blood group antigen on epithelial cells adjacent to healing wounds of the oral mucosa (Mackenzie and Dabelsteen, 1976). For these studies, linear wounds 1 mm wide were made in the keratinizing epithelium of the palate and gingiva and in the non-keratinizing buccal mucosa of adult Rhesus monkeys. At various intervals up to six days, proliferating cells adjacent to the healing wounds were labeled by local injection of tritiated thymidine and biopsies were taken and sectioned for: (a) autoradiography and (b) examination of a cell-surface antigen cross-reacting with human group B by a double layer immunofluorescence technique. The altered distribution of blood group antigen found in these biopsies showed a similar pattern in each of the tissues studied. Within three—six hours the strong blood group reactivity found on the surfaces of cells in the normal epithelium was lost from the region 100-200 μm from the edge of the wound. Antigen reactivity was also absent from the surfaces of cells forming the epithelial outgrowths into the healing wounds which were present at subsequent times. However, antigen activity was found in all specimens in which contact had become established between the opposing outgrowths of epithelium from either side of the wound.

Cell proliferation appeared to be neither temporary nor spatially related to the region of antigen loss. Increased cell proliferation was not observed until 24 hours or more after loss of antigen and it was then seen in the area lying adjacent to, but outside of, the region lacking antigen activity. The rate of cell labeling also remained high outside the wounded area even after restoration of antigen reactivity following establishment of epithelial continuity. These findings suggest that loss of epithelial antigen reactivity adjacent to healing wounds is some way associated with cell movement. At present, it is not known whether the type of cell-surface changes indicated by loss of antigen reactivity are produced by additions or deletions from the reactive groups or by masking. It is also uncertain whether such changes may be primarily related to altered adhesion of cells or to patterns of cell to cell recognition. However, the

finding that blood group antigen activity is lost during cell movement and regained when epithelial contact is re-established, provides some general evidence to support the concept that the type of alterations in cell-surface properties believed to affect cell movement in vitro (Hakomori, 1973) may also function to control epithelial movement following wounding in vivo.

Much of the recent interest in the role of the cell-surface components has focused on the behavior of neoplastic cells. The invasive properties of malignant cells may be related in some way to altered surface adhesiveness (Martz and Steinberg, 1973) or to failure to respond to surface information present on adjacent normal cells and therefore to show contact inhibition of movement (Abercrombie, 1962). There is also a considerable body of work pointing to the function of cell-surface properties during morphogenesis and indicating the tissue specificity of such interactions (Moscona, 1968). Given this putative background of evidence it therefore seems relevant to ask whether the surface properties of cells of epithelia of differing embryological origin may be such that contact between them would not lead to inhibition of movement. What then would be the effect of creating a wound between two epithelia of differing origin? Would normal surface interactions which lead to normal inhibition of further movement following wound closure fail to function leading to the continuous migration of the more active epithelium at the expense of the other?

The dissimilar epithelia abutting at embryologically-determined junctions appear to possess mutually interacting surfaces: such patterns of recognition would appear necessary to explain the observed stability of such junctions. The concept of "affinative" behavior, the ability to form a smooth organized junction between epithelia reacting in wound healing, has been discussed by Chiakkulas (1952). In amphibian grafting experiments, he found (a) affinitive behavior between epidermis and the epidermis of other body sites and corneal and oral epithelium but (b) disaffinitive behavior between epidermis and epithelia from the esophagus, intestine, gall bladder and other epithelia which were not normally contiguous. In disaffinitive situations the epidermis continued to move after contact was established with the transplanted epithelium, and the epidermal cells undermined and wedged themselves between the mucosal cells of the graft and their underlying connective tissue. He concluded that fusion between two epithelia to form a stable junction occurs only if normally there is continuity between these epithelia in the intact organism. The behavior of mammalian tissues may not be entirely analogous, and Cameron, Flaxman, and Yanoff (1974) have shown an endothelial inhibition of migration of the rabbit corneal epithelium.

Uterine Implantation of Epidermis as a Model for Study of Epithelial Growth

Recently we have used the system of implantation of pieces of skin to the uterus developed by Beer and Billingham (1970 and 1972) to examine connective tissue factors affecting the differentiation and structure of keratinizing epithelia. The following brief account of some aspects of the behavior of epithelium in this system is taken partly from the reported work of Beer and Billingham and partly from our own published (Mackenzie and Smith, 1976) and unpublished observations. If small pieces of ear skin are introduced surgically into the lumen of the upper part of the rat uterus and the rat treated postoperatively with estrogens, the piece of skin passes down the uterine lumen to become implanted into the uterine wall, apparently at one of the sites specialized normally to receive the conceptus. These implants appear to maintain an essentially normal structure and a junction between the keratinizing epidermis and the columnar epithelium of the normal uterine lining is formed. However, if the rat is subsequently treated systemically with estrogen, cells at the edge of the keratinizing epithelium of the skin implant migrate out to displace the normal uterine lining. If estrogen treatment is maintained, the entire columnar epithelial lining the uterus may be

replaced in this way. The keratinizing epithelial lining of the uterus so produced appears to be quite stable and upon cessation of estrogen treatment further migration ceases, but the epithelium maintains its established position and continues to keratinize and proliferate in a fairly normal manner (Fig. 32). Normal site-specific patterns of epidermal cellular architecture are maintained within the epidermis overlying the originally implanted dermis but are absent from the epidermis which has migrated onto the uterine connective tissue. In these areas a thicker epithelium more resembling plantar epidermis is formed. A similar epithelium results from sheets of pure ear epidermis which are separated from the dermis prior to implantation. Essentially similar results have been observed following implantation of pieces of tongue mucosa when there is retention of normal papillary patterns of epithelial architecture in the area of the original implant but loss of such patterns from the epithelial outgrowth onto the uterine connective tissue. Irrespective of the type of keratinizing epithelium implanted, the continuing proliferation of the new keratinizing lining of the uterus leads to a cystic appearance with progressive accumulation of keratin and gross distention of the uterine lumen (Figs. 33 and 34).

The mechanism of outgrowth of the keratinizing epithelium appears to be of interest. Figure 35 shows a junction between columnar uterine epithelium and an outgrowth from the stratified squamous epithelium of an implant. It can be seen that the advancing edge of stratified squamous epithelium has an appearance very similar to the outgrowth which occurs from the margin of a healing wound and that the leading epithelial cells appear to burrow under and lift off the adjacent cells of the columnar epithelium. This appearance is quite similar to that of the junction between the cuboidal epithelial lining of the middle ear and the keratinizing epithelium of a cholesteatoma (Friedmann, 1974 and Lim and Saunders, 1973).

The Effects of Estrogen and Inflammation on Epithelial Proliferation

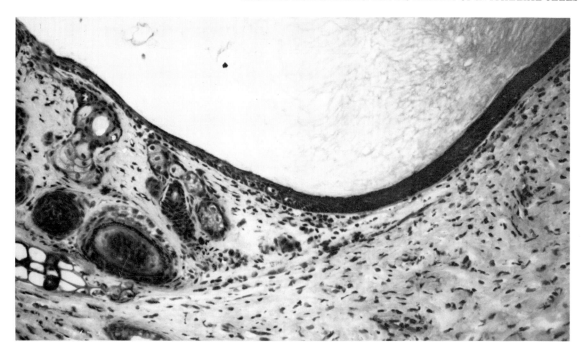

Fig. 32: Photomicrograph of a rat uterus implanted with ear skin. To the left, the originally implanted skin specimen can be recognized by the presence of cartilage and hair follicles. Under the influence of estrogen the epidermis has grown out to replace the columnar epithelial lining of the uterus. The epidermis growing on the uterine connective tissue (to the right) has continued to proliferate, but is thicker and the accumulated keratin filling the uterine lumen has a different appearance over this region.

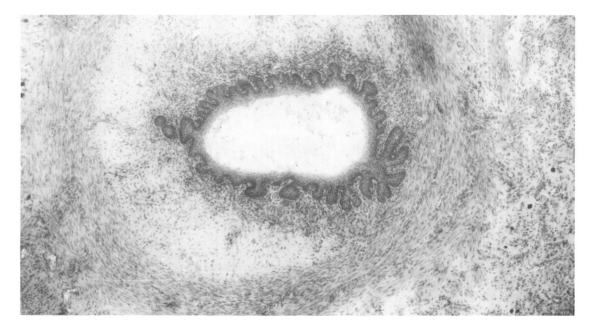

Fig. 33: Rat uterus implanted with ear skin and sectioned through an area where the uterine lining has been replaced by the outgrowth of epidermis from the transplant. A cyst-like appearance is seen with only limited keratinization of the epithelial lining.

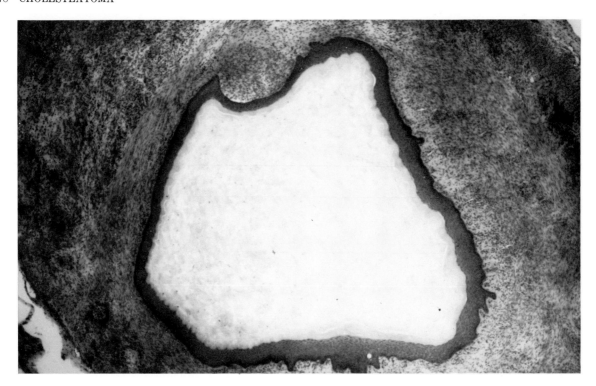

Fig. 34: A similar region to Figure 33 with further epithelial proliferation. The lumen of the uterus has been grossly extended by a mass of keratin and the epithelium of the lining has a flatter epithelial connective tissue interface.

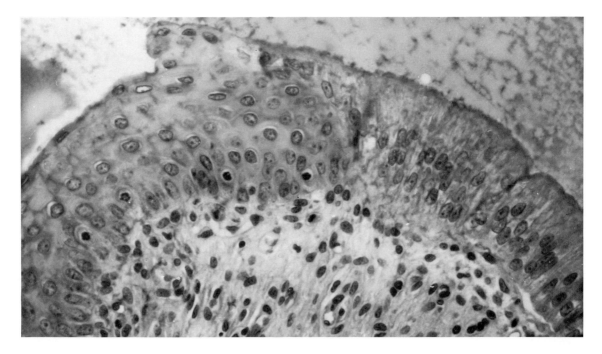

Fig. 35: A region showing the junction between the normal columnar epithelial lining of the uterus and the epidermal outgrowth. A high rate of cell proliferation in the epidermis is seen. The advancing edge of the epidermis appears similar to that of a healing wound and seems to burrow under and lift off the columnar epithelium.

In several respects the behavior of epithelium in the experimental model system obtained by implantation of epidermis into the uterus appears analogous to that described during the pathogenesis of cholesteatoma; there is invasion and replacement of a columnar epithelium by a keratinizing one and the keratinizing epithelium continues to proliferate leading to the accumulation of sloughed keratin and distention of the cavity it surrounds. In respect of the dependence of epithelial migration in the uterus on systemic estrogen levels, the uterine system differs from that found in cholesteatoma. However, the effects of subepithelial inflammation appear to be similar to those of estrogen in stimulating hyperplasia of keratinizing epithelia.

The observed effects of increased proliferation and thickening of keratinizing epithelia growing in the uterus appear similar to those reported by Lansing and Opdyke (1950), following topical estrogen application to guinea pig epidermis. A similar estrogen-related response of rat epidermis has been reported by Young (1968) and an increased rate of cell proliferation in oral epithelia has been associated with increased estrogen levels (Beagrie, 1966). The response of the epidermis to dermal inflammation by thickening and increased proliferative activity (Schellander and Marks, 1973) is therefore similar, as is the effect of inflammation on the keratinized epithelium of the gingiva (Demetrious, et al, 1971; Johnson and Hopps, 1974; and Lainson and Mackenzie, 1976). It is possible therefore that the chronic inflammation frequently associated with the pathogeneses of cholesteatoma could act to stimulate the growth and migration to its keratinized lining and the replacement of the columnar epithelium of the ear. The probable important role of inflammation in stimulating the epidermal growth observed in cholesteatoma has previously been heavily emphasized by Ruedi (1958).

Summary

The observations which have been made in this paper do not favor any one of the hypotheses of the etiology of cholesteatoma. However, as has been previously noted by many others, the anatomy of the ear appears unusual in respect of the close proximity of the keratinized stratified squamous epithelium lining the external auditory meatus to the cuboidal epithelium lining the middle ear. These epithelia arise embryologically from different sources, and do not normally contact one another. Establishment of continuity between these epithelia through perforation or basal ingrowth could therefore lead to a junction between epithelia at which no mechanism existed for the inhibition of the growth of one epithelium by the other. The situation described by Friedmann (1974) and by Lim and Saunders (1973) of a stratified squamous epithelium abutting, undermining and invading the columnar epithelium of the middle ear appears to show such a pattern. This concept of failure of inhibition of growth of the keratinized epithelium depends upon a considerable degree of speculation concerning the control of migratory behavior of epithelium. However, in the experimental model systems described a very similar invasion and replacement of columnar epithelium by stratified squamous epithelium of distant origin can be observed and it appears that, at present, the best explanation of this phenomenon is in terms of a failure of one epithelium to inhibit the normal wound healing behavior of the other.

Acknowledgements

The financial support for the studies described in this paper was provided by the John A. Hartford Foundation, Inc.

References

1. Abercrombie, M. and Ambrose, E. J.: The surface properties of cancer cells. A review. *Cancer Res.*, 22: 525, 1962.

2. Abercrombie, M: Behavior of cells toward one another. In Montagna, W. and Billingham, R.: (Eds.). *Advances in Biology of Skin*, Vol. 5. Pergamon Press, New York, New York, 1964, pp. 95.

3. Abercrombie, M. and Middleton, C. A.: Epithelial-mesenchymal interactions affecting locomotion of cells in culture. In Fleischmajer, R. and Billingham, R. E.: (Eds.). *Epithelial-Mesenchymal Interactions. 18th Habermann Symposium.* Williams and Wilkins, Baltimore, Maryland, 1968, p. 56.

4. Beagrie, G. S.: Observations on cell biology of gingival tissues of mice. *Br. Dent. J.*, 121: 417, 1966.

5. Beer, A. E. and Billingham, R. E.: Implantation, transplantation and epithelial-mesenchymal relationships in the rat uterus. *J. Exp. Med.*, 132: 721, 1970.

6. Beer, A. E. and Billingham, R. E.: In vivo approaches to the analysis of the conservation of epidermal specificities. In Maibach, H. and Rovee, D.: (Eds.). *Epidermal Wound Healing.* Year Book Medical Publishers, Inc., Chicago, Illinois, 1972.

7. Billingham, R. E. and Silvers, W. K.: Studies on the conservation of epidermal specificities of skin and certain mucosas in adult mammals. *J. Exp. Med.*, 125: 429, 1967.

8. Billingham, R. E. and Silvers, W. K.: Dermoepidermal interactions and epithelial specificity. In Fleischmajer, R. and Billingham, R. E.: (Eds.). *Epithelial-Mesenchymal Interactions, 18th Habermann Symposium.* Williams and Wilkins, Baltimore, Maryland, 1968, pp. 252.

9. Cairns, J.: Mutation selection and the natural history of cancer. *Nature*, 255 (5505): 197, 1975.

10. Cameron, I. L.: Cell proliferation, migration and specialization in the epithelium of the mouse tongue. *J. Exp. Zool.*, 163: 271, 1966.

11. Cameron, J. D.; Flaxman, A.; and Yanoff, M.: In vitro studies of corneal wound healing; epithelial-endothelial interactions. *Invest. Ophthalmol.*, 13: 575, 1974.

12. Chiakkulas, J. J.: The role of tissue specificity in the healing of epithelial wounds. *J. Exp. Zool.*, 121: 383, 1952.

13. Christophers, E.: Cellular architecture of the stratum corneum. *J. Invest. Dermatol.*, 56: 165, 1971.

14. Christophers, E.: Correlation between column formation, thickness and rate of new cell production in guinea pig epidermis. *Virhows Arch. (Zellpathol.)*, 10: 286, 1972.

15. Cohen, J.: Dermis, epidermis and dermal papillae interacting. *Adv. Biol. Skin*, 9: 1, 1969.

16. Cowan, W. K.: Blood group antigens on human gastrointestinal carcinoma cells. *Br. J. Cancer*, 16: 535, 1962.

17. Dabelsteen, E. and Pindborg, J. J.: Loss of epithelial blood group substances A in oral carcinomas. *Acta. Pathol. Microbiol. Scand. (A)*, 81: 435, 1973.

18. Dabelsteen, E. and Fejerskov, O.: Loss of epithelial blood group antigen-A during wound healing in oral mucous membrane. *Acta. Pathol. Microbiol. Scand. (A)*, 82: 431, 1974.

19. Dabelsteen, E. and Fejerskov, O.: Distribution of blood group antigen-A in human oral epithelium. *Scand. J. Dent. Res.*, 82: 206, 1974.

20. Dabelsteen, E.; Roed-Petersen, B.; and Pindborg, J. J.: Loss of blood group antigens A and B in oral premalignant lesions. *Acta. Pathol. Microbiol. Scand. (A)*, 83: 292, 1975.

21. Davidsohn, E.; Kovarik, S.; and Ni, L. Y.: Isoantigens A, B, and H in benign and malignant lesions of the cervix. *Arch. Pathol.*, 87: 306, 1969.

22. Demetrious, N. A.; Ramfjord, S. P.; and Ash, M. M.: Keratinization related to premitotic labeling and inflammation of gingiva and alveolar mucosa in rhesus monkeys. *J. Periodontol.*, 42: 338, 1971.

23. Edelman, G. M.: Surface modulation in cell recognition and cell growth. *Science*, 192: 218, 1976.

24. Friedmann, I.: *Pathology of the Ear.* Blackwell Scientific Publications, Oxford, England, 1974.

25. Gahmberg, C. G. and Hakomori, S.: Organization of glycolipids and glycoproteins in surface membranes: dependency of cell cycle and on transformation. *Biochem. Biophys. Res. Commun.*, 59: 283, 1974.

26. Gillman, T. and Penn, J.: Re-examination of certain aspects of histogenesis of healing of cutaneous wounds; preliminary report. *Brit. J. Surg.*, 43: 141, 1955.

27. Goodhill, V.: A cholesteatoma chronicle. *Arch. Otolaryngol.*, 97: 183, 1973.

28. Ham, A. W.: *Histology.* (Ed. 6). J. B. Lippincott Company, Philadelphia, Pennsylvania, 1969.

29. Hakomori, S.: Glycolipids of tumour cell membrane. In Klein, G. and Weinhouse, S.: (Eds.). *Advances in Cancer Research*, No. 18. Academic Press, New York, New York, 1973.

30. Hellman, K., cited by Friedmann, I.: *Pathology of the Ear*. Blackwell Scientific Publications, Oxford, England, 1974.

31. Hynes, R. O.: Role of surface alterations in cells transformation: the importance of proteases and surface proteins. *Cell*, 1: 147, 1974.

32. Johnson, N. W. and Hopps, R. M.: Epithelial cell proliferation in gingiva of macaque monkeys studied by local injections of ^{3}H-Thymidine. *Arch. Oral Biol.*, 19: 265, 1974.

33. Johnson, F. R. and McMinn, R. M.: The cytology of wound healing of body surfaces in mammals. *Biol. Rev.*, 35: 364, 1960.

34. Kim, Y. S. and Isaacs, R.: Glycoprotein metabolism in inflammatory neoplastic diseases of human colon. *Cancer Res.*, 35: 2092, 1975.

35. Lainson, P. and Mackenzie, I. C.: An examination of the cytology of uninflamed and inflamed gingiva using a filter imprint technique. *J. Periodontol.*, 47: 477, 1976.

36. Lansing, A. I. and Opdyke, D. L.: Histological and histochemical studies of the nipples of oestrogen treated guinea pigs with special reference to keratohyalin granules. *Anat. Rec.*, 107: 379, 1950.

37. Lim, D. J. and Saunders, W. H.: Acquired cholesteatoma: light and electron microscopic observations. *Ann. Otol. Rhinol. Laryngol.*, 81: 1, 1972.

38. Lozdan, J. and Squier, C. A.: The histology of the muco-gingival junction. *J. Periodontol. Res.*, 4: 83, 1969.

39. Mackenzie, I. C.: Ordered structure of the stratum corneum of mammalian skin. *Nature*, 222: 881, 1969.

40. Mackenzie, I. C.: The ordered structure of mammalian epidermis. In Mailbach, H. and Rovee, D.: (Eds.). *Epidermal Wound Healing*. Year Book Medical Publishers, Inc., Chicago, Illinois, 1972.

41. Mackenzie, I. C.: Ordered structure of the epidermis. *Proc. 24th Ann. Symp. on Biol. of Skin. J. Invest. Dermatol.*, 65: 45, 1975.

42. Mackenzie, I. C. and Dabelsteen, E.: Selective loss of epithelial blood group antigens in wound healing. *J. Dent. Res.*, Supp. #55(B), Abstract #810, P. 3264, 1976.

43. Mackenzie, I. C. and Smith, M. L.: Organization and differentiation of epithelia transplanted to the uterus. *J. Dent. Res.*, Supp. #55(B), Abstract #628, B218, 1976.

44. Martz, E. and Steinberg, M. S.: Contact inhibition of what? An analytical review. *J. Cell Physiol.*, 81: 25, 1973.

45. Marx, J. O.: Cell biology: cell surfaces and the regulation of mitosis. *Science*, 192: 455, 1976.

46. Mawson, S. R.: *Diseases of the Ear*. (Ed. 3). Williams and Wilkins Company, Baltimore, Maryland, 1974.

47. McKenzie, D.: Pathogeny of aural cholesteatoma. *J. Laryngol. Otol.*, 46: 163, 1931. Also, *Proc. R. Soc. Med. (Sect. Otol.)* 24: 6, 1931.

48. McLoughlin, C. B.: Mesenchymal influences on epithelial differentiation. *Symp. Soc. Exp. Biol.*, 17: 359, 1963.

49. Menton, D. N.: The minimum-surface mechanism to account for the organization of cells into columns in the mammalian epidermis. *Amer. J. Anat.*, 145: 1, 1976.

50. Mercer, E. H.: *Keratin and Keratinization. An Essay in Molecular Biology*. Pergamon Press, New York, New York, 1961.

51. Moscona, A. A.: Cell aggregation: properties of specific cell-ligands and their role in the formation of multicellular systems. *Biol.*, 18: 250, 1968.

52. Prendergast, R. C.; Toto, P. D.; and Garguilo, A. W.: Reactivity of blood group substances of neoplastic oral epithelium. *J. Dent. Res.*, 47: 306, 1968.

53. Rand, H. W.: Wound closure in actinian tentacles with reference to the problem of organization. *Arch. f. Entwcklngsmechn d. Organ., Leipz.*, 41: 159, 1915.

54. Robbins, P. W. and Macpherson, I. A.: Glycolipid synthesis in normal and transformed animal cells. *Proc. R. Soc. Lond. (Biol.)*, 177: 49, 1971.

55. Ruedi, L.: Cholesteatosis of the attic. *J. Laryngol. Otol.* 72: 593, 1958.

56. Schellander, F. and Marks, R.: The epidermal response to subepidermal inflammation. An experimental study. *Br. J. Dermatol.*, 88: 363, 1973.

57. Sengel, P.: The determinism of the differentiation of the skin and the cutaneous appendages of the chick embryo. In Montagna, W. and Lobitz, W. C.: (Eds.). *The Epidermis*, Academic Press, Inc., New York, New York, 1964, pp. 15-34.

58. Wallach, D. F. H.: *Membrane Molecular Biology of Neoplastic Cells*. Elsevier, New York, New York, 1975.

59. Young, W. G.: Mitotic activity in the oral epithelium of the female rat. *J. Periodont. Res.*, 3: 51, 1968.

FACTORS IN THE GROWTH OF CYSTIC LESIONS

Paul Toller, F.D.S.R.C.S.

My assignment is to discuss the hypothesis that epithelial cystic expansion in bone can be due to hydrostatic pressure and how that pressure originates. Epithelial cysts of the jaws are not uncommon, and very broadly may be divided into various categories. The dental root cysts or apical cysts are invariably associated with an initiating infective process, although as they mature the infective element dies out and the lesion continues to grow in its absence, and even in the absence of the initiating tooth. Then there is the dentigerous or follicular cyst, which by definition is a cyst which includes the crown of a tooth or denticle in its lumen, and is not at any point in its early history demonstrably connected with infection. Both these types are lined with simple ill-differentiated epithelium, not usually keratinized, and they tend to increase in size until terminated by the surgeon or by natural rupture and exteriorization. When treated they do not tend to recur. Histologically they are practically always associated with large amounts of retained cholesterol both in the lumen and in the walls, and sometimes are virtually solid with it. These non-keratinizing cysts bear some comparison with cholesterol granuloma of the middle ear (Friedmann, 1974).

The third main type of cyst, about 7% of the total number of all jaw cysts, are the keratinizing cysts, usually called odontogenic keratocysts. They are not primarily associated with any infective process. They seem to develop spontaneously, with no recognizable stimulus, from epithelial cell rests of the primitive dental lamina. These odontogenic keratocysts behave clinically in a manner different from the more common apical cyst and are comparatively aggressive. They may reach a large size before being discovered. After treatment by conventional surgical means they have a remarkably high recurrence rate, as high as 40%. Indeed, the recurrence rate following local enucleation seems to be very comparable with that of the ameloblastoma, which is an undoubted odontogenic neoplasm. This first led me to the hypothesis that the keratocyst may indeed be considered as a hollow benign neoplasm. There is much evidence to show that if any viable epithelial lining cells are left in the bone, or even in the soft tissues, then a recurrence will take place. Several cases have now been reported of recurrence in a bone-graft after attempted total resection of the lesion, and a few cases have even recurred in the soft tissues of the neck following operation on very large keratocysts of the jaws. This unpleasant clinical behavior gave rise to a study of their cellular characteristics and comparison with those jaw cysts which do not recur, and to the likely mechanism of cystic enlargement, and here is where our studies of jaws and ears may usefully coincide.

We believe the mechanisms whereby jaw cysts continue to enlarge, once formed, can be divided into these three groups:

(A) Mural growth
    (1) Peripheral cell division
    (2) Accumulation of cellular contents
(B) Hydrostatic expansion
    (1) Secretion
    (2) Transudation and exudation
    (3) Dialysis of osmotic expansion
(C) Bone resorption factor

Hydrostatic Expansion

I shall discuss hydrostatic expansion first. There is little to support the theory that either secretion or transudation contributes much to the increase in size of jaw cysts, but it was suggested as far back as 1926 that osmosis was an important factor. It might be assumed that in an established cyst the most centrally-placed cells, epithelial or not, will have completed their life cycle and will degenerate, or they will die through their remoteness from adequate nutrition and their autolysis will liberate into the cyst contents a mass of molecules less complex and of greater number than the vital proteins comprising the living tissues. This process of accumulation of an increased number of molecular particles might contrive a cyst fluid of higher osmolality than the surrounding tissue fluid. In order to attempt to achieve an osmotic balance, water from the surrounding tissue fluid will be drawn into the cyst cavity and this will raise the hydrostatic pressure. Physical measurements have shown that intracystic pressure in jaw cysts can be surprisingly high—40 to 80 cms of water—higher than what could be expected from the pressure exerted by the surrounding capillary bed.

Measurements have also been made directly to compare the osmolality of cyst fluids with that of the patient's own plasma, both by "depression of freezing point" method, and also by vapor pressure osmometry, and results showed that the mean osmolality of 44 cyst fluids was over 10 milliosmoles higher than that of serum (Toller, 1970). The consequence could be the net entry of fluid from the capsule capillaries into the lumen, but only if the cyst wall itself was semi-permeable.

So, a number of in vivo experiments have been carried out in which all fluids were evacuated from the cyst cavities, and were replaced immediately with an isotonic saline solution containing known amounts of both radioactive crystalloid in the form of 24 NaCl and a radioactive colloid, human serum albumin tagged with I 131. By using a gamma-spectrometer at intervals of time over the lesion, it was possible to study the rates of diffusion of both these substances, concurrently during the same periods of observation and through the intact cyst walls up to 24 hours before operation. In each case the diffusion rate of the crystalloid was rapid, but the colloid tended to be

retained, and so the semi-permeable properties of cyst walls in vivo seemed to be confirmed by these experiments (Fig. 36), (Toller, 1966).

The Principle of Lymphatic Access

These observations led me to postulate what indeed might be a fundamental concept in the occurrence of cysts of any type, anywhere in the body. Namely, that all closed physiological cavities are normally in connection with the lymphatic system which regulates their fluid balance (the central nervous system having a different arrangement), but any cavity in the body which becomes separated from lymphatic access, such as a cyst cavity, may be subject to an osmotic imbalance with the surrounding tissues, and may be liable to alteration in size due to hydrostatic pressure differences. I rather pompously termed this the "principle of lymphatic access." (Toller, 1967).

It seemed capable of fairly objective verification, and another harmless in vivo experiment was devised. A certain large-moleculed blue dye (Patent Blue) has for some years been used by my plastic surgery colleagues to inject into the tissues of the feet and legs in order to identify the lymphatics during later dissection in the procedure for lymphangiography. An 11% sterile isotonic aqueous solution of this dye was introduced into several cases of jaw cysts after emptying them by aspiration. At operation up to 24 hours afterwards, the dye was found to be retained within the cysts and it was not possible to identify any of the dye in the adjacent tissues. It appeared that no dye entered the lymphatics from the lumen of the cysts, and that the intrinsic isolation of the cyst cavities from the lymphatics seemed to be confirmed.

If an area in the bone of the jaws is subject long enough to a chronic infective process, the epithelial rests within the periodontal membrane which are the normal and numerous left-overs from the tooth-forming mechanisms, will be stimulated to proliferate and form little epithelial enclaves around the original granuloma. If the rate of epithelial growth exceeds any antagonistic

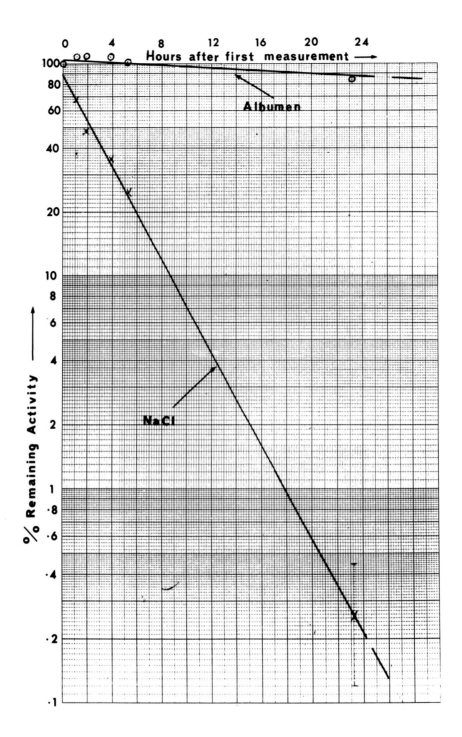

Fig. 36: Graphs obtained from double tracer experiment (gamma spectrometry) showing concurrent rates of diffusion of radio-iodated albumen (colloid) and radioactive sodium chloride (crystalloid) from within the lumen of a large dental cyst in vivo. The high rate of diffusion of crystalloid is to be compared with the slow diffusion of the large moleculed albumen, suggesting semi-permeable properties of the undisturbed cyst wall.

process, and the central area becomes isolated from lymphatic access, then a cystic process based upon osmotic disequilibrium can be initiated, which would then be entirely independent of the original infective process. It will be seen that an operation for the removal of the lining, or for the opening of the lumen permanently to a body surface, providing that opening is kept patent, will bring about a cure of the condition; and this is what successfully can be done with all non-keratinizing cysts of the jaws, although total enucleation of the lesion is a more common and convenient surgical approach. Alternatively the introduction of a substance which would destroy the lining and/or allow lymphatic access to the cavity and so render the maintenance of a raised osmotic pressure impossible, might conceivably bring about a cure. Thus I might provocatively suggest that the removal of only half a non-keratinizing dental cyst, which would allow the ingress of normal lymphatic-containing tissues to its lumen, would comprise a cure (Toller, 1972). This suggestion however might not work if the lining membrane was keratinizing, since, as I hope to demonstrate, we would then be dealing with an independently aggressive type of epithelial cell.

Indeed, very germane to the essence of today's meeting seems to be the clinical observation of what follows the operation for exteriorization of both types of jaw cysts. If a simple non-keratinizing cyst of any type is surgically opened to the mouth, and that opening is kept patent, then a positive intracystic pressure cannot be maintained and the entire lesion not only ceases to expand, but it immediately starts to contract. The rate of contraction is such that a lesion of 5ml volume will usually become totally obliterated with reformation of normal contour of the jaw bone in 9-18 months. It will not recur. This is strong evidence that its initial expansion was caused by pressure absorption of bone, as it is entirely reversible. This pressure which causes absorption of bone is of the same order as that used by orthodontists for the movement of teeth

through the same bone, assisted by the osteoclasts as elegantly demonstrated by Dr. Krane.

The odontogenic keratocysts do not behave exactly in a similar manner to similar treatment. After exteriorization they regress at a slower rate and not all of them disappear completely, although most of them do. Recurrence can occur, possibly from satellite or daughter cysts in their walls. I feel that with these lesions there is strong evidence that internal pressure exerts only some influence and this is probably of an osmotic character (especially as their fluids have been shown to be of raised osmolality and their walls are indeed very impermeable), but that other factors are also at play causing bone resorption, and these are likely to be local tissue pressure due to interstitial growth of a very active epithelium, together with other bone resorptive factors which I shall discuss in a moment.

Simple poorly-differentiated epithelium, such as is found in apical or primary dentigerous cysts, breaks down centrally by true lysis of its primary components into a liquid or semi-liquid mass resulting in an osmotic imbalance. However, the epithelium which is found in odontogenic keratocysts is quite different, since the cells do not die a rather ambiguous death but they seem to complete their programmed life cycle and mature to form squames of keratin in the cyst cavity, usually in a fluid which is very lacking in soluble proteins. The fundamental difference seems to be that in simple dental cysts we are witnessing a degenerative process, but with keratocysts the epithelium exhibits an active process of maturation, no degeneration. Thus the process of enlargement of a keratocyst seems much more related to mural cell growth than to hydrostatic processes, but an osmotic component is not excluded.

The histological picture of keratocyst epithelium is very typical; there is always a very well differentiated basal layer of columnar or cuboidal cells with strong basophilic nucleii. There are no rete pegs. This is surmounted by a narrow stratum spinosum about two-five cells thick with frequent vacuolization of its upper layer (Fig. 37). Over this is the keratinized or parakeratinized surface which matures to shed its squames into the cyst cavity (Browne, 1972). Some of these cyst cavities are so packed with keratin squames that they are morphologically indistinguishable from cholesteatoma of the middle ear and exactly comparable with Dr. Abramson's observations recorded in his extremely elegant research, for instance on the production of collagenase in cholesteatoma or those shown in Dr. Friedmann's works (1974). There is invariably a layer of connective tissue or mesenchyma between the epithelial wall and the bone, which Abramson mentions being like granulation tissue, but in the jaw lesions like this only resemble granulation tissue in the secondarily infected cases. The subepithelial layer over the bone in the jaw lesions is free from inflammation, but there are aggregates of lymphoid or plasma cells as seen also in the walls of thyroglossal cysts. These I believe are not inflammatory zones in response to infection, but they are subepithelial aggregates of lymphoid cells, possibly lymphoid nodules with an immunological function (Toller and Nolborow, 1969). Even the occasional germinal center may be found. I shall only briefly mention these lymphoid aggregates as I feel they are more indicative of a host reaction to buried epithelium rather than an inflammatory reaction inducing bone resorption. The plasma cell population is very high, and furthermore, when examined by immunofluorescent techniques they are shown to be producing large quantities of IgA, less of IgG, less still of IgM. By using different fluorochrome conjugated to each immunoglobulin one can assess them quantitatively as well as

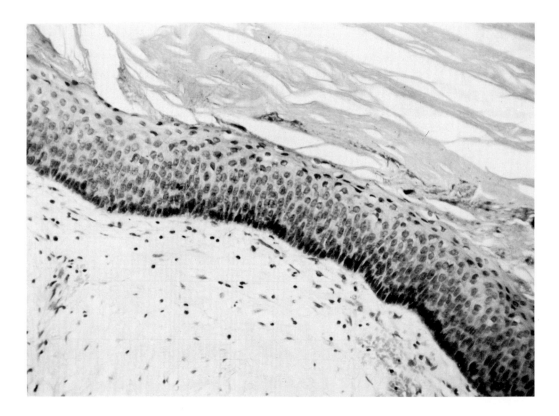

Fig. 37: Photomicrograph of the epithelial wall of a typical odontogenic keratocyst. Well-differentiated palisade layer of basal cells with a clear stratification up to the keratinous desquamation in the cyst lumen. Typical vacuolization in the prickle cell layer is shown.

qualitatively and also to demonstrate them rather prettily.

There are one or two very interesting differences between non-keratinizing cysts and keratocysts which have important clinical relevance. If the cyst contents of a keratocyst is sampled or aspirated before definitive operation, it is found that the total soluble protein content generally differs from that of all other jaw cysts (Toller, 1970). This is so significant that it can usefully be used in preoperative diagnosis of cyst types, with particular relevance to the fact that one's surgical approach has to be markedly different towards keratocysts whose recurrence rate can be as high as 40%. These lesions, if identifiable before operation, should be treated as having some of the potentialities of neoplasms, and absolutely all epithelial lining should be removed.

Although the increase in size of these lesions may be in part mediated by osmosis, I believe that their frequent tendency to non-spherical shape suggests that enlargement takes place largely by accumulation of keratin squares. Irregularities of shape seem to take place at sites where cellular proliferation is more active, and here these lesions may show close similarity with middle ear cholesteatoma.

Even if this epithelial proliferation together with an osmotic disequilibrium is accompanied by local expansion—what actually causes the bone to give way to accommodate its size? Well, we have quite a lot of recent evidence that cyst walls of all types in the jaws release a potent bone-resorbing factor. Vital cyst wall explants in tissue culture suggest this factor is predominantly a mixture of Prostaglandin E_2 and Prostaglandin E_3 (Manis, 1973). The source of this factor appears to be the capsule and not the epithelium. Indeed a quantitative difference of production of prostaglandins by different cysts is discernible, possibly being higher for keratocysts.

This osteoclast-stimulating factor has been very clearly demonstrated by in vitro experiments by Harris (1973) and at that time Donoff has demonstrated collagenase production in keratocyst walls, not unlike the very normal physiological process accompanying the necessary resorption of bone to allow an unerupted tooth to reach the surface as we cut our teeth in childhood. It is very significant that Abramson and Gross have demonstrated precisely the same process in the subepithelial connective tissue in cholesteatoma.

Indeed, Abramson, Asarch and Litton (1975) stated that the epidermis of cholesteatoma is not simply passive but plays an active role in bone absorption. Abramson (1971) did his work with explants from uninfected aural lesions. I (1971) also made some explants from jaw keratocysts, histologically indistinguishable from aural cholesteatoma and these were epithelial explants cultured for one hour in the presence of tritiated thymidine and later prepared by autoradiography to reveal the mitotic activity, and also compared directly with explants from the same patients normal mucous membrane of the mouth. In all cases the epithelial turnover was higher than normal mucous membrane, often much higher (Fig. 38). Certainly far higher than the more common and non-aggressive simple non-keratinizing jaw cysts. This work has been confirmed by others (Main, 1970 and Brown, 1972) using different techniques and it seems to lend support to the presumption that we are dealing with an epithelial activity disquietingly different from normal. I wonder whether this technique could usefully be applied to middle ear studies?

Finally, we in maxillofacial surgery now consider that odontogenic keratocysts arise spontaneously from dormant or resting remnants of the primitive dental lamina (which is the primitive invagination of oral epithelium which gave rise to tooth germs), but in this case no dento-formative function was complete, they seem to remain with an embryological potential for repeated cell division once they are awakened, but no demonstrable inflammatory stimulus has been identified and nothing seems to stop them once they are in an enclosed cystic modality, that is, in an undrained and endostial situation, even the surgeon does not find it very easy to stop them,

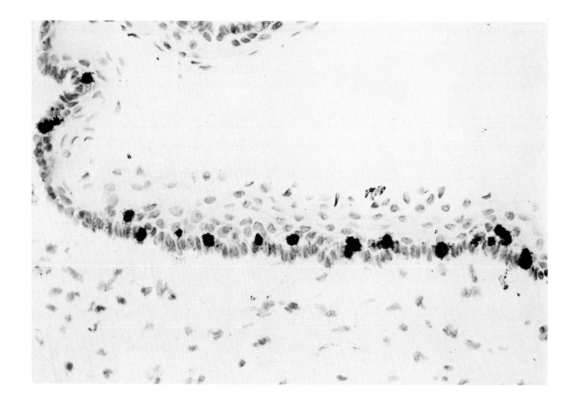

Fig. 38: Explant of odontogenic keratocyst wall cultured for one hour with tritiated thymidine. Proportion of labelled cells in mitosis is about twice that in the buccal mucosa of the same patient.

and it seems that neither does the otologist find it easy to stop his.

We do know that exteriorization to a body surface halts the growth of odontogenic keratocysts, would this be true of aural cholesteatoma? Some evidence may exist that osmosis may be one part of a group of factors in their growth, or at least in maintaining an inflated condition; this seems only to exist in addition to a free tendency of their epithelial cells to multiply on their own account in their totally enclosed context. Is this enclosed context, that is, a truly cystic mode, obligatory for their abnormal behaviour? In the jaw lesions, if this enclosed situation is negated by exteriorization, then the epithelial behavior becomes more normal, possibly completely normal—does this argue that the enclosed situation prevents the escape, or favors the accumulation of, an epithelial stimulating factor? How enclosed has the situation got to be? Is the anatomy of the middle ear itself a sufficiently restricted space to encourage the accumulation of epithelial stimulating factors? If lymphatic-carrying connective tissue can be introduced into an opened cholesteatoma cavity, will it cease to grow?

References

1. Abramson, M. and Gross, J.: Further studies on a collagenase in middle ear cholesteatoma. *Ann. Otol. Rhinol. Laryngol.*, 80: 177, 1971.

2. Browne, R. M.: The pathogenesis of odontogenic cysts. *J. Oral Pathol.*, 4(1): 31, 1975.

3. Donoff, R. B.; Harper, E.; and Guralnick, W. C.: Collagenolytic activity in keratocysts. *J. Oral Surg.*, 30: 879, 1972.

4. Friedmann, Imrich: *Pathology of the Ear.* Blackwell Scientific, Oxford, England, 1974.

5. Harris, M.; Jenkins, M. V.; Bennett, A.; and Wills, M. R.: Prostaglandin production and bone resorption by dental cysts. *Nature* (London), 245: 213, 1973.

6. Main, D. M. G.: Epithelial jaw cysts: A clinicopathological reappraisal. *Brit. J. Oral Surg.*, 8: 114, 1970.

7. Toller, P. A.: Experimental investigation into factors concerning growth of cysts in jaws. *Proc. R. Soc. Med.*, 41: 681, 1948.

8. Toller, P. A.: Epithelial discontinuities in cysts of the jaws. *Brit. Dent. J.*, 120: 74, 1966.

9. Toller, P. A.: Origin and growth of cysts of the jaws. *Ann. R. Coll. Surg. Engl.*, 40: 306, 1967.

10. Toller, P. A.: Protein substances in odontogenic cyst fluids. *Brit. Dent. J.*, 128: 317, 1970.

11. Toller, P. A.: Autoradiography of explants from odontogenic cysts. *Brit. Dent. J.*, 131: 57, 1971.

12. Toller, P. A.: Newer concepts of odontogenic cysts. *Int. J. Oral Surg.*, 1: 3, 1972.

13. Toller, P. A. and Holborow, E. J.: Immunoglobins and immunoglobulin-containing cells in cysts of the jaws. *Lancet*, 2: 178, 1969.

EPIDERMAL MIGRATION PATTERNS IN THE EAR AND POSSIBLE RELATIONSHIP TO CHOLESTEATOMA GENESIS

Ward B. Litton, M.D.

Introduction

Epidermal cysts of the ear have multiple origins; however, it is likely that the majority are lined by keratinizing stratified squamous epithelium derived from the epidermis of the tympanic membrane or nearby osseous canal wall. It will be the purpose of this presentation to review the normal migratory properties of this epithelium which makes it a unique organ system and to postulate abnormalities of migration leading to aural cholesteatoma as most commonly encountered.

Normal Epidermal Migration

Foreign substances placed on the outer keratinizing epidermal surface migrate radially outward from the center portion of the human tympanic membrane and thence over the osseous canal (Litton, 1963 and Alberti, 1964). This rate of migration over the tympanic membrane varies but has been measured as averaging .05 mm/day and .07 mm/day by two observers in normal volunteers. Sometimes the pattern is swirling with a curvilinear canalward movement (Alberti, 1964).

Observations of ink dot migrations have been made in the cat, dog and guinea pig ears. The latter was selected for detailed studies which revealed an outward pattern of migration originating inferiorly in the canal adjacent to the annulus. The rate of ink dot migration was about ten times that observed in humans.

Experiments employed thymidine (a substance incorporated in desoxyribinose nucleic acid) labelled with tritium to study the pattern of epidermal division at various intervals after its injection in guinea pigs (Litton, 1968). The tympanic membrane and adjacent canal skin were scanned for nuclear labels. A "label" of precipitated silver emulsion particles indicated that the cell was assembling nuclear material (in preparation for cell division) in the 60 minutes following injection of the tritiated thymidine. If the cell did not re-divide repeatedly in the post-injection period, the label was retained and the position change of divided cells could be inferred.

Labels initially were heaviest at the anatomic area from which ink dots were seen to migrate outward. At later intervals sacrificed animals showed this area clearing of labels which then moved outward in the direction and at the rate assumed by the ink dots. There was gradual loss of labels indicating later re-division of these cells and/or loss of the keratinized layer containing the radioactive material.

These experiments were interpreted to mean that the epidermal migration over the tympanic membrane and osseous canal was contributed to by a differential rate of cell division in the organ; the highest rate was at the "generation center". The epidermis of the external canal, then, is an organ system selected to provide this rigid cul-de-sac with a constantly renewed lining, but without obstruction by the cast-off outermost layer of renewing cells. Horizontal as well as vertical epidermal movement (observed on other external skin surfaces) occurs in the ear.

Postulated Abnormalities of Epidermal Migration in Aural Cholesteatoma

Most cholesteatomas originate in flaccid segments of tympanic membrane drawn into or pushed into the middle ear or attic. It is postulated that inflammation originating either in the middle ear or external canal (or both) results in an alteration of the normal equilibrium between vertical and horizontal migration of keratinizing epithelium in these indrawn segments. Vertical migration with differentiation to keratinization overwhelms the lateral migratory properties. Keratin then collects and serves to enhance or even start the inflammatory process and a cholesteatoma is born. Without an alteration in the balance between vertical and lateral migration a retraction pocket only is formed, not a cholesteatoma.

It has been shown that inflammation in the external canal slows the migration rate of ink dots in humans (Litton, 1963). This observation supports the above postulate. It also seems reasonable to expect the skin of the canal to produce more keratin as the result of inflammation by analogy with skin elsewhere. It is also reasonable to postulate a "de-differentiation" of this finely tuned organ system under the stress of inflammation. Horizontal migration slows or ceases and vertical migration increases.

Less commonly, squamous epithelium from the drumhead or canal may migrate through a perforation in response to an infection with subsequent tympanic membrane rupture denudement of middle ear mucosa, encystment and formation of a cholesteatoma. Under these abnormal circumstances we would not be surprised that the squamous epithelium once established as a cyst, lost its predecessors habit of orderly lateral migration.

Congenital and metaplastic origins of cholesteatoma have not been considered abnormalities of epidermal migration because their origin is not from epithelium possessing the lateral movement properties found in the normal external auditory canal.

References

1. Alberti, P. W.: Epithelial migration on the tympanic membrane. *J. Laryng.*, 78:808, 1964.
2. Litton, W. B.: Epithelial migration over tympanic membrane and external canal. *Arch. Otolaryng.*, 77:254, 1963.
3. Litton, W. B.: Epidermal migration in the ear: the location and characteristics of the generation center revealed by utilizing a radioactive desoxyribose nucleic acid precursor. *Acta. Otolaryng. Suppl.*, 1968, pp. 240.

QUESTIONS AND ANSWERS

Dr. Bradley: Dr. Lim, from the material you presented toward the end of the talk would the possibility be that the morphological basis for some of the clinical situations we see where an ingrowth of epithelium suddenly seems to become more invasive?

Dr. Lim: Cholesteatoma is not a true neoplasm in terms of invasiveness. In tumors, invasiveness resides in the epithelium, while the aggressiveness of a cholesteatoma is dictated by the inflammatory reaction surrounding it. It might become invasive or noninvasive and the type is entirely dependent on the perimatrix or the surrounding tissue. This is the dictating factor.

Dr. Bradley: Would Dr. Friedmann comment upon the effect of the connective tissue?

Dr. Friedmann: The principal tissue reaction responsible for the spread of the cholesteatoma is the surrounding inflammatory granulation tissue. This granulation tissue is responsible for absorption. Dr. Lim didn't mention osteoclasts, which are also a factor. He referred to the basal lamina, which is a dividing line between the matrix and underlying stroma. In tissue culture, exposure to protolytic enzymes like trypsin ruptures the basal lamina. The basal cells may collapse into the stroma, surrounding inflammatory granulation tissue. Certain elements of the cytoplasm are split off and these elements contain mitochondria, lysozymes and other particles. I wonder whether they might not also contribute to bone destruction.

Dr. Hawke: Dr. Friedmann showed a picture of what we have described in the literature as a keratin foreign body granuloma, that is, the presence of fairly large, irregular shaped cells containing keratin debris and surrounded by foreign body giant cells. Dr. Friedmann implied that this could be taken as evidence of an underlying cholesteatoma. I must disagree, as this is a general pathologic feature. It is commonly known to dermatopathologists where epidermoid cysts under the skin have been ruptured. In our series, all six cases arose in granulation tissue polyps in the external auditory canal which had been caused by a traumatic implantation of keratin under the skin, and there was a pyogenic granuloma containing the keratin formed granuloma as well. I would like to take a stab at your definition. One must look at cholesteatoma first from a histological point of view, which is the presence of stratified squamous keratinizing epithelium within the middle ear cleft, and Dr. Cody alluded to this definition. This is a two-phased definition. One phase is the presence of the keratinizing epithelium, but equally important is the location. In our laboratories we must be assured that this material came from the middle ear cleft. Occasionally there is a problem where you get what looks to all intents and purposes, like a cholesteatoma pearl, but, in fact, it is simply an inclusion cyst lateral to the tympanic membrane. Occasionally a malleus will be submitted, and I suppose when a malleus is submitted, you have evidence that major surgery has taken place, but if the epithelium is only on the external surface of the malleus, it could well be considered simply the outer layer of the tympanic membrane. Also, I must disagree with Dr. Cody on the presence of cholesterol. I think Dr. Friedmann would probably agree that cholesterol, itself, should not in any way be considered an essential part of the cholesteatoma.

Dr. Friedmann: I am very glad you caught on to what was presented, and so glad that Dr. Hawke could be here. I didn't really suggest that that slide showed a cholesteatoma. I was trying to illustrate some of the difficulties or limitations of morphology. I entirely agree about the clinicians giving us the site from which they remove a particular specimen. On your first point, I wouldn't entirely agree. You just said that the epidermis might rupture, and therefore, in some instances, that keratin surrounded by foreign body giant cells might in fact be a true cholesteatoma.

Dr. Bradley: Dr. Cody, would you like to comment regarding the other part of the discussion?

Dr. Cody: Our pathologists assure me that they usually find evidence of cholesterol in the specimens, so I included that in that subtitle. It usually is associated, but it could be dropped.

Dr. Lim: Dr. Laurence, where does the chalone come from?

Dr. Laurence: The chalone comes from the tissue that it acts on. So, for epidermal chalone, we extract it from epidermis. It is an endogenous substance, working by negative feedback circuit.

Dr. Friedmann: Would you expect it to be different in pathologic tissue?

Dr. Laurence: Do I expect or do I know? The answer is I don't know. I don't expect so because chalones have been found in every tumor. The cell membranes of the tumor we think have changed so that they "leak" out of the cells.

Dr. Friedmann: Dr. Trelstad, it has been suggested that the squamous epithelium or the cyst might be produced by the mesenchyme. You have referred to the record of Elizabeth Hay.

Dr. Trelstad: It is conceivable that mesenchyme cells can transform into squamous epithelial cells. From my experience of looking at adult tissues, I would strongly doubt that. What I am suggesting is that the mesenchyme does not have a corner on the market for making connective tissue, and that it is useful to look at the epithelial tissues on both sides of any structure and ask the question, is it conceivable they are contributing to the extracellular matrix?

To continue the discussion, Dr. Roth and Dr. Ehrlich commented upon the importance of the basal lamina. Dr. Lim showed us pictures of epidermal cells moving down into the substratum. Type IV collagen, the principal collagenous component of the basal membrane, is a molecule very rich in carbohydrates. It truly is a glycoprotein, and many of the glycosyl transferases that Dr. Roth is talking about may indeed, and this is Roth's speculation, be available for those cell surface glycosyl transferases that he is studying. It is conceivable that the pattern of cellular migration across that intact basal lamina is dependent on some kind of cell surface matrix interaction that is mediated by the glycosyl transferases very analogous to the kind of cell action that has been discussed.

Dr. Lim: We seldom have this opportunity to interact with the people who are dealing with the basic problems of the skin. My first question is that if there is a specific element somehow which makes the middle ear mucosa change into a mucosecreting system, or keratin secreting system, then we have to identify that element. What I gather from people who are studying mesenchymal epithelial interaction, they seem to say that they don't know, although they do suspect that something is going on.

Dr. Pulec: I was interested in some of the clinical possibilities of these discussions of Dr. Ehrlich and Dr. Roth. We have certain problems with wound healing, where we do not get migration where we would like it. Two of them are trying to get skin to grow over muscle, when we obliterate a cavity, and we have learned that we have to put fascia between muscle and the place where the skin should grow. The other is trying to get skin to grow over homograft bone. For some reason it grows up to it, and is inhibited by possibly some of the processes we heard about. I wonder what the possibilities or the rationale might be to soak these ears or cover them with vitamin A?

Dr. Palva: We have been hearing very much today about vitamin A, its effect upon the squamous epithelium, and Dr. Pulec just pointed out that it might be of clinical importance. Now, I wonder whether we really have any answers to these questions. I have been doing some organ culture work with vitamin A, starting with the work of Fell and Mellanby, where they showed that the squamous epithelium can be changed into mucous epithelium, but if you take a cholesteatoma membrane matrix, or an ear canal skin, and put vitamin A into the culture medium, you will still have the keratinizing properties as they ordinarily are. You have to go back, at least I had to go back, to the chick embryo. There you can have this change from the squamous epithelium into the other type of epithelium. It would be very fine from the clinical point of view if we could apply vitamin A to the middle ear, and see if we could treat epithelial tissue like this, but I don't think that would work.

Another thing I would like to ask here is about the actual mesenchyme. You certainly are aware of the work of Dr. McLaughlin in England, who grew squamous epithelium on heart fibroblasts and heart myoblasts. On fibroblasts it keratinizes in abundance, but if put on myoblasts, then you have an endothelium-like cover instead of a keratinizing epithelium. I thought this might be a fine idea to work with, and I put these things, also, into organ culture, and I didn't use the heart myoblasts, of course, because they are difficult to get from a patient, but I took muscle and I took fascia, but it was a very disappointing experience because on both of them we had the same keratinization as the squamous epithelium—no action from the mesenchyme. Do you have any explanation why this doesn't work? Is that just because we have this adult animal human being that the system that works in embryos doesn't work on human beings?

Dr. Ehrlich: This could be a very difficult technical problem because vitamin A is so easily oxidized that you have to be very, very careful when you put your vitamin A in the organ cultures.

Dr. Palva: If it works with chick embryos, it should work with the other species, too. Sure there are technical problems, where you must have your controls. We have had our controls, and it doesn't work with the human ear canal skin or cholesteatoma matrix.

Dr. Sadé: Tauno, I have two pieces of information in order: one to complicate matters and another to comfort you. The one to comfort is that we have sneaked in a lecture about the treatment of cholesteatoma with vitamin A that will be a surprise, and the one to complicate matters is the following. The following sources, all surgeons, Dr. McCabe, Dr. Gordon Smyth, Dr. Blair Simmons, Dr. Arnie Schering and Dr. Michael Glasscock— five surgeons—each told me independently that they have left stratified squamous epithelium in the middle ear, using a closed technique, and when they returned for a second look, this had disappeared. One of them even has a biopsy, so we realize how intricate and complicated the problem is.

Dr. Palva: It really is complicated, because I started from the clinical fact that I left squamous epithelium into the oval window niche, and covered that with crushed muscle, and when I went back there wasn't any squamous epithelium. Then, I thought I should be able to fit this into tissue or organ culture, but I wasn't able to do it.

Dr. Sadé: So, you are number six.

Dr. Toohill: Perhaps Dr. Trelstad answered this question, but I would like to ask it again anyway. Does he feel that the fascia that we use in grafting these eardrums could be induced to develop squamous epithelium?

Dr. Trelstad: No, I don't think that the fully differentiated connective tissues have the capacity to become true epithelial structures, either the squamous or the simple cuboidal epithelium that is on either side of the cyst. I think they are pretty well locked into being a connective tissue type cell, once they are at the state that you are dealing with them.

Dr. Toller: I would like to comment that Dr. Roth has made one of the most significant remarks of the day. He said cholesteatoma may be a disease of growth control. Disease of growth control is only four words, but it is a profound remark. May I ask whether he feels that he could culture middle ear epithelium and external ear epithelium, and allow them to contact each other in tissue culture? Could he culture cholesteatoma epithelium in this system to allow us to answer one or two of our questions?

Dr. Roth: I don't know whether it is possible. I

have never tried, but offhand, I don't see why not. Many cell types can be cultured. Can someone here tell me if an attempt has been made to culture the outer ear epithelium on top of the middle ear epithelium, and vice versa? It would be interesting to see if the results were asymmetrical. One might predict that outer ear epithelium would grow very well on the mucous epithelium of the middle ear, but not the other way around. I don't see why it could not be done.

Dr. Sadé: It was done, and it is part of a lecture tomorrow.

I'd like to ask a question of the panel. There is no doubt today that vitamin A can really switch an epithelial cell into a mucus producing cell. If this cell will be deprived of vitamin A, then that cell was thought to produce keratin. We also know that this is not a specific inducer. Can any of our lecturers tell us if we know how this comes about? What is the molecular basis for it?

Dr. Roth: I can't. It is difficult to be definite. There is a very rapidly growing body of evidence now that vitamin A has many functions. One of the functions clearly is in, perhaps, glycoprotein, but not necessarily glycolipid biosynthesis. The basic problem that one faces when one is trying to make glycoprotein is that the product is always on the wrong side of the membranes from the substrates, that is the sugar nucleotides that are the precursors to the sugars, are always topologically inside a cell, regardless of whether we are talking about a Golgi membrane or a plasma membrane, and the product is always topologically outside the cell, and the sugar nucleotides themselves, as far as anyone knows, never permeate cell membranes. As a result, only recently has vitamin A also been implicated as a carrier. It is clear that vitamin A, in some cases, can accept a sugar phosphate and carry it across the membrane where the enzyme can attach the sugar to the appropriate substrate. That is how all of the glycoproteins are built—that is the blood group antigens and the glycosulated collagens, and all of the mucopolysaccharides. The difficulty is that vitamin A is not the only compound of its type. There are a wide variety, and

there seems to be a sort of a specificity, although exactly what that specificity is, no one knows. These are only now being worked out. Only now the methods are available to even think about working them out. So, that is one known function of vitamin A. Of course, it has an analogous function in the eye as a visual pigment, where it is also a carrier in a sense. So, I can't answer the question very well. I can just say that vitamin A has that function in some selective tissues, and that other vitamin A-like compounds probably have similar functions in other tissues, but exactly where and how and how much, is not known.

Dr. Sadé: Can Dr. Peck enlighten us on that?

Dr. Peck: This was mainly the work of Dr. Luigi DeLuca, who has postulated that the effect of vitamin A in epithelial differentiation may be at the post-translational level where vitamin A would act as the carrier of monosaccharide units and glycose-like pre-existing proteins. Trying to extrapolate from the vitamin A chick skin system makes it a little difficult to prove that point, because one would expect that all cell layers of the epidermis should be able to be affected by vitamin A and produce mucin, whereas right now it seems like it is the basal cells that have that ability. The mucus-containing cells that we see at the surface probably are derived from basal cells that have migrated to the surface. That would not be in accord with a post-translational theory of metaplasia induced by vitamin A, but rather a theory of vitamin A acting somehow on the gene-producing new messengers producing new glycoproteins. Dr. Roth has studied surface glycosyl transferases in the vitamin A chick skin system, and whether in general cells have to be capable of DNA synthesis to be transformed, or whether post-synthetic cells can show a post-translational effect through the glycosyl transferase reaction.

Dr. Roth: We have not looked at the effects of vitamin A on the chick's skin system at all. We simply have been doing very detailed and limited-scope experiments on the effects of vitamin A on the plasma membrane transferases themselves in fibroblasts, where they do have an effect. They only have an effect on the malignant cell plasma membrane, which seems to be relatively depleted of vitamin A, or vitamin A in the correct form. So, I don't know anything about the requirements for DNA for such a system.

Dr. Trelstad: It deserves to be emphasized that our real understanding of the way in which epithelial cells and mesenchymal cells interact in the embryo, in a way that we can talk of it in molecular terms is still very, very rudimentary. I brought to your attention this whole question of extracellular molecules as agents in this, because as of 1976, it is a subject that is being discussed a great deal in the embryological literature, and the fallout that comes in other literature is there. I find it still somewhat difficult to understand how these extracellular materials, which we think serve principally in the structural elements, may also serve to modulate cell activity, but it may well be that one of the components of the way in which the epithelium influences mesenchymal cell differentiation and vice versa is just simply a permissive one. It puts it into an environment such that the cell can go ahead and execute the things that it would normally want to do. If you take an epithelial cell out, and just try to grow it in a naked environment, it does very poorly. If you simply take a rat tail and put it on a culture dish, and then grow the epithelial cell on that, it does much better. It may be a function simply of being in an appropriate environment, and to allow the epithelial cell to simply exercise the things that it can do. So, the rule of the extracellular matrix in these interactions may be very, very permissive, not instructional in any sense of the word. The epithelium has a certain time clock that it is locked into, that it will, on the 33rd day of gestation, either become squamous or mucous because of some kind of either internal signal, or another signal that we do not understand, but absolutely requisite for it to be able to go through that period, that window in development, and execute the change either to mucous epithelium or squamous epithelium. It has to be happy. So, if you remove the connective tissue matrix from it, at that criti-

cal point in development, it will stop or it will do something aberrant. So, that may be the level at which the matrix really is interacting in these epithelial-mesenchymal interactions. It may well be that cell surface contacts between interacting tissues may be more important in these interactions in influencing a cell in which way to do, or it may be internal clocks that we really have no idea about.

Now, with respect to your experiment where you transplant a particular tissue and find it modulates, I think that the literature, both in the adult organisms and the embryo, is just replete with such examples, and we just don't understand them. I mean it is a phenomenology. I am sure you can reproduce that a hundred times, but we can't explain it.

Dr. Sadé: May I explain the strategy of planning of this portion of the meeting? You know that ear, nose and throat meetings usually cover large topics, and you might have been under the impression that the topic which we chose, cholesteatoma, is a very narrow one. In fact, it isn't. In fact, we have touched upon eight problems: mitosis, differentiation of epithelial cells, metaplasia of epithelial cells, interaction of epithelial cells with connective tissue or mesenchymal tissue, migration of epithelia in general, inhibition of migration, mainly contact inhibition, and last and not least, direction of epithelial migration. I really think that we only touched upon it, and we couldn't do more than that. Now we should discuss how we can relate these various basics to the central clinical question which interests us, namely cholesteatoma.

Dr. Abramson: We began with the concept that we probably weren't going to solve all the problems of cholesteatoma biology. As I think back on the day's events, I don't think we have solved any. In fact, we haven't even defined the disease. Everyone of us has a different opinion. To sort out the impressions of today will require a little time, and there is nothing wrong with coming back to our impressions of the interaction of basic science and possible models to this disease. This involution that Dr. Toller describes points up the very paradox of the problem and the complexity of the problem we are studying. We are studying a problem that has a progressive character. It is a tumor-like structure, and yet the models that we try to study it with are reversible processes. Metaplasia is a reversible process. The cysts that we implant grow slightly, and then usually go into involution, and yet the disease is so very independent. Would any of the speakers comment on the nature of this independence, or would they relate this to the early definitions that we attempted.

Dr. Palva: I am going to comment on the speakers' definition of cholesteatoma. This may have left many of us clinicians in a little bit of a mixed state, because if you define cholesteatoma as simply keratinizing epithelium in the middle ear, that definition is not always applicable or true. This should be made clear to everyone of us who is working as a clinician treating these cases of middle ears. You may have squamous epithelium. It may be non-keratinizing totally. It may show just slight keratinization, but this horizontal movement may take all of the keratin away. So, you don't have cholesteatoma there. If I may then comment on another thing that is important for the future. We, as clinicians, should like to have some ways to affect the squamous epithelium. We have been hearing quite a lot about vitamin A and cortisone that suppresses the action of fibroblasts. We should have something developed along these lines, such as the different enzymes. These have not been discussed but we can take, for instance, one enzyme, alkaline phosphatase, which does not appear in the squamous epithelium. If we block a certain system in the stratified squamous epithelia, it appears. So, what happens to squamous epithelium if we subject it to alkaline phosphatase? Another one is esterase which we can find sometimes in children's cholesteatoma, in large amounts, in the submucous layer.

Dr. Abramson: Bob, do you wish to comment?

Dr. Trelstad: Well, as a neophyte in ENT pathology, I can't comment, but will leave that to Dr. Lim. In freely associating and thinking of the many things that I have heard today, I am asking myself in what other clinical situations do we see a structural weakness of connective tissue. If, for example, we take and synthesize the discussion that Dr. Bluestone gave us, and the discussions that we have had about migration of epithelium, and we think of how this entity may derive, under what circumstances do you see pouchy, patulous-like connective tissues, and I am reminded of things like the Floppy Valve Syndrome. I am wondering when you see a subset of people come in with middle ear disease, what other problems do they have? Do they have other associated connective tissue problems? I would doubt that, but perhaps it hasn't been looked for. I mean floppy valves, mitral valve prolapse, is something that we didn't even think about ten years ago, and now I would suspect that 20% of the people that come to mitral valve surgery are in for either coronary artery bypass graft, or a floppy valve. Mitral valve disease is becoming more floppy and less rheumatic these days. Do these people already have insufficient amount of elastic or connective tissue in their drum that makes them particularly prone or susceptible to negative pressures in the eustachian tube? Perhaps, that is free association sub-one.

Free association sub-two relates to the young people in our respiratory intensive care unit, who have come to the hospital in acute respiratory failure. Many of these people are admitted after a mild viral illness, and have essentially a destruction of their normal alveolar architecture, which we can examine ultrastructurally. One fascinating finding in the biopsies that we have examined in these people is that there seems to be an enormous loss of elastin. So, their alveolar septum has sustained a complete loss of elastin, and most of these people die in acute respiratory failure. The question is again, are there trivial middle ear infections which lead to an inflammatory response which are either subclinical or don't really come to your attention that antedate these events, such that there is some kind of mild, inflammatory lesion in the tympanum that is inappropriate, and leads to some destruction of the tissue, which then, two years later results in its rupture and subsequent development of these other sequelae?

Dr. Lim: The tympanic membrane in guinea pigs which Dr. Litton used is quite unique. It is different from human or cat and the animals that we use, in that the migration pattern in tympanic membrane is going across the whole membrane, which is quite different from human where from umbo it goes out in a radial direction. In the guinea pig tympanic membrane, there is a large fiber which goes across the whole membrane, which is quite unique from the other species. That fiber is the essential guiding system for the migratory pattern, and the way the cell migrates is dictated by contact guidance system, which is established in all of the biological systems. I don't see why it shouldn't be applied in the ear or even cholesteatoma.

So, in a sense, when we have a pole formation or cystic formation, it is a system where a cell is enlarged in connection to the fibrin, and the fibrin or fiber will arrange this way. It will shrink like in the wound healing, then the fibrin will orient itself toward the center of the wound, and it is a pretty well accepted concept, and it is a nice concept in understanding wound healing or epithelial migration.

In the pars tensa, the fibers are made of reticulin. In fact, in guinea pigs there is no collagen. The tympanic membrane is formed of reticular fibers and would have little elasticity. This is what happens in retraction pockets—a loss of elasticity.

Dr. Trelstad: If there is an important distinction between the presence of collagen and reticulum in tympanic membranes then some biochemical correlations are in order. In the old days we felt that reticulin might be a different and immature form of collagen. The data that are now being evolved using antibodies derived from those four different types of collagen that I noted on the board, suggest that Type III collagen is probably

reticulin, or is found abundantly in reticulin rich tissues. If that holds, and that should be possible to document rather clearly, it would suggest that the tympanic membrane is really made up of, as far as the collagenous components are concerned, of two different species, Type I which is usually the fiber stuff that you see in tendons or dermis, and Type III which you see in reticulin-rich tissues. Now, these two different molecules have different properties in respect to their stability, probably, perhaps in respect to the turnover, and it may be that there actually is some substantial difference in the composition of the drum, at that one particular point which may relate to the pathogenesis of drum weakness.

Dr. Abramson: With reference to the complications of the mode for contact guidance that David has described, there are many situations when we see retractions and reorientation of the connective tissue fibers in a medial direction, and yet they do not form an independent growth process. They do not form an active and expanding cholesteatoma. There are many things we haven't considered. Will Dr. Cody comment on when is a retraction pocket a cholesteatoma?

Dr. Cody: Well, Max, you can start out at one extreme and say, look here, we have a well healed modified radical mastoid cavity, and it is lined by skin, and no one is going to call that a cholesteatoma, the reason being it is exteriorized. It is not trapped in the temporal bone. Similarly if there is a posterior tympanic membrane retraction pocket, where the skin is against the medial wall of the middle ear, the drum is atelectatic, may even be protruding a little bit into the facial recess or sinus tympani but it is a clean pocket, it is self-cleaning because it is exteriorized, and I don't consider that a cholesteatoma. I don't consider the clean retraction pocket, particularly when it is not communicating with the epithelium, a cholesteatoma. Once you get a retraction pocket, however, that is communicating directly with the interior of the epitympanum, the mastoid process is expanding. It is forming the typical tumor mass that I described earlier this morning, and then I think it becomes a cholesteatoma. I think the important words here are trapped in the temporal bone and exteriorized skin in the temporal bone. I won't go any further.

Dr. Abramson: Does anyone wish to comment on this definition between retraction and cholesteatoma? Does anyone in this audience have an idea on this question? It is something that we have to decide every day in practice. All of us are experts at this. Dr. Kirchner?

Dr. Kirchner: This question will possibly come to an answer tomorrow. In retraction pockets there may be infection. Has anybody done any studies, any smears, during the active stages, and correlate it with the bacteriology in the pocket? I classify an active retraction pocket cholesteatoma when there is entrapment.

Dr. Austin: I'd like to answer your question in a backwards manner. I intend to answer it more fully later, but there are a couple of aspects of the disease definition which have not been covered, and of course it is difficult to create hypotheses unless we can define what we are talking about. One obvious answer to your question on what is the difference between a retraction pocket and cholesteatoma, is how it behaves over time, and how it responds to treatment. If a retraction pocket becomes a cholesteatoma, then it is a precursor of a cholesteatoma. If it does not, then it is different and not related to a cholesteatoma. One fact that has been ignored, though it was referred to this morning by Dr. Cody, is that cholesteatoma has a strong tendency to recur. If treated in such a way that permits recurrence, it will recur over and over again. It will never end. Dr. Cody reports recurrence in 50% of patients after eight years. That is a good reason to believe that the disease will recur over a long period of time in most individuals. In mine, it is only 20%, but that is only a 3½ year mean observation period versus a five year period. So, recurrence is a part of this disease. I intend to suggest later in the week that indeed it is very possible that the tendency to recurrence is the primary feature of the disease, and should be regarded as such, and not a feature sec-

ondary to negative pressure or inadequate surgery, or to other factors, and should be a part of the definition of the disease itself.

Dr. Pulec: Discussing some of the fine points of definition, this morning I was struck by two main points. One is that when we talk about tumor and the relationship of it to cholesteatoma, a cholesteatoma is a tumor. It is a true tumor, if you use a dictionary definition of tumor. Tumor is a lump, a swelling. It is not a neoplasm, and if we use the common lay person definition of tumor, we are thinking neoplasm, but that is not what tumor means. Secondly, we talked a lot this morning about middle ear cleft, and if we are doing that we are confining the cholesteatoma to a specific type. The congenital cholesteatoma often is not in the middle ear cleft. It is in the petrous apex or the angle, and if we are going to define our terms or areas, this little difference has to be kept in mind. About the etiology or pathogenesis of the attic cholesteatoma, I didn't hear, possibly it was said and I didn't hear it, that this retraction can take place for at least three different reasons, probably more. One might be a vacuum, but this vacuum is relative, and has to do with the diameter of the stretched pars flaccida or the artificially repaired attic defect, and we have learned surgically that if you reduce that size, in other words put in a piece of bone or cartilage over the big attic defect, you will prevent this retraction. Second, attic block which was alluded to a moment ago is possibly a subclinical or minor inflammation in the attic which produces a situation that acts as a pulsion.

Dr. Bernstein: Today we have concentrated on squamous epithelium and keratin, and although Dr. Cody alluded to it in his definition, it seems to me we should not walk away from today's papers without thinking about something which I am sure is a prelude to tomorrow, but I think it should be emphasized, and that is the subepithelial inflammatory tissue or granulation tissue. As clinicians, we are concerned about destruction of tissue, particularly bone and soft tissue underlying the cholesteatoma, and we must not forget that there are lysosomal enzymes in inflammatory cells which may be responsible for the destruction that occurs, and it seems that nobody today really has alluded to the inflammatory tissue that is underneath the cholesteatoma. As far as I know, the squamous epithelium and/or the keratin is not really responsible for the serious problems that arise from cholesteatoma.

Dr. Abramson: Dr. Plester, would you like to make a comment on your conception of cholesteatoma?

Dr. Plester: As long as retraction has preserved its capacity to clean itself, it is a retraction. Once it has lost this capacity, we have a cholesteatoma

with all its sequences.

Dr. Abramson: Do you think you can develop any of the complications of cholesteatoma in spite of a lack of accumulation of epithelial debris? For example, can you develop bone resorption under this pocket?

Dr. Plester: I don't think so.

Dr. Abramson: Dr. Trelstad gave us a very nice paradigm of this meeting. He was talking about the epithelial-mesenchymal interaction. Well, we here had an otologist-scientist interaction, and I think there is much more that can be done and more to be learned.

Chapter 2

Bone Resorption

ASPECTS OF BONE RESORPTION

Stephen M. Krane, M.D.
Jean-Michel Dayer, M.D.
Steven R. Goldring, M.D.

Pathological bone resorption is a feature of a number of seemingly unrelated disorders. In a conference such as this one, it is appropriate to consider general aspects of the biology of the resorption process that could pertain to the interpretation of the findings in patients with cholesteatoma.

Bone Structure

Normal bone is a living tissue which is constantly being remodeled. Resorption is carried out by osteoclasts and new bone is deposited through the action of osteoblasts which, as they become encased in the bone they have produced, become osteocytes. The osteocytes are connected with each other and to their blood supply through an interlacing network of canaliculi. The extracellular fraction of bone consists of a mineral phase and an organic phase. The organic material is 90-95% collagen in addition to glycoproteins and other acidic proteins (Glimcher and Krane, 1968). It has been found recently that the acidic proteins extractable with EDTA have a unique post-translational modification, the gamma carboxylation of specific glutamic acid residues (Hauschka, et al, 1975) and it is possible that they may have specific functions, for example, in calcification. The collagen molecules of bone consists of three α chains of composition $[\alpha 1(I)]_2 \alpha 2$ (Miller, 1973). The collagen fibrils and fibers of bone are comprised of molecules which are organized in a pattern that is unique for this tissue. The mineral phase (Posner and Betts, 1976) which consists of so-called amorphous calcium phosphate and poorly crystalline hydroxyapatite is highly organized with respect to the collagen (Glimcher and Krane,

1968); it is the two phase material which gives bone its unique mechanical properties. The presence of the mineral phase predominantly within the "hole" zones produced by the quarter-stagger arrangement of the collagen molecules within the fibril is such that the physical-chemical properties of the collagen are altered. All collagens are denatured by heating and when the collagen is in the insoluble fibrillar form the extent of denaturation can be assessed by measuring shrinkage of the fibers or by assessing alteration in the characteristic low- and wide-angle x-ray diffraction pattern. Mineralized bone can be heated to temperatures of 70°C and if cooled, and then demineralized, evidence of ordered structure remains. Whereas if the bone is first demineralized, heating to 70°C abolishes the higher order collagen structure (Glimcher and Krane, 1968 and Bonar and Glimcher, 1970). Collagenolytic enzymes, even those from clostridial species, which can readily attack bone collagen if the mineral is first removed, cannot degrade bone collagen if the mineral phase is intact (Neuman, et al, 1960; Stern, et al, 1970; and Krane, 1975). The mineral thus protects the collagen from both thermal denaturation and proteolytic attack. Therefore, some mechanism for prior removal of mineral ions must be operative in both normal and pathological situations to permit degradation of the collagenous matrix. The process of demineralization must be closely followed by matrix resorption since extensive denuding of the collagen is not observed.

Bone Resorption

The resorption of bone requires the action of

living cells. Dead bone can remain in situ for years without being resorbed, as illustrated by the sequestrum of chronic osteomyelitis. Some osteolysis is accomplished by the osteocyte in a localized region surrounding each cell (Bélanger, 1969 and Shea, et al, 1968) although it is still not certain how important osteocytic osteolysis is in physiological bone resorption. Most resorption is carried out by osteoclasts, cells normally derived from primitive precursors (Owen, 1971). These osteoclasts must have the machinery necessary to resorb both the mineral and the matrix. The mineral phase could be removed by (1) local decreases in pH; (2) production of substances which could bind calcium ions and reduce ion activity producing a downhill gradient between the precipitated phase and solution; (3) pumping calcium ions unidirectionally away from the resorbing site similarly resulting in a gradient from solid to solution. Dissolution of the precipitated mineral and organic phases is largely an extracellular event (Birkedal-Hansen, 1974), although in other situations where resorption of connective tissue is intense phagocytosis of collagen fibers can be observed (Parakkal, 1969). The osteoclasts would therefore have to release extracellular enzymes, particularly collagenases, capable of degrading the undenatured collagen matrix (Harris and Krane, 1974 and Gross, 1974). The possible role lysosomal enzymes such as acid phosphatase, β-glucuronidase or aryl sulfatase remains unclear. Although such acid hydrolases may be released extracellularly in bone resorbing systems (Vaes, 1969 and Reynolds, 1970) the precise reactions that these enzymes catalyze in vivo have not been established. Cathepsins acting at acid or neutral pH may have a function in degradation of the proteoglycans of cartilage matrix (Barrett, 1975) but proteoglycans are only minor constituents of the extracellular matrix of bone (Glimcher and Krane, 1968).

Pathological Bone Resorption

In human disease there are many disorders accompanied by pathological bone resorption. It would be worthwhile to consider several different conditions which would illustrate certain biological features of the resorption process in general. Eventually, we might be able to obtain answers to a number of questions that are critical to our understanding of the problem and our ability to devise rational therapy. We can pose the questions but will have few answers.

(1) Are the cells involved in pathological bone resorption the same as those involved in normal remodeling?

(2) Are the osteoprogenitor cells of normal bone also the precursors in pathological conditions?

(3) Must a cell undergo mitotic division and differentiation prior to assuming a bone resorbing function, or can the function of already existing cells be modified? Does increasing function always necessitate increasing numbers of cells? What is the function of the increased number of nuclei in osteoclasts?

(4) Are all cells in a resorbing area in different pathological conditions responsive to physiological control?

(5) Are the mediators responsible for pathological bone resorption unique?

(6) Do the cells involved in pathological resorption share common receptors with normal cells?

(7) If there are different mediators to which the cells from different conditions respond are the subsequent biological events similar?

(8) In the various pathological states, is bone resorption carried out through the same biochemical effectors?

(9) What is the fate of the resorbing cell?

We may obtain some of the answers to some of these questions in this symposium, but it is more likely that there will be enough for us to do in the future.

Bone Resorption Associated with Hyperparathyroidism

Excessive bone resorption with increased numbers of active osteoclasts (osteitis fibrosa cystica) is a classical finding in primary hyperparathyroidism, but is found in less than 20% of patients with proven disease (Fig. 39). It is of interest to speculate why osteitis fibrosa is not found with greater frequency. Under experimental conditions in rats given large amounts of parathyroid hormone (PTH), in all animals there is a prompt increase in the number of osteoclasts in bone reaching a maximum within 24 hours (Talmage, 1967); these osteoclasts are presumably derived from proliferation of progenitor cells in a specialized precursor pool. It has been suggested that the degree of osteoclastic activity in human cases of hyperparathyroidism is proportional to the severity and duration of the hyperparathyroidism (Bordier, et al, 1973). However, there are indications that there are two popula-

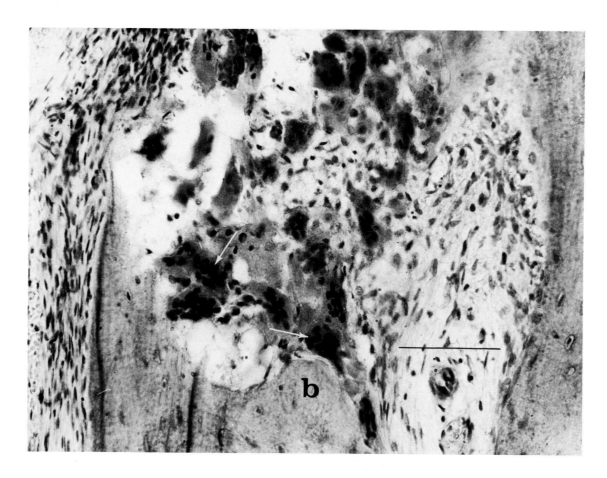

Fig. 39: Biopsy from the tibia from a patient with primary hyperparathyroidism and osteitis fibrosa cystica. Region of lamellar bone (b) shows active resorption with abundant multinucleated osteoclasts (arrows). Bar = 100 μm.

tions of patients, those with bone disease and those without, and not a continuous spectrum of osteoclasts (Hellstrom and Ivemark, 1962). When osteitis fibrosa does occur, it is a generalized phenomenon throughout the skeleton although only local manifestations may be evident clinically. There is no evidence that the presence or absence of osteitis fibrosa is influenced by the levels of calcitonin, a hormone that inhibits bone resorption. It is also possible that there are factors other than the intensity of the hyperparathyroidism that determine whether or not osteoclastic resorption is prominent. These might include genetically determined responses of precursor cells, variations in the pool size of precursor cells, or variations in levels of substances that could inhibit or amplify the response to PTH.

The cells that respond to PTH must have receptors on their surface for that hormone. In the case of another polypeptide hormone such as thryotropin-releasing hormone (TRH), it has been demonstrated that TRH itself induces loss of its own receptors (Hinkle and Tashjian, 1975 and Raff, 1976). This has also been shown for calcitonin (Wright, et al, 1976). It is thus possible that the response to PTH could be influenced by this sort of variation in number of receptors or their affinity for the specific ligand.

It has been proposed that PTH like other peptide hormones acts by stimulating the adenyl cyclase system in its target cells, thus increasing the concentration of cyclic adenosine 3'-5' monophosphate (cAMP). This effect was shown first by Chase, et al (1969) in whole fetal rat calvaria and subsequently by Peck, et al (1973) in isolated cells cultured from similar tissue. In the heterogeneous population derived from such bones it could not be determined which cell(s) was the responsive one. Subsequently it was demonstrated by Smith and Johnston (1974) that populations of bone cells could be separated into different groups, each of which responded differently to calcitonin and PTH. Wong and Cohn (1975) were able to separate and enrich populations of cells from mouse calvaria which responded predominantly to either PTH or calcitonin.

We have begun to examine human cells in an attempt to demonstrate responses to various hormones and other substances seeking answers to several questions. Could the presence of a response to a specific hormone such as PTH serve as a cell marker? If present, would this marker persist in culture after many months and several passages? Would the cells presumably responsible for focal pathological resorption have similar specific hormonal receptors? Is the response of cells in increasing cAMP levels directly related to the hormone's physiologic effects and how could this relate to effects on cell growth?

Bone Resorption with Giant Cell Tumors of Bone

We have obtained some preliminary data which are pertinent to this discussion. Human giant cell tumors of bone are comprised of multinucleated giant cells interspersed among so-called stromal cells (Jaffe, et al, 1940 and Steiner, et al, 1972). The giant cells are rich in acid phosphatase activity and have ultrastructural features resembling those of osteoclasts (Hanaoka, et al, 1970; Schajowicz, 1961; and Kuhlman and McNamee, 1970). These tumors tend to produce bone resorption predominantly and have been considered by several pathologists to be neoplasms of osteoclasts

(Stewart, 1922; Wills, 1967; and Aegerter and Kirkpatrick, 1968) (Fig. 40). In areas of bone resorption adjacent to the tumor it may be difficult to determine the derivation of the resorbing cells whether from tumor or bone. Our involvement with these tumors was stimulated by Dr. H. J. Mankin who has been particularly interested in their biology and who has been treating a number of patients with bone allografts. Dr. Mankin provided us with the tumors as well as skin and synovium from the same patients. The cells were dispersed with trypsin-EDTA. A heterogeneous population consisting predominantly of multinucleated (giant) and mononucleated (?stromal) cells adhered to the plastic surface of the culture vessels. The multinucleated cells survived for only 7-10 days whereas the mononucleated cells replicated and have been carried through several passages to date. Examples of some of our preliminary findings are as follows: in cells from one tumor, levels of cAMP in primary culture increased from basal levels of 0.96 ± 0.23 to 8.16 ± 1.32 pmoles/μg DNA when exposed to 2 μg/ml of bovine PTH for 5 minutes, whereas PGE$_2$ (2 μg/ml) increased these levels to 12.40 pmoles/μg DNA. In contrast, skin cells from the same patient at the same stage of culture showed little change in cAMP in the presence of PTH (basal levels of 0.91 ± 0.26 to 0.71 ± 0.07) whereas with PGE$_2$ the levels increased to 17.89 ± 0.78 pmoles/μg DNA. None of these cultured cells showed an increase in levels of cAMP when exposed to calcitonin. Thus these neoplastic cells respond to PTH consistent with an osteoclast phenotype. In addition the non-tumor cells from the same individual had a different pattern of response. Not all of the giant cell tumors studied responded in the same manner, and the sensitivity of the response declined with age and passage of the cells in culture. However, using these techniques it should be possible to characterize the hormone receptors in cells from different conditions in order to devise ways to modulate their activity.

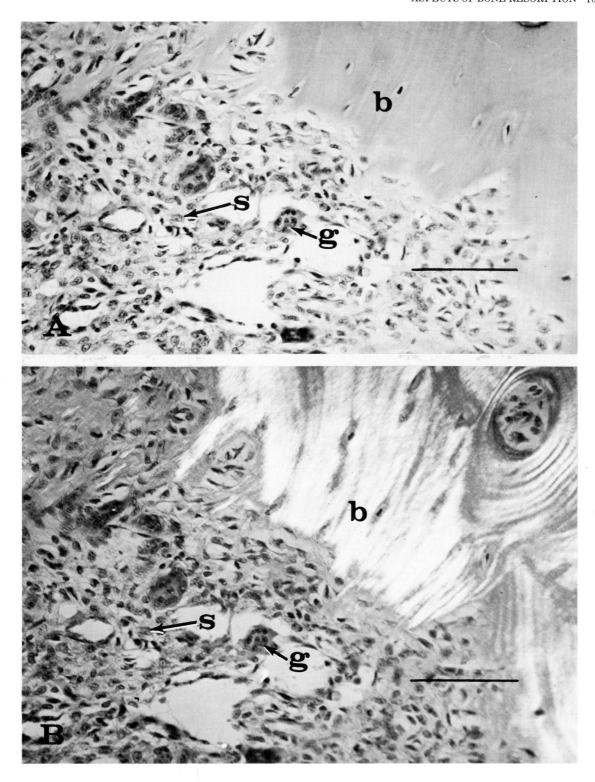

Fig. 40: Sections near the margin of a giant cell tumor of bone. (**A**) The two types of cells in the tumor are the giant cells (g) and the stromal cells (s). The tumor has grown up to the edge of the surrounding bone (b). There is no distinction between the cells in the resorption spaces and the tumor cells. (**B**) Same sections viewed under polarized light. The birefringent collagen fibers of the lamellar bone (b) appear bright on the gray background. The tumor cells are in close contact with the bone. Bar = 100 μm.

Bone Resorption with Rheumatoid Arthritis

Another type of pathological bone resorption is the local erosion that accompanies persistent synovitis in rheumatoid arthritis (Collins, 1949) (Fig. 41). Occasionally the process is so intense that a large section of bone such as a femoral head may be destroyed over a period of 6 to 8 months (Krane, 1975). The histological appearance of the resorbing bone reflects the severity of the process. The bone as well as the adjacent cartilage may be undergoing resorption in contact with the mass of inflammatory cells. In such instances one could hardly be certain whether the cells responsible for resorption would be derived from the bone itself or the inflammatory mass invading the bone.

Evanson, et al (1967) demonstrated that the hypercellular synovium in rheumatoid arthritis produces collagenase in culture and showed in a series of studies that collagenase is likely to be involved in the pathogenesis of the joint destruction (Krane, 1975; Harris and Krane, 1974; and Krane 1975). We have recently been successful in culturing cells dispersed from rheumatoid synovium with proteolytic enzymes which produce large amounts of collagenase initially and continue to do so for weeks to months even after several passages (Dayer, et al, 1976). These cells do not have macrophage markers and are morphologically distinct from fibroblasts. We do not yet know if they are capable of bone resorption by themselves. In the one culture we have tested there was no change in basal cAMP in cells exposed to PTH for five minutes. However, there was a relatively small response to PGE_2 (2 μg/ml) from 1.69 $\pm$ 0.20 to 3.62 $\pm$ 0.12 pmoles/μg DNA. Furthermore, in one experiment neither PTH nor calcitonin altered collagenase production over a period of several days in culture.

On the other hand these synovial cells demonstrate a stimulation of collagenase production when exposed to products of blood lymphocytes (Dayer, et al, 1976). We initiated these experiments following the reports of Horton, et al (1972) and Mundy, et al (1974) on an osteoclast activating factor derived from lymphoid cells, and that of Wahl, et al (1975) on a soluble factor from guinea pig lymphocytes cultured in the presence of specific antigen which stimulated collagenase production by macrophages. In our hands macrophages derived from human blood monocytes produce levels of collagenase less than 0.1% of those found in our cultured synovial cells. Lymphocytes are usually abundant in the region just beneath the proliferating lining cells in rheumatoid arthritis and we had reasoned that products of these lymphocytes might affect the activity of adjacent cells. We therefore prepared peripheral blood lymphocytes from rheumatoid and control subjects by Ficoll-Hypaque gradients and incubated such cells in tissue culture at 37°C (Dayer, et al, 1976). We found that all samples of lymphocytes produced a factor capable of stimulating collagenase production by active and previously active synovial cells. The factor was not present in lymphocytes lysed by freezing and thawing, and its production was inhibited by incubation at 4°C.

Under proper conditions both concanavalin A and phytohemagglutinin can stimulate lymphocytes to produce the factor. It has been possible to assay the stimulating factor in eluates from gel filtration columns and obtain an apparent molecular weight of 8,000-12,000 daltons. The lymphocyte factor is not mitogenic for synovial cells and does not stimulate glycolysis. We are currently examining the specificity of production and response in different cells under different circumstances. For example, is the factor produced by T cells, the most abundant cell in the rheumatoid synovium (Van Boxel and Paget, 1975), or B cells? Are macrophages necessary? The molecular weight of this factor is different from that reported for osteoclast activating factor but whether or not these different lymphocyte derived substances are related remains to be shown.

The possible role of localized decrease in pH in promoting release of mineral from bone may also be important in the pathogenesis of bone resorption in rheumatoid arthritis. In rats, systemic acidosis increases and alkalosis decreases the rate

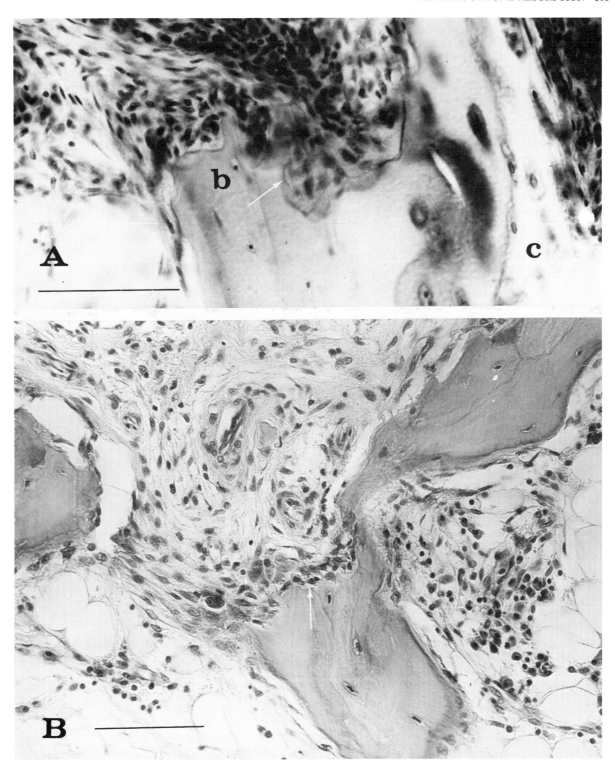

Fig. 41: Sections from metacarpal-phalangeal joints of patients with rheumatoid arthritis. **(A)** The mass of inflammatory cells (pannus) has moved under the articular surface and is in close contact with the subchondral bone (b) and articular cartilage. The cells are in contact with bone in resorption lacunae (arrow). There is no demarcation between the inflammatory cells and the cells in the resorption spaces. **(B)** An area deeper from the articular surface than the one above. Bone is undergoing resorption in regions of scalloping (arrow) occupied by cells which blend with the inflammatory cells. Bar = 100 μm.

of bone loss (Barzel and Jowsey, 1969). Raisz (1970) has shown that PTH-dependent bone resorption declines at high pH but very small reductions in pH within the physiological range can increase bone resorption. It has been shown that the rate of glycolysis is high in rheumatoid synovium (Barland and Hamerman, 1962 and Roberts, et al, 1967) and the resultant decrease in pH could act directly to leach mineral and indirectly to stimulate other bone-resorbing cells. The pH in rheumatoid effusions is lower than that in non-rheumatoid effusions but not below 6.8 (Falchuk, et al, 1970). However, it is possible that there are even more acid regions within the synovium and a gradient between these regions and the synovial fluid.

A possible effect of other substances on increasing bone resorption in rheumatoid arthritis has also been investigated. We found that cultured rheumatoid synovia release a factor even in the presence of indomethacin that can accelerate bone resorption (Krane, 1975) using the test system of Raisz and Niemann (1967) in which paired shafts of radius or ulna from 19-day rat embryos, labeled with ^{45}Ca by injecting the pregnant mother one day earlier, are incubated in tissue culture medium. The characteristics of this material were different from those of unmodified osteoclast activating factors and from prostaglandins as well.

Studies by Tashjian, et al (1972) and Voelkel, et al (1975) showed that a mouse fibrosarcoma and a rabbit carcinoma which produced hypercalcemia in tumor bearing animals also released large amounts of prostaglandin E_2 (PGE$_2$) in culture. Prostaglandins have also been implicated in the bone resorption associated with human neoplasms (Seyberth, et al 1975). Robinson, et al (1975) found that culture media from rheumatoid synovial explants released large quantities of PGE$_2$ and that these culture media contained potent bone resorbing activity when tested in a mouse calvaria system. Under the conditions of their experiments, it was concluded that PGE$_2$ was primarily responsible for the bone resorbing activity in view of the following: (1) both the bone resorbing

activity and PGE$_2$ production were inhibited by indomethacin, an inhibitor of the prostaglandin synthetase system; (2) the bone resorbing activity was extracted into ether at low pH as was the PGE$_2$; (3) finally, the bone resorbing activity in the media paralleled the PGE$_2$ concentration measured independently by radioimmunoassay. The PGE$_2$ produced by the synovial cells could thus act on other bone resorbing cells to stimulate their activity.

The interactions of synovial cells with the prostaglandins are complex. The isolated adherent synovial cells described above (Dayer, et al, 1976) produce large amounts of PGE$_2$ early in culture, but the levels decline with continued culture much more rapidly than those of collagenase. Colchicine which stimulates collagenase production in synovial tissue (Harris and Krane, 1971) also stimulates production of PGE$_2$ (Robinson, et al, 1975). Glucocorticoids decrease both collagenase and PGE$_2$ (Dayer, et al, 1976 and Kantrowitz, et al, 1975). However, indomethacin while inhibiting prostaglandin production, stimulates collagenase production (Dayer, et al, 1976). In preliminary experiments with Dr. D. R. Robinson, we found that the lymphocyte factor which stimulates collagenase production by synovial cells also stimulates production of PGE$_2$. As noted, the cultured synovial cells also have an increase in the levels of cAMP when exposed to PGE$_2$. Because we are dealing with a heterogeneous cell population in the synovial cell cultures, it is quite possible that some cells in the same cultures produce prostaglandins and different cells respond to these hormones.

The etiology of rheumatoid arthritis is unknown. It is remarkable, however, that in a chronic inflammatory condition in which the etiology is known, i.e. tuberculosis, the histological features of bone resorption are similar to those of rheumatoid arthritis (Fig. 42). The pathologists can readily distinguish these different disorders, but one can raise similar questions about the bone resorption such as: (1) are the inflammatory cells responsible for the bone resorption, or are they

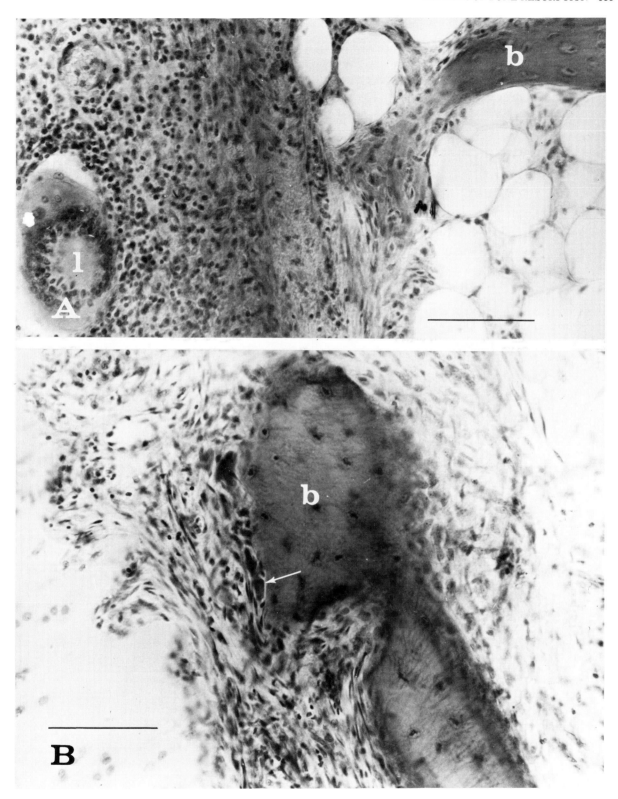

Fig. 42: Section from the wrist of a patient with tuberculous arthritis. (**A**) Region at the edge of the granuloma showing mononuclear infiltrate and a Langhans giant cell (1). A spicule of bone (b) is undergoing resorption. (**B**) An area deep from that shown above. An isolated bone spicule (b) is being resorbed with large cells in a lacuna (arrow) which blend with surrounding inflammatory cells. Bar = 100 μm.

derived from the bone? (2) Are lymphocytes (particularly T lymphocytes) stimulated by specific mycobacterial antigens to produce factors which turn on other cells? (3) Do hormones such as prostaglandins play a permissive role in the function of the involved cells?

Conclusion

The interactions of the mineral and organic phases of bone are such that the matrix cannot be resorbed without first removing the mineral ions. We do not know how this is accomplished, but living cells in close contact with the resorbing surface are essential. There are many similarities between physiological bone remodeling and pathological bone resorption, but we are not certain whether the resorbing cells in these different conditions are derived from the same precursors, have similar receptors and are subject to the same modifying influences. We can identify some of these influences and others we have not even discussed. It is possible that the generalized bone resorption such as that associated with parathyroid hormone excess is a different process from the focal resorption seen in rheumatoid arthritis or that in cholesteatoma. It was our purpose here to describe several conditions in which information has been obtained using a variety of approaches which may help to understand the basic phenomenon and devise appropriate control measures.

References

1. Aegerter, E. and Kirkpatrick, J. A., Jr.: *Orthopedic Diseases.* Saunders Company, Philadelphia, Pennsylvania, 1968, p. 620.
2. Barland, P. and Hamerman, D.: Studies on oxidative and hydrolytic enzymes in synovial membrane of normal and arthritic patients. *Bull. N. Y. Acad. Med.*, 38: 507, 1962.
3. Barrett. A. J.: The enzymatic degradation of cartilage matrix. In Burleigh, P. M. C. and Poole, A. R.: (Eds.). *Dynamics of Connective Tissue Macromolecules.* North-Holland Publishing Company, Amsterdam, Holland, 1975, p. 189.
4. Barzel, U. S. and Jowsey, J.: The effects of chronic acid and alkali administration on bone turnover in adult rats. *Clin. Sci.*, 36: 517, 1969.
5. Belanger, L. F.: Osteocytic osteolysis. *Calcif. Tissue Res.*, 4: 1, 1969.
6. Birkedal-Hansen, H.: Osteoclastic resorption of ^{3}H-proline labelled bone, denine and cementum in the rat. *Calcif. Tissue Res.*, 15: 77, 1974.
7. Bonar, L. C. and Glimcher, M. J.: Thermal denaturation of mineralized and demineralized bone collagens. *J. Ultrastruct. Res.*, 32: 545, 1970.
8. Bordier, P. J.; Arnaud, C.; Hawker, C. et al: Relationship between serum immunoreactive parathyroid hormone, osteoclastic and osteocytic bone resorptions and serum calcium in primary hyperparathyroidism and osteomalacia. In Frame, B.; Parfitt, A. M.; and Duncan, H.: (Eds.). *Clinical Aspects of Metabolic Bone Disease.* Excerpta Medica, Amsterdam, Holland, 1973, p. 222.
9. Chase, L. R.; Fedak, S. A.; and Aurbach, G. D.: Activation of skeletal adenyl cyclase by parathyroid hormone in vitro. *Endocrinology*, 84: 761, 1969.
10. Collins, D. H.: *The Pathology of Articular and Spinal Diseases.* Edward Arnold and Company, London, England, 1949.
11. Dayer, J. M.; Krane, S. M.; Russell, R. G. G. et al: Production of collagenase and prostaglandins by isolated adherent rheumatoid synovial cells. *Proc. Nat. Acad. Sci.*, 73: 945, 1976.
12. Dayer, J. M.; Russell, R. G. G.; and Krane, S. M.: Collagenase production by isolated, adherent rheumatoid synovial cells: stimulation by a lymphocyte factor. *Clin. Res.*, 24: 445A, 1976.
13. Evanson, J. M.; Jeffrey, J. J.; and Krane, S. M.: Human collagenase: identification and characterization of an enzyme from rheumatoid synovium

in culture. *Science,* 158: 499, 1967.

14. Falchuk, K. H.; Goetzl, E. J.; and Kulka, P. J.: Respiratory gases of synovial fluids. An approach to synovial tissue circulatory-metabolic imbalance in rheumatoid arthritis. *Amer. J. Med.,* 49: 223, 1970.

15. Glimcher, M. J. and Krane, S. M.: The organization and the structure of bone and the mechanism of calcification. In Gould, B.S.: (Ed.). *Treatise on Collagen,* Vol. 2, Part B. Academic Press, London, England, 1968, p. 68.

16. Gross, J.: Collagen biology: structure, degradation and disease. *Harvey Lect.,* 68: 351, 1974.

17. Hanaoka, H.; Friedman, B.; and Mack, R. P. Ultrastructure and histogenesis of giant-cell tumor of bone. *Cancer,* 25: 1408, 1970.

18. Harris, E. D., Jr. and Krane, S. M.: Effects of colchicine on collagenase in cultures of rheumatoid synovium. *Arthritis Rheum.,* 14: 669, 1971.

19. Harris, E. D., Jr. and Krane, S. M.: Collagenases. (First, second, and third of three parts.) *N. Engl. J. Med.,* 291: 557; 605; 652, 1974.

20. Hauschka, P. V.; Lian, J. B.; and Gallop, P. M.: Direct identification of the calcium-binding amino acid gamma-carboxyglutamate, in mineralized tissue. *Proc. Natl. Acad. Sci., USA,* 72(10): 3925, 1975.

21. Hellstrom, J. and Ivemark, B. I.: Primary hyperparathyroidism. Clinical and structural findings in 138 cases. *Acta Chir. Scand., Suppl.,* 294: 1, 1962.

22. Hinkle, P. M. and Tashjian, A. H., Jr.: Thyrotropin-releasing hormone regulates the number of its own receptors in the GH$_3$ strain of pituitary cells in culture. *Biochemistry,* 14 (17): 3845, 1975.

23. Horton, J. E.; Raisz, L. G.; Simmons, H. A. et al: Bone resorbing activity in supernatant fluid from cultured human peripheral blood leukocytes. *Science,* 177: 793, 1972.

24. Jaffe, H. L.; Lichtenstein, L.; and Portis, R. B.: Giant cell tumor of bone: its pathologic appearance, grading, supposed variants and treatment. *Arch. Pathol.,* 30: 993, 1940.

25. Kantrowitz, F.; Robinson, D. R.; and McGuire, M. B.: Corticosteroids inhibit prostaglandin production by rheumatoid synovia. *Nature,* 258: 737, 1975.

26. Krane, S. M.: Collagenase production by human synovial tissues. *Ann. N.Y. Acad. Sci.,* 256: 289, 1975.

27. Krane, S. M.: Degradation of collagen in connective tissue diseases. Rheumatoid arthritis. In Burleigh, P. M. C. and Poole, A. R.: (Eds.). *Dynamics of Connective Tissue Macromolecules.* North-Holland Publishing Company, Amsterdam, Holland, 1975, p. 309.

28. Kuhlman, R. E. and McNamee, M. J.: Quantitative microchemical studies of chondroblastoma, giant-cell tumor, chondromyxoid fibroma and desmoplastic fibroma. *Clin. Orthop.,* 69: 264, 1970.

29. Miller, E. J.: A review of biochemical studies on the genetically distinct collagens of the skeletal system. *Clin. Orthop.,* 92: 260, 1973.

30. Mundy, G. R.; Raisz, L. G.; Cooper, R. A. et al: Evidence for the secretion of an osteoclast stimulating factor in myeloma. *New Engl. J. Med.,* 291: 1041, 1974.

31. Neuman, W. F.; Mulryan, B. J.; and Martin, G. R.: A chemical view of osteoclasis based on studies with yttrium. *Clin. Orthop.,* 17: 124, 1960.

32. Owen, M.: Cellular dynamics of bone. In Bourne, G. H.: (Ed.). *The Biochemistry and Physiology of Bone,* Vol. III. Academic Press, New York, New York, 1971, p. 271.

33. Parakkal, P. F.: Involvement of macrophages in collagen resorption. *J. Cell Biol.,* 41: 345, 1969.

34. Peck, W. A.; Carpenter, J.; Messinger, K., et al: Cyclic 3'5' adenosine monophosphate in isolated bone cells. Response to low concentrations of parathyroid hormone. *Endocrinology,* 92: 692, 1973.

35. Posner, A. S. and Betts, F.: Synthetic amorphous calcium phosphate and its relation to bone mineral structures. *Accounts of Chem. Res.,* In press, 1976.

36. Raff, M.: Self regulation of membrane receptors. *Nature,* 259: 265, 1976.

37. Raisz, L. G.: Physiologic and pharmacologic regulation of bone resorption. *New Engl. J. Med.,* 282: 909, 1970.

38. Raisz, L. G. and Niemann, I.: Early effects of parathyroid hormone and thyrocalcitonin on bone in organ culture. *Nature (London),* 214: 486, 1967.

39. Reynolds, J. J.: Degradation processes in bone and cartilage. *Calcif, Tissue Res.,* (Suppl): 52:, 1970.

40. Roberts, J. E.; McLees, B. D.; and Kerby, G. P.: Pathways of glucose metabolism in rheumatoid and nonrheumatoid synovial membrane. *J. Lab. Clin. Med.,* 70: 503, 1967.

41. Robinson, D. R.; Smith, H.; McGuire, M. B. et al: Prostaglandin synthesis by rheumatoid synovium and its stimulation by colchicine. *Prostaglandins,* 10 (1): 67, 1975.

42. Robinson, D. R.; Tashjian, A. H., Jr.; and Levine, L.: Prostaglandin-stimulated bone resorption by rheumatoid synovia. A possible mechanism for bone destruction in rheumatoid arthritis. *J. Clin. Invest.,* 56: 1181, 1975.

43. Schajowicz, F.: Giant-cell tumors of bone (osteoclastoma). A pathological and histochemical study. *J. Bone Joint Surg.,* 43A: 1, 1961.

44. Seyberth, H. W.; Segre, G. V.; Morgan, J. C. et al: Prostaglandins as mediators of hypercalcemia associated with certain types of cancer. *New Engl. J. Med.,* 293 (25): 1278, 1975.

45. Shea, J. F.; Yeager, V. L.; and Taylor, J. J.: Bone

resorption by osteocytes. *Proc. Soc. Exp. Biol. Med.*, 129: 41, 1968.

46. Smith, D. M. and Johnston, C. C., Jr.: Hormonal responsiveness of adenylate cyclase activity from separate bone cells. *Endocrinology*, 95: 130, 1974.

47. Steiner, G. C.; Ghosh, L.; and Dorfman, H. D.: Ultrastructure of giant cell tumors of bone. *Human Pathol.*, 3: 569, 1972.

48. Stern, B.; Golub, L.; and Goldhaber, P.: Effects of demineralization and parathyroid hormone on the availability of bone collagen to degradation by collagenase. *J. Periodont. Res.*, 5: 116, 1970.

49. Stewart, M. J.: The histogenesis of myeloid sarcoma. *Lancet*, 2: 1106, 1922.

50. Talmage, R. V.: A study of the effect of parathyroid hormone on bone remodeling and on calcium homeostasis. *Clin. Orthop.*, 54: 163, 1967.

51. Tashjian, A. H., Jr.; Voelkel, E. F.; Levine, L. et al: Evidence that the bone resorption-stimulating factor produced by mouse fibrosarcoma cells is prostaglandin E_2. A new model for the hypercalcemia of cancer. *J. Exp. Med.*, 136: 1329, 1972.

52. Vaes, G.: Lysosomes and the cellular physiology of bone resorption. In Dingle, J. T. and Fell, H. B.: (Eds.). *Lysosomes in Biology and Pathology*. Vol. I.

North-Holland Publishing Company, Amsterdam, Holland, 1969, p. 217.

53. Van Boxel, J. A. and Paget, S. A.: Predominantly T-cell infiltrate in rheumatoid synovial membranes. *New Engl. J. Med.*, 292: 517, 1975.

54. Voelkel, E. F.; Tashjian, A. H., Jr.; Franklin, R. et al: Hypercalcemia and tumor prostaglandins: the VX_2 carcinoma model in the rabbit. *Metabolism*, 24 (8): 973, 1975.

55. Wahl, L. M.; Wahl, S. M.; Mergenhagen, S. E. et al: Collagenase production by lymphokine-activated macrophages. *Science*, 187 (4173): 261, 1975.

56. Willis, R. A.: Osteoclastoma. In *Pathology of Tumours*, 4th Ed. Butterworths and Company, Ltd., London, England, 1967, p. 696.

57. Wong, G. L. and Cohn, D. V.: Target cells in bone for parathormone and calcitonin are different: enrichment for each cell type by sequential digestion of mouse calvaria and selective adhesion to polymeric surfaces. *Proc. Nat. Acad. Sci.*, 72: 3167, 1975.

58. Wright, D. R.; Ivey, J. L.; and Tashjian, A. H., Jr.: Self-induced loss of calcitonin receptors in bone: a possible explanation for "escape". *Clin. Res.*, 24: 461A, 1976.

CONTROL OF HUMAN SKIN COLLAGENASE ACTIVITY

Arthur Z. Eisen, M.D.
Eugene A. Bauer, M.D.
George P. Stricklin
Jo L. Seltzer, Ph.D.
Thomas J. Koob
John J. Jeffrey, Ph.D.

The maintenance of the normal architecture of human skin requires the elaboration and precise regulation of the enzyme collagenase which is the specific enzyme required for the initiation of collagen degradation. It is the function of the dermal cellular components to correctly oversee the relatively slow collagen breakdown occurring during normal turnover as well as to react to acute requirements for degradation as, for example, in the wound healing process. Our laboratory has been concerned with the nature of these processes for a number of years. From the beginning, our studies have centered on the regulation of a collagenase produced by cultured explants of human skin (Eisen, et al, 1970). More recently, lines of human skin fibroblasts have been developed which produce collagenase as a major secretory product (Bauer, et al, 1975). Both systems have unique advantages, and it is our hope, that combined studies using both the monolayer cell culture and the organized tissue explant system will enable us to describe precisely the nature of the regulation of collagenase activity in vivo.

Human skin collagenase (HSC) was first isolated from the culture medium in which living skin explants were grown and appeared to be synthesized de novo from viable cells in tissue culture (Eisen, et al, 1968). Such an organ culture system was required since extracts of skin consistently failed to yield an enzyme with collagenase activity. If, however, tissue extracts were subjected to specialized techniques which separated active enzyme from serum and possibly tissue inhibitors,

then small amounts of collagenase could be obtained but recovery was laborious and not quantitative (Eisen, et al, 1971). HSC obtained from culture medium degrades collagen at physiologic pH and temperature by cleaving the native molecule across its three constituent polypeptide chains producing two fragments, one three-quarters and the other one-quarter the length of the molecule. Studies using animal collagenases have shown that they specifically cleave $\alpha 1$ (Eisen, et al, 1970) at a Gly-Ile bond (residues 772-773 of this chain) and $\alpha 2$ at a Gly-Leu bond in the homologous region of the chain (Gross, et al, 1974 and Miller, et al, 1976). This appears to be a susceptible region in the collagen molecule and it is presumed that the human enzymes, when examined, will attack the same site.

Because of the difficulties in detecting collagenase activity in vivo in human skin it was important to establish whether the enzyme activity present in the culture medium accurately reflected the in vivo synthetic activity of the tissue. The presence of collagenase in human skin in vivo, i.e. in tissue extracts, was first demonstrated using functionally monospecific antisera against HSC purified from culture medium (Eisen, et al, 1971). In addition, human synovial, gingival and granulocyte collagenases were identical in their immunologic cross reactivity to HSC supporting the concept that extensive homologies probably exist among collagenases from various human organs (Bauer, et al, 1970 and 1972). Collagenases from distantly related species (rat, mouse, tadpole) cross reacted poorly if at all with HSC suggesting fewer structural similarities to the human enzymes. The major significance of these studies was the demonstration that readily detectable levels of collagenase exist in vivo and that the in vivo enzyme is immunologically identical to collagenase obtained from tissue culture.

Whether the failure to detect enzymatic activity directly in skin extracts in the presence of immunoreactive collagenase is due (1) to the presence of serum antiproteases or perhaps other tissue inhibitors (Eisen, et al, 1970; Bauer et al, 1972; and Bauer, et al, 1975 (2) to the high affinity of the enzyme for its substrate, collagen (Ryan and Woessner, 1971 and Pardo and Tamayo, 1975) or (3) perhaps to the existence of a precursor or zymogen form of the enzyme (Harper, et al, 1971; Vaes, 1972; and Bauer, et al, 1975) is not known. It is clear, however, that insight into the mechanisms for controlling collagenase biosynthesis and subsequent activity are essential if the regulation of collagen remodeling at the molecular level in both normal and pathologic states is to be understood.

Regulation of Collagenase by Serum Antiproteases

The alpha globulin fraction of human serum, which contains both alpha$_2$-macroglobulin (α_2M) and alpha$_1$-antitrypsin (α_1-at) has been shown to be an effective inhibitor of HSC (Eisen, et al, 1970; Bauer, et al, 1972; and Eisen, et al, 1970). It is now clear that the major collagenase inhibitor in this serum component is alpha$_2$-M. Alpha$_2$-M, a glycoprotein having a molecular weight of approximately 725,000, reacts on a mole for mole basis with collagenase to form an apparently irreversible enzyme-inhibitor complex (Abe and Nagai, 1972 and Werb, et al, 1974). Whether the major physiologic importance of α_2-M is to facilitate the clearing of inhibitor-enzyme complexes from the circulation (Ohlsson, 1971) or whether HSC might act freely near its site of production and that α_2-M prevents its action on collagen at distant sites (Eisen, et al, 1970) remains to be determined.

The role of α_1-at as a collagenase inhibitor is less clear. We initially reported that α_1-at was capable of inhibiting both human skin and rheumatoid synovial collagenases but clearly was a less potent inhibitor than α_2-M (Eisen, et al, 1970; Bauer, et al, 1972; Eisen, et al, 1970; and Bauer, 1971). Although it has been shown that α_1-at inhibits granulocyte collagenase (Ohlsson and Olsson, 1973) it apparently did not inhibit certain other human and animal collagenases (Werb, et al, 1974; Berman, et al, 1973; Sakamoto, et al, 1972; and Woolley, et al, 1975). Further studies in our laboratory indicated that the purer the preparation of α_1-at used the more effective was the inhibition, nonetheless, at best it was only a weak inhibitor of HSC. As shown (Table 10) when a known quantity of HSC, as determined accurately by radioimmunoassay of a crude enzyme solution, is reacted with a preparation of α_1-at purified to homogeneity (a gift from Dr. Jack Pierce) it is possible to attain almost complete inhibition of HSC. However, maximum inhibition occurs at approximately a 45-fold molar excess of inhibitor to enzyme indicating that α_1-at is a poor inhibitor of HSC. The failure of other investigators to obtain

TABLE 10

Inhibition of Human Skin Collagenase by Pure Alpha$_1$-Antitrypsin

iHSC (μg)	α_1-at (μg)	Cpm above blank	Inhibition (%)
1.3	-	462	-
1.3	15	373	19
1.3	30	291	27
1.3	60	33	93

Reaction mixtures contained 18.3 μg crude enzyme protein in a total volume of 225 μl. Incubation was carried out at 37°C in a shaker water bath for 3 hours. ^{14}C-glycine labeled collagen containing 1500 cpm was used as a substrate gel.

even limited inhibition of other collagenases (Woolley, et al, 1975) might well be related to the purity and concentrations α_1-at used relative to the enzyme preparations used.

Since the most recent preparation of α_1-at used in our laboratory had been purified to homogeneity, its ability to inhibit HSC cannot be due to contamination by the smaller serum collagenase inhibitor recently described by Wooley and associates (Woolley, et al, 1975). This protein has a molecular weight of approximately 40,000 and is an effective inhibitor of human collagenases but has no effect on trypsin. It is possible, however, that separation of HSC in crude tissue extracts from this inhibitor by gel filtration permitted us to detect collagenase activity in skin extracts (Eisen, et al, 1971). The relationship of this inhibitor to a collagenase inhibitor of roughly the same size that we recently have isolated from human skin fibroblasts (Bauer, et al, 1975) will be

discussed below.

Hormonal Regulation of HSC in Organ Culture

Corticosteroids exert major effects on the metabolism of protein in a variety of mammalian systems both in vitro and in vivo. In view of the profound effects exerted by these hormones it was of particular interest to determine whether steroids could affect in vitro collagen metabolism in human skin (Koob, et al, 1974). As shown in Table 11 both hydrocortisone at 10^{-7}M and dexamethasone at 10^{-8}M in culture medium reduces collagenase activity almost completely. The inhibition of collagenase activity is dependent on steroid concentration in the culture medium, with consistently detectable inhibition occurring at 10^{-8}M hydrocortisone and 10^{-12}M dexamethasone. Dexamethasone is more effective than the parent compound in producing inhibition of enzyme activity.

TABLE 11

Effect of Hydrocortisone and Dexamethasone on Collagenase Activity
and Collagen Degradation in Human Skin Cultures

Culture Conditions	Medium Collagenase*	% Inhibition	Medium Hydroxyproline+	% Inhibition
Control	4.05		115	
Hydrocortisone, 10^{-7}M	0.39	90	38	68
Hydrocortisone, 10^{-8}M	1.58	61	85	26
Hydrocortisone, 10^{-9}M	4.02	0	120	0
Control	10.49		290	
Dexamethasone, 10^{-8}M	1.51	86	76	74
Dexamethasone, 10^{-9}M	2.30	78	96	67
Dexamethasone, 10^{-10}M	4.89	54	222	23
Dexamethasone, 10^{-11}M	6.26	41	179	38
Dexamethasone, 10^{-12}M	9.10	14	298	0
Cycloheximide, 40 μg/ml	0.53	95		

Aliquots (150 μl) of crude culture medium on the third day of culture were incubated for 18 hrs with 200 μg native ^{14}C-glycine labeled collagen fibrils (3600 cpm).

---

*Results are expressed as μg collagen degraded per mg medium protein. +Medium hydroxyproline represents the total imino acid in the medium from two culture flasks (30 ml).

Cyclohexamide, as expected, inhibits protein synthesis in the cultured skin by 95-100% and also prevents the appearance of collagenase in the cultures. The reduction in enzyme activity by cyclohexamide is a direct result of the inhibition of overall protein synthesis in this tissue. In direct contrast, neither of the steroids effect overall protein synthesis, thus, hydrocortisone at 10^{-7}M and dexamethasone at 10^{-8}M in the culture medium, appear to selectively inhibit the production of active collagenase.

Concomitant with the inhibition by these steroids of collagenase activity is a cessation of collagen degradation in the tissue as measured by a marked reduction in the level of hydroxyproline containing peptides in the culture medium. This inhibition of collagen catabolism is dependent upon steroid concentration and is parallel with the inhibition of collagenase activity.

The low concentrations of steroids employed suggest that their effect on collagenase and collagen catabolism observed in vitro may be indicative of a physiologic regulatory role of corticosteroids on in vivo collagen metabolism in human skin. It is also important to note that similar results have been obtained in cultures of human rheumatoid synovium and postpartum rat uterus (Koob, et al, 1974).

Based on our previous observations that the reproductive steroid progesterone is of prime importance in the regulation of collagenase activity in the postpartum rat uterus (Jeffrey, et al, 1971; Jeffrey, et al, 1971; and Jeffrey, et al, 1975) we have examined the effect of progesterone on collagenase production by human skin in vitro. Progesterone when added to the culture medium also prevents the appearance of collagenase from skin explants in culture but at concentrations higher than that required to inhibit collagenase production by the uterus (Koob, et al, in preparation). The precise mechanism whereby progesterone inhibits collagenase production by human skin and its physiological significance is currently under investigation.

Of particular interest in regard to the control of collagenase in human skin are our observations on the effects of cyclic AMP (Jeffrey, et al, 1975). It has been demonstrated (Koob and Jeffrey, 1974) that cyclic AMP blocks the appearance of collagenase by rat uterus in vitro. As shown (Table 12), dibutyryl cyclic AMP, when added to organ cultures of human skin, produces a marked inhibition of collagenase activity found in the medium concentrations which do not significantly affect tissue protein synthesis. In the skin, as in the uterus, theophylline, an inhibitor of cyclic nucleotide phosphodiesterase, produced similar reductions in collagenase activity (Jeffrey, et al, 1975). In addition, both these compounds also block the production of collagenase which is tightly bound to the endogenous collagen of the skin tissue explants (Koob, et al, in preparation). These findings are further emphasized by the observations that both cyclic AMP and theophylline lowered the

TABLE 12

Effect of Dibutyryl Cyclic AMP and Theophylline on Collagenase Production by Human Skin

Culture additions	Collagenase activity cpm	Inhibition %
Control	1942	
DB-cAMP, 1 mM	198	90
DB-cAMP, 1 x 10^{-5}M	1650	15
Control	3672	
Theophylline, 2.5 mM	1504	58
Theophylline, 1 mM	2720	25

Organ cultures of human skin were initiated and incubated with the indicated concentration of either dibutyryl cyclic AMP or theophylline dissolved directly in the culture medium. On the third day of culture aliquots (150 μ1) of medium were incubated with native (^{14}C)glycine-labeled collagen fibrils, for 6 h and collagenase activity was determined by measuring solubilized (^{14}C)glycine-containing peptides.

levels of hydroxyproline containing peptides in the medium, indicating that endogenous collagen degradation was inhibited in parallel with the loss of collagenase activity.

Although this report deals principally with human skin, it is of general biologic interest to note that collagenase produced by the skin from another species, the tadpole, also appears to be hormonally regulated (Davis, et al, 1975). Explants of tadpole tailfin tissue (Rana pipiens or R. catesbeana) undergo complete re-epithelialization of the cut surfaces (healing) when cultured at 22°C. Healing does not occur when freshly cut explants are cultured at higher temperatures (37°C). After re-epithelialization, these healed explants maintain normal tissue organization in subsequent culture at either 22° or 37°C. When thyroxine was added to the medium of these healed explants, an organized resorption of the tissue occurred, characterized by a gradual loss of explant size and the loss of tissue collagen which was concomitant with the appearance of collagenase in the medium. Control re-epithelialized explants showed none of these changes and most importantly did not produce collagenase.

In contrast, tailfin tissue when placed directly in culture at 37°C not only failed to re-epithelialize but underwent massive resorption independent of hormonal conditions. Collagenase production in these explants may be one consequence of tissue wounding and that incubation of freshly wounded tissue at 37°C favors the continuous production of collagenase normally associated with hormone dependent tailfin resorption. These findings indicate that collagenase is involved in the physiological removal of collagen from the resorbing tadpole tailfin and that the expression of collagenase activity is regulated by thyroxine (Davis, et al, 1975).

Role of Metals in the Control of HSC Activity

For many neutral proteases, the presence of calcium (Ca^{2+}) has been shown to be essential for maintaining optimal activity under physiological conditions. The role of Ca^{2+} in the action of HSC,

rat skin and rat uterus collagenases have now been well defined (Seltzer, et al, 1976). The results of these studies indicate that the metal plays a dual role acting both as an enzyme activator and to prevent the irreversible loss of enzyme activity at 37°C and neutral pH, presumably by maintaining the required tertiary structure of the enzyme.

In the absence of extrusic Ca^{2+} these three mammalian collagenases lose activity in a two-step process which in the first stage is reversible and subsequently, with increasing length of Ca^{2+}-free incubation under physiological conditions, becomes irreversible. Calcium is necessary for thermostabilization both in the presence and absence of the collagen substrate. The collagenases from the three sources display an increase in enzyme activity with increasing Ca^{2+} concentration which is associated with an increase in thermostabilization. It seems probable that in the absence of extrinsic Ca^{2+} there is a progressive destabilization of the tertiary structure of the enzyme molecule, resulting in a loss of the enzymes catalytic ability. This initial loss of structure may lead either to autolysis or to nonspecific proteolysis of the collagenase by other neutral proteases in semi purified enzyme preparations. It should also be noted that rat uterus collagenase unlike the skin enzymes is more susceptible to loss of its specifically required tertiary structure. In addition barium and strontium are effective substitutes for Ca^{2+} in HSC but not in the collagenases from rat tissues. These findings suggest that although the basic mechanisms of collagenase activity are most likely the same for all three enzymes there are species and perhaps organ differences probably reflecting differences in enzyme structure.

It is also important to point out that Ca^{2+} plays no role in the binding of HSC or the rat collagenases to their collagen substrate (Seltzer, et al, 1976). This is unlike bacterial collagenase in which it has been proposed that Ca^{2+} is necessary for binding of this enzyme to its substrate (Gallop, et al, 1957).

In addition to its requirement for extrinsic

Ca^{2+} HSC as well as rat skin and uterus collagenases are inhibited by certain chelating agents in the presence of excess Ca^{2+}, indicating the involvement of a second metal ion in the activity of the enzyme. Zinc (Zn^{2+}) was the most effective ion able to prevent and reverse the inhibition of chelators (Seltzer, et al, submitted) indicating that, as has been suggested for bacterial (Harper and Seifter, 1974) and corneal (Berman and Manabe, 1973) collagenases as well, these enzymes contain Zn^{2+} as an intrinsic metal ion. Mammalian collagenases then, are most probably a part of a group of neutral proteases in which Zn^{2+} is the metal at the active site, and extrinsic Ca^{2+} is also required. Furthermore, from the standpoint of regulation, it is clear that any directive mechanisms in vivo which modulate the tissue calcium concentration could be affective in regulating collagenase activity.

Procollagenase and Collagenase Inhibitor from Human Skin Fibroblasts

As has already been discussed in detail, human skin in organ culture has served as an important means for examining some of the mechanisms involved in the regulation of collagenase production and activity. However, we felt that if the various parameters involved in the control of collagenase biosynthesis were to be adequately examined in both normal and diseased states it was necessary to develop a system that could be maintained for longer periods of time and be subjected to well defined changes.

To attain this goal we employed fibroblasts in monolayer culture and succeeded in localizing collagenase in human skin fibroblasts using immunohistochemical techniques (Reddick, et al, 1973 and 1974). Despite the immunologic evidence for the presence of collagenase we were unable to detect enzymatic activity in the fibroblast culture medium and initially attributed this to inhibition of the enzyme by whole serum in the medium. However, even when normal human skin fibroblasts were cultured in serum-free medium it was still not possible to detect collagenase ac-

tivity. This failure to detect active ᴉgenase in human skin fibroblast cultures, no\ ears to be due to the fact that the enzyme was secreted into the medium in an inactive form.

We have been able to show (Bauer, et al, 1975) that the enzyme in the crude serum-free medium obtained from cultured human skin fibroblasts could be activated by trypsin and, once activated, was identical in its mechanism of action to human skin collagenase obtained from organ cultures. It is also of considerable interest to note that the partially purified inactive collagenase obtained from these fibroblast cultures was capable of undergoing autoactivation. Thus the presence of a trypsin-activatable enzyme indicated that a zymogen (procollagenase) was produced by skin fibroblasts as had initially been suggested for the collagenases obtained from tadpole tailfin explants (and tissue homogenates) by Harper, et al (1971 and 1972) and by Vaes (1972) for mouse bone explants.

The zymogen of the tadpole (Harper, et al, 1971 and 1972) seems to differ from that of mouse bone (Vaes, 1972) and skin fibroblasts (Bauer, et al, 1975) in that it is activated by an apparent specific protease in the culture medium but not by trypsin. To date, we have not been able to identify a specific activator for procollagenase in skin fibroblast cultures. Of particular note is the fact that we have not, as yet, been successful in demonstrating collagenase in zymogen form in organ cultures of human skin. Differences between collagenase production by fibroblasts and by organ cultures are currently under active investigation in our laboratory.

The skin fibroblast procollagenase has been purified and partially characterized. Its properties will be presented in detail elsewhere (Stricklin, et al in preparation). Briefly the proenzyme has a molecular weight of 55,000-60,000 daltons and following trypsin treatment loses approximately 10,000 daltons to form the active enzyme. The purified proenzyme is still capable of autoactivation. It is not, however, complexed by whole serum or by alpha globulins and can, therefore, be obtained from serum containing culture medium. The presence of a procollagenase produced by skin fibroblasts in vitro provides yet another area for the regulation of collagenase biosynthesis and thus, ultimately the remodeling of collagen. If a zymogen is shown to be operative in vivo then any imbalance in this system could lead to abnormalities in collagen degradation in a variety of disease states.

Fibroblast Collagenase Inhibitor

An inhibitor of collagenase is also present in the medium of fibroblast cultures and all evidence to date indicates that it is produced by the cells (Bauer, et al, 1975). Although the molecular weight of the partially purified inhibitor has not as yet been precisely determined it is slightly heavier than active collagenase (45,000 daltons) on gel filtration. The inhibitor appears to be a glycoprotein capable of inhibiting active HSC or fibroblast enzyme with equimolar stoichiometry. The inhibitor does not inhibit trypsin and is devoid of material reacting with anti-bovine whole serum in gel diffusion indicating that the inhibitor is not derived from residual serum in the medium. Of considerable importance is the observation that the inhibitor binds preferentially to active collagenase and does not form a complex with the proenzyme (Stricklin, unpublished observations).

The existence of an apparently specific inhibitor of collagenase which is produced by fibroblasts in cell culture offers another potential control mechanism of collagen degradation. Whether this inhibitor is present in vivo is as yet unknown as is its possible relationship to the newly defined collagenase inhibitor present in human serum (Woolley, et al, 1975).

In summary then, we can now identify a number of specific loci in the pathway of collagenase biosynthesis where effective biological control can be exerted. These points at which collagenase activity might be modulated are illustrated schematically in Figure 43. It is clear that control of the activity of this enzyme can be a manifold process. Intracellularly, hormones can regulate m-

RNA levels, rates of translation, correct folding, insertion of metal ions and proper packaging; on the other hand, extracellular events such as proper activation, proper Ca^{++} levels and proper control over the concentrations of tissue and serum antiproteases all must be carefully managed. It would not be surprising ultimately to find that biology makes use of all of these avenues in the specification of the onset and duration of collagenase activity, the levels of enzyme activity at a given time and the geographical distribution of that activity within a tissue such as skin.

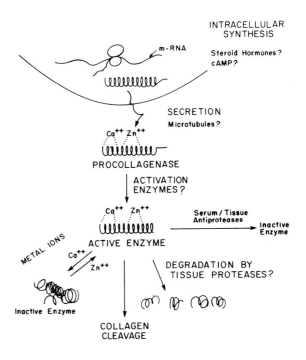

Fig. 43: Control points in the pathway of collagenase biosynthesis.

Acknowledgements
Supported by U.S.P.H.S. grants AM 12129, AM 05611, and HD 05291. Dr. Bauer is the recipient of Research Career Development Award 1 K04 AM 00077 from the National Institutes of Health.

References

1. Abe, S. and Nagai, Y.: Interaction between tadpole collagenase and human 2-macroglobulin. *Biochem. Biophys. Acta.*, 278: 125, 1972.
2. Bauer, E. A.; Eisen, A. Z.; and Jeffrey, J. J.: Immunologic relationship of a purified human skin collagenase to other human and animal collagenases. *Biochem. Biophys. Acta.*, 206: 152, 1970.
3. Bauer, E. A.; Eisen, A. Z.; and Jeffrey, J. J.: Studies on purified rheumatoid synovial collagenase in vitro and in vivo. *J. Clin. Invest.*, 50: 2056, 1971.
4. Bauer, E. A.; Eisen, A. Z.; and Jeffrey, J. J.: Radioimmunoassay of human collagenase. Specificity of the assay and quantitative determination of in vivo and in vitro human skin collagenase. *J. Biol. Chem.*, 247: 6679, 1972.
5. Bauer, E. A.; Eisen, A. Z.; and Jeffrey, J. J.: Regulation of vertebrate collagenase activity in vivo and in vitro. *J. Invest. Dermatol.*, 59: 50, 1972.
6. Bauer, E. A.; Stricklin, G. P.; Jeffrey, J. J. et al: Collagenase production by human skin fibroblasts. *Biophys. Res. Commun.*, 64: 232, 1975.
7. Berman, M. B.; Barber, J. C.; Talamo, R. C. et al: Corneal ulceration and the serum antiproteases. I. Alpha 1-antitrypsin. *Invest. Ophthalmol.*, 12: 759, 1973.
8. Berman, M. B. and Manabe, R.: Corneal collagenases: Evidence for zinc metalloenzymes. *Ann. Ophthalmol.*, 5: 1193, 1973.
9. Davis, D. P.; Jeffrey, J. J.; Eisen, A. Z. et al: The induction of collagenase by thyroxine in resorbing tadpole tailfin in vitro. *Develop. Biol.*, 44: 217, 1975.
10. Eisen, A. Z.; Bauer, E. A.; and Jeffrey, J. J.: Animal and human collagenases. *J. Invest. Dermatol.*, 55: 359, 1970.
11. Eisen, A. Z.; Bauer, E. A.; and Jeffrey, J. J.: Human skin collagenase. The role of serum alpha-globulins in the control of activity in vivo and in vitro. *Proc. Natl. Acad. Sci.*, 68: 248, 1971.
12. Eisen, A. Z.; Bloch, K. J.; and Sakai, T.: Inhibition of human skin collagenase by human serum. *J. Lab. Clin. Med.*, 75: 258, 1970.
13. Eisen, A. Z.; Jeffrey, J. J.; and Gross, J.: Human skin collagenase. Isolation and mechanism of attack on the collagen molecule. *Biochem. Biophys. Acta.*, 151: 637, 1968.
14. Gallop, P. M.; Seifter, S.; and Meilman, E.: Studies on collagen. I. The partial purification, assay and mode of activation of bacterial collagenase. *J. Biol. Chem.*, 227: 891, 1957.
15. Gross, J.; Harper, E.; Harris, E. D. et al: Animal collagenases: specificity of action and structures of the substrate cleavage site. *Biochem. Biophys. Res. Commun.*, 61 (2): 605, 1974.
16. Harper, E.; Bloch, K. J.; and Gross, J.: The zymogen of tadpole collagenase. *Biochemistry*, 10: 3035, 1971.
17. Harper, E. and Gross, J.: Collagenase, procollagenase and activator relationships in tadpole tissue cultures. *Biochem. Biophys. Res. Commun.*, 48: 1147, 1972.
18. Harper, E. and Seifter, S.: Studies on the mechanism of action of collagenase: inhibition by cysteine and other chelating agents. *Isr. J. Chem.*, 12: 515, 1974.
19. Jeffrey, J. J.; Coffey, R. J.; and Eisen, A. Z.: Studies on uterine collagenase in tissue culture. I. Relationship of enzyme production to collagen metabolism. *Biochem. Biophys. Acta.*, 252: 136, 1971.
20. Jeffrey, J. J.; Coffey, R. J.; and Eisen, A. Z.: Studies on uterine collagenase in tissue culture. II. Effect of steroid hormones on enzyme production. *Biochem. Biophys. Acta.*, 252: 142, 1971.
21. Jeffrey, J. J.; Koob, T. J.; and Eisen, A. Z.: Hormonal regulation of mammalian collagenases. In Burleigh, P. M. C. and Poole, A. R.: (Eds.). *Dynamics of Connective Tissue Macromolecules.* North-Holland Publishing Company, Amsterdam, Holland, 1975, p. 147.
22. Koob, T. J. and Jeffrey, J. J.: Hormonal regulation

of collagen degradation in the uterus: inhibition of collagenase expression by progesterone and cyclic AMP. *Biochem. Biophys. Acta.*, 354: 61, 1974.

23. Koob, T. J.; Jeffrey, J. J.; and Eisen, A. Z.: Regulation of human skin collagenase activity by hydrocortisone and dexamethasone in organ culture. *Biochem. Biophys. Res. Commun.*, 61: 1083, 1974.

24. Miller, E. J.; Harris, E. D.; Chung, E. et al: Cleavage of Type I and II collagens with mammalian collagenase: site of cleavage and primary structure at the NH-2 terminal portion of the smaller fragment released from both collagens. *Biochemistry*, 15(4): 787, 1976.

25. Ohlsson, K.: Interactions in vitro and in vivo between dog trypsin and dog plasma protease inhibitors. *Scand. J. Clin. Lab. Invest.*, 28: 220, 1971.

26. Ohlsson, K. and Olsson, I.: The neutral proteases of human granulocytes. Isolation and partial characterization of two granulocyte collagenases. *Eur. J. Biochem.*, 36: 473, 1973.

27. Pardo, A. and Tamayo, R. P.: The presence of collagenase in collagen preparations. *Biochem. Biophys. Acta*, 393: 121, 1975.

28. Reddick, M. E.; Bauer, E. A.; and Eisen, A. Z.: Immunocytochemical localization of collagenase in human skin and fibroblasts in monolayer culture. *Clin. Res.*, 21: 481A, 1973.

29. Reddick, M. E.; Bauer, E. A.; and Eisen, A. Z.: Immunocytochemical localization of collagenase in human skin and fibroblasts in monolayer culture. *J. Invest. Dermatol.*, 62: 361, 1974.

30. Ryan, J. N. and Woessner, J. F.: Mammalian collagenase: direct demonstration in homogenates of involuting rat uterus. *Biochem. Biophys. Res. Commun.*, 44: 144, 1971.

31. Sakamoto, S.; Goldhaber, P.; and Glimcher, M. J.: Further studies on the nature of the components in serum which inhibit mouse bone collagenase. *Calc. Tissue Res.*, 10: 280, 1972.

32. Seltzer, J. L.; Welgus, H. G.; Jeffrey, J. J. et al: The function of Ca^2 in the action of mammalian collagenases. *Archives Biochem. Biophys.*, 173: 355, 1976.

33. Vaes, G.: The release of collagenase as an inactive proenzyme by bone explants in culture. *Biochem. J.*, 126: 275, 1972.

34. Werb, Z.; Burleigh, M. C.; Barret, A. J. et al: The interaction of alpha 2-macroglobulin with proteinases. Binding and inhibition of mammalian collagenases and other metal proteinases. *Biochem. J.*, 139: 359, 1974.

35. Woolley, D. E.; Roberts, D. R.; and Evanson, J. M.: Inhibition of human collagenase activity by a small molecular weight serum protein. *Biochem. Biophys. Res. Commun.*, 66: 747, 1975.

THE LIFE-CYCLE OF EPIDERMOID IMPLANTATION CYSTS IN THE HUMAN

Paul Toller, F.D.S.R.C.S.

The surgical technique employing the buried dermis graft has been used in the past by plastic surgeons for correcting deficiencies of tissue bulk in some situations, where synthetic implants have been unsuitable. In such cases an area of skin on the abdomen was shaved by dermatome to expose the dermis, and then a portion of this dermis, together with some underlying fat was excised to be inserted into the connective tissues at the site where bulking was required.

Over the years in a busy center it has been found necessary to reopen a few of these sites in order to trim the grafts where slight adjustments have been necessary to achieve more perfect results. My colleagues kindly made available to me any tissues which were removed, since I realized that it must contain epithelial structures which had been buried for known periods of time. Fortunately for the patients such material is very scarce, but what I am briefly presenting here is derived from these sources of a few years ago.

As is very well known, buried epithelium tends to give rise to epidermoid cysts, and in the present material we have observed cysts derived from either the hair-follicles or from little bits of epidermis remaining on the graft having escaped the initial dermatome shave.

In a single case, small cysts derived from hair-follicles were observed at the end of one week, and other minute whorls of epithelial cells were apparent in the receptor site. In another case, after two weeks burial (Fig. 44A) minute epidermoid cysts containing keratinous desquamation had formed.

At three weeks, in addition to the hair-follicle lesions, there could be seen larger cysts, not formed intra-epidermally, but by a peripheral outgrowth from small implanted epithelial islands, the outgrowth encircling spaces within the mesoderm, and resembling those lesions which have long been termed "epidermoid implantation cysts."

At six weeks (Fig. 44B) all the cysts were showing a considerable surrounding fibrotic reaction and they were beginning to be associated with a conspicuous monocytic infiltration. There was evidence of a decline in activity in all the epithelial cells in walls of cysts from whatever epithelial origin. At this stage there was no evidence that any microcyst was increasing in size. Hair-follicle cysts usually attained no larger diameter than one millimeter, but the size of flattened epidermoid inclusion cysts depended upon the area of the embedded pieces of epithelium.

At twelve weeks (three months) all cysts were showing greatly diminished epithelial activity, the basal layer of these cells being thinned. There was some surrounding fibrosis, but adjacent inflammatory reaction had diminished. In general there was a loss of typical definition of basal cells and complete loss of stratum spinosum. No cysts were larger than those found at six weeks. They all appeared to be from one quarter to one millimeter in diameter at three months. By comparison, the normal surface skin from the same original abdominal area of the same individual showed a normal granular layer, no flattening of basal cells, the whole epithelial layer was thicker, and there was a well marked prickle-cell layer.

At twenty weeks, epidermoid cysts had not increased in size and all had greatly thinned epithelial cellular layers with signs of surface cell degeneration. There were epithelial discontinuities in some of these cysts. There was often a heavy pericystic fibrosis, possibly restricting the nutrient supply, and the whole lesion was surrounded by a monocytic infiltration which was not immediately adjacent to the basal cells of the epithelium but lay outside the fibrotic layer.

At one year (Fig. 44C) no true epithelium could be recognized in the microcysts. Its previous position was represented by an amorphous thick eosinophilic layer which was surrounded by many giant cells, and enclosing a mass of desquamatory material. These structures were still clearly recognizable as old cysts. The areas were surrounded by mature fibrosis, and only a low-grade inflammatory reaction was present around some of them.

At eighteen months few cystic epithelial ele-

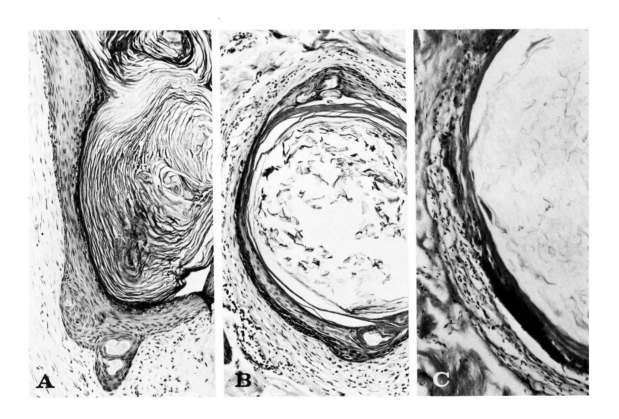

Fig. 44: Epidermoid cysts following burial of autologous skin in the human. (A) At two weeks active epithelium producing keratin desquamation in cyst cavity. (B) At six weeks, diminishing epithelial activity, and commencement of surrounding fibrosis. (C) At one year the epithelial cells cannot clearly be recognized, and the lesion is becoming surrounded by giant cells. No longer active production of keratin.

ments were found. Some small spaces were filled with amorphous material and surrounded by a foreign body reaction represented largely by many giant cells, and similar sites with fragments of hair shafts were seen, but no recognizable epithelium was associated with any of these areas which are presumed to be the final state of the cystic units at this stage.

At two years only a few regions of foreign body reaction around hair shaft fragments remain, and no sign of any epithelial cysts were found.

At four years no recognizable hair keratin nor any sign of epithelial cysts could be found and no inflammatory reaction in the areas where the epithelial elements had been buried.

Discussion

Minute epidermoid cysts which appeared after deliberate implantation of epithelium presented histological appearances which were very similar to the small epithelial cysts which are found around the mouth in the fetus just before birth, and which are commonly located along the embryological fusion lines of the face and jaws (Fig. 45) (Scott, 1955). Both types are generally present for a limited period of a year or so, before their involution and total disappearance. Although at first their histological appearance is very similar to early keratocysts derived from the dental lamina in the jaws and early congenital cholesteatoma, they behave very differently. The difference in behavior may be related to the derivation of their epithelial cells rather than their environment. The awakened epithelial cell rests in the jaws seem to give rise in the odontogenic keratocysts to an epithelium which retains a more embryological potential and multiplication occurs in the absence of any discernible stimulus, and continues under conditions in which the multiplication of the normal cell ceases. I wonder how closely the odontogenic keratocyst and the congenital epidermoid cholesteatoma resemble each other? Or is it that the same original stem-cell has received a different local instruction to multiply repeatedly and in a rather uncontrolled manner, and to synthesize keratin continually?

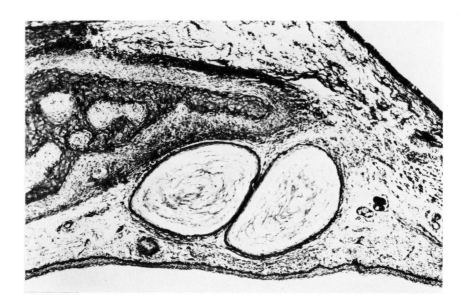

Fig. 45: Two epithelial cysts in midline of palate in 85 mm C.R. foetus, saggital section. These cysts will have disappeared spontaneously within three months of birth. Their size and life-history seems similar to most implantation dermoids in adults.

Reference

1. Scott, J. H.: Early development of oral cysts in man. *Brit. Dent. J.*, 98:109, 1955.

BONE RESORPTION IN CHRONIC OTITIS MEDIA WITH AND WITHOUT CHOLESTEATOMA

J. Sadé, M.D.
E. Berco, M.D.
A. Halevy, M.D.
I. Yarowitzkaya, M.D.

Bone resorption or bone destruction associated with chronic otitis media is usually related pathogenetically to cholesteatoma (McKenzie, 1931; Day, 1934; and Ritter, 1970); in fact, otologists believe that cholesteatomatous epithelium has specific bone destruction capabilities, but does occur in chronic otitis media without cholesteatoma. This communication, an extension of our previous studies (Sadé and Halevy, 1974 and Sadé and Berko, 1974), compares bone destruction in these two entities and examines the specificity of bony lesions in cholesteatomatous ears.

Methods and Material

Macroscopic: We have tried to answer the following questions in analyzing 100 consecutive chronic otitis media ears which have undergone tympanoplasty:

(1) How often was the ossicular chain damaged and which of the ossicles showed bone absorption?

(2) Was there bone destruction in addition to the ossicular chain involvement?

(3) What was the relationship between the bone lesions, the cholesteatoma epithelium, and the infected state of the ear?

These 100 ears comprised two groups: (1) 25 patients suffering from chronic otitis media with cholesteatoma, and (2) 75 patients suffering from simple non-cholesteatomatous chronic otitis media.

Microscopic: Eighty ossicles removed at tympanoplasty because of bone defect were processed for histologic examination; 39 ossicles were from ears exhibiting chronic otitis media with cholesteatoma (Group A) and 41 were from cases of simple chronic otitis media (Group B). The ossicles were fixed in formalin and decalcified in 2% nitric acid. Specimens were embedded in paraffin after dehydration in alcohol and xylol. Serial sections were stained with hematoxylin eosin as well as PAS.

The following histologic features were looked for: (a) connective tissue, (b) granulation tissue, (c) connective tissue plus granulation tissue, (d) intraossicular inflammatory infiltration, (e) glands, (f) normal middle ear mucosa (flat, cuboidal or respiratory epithelium), (g) stratified squamous epithelium, i.e., cholesteatoma, (h) bone destruction.

Results

Macroscopic Findings

(1) Bone destruction was usually found to be confined to the ossicular chain where the ossicles showed partial or total resorption: only in six cases was there bone resorption of the middle ear framework—when it was limited to the scutum (which is in the vicinity of the ossicular chain). Scutum erosion was found in five cases with cholesteatoma and in one without.

(2) Ossicular destruction was seen in 84% of the cholesteatomatous ears and in 42.3% of the chronic ears without cholesteatoma. Approximately two-thirds of the ossicles from either group showed granulation tissue bordering the ossicular lesion (Table 13).

TABLE 13

| | Group A - 25 Cases | | Group B - 75 Cases | |
	%	No.	%	No.
Lesion of ossicular chain	84%	21	42.3%	32
Malleus	33.3%	7	25%	8
Incus	95%	20	75%	24
Stapes	33.3%	7	28%	9
Granulation tissue around ossicular lesion	71.5%	15	62.5%	20
Destruction of middle-ear frame, i.e., above notch of Rivinus		5		1

Group A: Chronic otitis media with cholesteatoma
Group B: Simple chronic otitis media without cholesteatoma

Histologic Findings

(1) Bone destruction was demonstrated in 85% of the ossicles removed from cholesteatomatous ears and in 83% of the non-cholesteatomatous ears. The free margin of the destroyed bone showed in most cases (in both groups) an osteoid reaction (Fig. 46) similar to that seen in chronic inflammatory bone conditions.

(2) Lining the bone defect (destroyed area)—in all specimens—either granulation tissue (Figs. 46, 47, & 48) or connective tissues or both were found (Table 14).

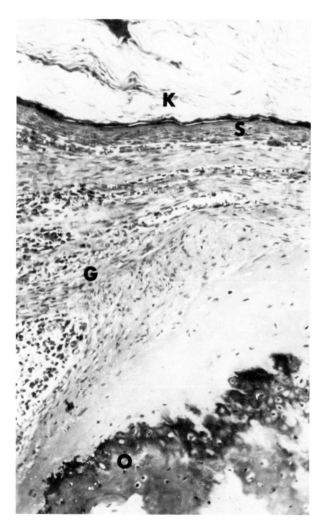

Fig. 46: Cholesteatoma (s); keratin (k); separated by granulation tissue (g) from bone, showing osteoid (o) reaction.

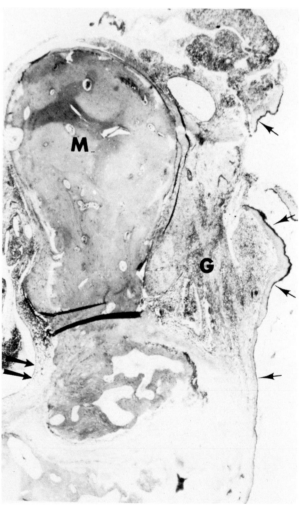

Fig. 47: Malleus (m) bordered on one side by respiratory mucosa (heavy arrow) and on the other by cholesteatoma (thin arrow). Note granulation tissue (g) separating the cholesteatoma from the bone.

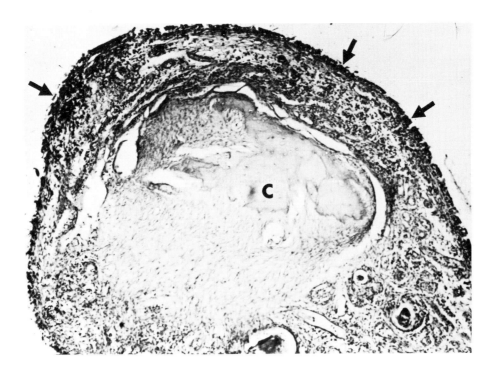

Fig. 48: Incus partially destroyed (c) surrounded by respiratory epithelium (arrows)—the two separated by granulation tissue.

TABLE 14

Tissue in Direct Contact with Areas of Bone Destruction

	Group A (39 cases)	Group B (41 cases)
Connective tissue	53%	39%
Granulation tissue	27%	51%
Connective and granulation tissue	20%	10%
Cholesteatoma	0%	0%
Osteomyelitis	17%	20%

Group A - Chronic otitis media with cholesteatoma
Group B - Simple chronic otitis media

(3) Stratified squamous epithelium was present in all cases where the ossicles were removed from cholesteatomatous ears, but this epithelium was never found lining the bone lesions directly. Wherever bone destruction was present in cholesteatomatous ears, granulation tissue or connective tissue, or both, were found between the bone defect and the stratified squamous epithelium (Figs. 46 & 47). Stratified squamous epithelium also covered healthy bone but here again, some connective tissue separated the two.

(4) Ossicles from ears with simple chronic otitis media, as well as limited areas in cholesteatomatous ossicles, showed cuboidal or respiratory epithelium covering the granulation or connective tissue which lined the bone defect (Fig. 48). This epithelium was also seen over intact bone but never in direct contact with it; some connective tissue always separated the two.

(5) In no case did we find superimposed layers of normal middle ear mucosa and stratified squamous epithelium; every specimen showed at one point either the one or the other (Fig. 47); that is, whenever stratified squamous epithelium was seen, it replaced the normal mucosa. In no instance was there normal mucosa between stratified squamous epithelium and bone.

(6) Seventeen to 20% of the ossicles in both groups showed an inflammatory reaction deep in the bony spaces (osteomyelitis) in conjunction with bone destruction (Table 15).

(7) The relation of glands to ossicles was

TABLE 15

Effect of Cholesteatoma Culture Medium and Corresponding Canal Skin Culture Medium on ^{45}Ca Release by Embryonic Bones During Organ Culture

		^{45}Ca Release Ratio (48 hrs.)		
Sample	Cholesteatoma	Canal	Skin	
1	1.29±0.08	p > 0.05	1.07±0.06	N.S.
2	1.55±0.30	*N.S.	**N.D.	
3	1.37±0.10	p > 0.02	0.97±0.06	N.S.
4	1.61±0.19	p > 0.05	N.D.	
5	1.41±0.09	p > 0.02	0.91±0.10	N.S.
6	4.07±0.20	p > 0.001	N.D.	
7	1.78±0.22	p > 0.02	N.D.	

* N.S. = Not Significant
**N.D. = Not Done

^{45}Ca release ratios are mean± S.E. for six pairs of cultures in each experiment; 24-hour preculture was used.

described elsewhere (Sadé, 1972).

Discussion

Our macroscopic and microscopic findings show bone resorption to occur in chronic otitis media whether stratified squamous epithelium is or is not present; i.e., cholesteatoma. Consequently, bone destruction is not necessarily related to the presence of cholesteatoma. Stratified squamous epithelium was not found in direct contact with resorbed bone in any of our patients. The common finding in both groups, as far as bone resorption is concerned, is an inflammatory reaction near the destroyed bone. Bone resorption in the presence of cholesteatoma can therefore be viewed as an aftermath of a non-specific inflammatory lesion. This observation was also made by Gippaudu (1958); Harris (1962); and Thomsen, et al (1974). Yet, bone destruction is twice as frequent in cholesteatomatous ears as in simple chronic otitis media. This could be due to infection which is found in the majority of cholesteatomatous ears. Only 58% of the patients with chronic otitis media without cholesteatoma had a "wet" infected ear. However, the rate of ossicular interruption was twice as high than in the other 42% "dry" ears.

Bone resorption associated with cholesteatoma is usually accompanied by bacterial infection whether acute or chronic. Probably, the frequency of an inflammatory process is due to the local condition which is a non-self-cleansing pocket. Here the cellular and keratin debris are an ideal culture media for bacteria. However, at times the connective tissue underlying the stratified squamous epithelium is inflamed without obvious infective process, as in silent epidermoid post-tympanoplasty inclusion graft cysts (Fig. 49). Such a reaction could explain bone resorption in the so-called "congenital cholesteatomas" in the absence of perforation or of infection (when pressure should obviously also be taken into account). Bony defects of the various silent "nature's mastoidectomies" could also be explained in a similar manner. Probably, such bone resorption is in relatively

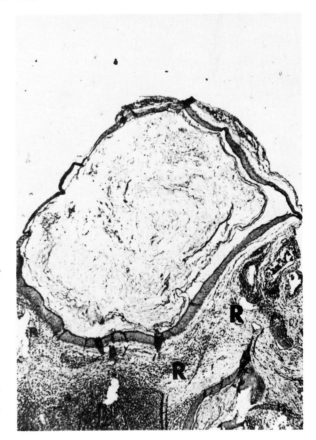

Fig. 49: Small epidermoid cyst—with an inflammatory reaction (r) underlying it.

slow progressive process when compared to bone resorption accompanied by vigorous infection. This may explain the rarity of accompanying bone destruction in recurrent non-infected postoperative cholesteatoma behind a non-perforated drum—and the actual difficulty in detecting such recurrences. Such recurrences are probably more frequent than may be realized, but their slow growth and minimal effect as long as secondary infection is absent, masks their quiet presence.

The detailed mechanism of inflammatory bone destruction is still obscure. This should probably entail first demineralization and thereafter degradation of the organic matrix (Sadé and Halevy, 1974; Sadé and Berko, 1974; Abramson, et al, 1975; and Abramson and Gross, 1971) both of which are mesenchymal, not epithelial phenomena. There is actually no evidence that stratified squamous epithelium has any direct "lytic" effect on bone.

Bone, like certain other tissues, shows a constant turnover under physiological conditions, a remodeling which entails breakdown and buildup. It would be plausible that the same modus operandi holds true in disease as in health—the difference being that under pathological conditions, the harmonious equilibrium is disturbed. One of the central questions, therefore, is understanding the change in direction of these reactions under inflammatory conditions which cause thereby more bone destruction than bone buildup.

Bone destruction in chronic otitis media was apparently much more extensive in days gone by—as seen from the greater frequency of intracranial breakthroughs and bone destruction seen on mastoid x-rays. Today, both are rare— only the scutum is at times seen to be eroded. This turn of events has its origin in antibiotic influence on inflammation, especially in its acute phase. In acute flareups of chronic ears much more bone is being destroyed and more complications occur. While infection has changed its character and is seen today in chronic ears more as a quiet smoldering process, it still is probably realistic to view destructive middle ear disease as usually of bacterial origin.

This study indicates that "running ears", now much less dangerous to life, can destroy the ossicular chain and lose the patient's hearing, whether or not cholesteatoma is present. The presence of stratified squamous epithelium by itself is less ominous than usually thought—its greatest danger is when it is topographically situated in such a fashion (pocket or cyst) that it cannot cleanse itself of debris and becomes secondarily infected.

Summary

We have attempted to clarify the mechanisms of bone destruction in chronic otitis media. A comparison of bone destruction in chronic otitis media in the presence of and absence of cholesteatoma was made. Macroscopically ossicular destruction was found in 84% of cholesteatomatous ears and 42.3% of chronic otitis media ears without cholesteatoma. Granulation tissue was usually associated with the ossicular lesion. Infected simple chronic otitis media ear without cholesteatoma showed twofold incidence of ossicular lesions compared with dry perforation. Microscopic granulation or connective tissue was also found with the bony defect whether or not cholesteatoma was present. Osteomyelitis occurred in about one-fifth of the ossicles of both groups. In no case was stratified squamous epithelium found to associate directly with bone destruction—inflammatory connective tissue was always interposed between the two. This study demonstrates that bone destruction in chronic otitis media occurs with and without cholesteatoma and is caused in both instances by an adjacent infected inflammatory reaction. At the same time, cholesteatoma can be associated with mild inflammatory reaction, not obviously of infective origin. Stratified squamous epithelium by itself is probably not a bone-absorbing agent, yet when topographically forming a cyst or a non-self-cleansing pocket, secondary infection might set in. While danger to life from chronic otitis media hardly exists, an infected "running ear", with or without cholesteatoma, does compromise the ossicular integrity, requiring special care.

References

1. Abramson, M. and Gross, J.: Further studies on collagenase in middle ear cholesteatoma. *Ann. Otol. Rhinol. Laryng.*, 80:177, 1971.

2. Abramson, M.; Asarch, R. G.; and Litton, W. B.: Experimental aural cholesteatoma causing bone resorption. *Ann. Otol. Rhinol. Laryng.*, 84:425,

1975.

3. Day, K. M.: The etiological factors in formation of cholesteatoma. *Ann. Otol. Rhinol Laryng.*, 43:837, 1934.

4. Gippaudu, M.: Histopathological studies of the ossicles in chronic otitis media. *J. Laryng. Otol.*, 72:177, 1958.

5. Harris, H. J.: Cholesteatosis and chronic otitis media. *Laryngoscope*, 72:954, 1962.

6. McKenzie, D.: The pathology of aural cholesteatoma. *J. Laryng. Otol.*, 46:163, 1931.

7. Ritter, F. N.: Chronic suppurative otitis media and the pathologic labyrinthine fistula. *Laryngoscope*, 80:1025, 1970.

8. Sade, J.: Epithelial invasion of intraossicular spaces. *J. Laryng. Otol.*, 86:15, 1972.

9. Sade, J. and Halevy, A.: The etiology of bone destruction in chronic otitis media. *J. Laryng. Otol.*, 88:139, 1974.

10. Sade, J. and Berko, E.: The inflammatory factor in bone destruction in chronic otitis media. *J. Laryng. Otol.*, 88:413, 1974.

11. Thomsen, J.; Jørgensen, M. B.; Bretlau, P.; and Kristensen, H. K.: Bone resorption in chronic otitis media. A histological and ultrastructural study. *J. Laryng. Otol.*, 88.975, 1974.

BONE RESORPTION IN CHRONIC OTITIS MEDIA

Jens Thomsen, M.D.
P. Bretlau, M.D.
M. B. Jørgensen, M.D.
H. K. Kristensen, M.D.

Ever since Cruveilhier (1829) described the "pearly" tumor of the middle ear, and Müller (1838) named it cholesteatoma, there has been discussion—at times heated—as to the origin and pathogenesis of cholesteatoma. The prevailing theories have been the following: (1) epidermoid or congenital, (2) traumatic, (3) metaplasia of middle ear epithelium, or (4) immigration of canal epidermis into the middle ear. However, discussion continues, and perhaps the origin of cholesteatoma is not from one of these causes, but from several (Karma, 1972).

Just as there has been discussion as to the origin of cholesteatoma, so there has been confusion regarding the activity of cholesteatoma, especially its seeming ability to erode bone. The usual explanation for the action of cholesteatoma on bone is that the exfoliated epithelial debris becomes trapped inside the epithelial cyst which swells, exerting pressure against the surrounding bone; the pressure then causes bone erosion by disrupting the blood supply. This has been repeatedly stated, but as yet there has been no experimental support for this theory.

To study bone resorption one must look where this resorption takes place: that is, the surface of bone in the middle ear. The following is a report of our investigations (light microscopical, electron microscopical and histochemical) of the subepithelial bone marginal zone in patients with chronic otitis media. We present evidence against the pressure-anoxia theory, and advance a new theory concerning the mechanism of bone resorption in the middle ear in chronic otitis media.

Methods and Material

(1) Light microscopical and electron microscopical examinations. Biopsies from various parts of the middle ear, wherever bone destruction was evident macroscopically, were taken with a fine chisel. Each biopsy was intended to include both cholesteatoma itself as well as underlying bone. The specimens were divided in 1-2 mm small pieces, fixed immediately in glutaraldehyde, decalcified in EDTA, post-fixed in osmium tetraoxide and embedded in EPON 812. For further information about details, see Thomsen et al (1974). Semi-thin survey sections were used for light microscopic examinations, and the ultra-thin sections examined with a Zeiss EM 9-S electron examination.

(2) Histochemical examinations. In each biopsy we attempted to include the cholesteatomatous membrane with the underlying subepithelial tissue and bone. The whole block was gently removed with a fine chisel. The biopsies were fixed in cold (4° C) formol-calcium, (4% formaldehyde containing 1% calcium chloride adjusted to pH 7,2 with sodium hydroxide). Decalcification was obtained with EDTA for 2-8 days, with storage at 4° C, depending upon the size of the biopsy. The specimens were then stored at 4° C in gum arabic (1% gum acacia in 0,88 M sucrose). Just before sectioning, the specimens were frozen in isopentane in a freezing mixture of acetone and solid carbon dioxide ($-80°$ C).

After mounting in the microtome, six sections were made from each specimen, the thickness alternating from 8-10 μm to 50 μm. Two of the thin sections (8-10 μm) were stained according to Barka and Anderson's method (1963) for demonstrating acid phosphatase using alpha-naphtyl phospate as substrate and pararosanilin as indicator, at pH 6,5 and room temperature. Staining times were 20 minutes and 30 minutes. The third section was used as a control of the staining specificity, either by avoiding the substrate or by applying sodium floride as an enzyme inhibitor. The specimens were mounted on glass slides and covered with a cover slip.

Ten biopsies from ten patients with otosclerosis served as normal material. These biopsies were taken from the promontory or the deepest part of the bony ear canal, where no macroscopic

otosclerotic foci were present, and prepared as described above.

As a control of the staining properties of the dye, a specimen of either mouse kidney or lung was stained the same day with the same solution of the pararosanilin as used for demonstration of acid phosphatase activity in our specimens.

Results

In the light microscope the cholesteatoma matrix was formed by typical keratinizing squamous epithelial cells. Whenever cholesteatoma was present the picture was as seen in Figure 50. Even if it macroscopically looked as if the cholesteatomatous membrane was lying directly upon

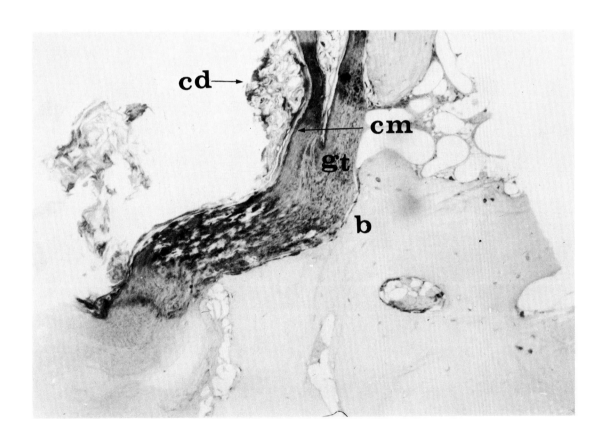

Fig. 50: Light microscopic picture of biopsy from patient with chronic otitis media, with cholesteatoma. The picture illustrates that cholesteatoma membrane (cm) is separated from underlying bone (b) by a subepithelial granulation tissue (gt). Cholesteatoma cyst with debris (cd).

the bone, it was clearly demonstrated in the light microscope that there was always a layer of subepithelial granulation tissue between the cholesteatoma cyst and membrane and the bone. This layer was formed by loose connective tissue containing collagen fibers and a cellularity varying from the specimen to specimen. In the marginal zone it was apparent that erosion of bone was found in close relation to a capillary surrounded by numerous, rather irregularly shaped cells (Fig. 51). The overall picture of the marginal zone was that of capillary proliferation (Figs. 51 and 52).

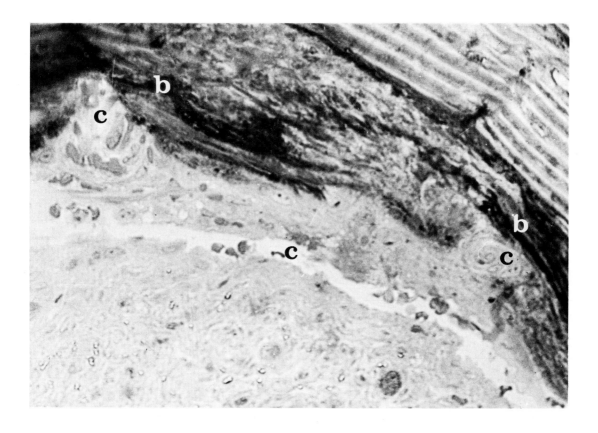

Fig. 51: Light microscopic picture of semi-thin survey section of biopsy from patient with chronic otitis media, with cholesteatoma. The picture shows the subepithelial-bone marginal zone. The bone (b) is eroded and there is a marked capillary and cellular proliferation. The capillaries (c) are in close relation to the bone.

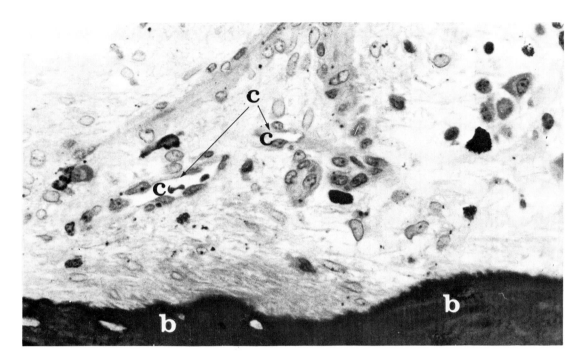

Fig. 52: Light microscopic picture of subepithelial granulation tissue in close relation to the bone
(b). Capillary (c).

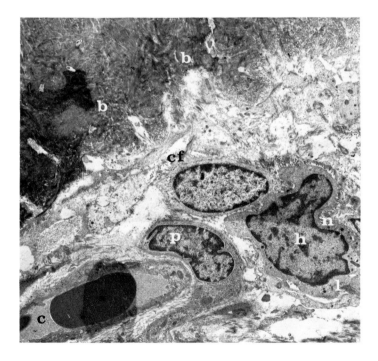

Fig. 53: Electron-microscopic picture of the subepithelial-bone marginal zone. The decalcified bone (b) is irregular and
eroded. The capillary (c) is displaying pinocytosis, and is lined by a pericyte (p) probably transforming into a
histiocyte. The characteristic finding is the histiocyte (h) with notches (n) and lysosomes (l). The stroma is a loose connective tissue, with collagen fibers (cf).

In the electron microscope the subepithelial layer presents a marked proliferation of fibrocytes and fibroblasts, with proliferation of capillaries, surrounded with pericytes in different shapes, some of them transforming into histiocytes. The capillaries were obviously of the "active" type, displaying pinocytosis and marginal folds (Fig. 53). Infiltration of inflammatory cells (neutrophillic leucocytes), often in a necrotic state, was evident. Occasional plasma cells, lymphocytes and a few mast cells were noted. The above mentioned histiocyte was the dominating cell in the marginal zone, close to the bone. Its electron microscopic appearance (Figs. 53 and 54) showed a cell 8-10 μ m in size, with relatively dark cytoplasm, containing dense cytoplasmatic bodies, called lysosomes (Figs. 53, 54, and 55). Ribosomes were numerous, and the number of mitochondria was greater than found in osteocytes. Endoplasmatic reticulum was scarce.

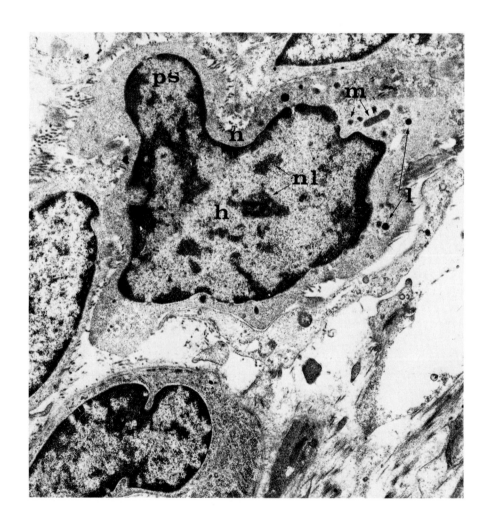

Fig. 54: Electron-microscopic picture of same cell as seen in Figure 53. This histiocyte (h) measures 9 μ m, is irregular with notches (n), pseudopodia (ps), mitochrondria (m) and lysosomes (1). The nucleus contains nucleoli (nl).

The cytoplasm contained vacuoles. The nucleus was dark and fairly large, though varied in shape, containing one or two nucleoli. A notching in one side of the nuclear membrane was a characteristic finding, the notching often corresponding to the vacuoles. The cell displayed pseudopodia of different sizes and shapes. The cell was usually found near proliferating capillaries, but could also be found scattered along the surface of the bone.

The results of the histochemical examinations were rather uniform: all biopsies containing macroscopically eroded bone as well as granulation tissue showed a marked acid phosphatase activity in the resorbing margin of bone. The activity with the Barka and Anderson (1963) simultaneous coupling azo dye method, using alpha-naphtyl phosphate as substrate and pararosanilin as the coupler, is indicated with a red or reddish-brown dye deposit. The dye was localized in some specimens as a rather homogeneous deposit

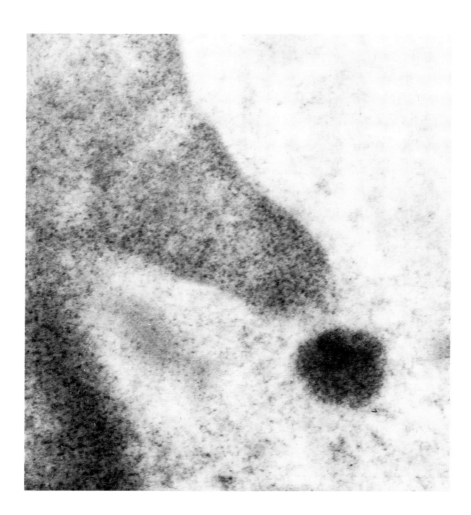

Fig. 55: High power view of the dense cytoplasmatic body, called a lysosome, found in high numbers in the histiocyte.

spread along the entire surface of the bone (Fig. 56). In other parts it was seen in isolated erosions of the bone (Fig. 57), in relation to the proliferated capillaries, here too, as a rather homogeneous deposit. Furthermore, it was clear that some cells, either spread along the bony surface or at some distance from the bone, displayed acid phosphatase activity (Fig. 58). This activity was not uniformly spread in the cytoplasm, but was concentrated in small particles. The cells had only one nucleus, and this nucleus was not stained. These cells could very well be histiocytes. On examining the normal material it was demonstrated that none of these biopsies showed any activity either in the subepithelial layer or in the bone, when using the fixation, decalcification and staining methods described above.

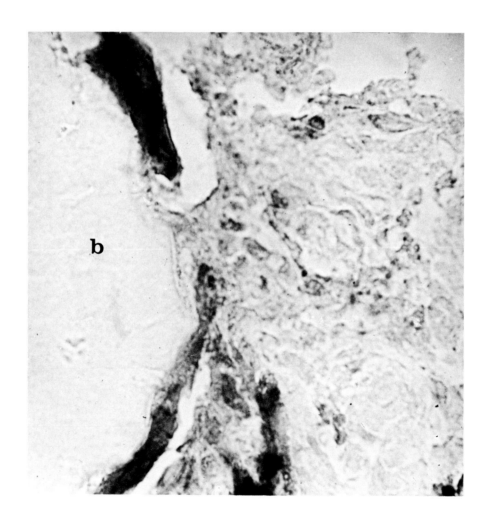

Fig. 56: Light-microscopic picture of the subepithelial-bone marginal zone in biopsy from the middle ear, in a patient with chronic cholesteatomatous otitis media. The dye deposit is due to acid phosphatase activity, spread over the entire eroded surface of the bone.

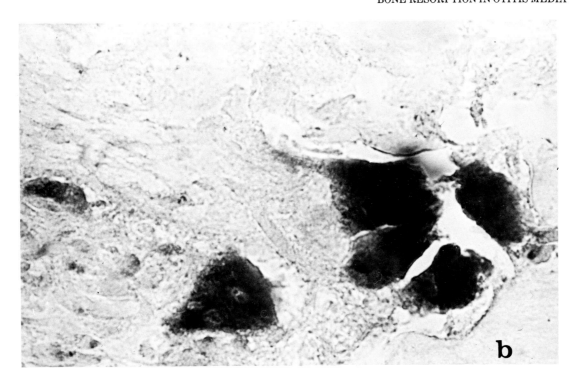

Fig. 57: Acid phosphatase activity, represented by a reddish hexaxonium pararosanilin, a homogeneous deposit in a localized erosion of the bone.

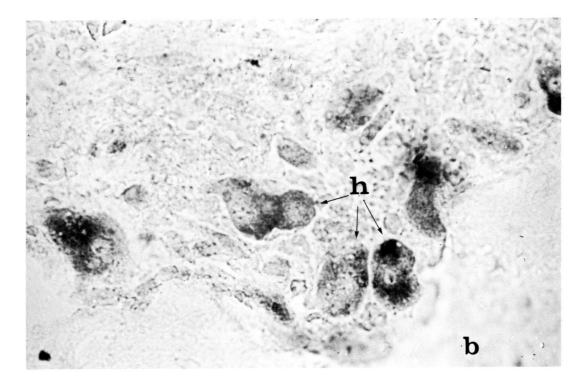

Fig. 58: Acid phosphatase activity is seen in mononuclear cells, possibly histiocytes (h), spread along the eroded surface of the bone (b).

Discussion

With regard to the role of cholesteatoma in bone resorption in patients with chronic otitis media, we have demonstrated in previous papers that cholesteatoma itself is not necessary for bone resorption (Thomsen et al, 1974). These findings have been supported by observations by Sade and Halevy (1974), and Abramson et al (1975). We have shown that the cellular population of the submucosa bone marginal zone is essentially the same whether cholesteatoma is present or not. We have demonstrated that capillary proliferation is a cardinal finding in the resorbing margin of bone, emphasizing the improbability of the anoxia theory in middle ear bone resorption. The dominating cell in the eroded marginal zone is a mononuclear, histocyte-like cell, with dense cytoplasmatic bodies, of lysosomatic character.

The term lysosome was first introduced by DeDuve and co-workers (Appelmans et al, 1955), for a fraction of cell particles, distinct from mitochondria, being rich in lytic enzymes. About 40 hydrolytic enzymes, most of them hydrolases, have been demonstrated so far (DeDuve, 1969).

The first report of enzymatic activity in chronic otitis media was published by Harris (1962). He found acid phosphatase to have a distinct localization in the stratum granulosum of the cholesteatoma epidermis, but no activity was found in the deeper layers of the epidermis or throughout all the subepithelial connective tissues. No reaction was found in bone. Paparella and Dito (1964) examined the enzyme content of serous middle ear effusions. The normal middle ear mucosa was examined histochemically by Lim and Hussl (1969) and Hiraide and Paparella (1971 and 1972). Maeda, et al (1967) and Palva, et al (1970) also localized the acid phosphatase activity to the stratum granulosum, but did not examine the submucosa bone area. Furthermore, Palva, et al (1970) investigated the lactate dehydrogenase pattern of the middle ear mucosa in chronic otitis with cholesteatoma as well as the esterases (Palva, et al, 1971).

Abramson (1969) and Abramson and Gross (1971) studied the activity of collagenase in middle ear cholesteatoma. They found the highest collagenolytic activity when granulation tissue was present, and that granulation tissue in itself could lyse the collagen.

In contrast to the finding of Harris (1962) Zechner, et al (1968) demonstrated that highly positive acid phosphatase activity was visible when studying bone trabeculae obtained at tympanotomy. The strongest ferment activity was noticeable in the granulation tissue lying closest to the bone. Until now, this observation has remained unnoticed.

In order to discuss bone resorption in general, one must have in mind the composition of bone. According to Eastoe (1956), bone consists of inorganic material, mostly calcium phosphatate, collagen, water (about 20%), mucopolysaccharide and resistant protein.

Under resorptive stimulus the bone cells produce considerable amounts of acids, mostly lactic, and to a lesser extent citric acid, due to glycolytic activity (Borle, et al, 1960 and Nichols, 1963). The lowering of the pH makes the calcium phosphate salts of the mineral easily soluble.

There are two possible mechanisms for the removal of the decalcified collagen matrix: degradation by a specific collagenase active, at neutral pH, of the native collagen molecule, or digestion by non-specific, possibly lysosomal, acid hydrolases after denaturation of the molecule by local accumulations of metabolic acid.

Collagenolytic activity at neutral pH has been shown to exist in isolated bone cells from animals and man (Walker, et al, 1964; Woods and Nichols, 1965; Abramson, 1969; and Abramson and Gross, 1971).

Likewise, Vaes (1969) has shown that bone cells contain lysosomes, and that the rate of synthesis and release of typical acid hydrolases are markedly increased by parathyroid hormone in tissue culture. Thus both mechanisms for collagen breakdown seem to exist in bone. Vaes (1965) and Vaes and Jacques (1965) have furthermore demonstrated that lysosomal hydrolytic enzymes are capable of degrading mucopolysaccharides. The same lysosomal enzyme would presumably be able to remove bone cells. But which cells are responsible for the bone resorption? It is generally accepted that the multinuclear osteoclast, with its lysosomal hydrolases, is capable and responsible for the normal resorption (Gonzales and Karnovsky, 1961; Hancox and Boothroyd, 1963; Young, 1963; and Irving and Heeley, 1970). Several authors have presented evidence suggesting that the osteocytes are capable of resorbing their lacunar walls (Jaffe, 1933; Heller-Steinberg, 1951; Bélanger, et al, 1963; Bélanger, 1965; Bélanger, et al, 1966; and Frost, et al, 1960). Jaffee (1933) and Cameron (1961) have indicated that endothelial cells may be implicated in resorption. Muhlethaler (1953); Goldhaber (1961); Andersen and Mathiessen (1966); Chevance, et al (1970); and Bretlau, et al (1971) have suggested that histiocytes are capable of bone resorption, or they can serve as precursors of osteoclasts (Hancox, 1963 and Jee and Nolan, 1962).

Conceivably, these cells represent mesenchymal specializations which have retained their capacity to resorb and are capable of doing this under suitable circumstances (Young, 1963). Goldhaber (1961 and 1963) demonstrated that high oxygen tensions induced an osteoclastic type of bone resorption with increased collagenolysis (Stern, et al, 1966). Sledge (1966) and Sledge and Dingle (1965) could release and activate the lysosomes by hyperoxia in cartilage resorption. Allison (1965) could also activate the lysosomes of marcrophages by excess oxygen. It is therefore conceivable that increased oxygen tensions could play a significant role in the release of hydrolytic, lysosomal enzymes from the mononuclear, histiocyte-like cell with subsequent bone resorption in chronic otitis media.

Apart from high oxygen tensions, other factors may have an influence on bone resorption. Stern (1971) could induce resorption of living bone with the presence of serum albumin, and the effect was concentration dependent. Hausmann, et al (1972) could stimulate bone resorption with highly purified lipopolysaccharides, and Hausmann, et al (1973) increased resorption in tissue culture by adding unheated normal serum. Puche, et al (1973) concluded that insulin stimulates bone resorption.

In this presentation we have demonstrated that the marker enzyme for lysosomal activity, the acid phophatase, is present in large quantities along the eroded bone in the middle ear, both intracellularly in mononuclear cells as well as extracellularly. As stated by Vaes (1969) it appears difficult to avoid the conclusion that the lysosomes and their enzymes are directly involved in the processes of bone resorption. However, in chronic otitis media, the enzymatic activity seems to originate from a histiocyte-like cell, rather than from a multinucleated, giant cell, osteoclast, normally found in resorptive zones. We have not been able to demonstrate any of these giant cells, a finding which is supported by the examinations of Abramson, et al (1975), who could not either demonstrate osteoclasts at the resorbing margin of bone. This finding corresponds to the observations of Chevance, et al (1970), that on the active, otosclerotic front they could not find a single osteoclast, but the picture was dominated by mononuclear, histiocyte-like cells, showing acid phosphatase activity in the lysosomal-like bodies in the cytoplasm. Even though the etiology of otosclerosis is entirely different from that of middle ear infection, there is no reason to believe that the absorption of bone, on a cellular basis, should differ in any way.

The following working theory concerning the mechanism of bone resorption is therefore proposed: some inflammatory stimulus that may be sepsis, a foreign body reaction or a migrating epithelial layer, entails capillary proliferation. This is followed by a progressing differentiation of the pericyte which assumes a more roundish shape, and migrates away from the capillary as a mature histiocyte, now containing lysosomal enzymes capable of destroying bone. The release of the lysosomal enzymes is enhanced by the presence of high oxygen tensions, due to the capillary proliferation.

Summary

Even though Cruveilhier described cholesteatoma, the pearly tumor of the ear, in 1829, it is still unknown how it erodes the bone of the middle ear. It is not necessary for cholesteatoma to be present for bone resorption in chronic otitis media. When it is present, there is always a subepithelial layer of granulation tissue between the cholesteatomatous membrane and the underlying bone, with domination of capillary and cellular proliferation. Both light microscopically as well as electron microscopically, the dominating cell is a histiocyte-like cell, with a content of dense cytoplasmatic bodies, called lysosomes. The marker enzyme for lysosomal enzymatic activity, the acid phosphatase, is present in large quantities along the eroded bone as well as localized in small particles in a histiocyte-like cell found in the resorbing margin of bone. The authors believe the evidence is conclusive that these lysosomes, with their enzymes are directly involved in the process of bone resorption in chronic otitis media.

References

1. Abramson, M.: Collagenolytic activity in middle ear cholesteatoma. *Ann. Otol. Rhinol. Laryngol.*, 78: 112, 1969.

2. Abramson, M. and Gross, J.: Further studies on a collagenase in middle ear cholesteatoma. *Ann. Otol. Rhinol. Laryngol.*, 80: 177, 1971.

3. Abramson, M.; Asarch, R. G.; and Litton, W. B.: Experimental aural cholesteatoma causing bone resorption. *Ann. Otol. Rhinol. Laryngol.*, 84 (4 Pt. 1): 425, 1975.

4. Allison, A. C.: Role of lysosomes in oxygen toxicity. *Nature* (London), 205: 141, 1965.

5. Andersen, H. and Mathiessen, M. E.: The histiocyte in human foetal tissues. Its morphology, cytochemistry and origin, function and fate. *Z Zellforsch. Mikrosk. Anat.*, 72: 193, 1966.

6. Appelmans, F.; Wattiaux, R.; and DeDuve, C.: Tissue fractionation studies 5. The association of acid phosphatase with a special class of cytoplasmatic granules in the liver. *Biochem. J.*, 59: 438, 1955.

7. Barka, T.: *Histochemistry, Theory, Practice and Bibliography.* Hoeber Medical Division, New York, New York, 1963.

8. Bélanger, L. F.: Osteolysis: An outlook on its mechanism and causation. In Gaillard, P. J.; Talmage, R. V.; and Budy, A. M.: (Eds.). *The Parathyroid Glands: Ultrastructure, Secretion and Function.* The University of Chicago Press, Chicago, Illinois, 1965, p. 140.

9. Bélanger, L. F.; Robichon, J.; Migicovsky, B. B., et al: Resorption without osteoclasts (osteolysis). In Sognnaes, R.: (Ed.). *Mechanisms of Hard Tissue Destruction.* American Association for Advancement of Science, Publication No. 75, Washington, D.C., 1963, p. 531.

10. Bélanger, L. F.; Semba, T.; Tolnai, S. et al: The two faces of resorption. In Fleisch, H.; Blackwood, H. J.; and Owen, M.: (Ed.). *Calcified Tissues 1965 Proceedings of the Third European Symposium on Calcified Tissues held at Davos.* Springer Verlag, New York, New York, 1966, p. 1-10.

11. Borle, A. B.; Nichols, N.; and Nichols G. Jr.: Metabolic studies of bone in vitro. II. The metabolic patterns of accretion and resorption. *J. Biol. Chem.*, 235: 1211, 1960.

12. Bretlau, P.; Causse, J.; Balslev Jørgensen, M. et al: Histiocytic activity in otosclerotic bone. *Arch. Klin. Exp. Ohren. Nasen Kehlkopfheilkd.*, 198: 301, 1971.

13. Cameron, D. A.: Erosion of the epiphysis of the rat tibia by capillaris. *J. Bone Joint Surg. (Br)* 43B: 590, 1961.

14. Chevance, L. G.; Bretlau, P.; Balslev Jørgensen, M. et al: Otosclerosis. An electron microscopic and cytochemical study. *Acta Otolaryngol, Suppl. (Stockh)*, 272: 1+, 1970.

15. Cruveilhier, J.: *Anatomie Pathologigue du Corps Human.* Vol. 1. J. B. Bailliere, Paris, France, 1829, p. 349.

16. DeDuve, C.: The lysosomes in retrospect. In Dingle, J. T. and Fell, H. B.: (Ed.). *Lysosomes in Biology and Pathology*, Vol. 1. North Holland Publishing Company, New York, New York, 1969, p. 1.

17. Eastoe, J. E.: The organic matrix of bone. In Bourne, G. H.: (Ed.). *The Biochemistry and Physiology of Bone.* Academic Press, New York,

New York, 1956, p. 81.

18. Frost, H. M.; Villaneuva, A. R.; and Roth, H.: Halo volume. *Henry Ford Hosp. Med. Bull.* 8: 228, 1960.

19. Goldhaber, P.: Oxygen-dependent bone resorption in tissue culture. In Greep, R. O. and Talmage, R. V.: (Eds.). *Parathyroids. Proceedings of a Symposium on Advances in Parathyroid Research.* Charles C Thomas, Springfield, Illinois, 1961, p. 243.

20. Goldhaber, P.: Some chemical factors influencing bone resorption in tissue culture. In Sognnaes, R.: (Ed.). *Mechanisms of Hard Tissue Destruction.* American Association for Advancement of Science, Publication No. 75, Washington, D.C., 1963, p. 609.

21. Gonzales, F. and Karnovsky, M. J.: Electron microscopy of osteoclasts in healing fractures of rat bone. *J. Biophys. Biochem. Cytol.,* 9: 299, 1961.

22. Hancox, N. M. and Boothroyd, B.: Structure-function relationships in the osteoclasts. In Sognnaes, R.: (Ed.). *Mechanisms of Hard Tissue Destruction.* American Association for Advancement of Science, Publication No. 75, Washington, D.C., 1963, p. 497.

23. Harris, A. J.: Cholesteatosis and chronic otitis media. The histopathology of osseous and soft tissue. *Laryngoscope,* 72: 954, 1962.

24. Hausmann, E.; Genco, R.; Weinfeld, N. et al: Effects of sera on bone resorption in tissue culture. *Calcif. Tissue Res.,* 13: 311, 1973.

25. Hausmann, E.; Weinfeld, N.; and Miller, W. A.: Effects of lipopolysaccharides on bone resorption in tissue culture. *Calcif. Tissue Res.,* 9: 272, 1972.

26. Heller-Steinberg, M.: Ground substance, bone salts and cellular activity in bone formation and destruction. *Am. J. Anat.* 89: 347, 1951.

27. Hiraide, F. and Paparella, M. M.: Histochemistry of the normal eustachian tube. *Acta Otolaryngol. (Stockh),* 72: 310, 1971.

28. Hiraide, F. and Paparella, M. M.: Histochemical characteristics of normal ear mucosa. *Acta Otolaryngol, (Stockh).,* 74: 45 1972.

29. Irving, J. T. and Heeley, J. D.: Resorption of bone collagen by multi-nucleated cells. *Calcif. Tissue Res.,* 6: 254, 1970.

30. Jaffe, H. L.: Hyperparathyroidism (Recklinghausens' disease of bone). *Arch. Pathol.,* 16: 63, July and 236, August; 1933.

31. Jee, W. S. S. and Nolan, P.: Origin of osteoclasts from coalescence of histiocytes. *Anat. Rec.,* 142: 310, 1962.

32. Karma, P.: Middle ear epithelium and chronic ear disease. *Acta Otolaryngol. Suppl.,* 307: 7, 1972.

33. Lim, D. J. and Hussl, B.: Human middle ear epithelium. An ultrastructural and cytochemical study. *Arch. Otolaryngol, (Chicago),* 89: 835, 1969.

34. Maeda, M.; Tabata, T.; Shimada, T. et al: Histological and histochemical studies on cholesteatoma epidermis. *Ann. Otol. Rhinol. Laryngol.,* 76: 1043,

1967.

35. Muhlethaler, J. P.: La resorption de l'os mort etudiée par la methode de culture des tissus. *Z. Zellforsch. Mikrosk. Anat.,* 38: 69, 1953.

36. Müller, J.: *Uber den feinern Bau und die Formen der krankhaften Geschwulste.* G. Reimer, Berlin, Germany, 1838, p. 50.

37. Nichols, G. Jr.: In vitro studies of bone resorptive mechanisms. In Sognnaes, R.: (Ed.). *Mechanisms of Hard Tissue Destruction.* American Association for Advancement of Science, Publication No. 75, Washington, D.C., 1963, p. 557.

38. Palva, T.; Forsén, R.; Raunio, V. et al: Lactate dehydrogenase pattern of middle ear mucosa. *Pract. Otorhinolaryngol, (Basel),* 32: 129, 1970.

39. Palva, T.; Palva, A.; and Dammert, L.: Middle ear mucosa and chronic ear disease. II. Enzyme studies. *Arch. Otolaryngol.,* 91: 50, 1970.

40. Palva, T.; Raunio, V.; Forsén, R. et al: Esterases of postauricular and ear canal skin, compared with cholesteatoma epithelium. *Acta Otolaryngol. (Stockh).,* 72: 329, 1971.

41. Paparella, M. M. and Dito, W. R.: Enzyme studies in serous otitis media. *Arch. Otolaryngol. (Chicago),* 79: 393, 1964.

42. Puche, R. C.; Romano, M. C.; Locatto, M. E. et al: The effect of insulin on bone resorption. *Calcif. Tissue Res.,* 12: 8, 1973.

43. Sadé, J. and Halevy, A.: The aetiology of bone destruction in chronic otitis media. *J. Laryngol. Otol.,* 88: 139, 1974.

44. Sledge, C. B.: Lysosomes and cartilage resorption on organ culture. In Fleisch, H. F.; Blackwood, H. J. J.; and Owen, M.: (Eds.). *Calcified Tissues 1965 Proceedings of the Third European Symposium on Calcified Tissues held at Davos.* Springer-Verlag, New York, New York, 1966, p. 52.

45. Sledge, C. B. and Dingle, J. T.: Activation of lysosomes by oxygen: Oxygen-induced resorption of cartilage in organ culture. *Nature (London),* 205: 140, 1965.

46. Stern, B.; Glimacher, M. J.; and Goldhaber, P.: The effect of various oxygen tensions on the synthesis and degradation of bone collagen in tissue culture. *Proc. Soc. Exp. Biol. Med.,* 121: 869, 1966.

47. Stern, P. H.: Albumin-induced resorption of fetal rat bone in vitro. *Calcif. Tissue Res.,* 7: 67, 1971.

48. Thomsen, J.; Balslev Jørgensen, M.; Bretlau, P. et al: Bone resorption in chronic otitis media. A histological and ultrastructural study. I. Ossicular necrosis. *J. Laryngol. Otol.,* 88: 975, 1974.

49. Thomsen, J.; Balslev Jørgensen, M.; Bretlau, P. et al: Bone resorption in chronic otitis media. A histological and ultrastructural study. II. Cholesteatoma. *J. Laryngol. Otol.,* 88: 983, 1974.

50. Vaes, G.: Hydrolytic enzymes and lysosomes in

bone cells. In Richelle, L. J. and Dallemagne, M. J.: (Ed.). *Proceedings of the Second European Symposium on Calcified Tissues, Liege.* University of Liege, Liege, Belgium, 1965, p. 51.

51. Vaes, G.: Lysosomes and bone resorption. In Dingle, J. T. and Fell, H. B.: (Eds.). *Lysosomes in Biology and Pathology.* Vol. 1. North-Holland Publishing Company, New York, New York, 1969, p. 247.

52. Vaes, G. and Jacques, P.: Studies on bone enzymes. The assay of acid hydrolases and other enzymes in bone tissue. *Biochem. J.,* 97: 380, 1965.

53. Walker, D. G.; Lapiere, C. M.; and Gross, J.: A collagenolytic factor in rat bone promoted by parathyroid extract. *Biochem. Biophys. Res. Commun.,* 15: 397, 1964.

54. Woods, J. F. and Nichols, G. Jr.: Collagenolytic activity in rat bone cells. Characteristics and intracellular location. *J. Cell Biol.,* 26: 747, 1965.

55. Young, R. W.: Histophysical studies on bone cells and bone resorption. In Sognnaes, R.: (Ed.). *Mechanisms of Hard Tissue Destruction.* American Association for Advancement of Science, Publication No. 75, Washington, D.C., 1963, p. 471.

56. Zechner, G.; Tarkkanen, J.; and Holopainen, E.: Histomorphological and histochemical studies of chronically infected middle ear mucous membrane. *Ann. Otol.,* 77: 54, 1968.

OSTEOCLAST ACTIVATING FACTOR

Gregory R. Mundy, M.D.
Lawrence G. Raisz, M.D.

Localized bone resorption is often found adjacent to collections of chronic inflammatory cells or tumor cells. This occurs in diseases such as rheumatoid arthritis where lytic bone lesions occur adjacent to involved joints; in chronic osteomyelitis where bone is resorbed to form sequestra and limit the spread of infection; and in periodontal disease of the gingiva where alveolar bone is resorbed and the teeth fall out. Malignant disease also frequently involves the skeleton, either in the form of bone metastases or in the production of hypercalcemia.

Bone resorption is a very specialized process which involves both the release of mineral from bone and the breakdown of bone matrix, probably by a series of lysosomal enzymes working at acid pH, and collagenase. The major cell responsible for bone resorption is the osteoclast, which has all the intracellular machinery necessary to accomplish this complex process. It is our hypothesis that the localized bone resorption which occurs in chronic inflammatory disease and in neoplasia is due to the stimulation of osteoclasts by humoral mediators which are released by chronic inflammatory cells or neoplastic cells. There are five known humoral agents which stimulate osteoclastic activity and bone resorption. These are parathyroid hormone (PTH) (Raisz, 1965), the active metabolites of vitamin D (Raisz, et al, 1972), the thyroid hormones (Mundy, et al, 1976), prostaglandins (Klein and Raisz, 1970), and osteoclast activating factor (OAF) (Horton, et al, 1972). Both OAF and the prostaglandins are likely mediators of the localized bone resorption which occurs in chronic inflammation and in neoplasia. The role of prostaglandins has recently been reviewed (Dietrich and Raisz, 1975).

OAF is a potent bone resorbing factor which is released by normal human peripheral blood leukocytes when they are activated by an antigen to which they have previously been exposed, or by a mitogen such as phytohemagglutinin (Horton, et al, 1972). Over the last few years, the biological effects of OAF in vitro have been described (Raisz, et al, 1975), and OAF has been partially characterized chemically (Luben, et al, 1974). OAF is one of a series of biologically active mediators which are released by stimulated leukocytes after activation as part of the cell-mediated immune defense mechanism.

The biological effects of OAF have been assessed using a sensitive bioassay for bone resorption which has been described in detail previously (Raisz, 1965 and Raisz, et al, 1975). This assay involves the release of previously incorporated ^{45}Ca from fetal rat long bones organ culture. At the 18th day of gestation, pregnant rats are injected with 0.2 millicuries of ^{45}Ca. The following day the mother is sacrificed, the uterus sectioned, and the mineralized shafts of the fetal radius and ulna are dissected free. These mineralized shafts are precultured for 24 hours to allow for the exchange of loosely-complexed ^{45}Ca with stable calcium in the culture medium. During the following 48 hours the bones are cultured in the presence of the mediator of bone resorption being assessed. Bone resorbing activity is quantitated by the ratio of the release of ^{45}Ca from paired test and control bones, or the percent total radioactivity released from individual bones. The significance of differences between test and control is assessed using Student's t-test.

When OAF containing leukocyte culture supernatants are cultured with fetal rat long bones, histologic sections of the bones show increased osteoclast activity compared with control bones (Horton, et al, 1972). OAF treated bones contain numerous osteoclasts with foamy vaculated cytoplasm, multiple nuclei, and decreased mineralized matrix. Electron microscopy of these bones show an increased area of osteoclast ruffled borders and clear zones (Holtrop, Raisz and Simmons, unpublished observations). These findings are relatively nonspecific. Similar findings are seen when bones are cultured in the presence of parathyroid hormone or prostaglandins.

Studies on the cell source of origin of OAF have shown that both lymphocytes and monocytes are necessary for OAF production (Horton, et al, 1974). When unseparated normal human peripheral blood leukocytes containing neutrophils, lymphocytes and monocytes were stimulated with phytohemagglutinin, potent bone resorbing activity was found in the leukocyte culture supernatants. When neutrophils were removed from the cell preparation by ficoll-hypaque gravity sedimentation, there was no decrease in bone resorbing activity after PHA activation. When monocytes were removed by passing the leukocytes through a glass-bead column, purified lymphocytes produced no bone resorbing activity after activation. Peritoneal macrophages alone produced no bone resorbing activity. However, when macrophages were added back to lymphocytes, OAF was produced by the activated lymphocyte-monocyte cell population. Thus, it was concluded that lymphocyte-monocyte synergy is necessary for normal OAF production.

Most of the OAF like activity in activated leukocyte culture supernatants can be chromatographed on Sephadex G100 columns to elute between the molecular weight markers, Chymotrypsinogen (25,000 daltons) and Ribonuclease A (13,700 daltons) (Luben, et al, 1974). The biological activity eluting between these two molecular weight markers is now called "Big OAF", because there is another peak of biological activity which

elutes from Sephadex G50 columns in the same area as ^{3}H-proline (molecular weight 140 daltons). The biological activity eluting in this area has been called "Little OAF" (Mundy, et al, 1976). Big OAF and Little OAF are related. When Big OAF was equilibrated in 1M sodium chloride or 2M urea and chromatographed again on a Sephadex G50 column, the biological activity eluted in the Little OAF area. This indicates that Big OAF is converted to Little OAF under dissociating conditions. When Little OAF was equilibrated with Tris-HCl buffer at ionic strength .005M, the biological activity eluted from Sephadex G50 columns in the Big OAF area. Thus under conditions favoring reaggregation, Little OAF is converted back to Big OAF. The biological activity produced by leukocyte culture supernatants can also be transferred across an Amicon PM10 membrane (assigned molecular weight cutoff 10,000 daltons) by equilibrating the media in buffers favoring dissociation (higher ionic strength) while it is retained by such membranes in buffers favoring reaggregation (lower ionic strength).

The biological activity produced by activated leukocyte culture supernatants is separate from PTH, prostaglandins and the vitamin D metabolites (Luben, et al, 1974). PTH and PGE immunoassays on biologically active leukocyte culture supernatants do not contain enough immuno-reactive material to account for the biological activity in the culture supernatants. Similarly, extraction of the leukocyte culture supernatants in organic solvents which extract vitamin D metabolites and prostaglandins do not extract the biological activity.

Although Big OAF is not extracted in organic solvents which extract prostaglandins (acidified ethyl acetate), we have found recently that Little OAF is extracted in ethyl acetate acidified to pH 3.5. It is unlikely however, that Little OAF is a prostaglandin, prostaglandin metabolite or prostaglandin analog because of the reaggregation phenomena. It is more likely that Little OAF is either a small peptide or other lipid-soluble compound which is a potent stimulator of bone resorption.

There are a number of ways in which OAF could be involved in the bone resorption which occurs in chronic inflammation and in malignant disease. Firstly, in disease where chronic inflammatory cells accumulate, activated leukocytes may release OAF which stimulates osteoclasts locally to resorb bone. This could account in part for the bone resorption which occurs in diseases such as rheumatoid arthritis, periodontal disease, or chronic osteomyelitis. Secondly, in neoplastic disease, OAF may be responsible for localized bone resorption in several ways. It could be released by normal leukocytes as part of the cellular immune response to a tumor. It could also be released directly by the malignant cells themselves. This is the mechanism for which we have the most evidence at present. In myeloma and other hematologic neoplasms, bone resorption and hypercalcemia occur very frequently. We have now gathered evidence that the cellular mechanism of bone resorption in myeloma is osteoclastic and that the myeloma cells themselves secrete a bone resorbing factor with similar chemical and biological characteristics to OAF (Mundy, et al, 1974; Mundy, et al, 1974).

References

1. Dietrich, J. W. and Raisz, L. G.: Prostaglandin in calcium and bone metabolism. *Clin. Orthopedics and Related Research*, 111:228, 1975.

2. Horton, J. E.; Raisz, L. G.; Simmons, H. A.; Oppenheim, J. J.; and Mergenhagen, S. E.: Bone resorbing activity in supernatant fluid from cultured human peripheral blood leukocytes. *Science*, 177:793, 1972.

3. Horton, J. E.; Oppenheim, J. J.; Mergenhagen, S. E.; and Raisz, L. G.: Macrophage-lymphocyte synergy in the production of osteoclast activating factor. *J. Immunol.*, 113:1278, 1974.

4. Klein, D. C. and Raisz, L. G.: Prostaglandins: Stimulation of bone resorption in tissue culture. *Endocrinology*, 86:1436, 1970.

5. Luben, R. A.; Mundy, G. R.; Trummel, C. L.; and Raisz, L. G.: Partial purification of osteoclast activating factor from phytohemagglutinin-stimulated human leukocytes. *J. Clin. Invest.*, 53:1473, 1974.

6. Mundy, G. R.; Luben, R. A.; Raisz, L. G.; Oppenheim, J. J.; and Buell, D. N.: Bone resorbing activity in supernatants from lymphoid cell lines. *New Engl. J. Med.*, 290:867, 1974.

7. Mundy, G. R.; Raisz, L. G.; Cooper, R. A.; Schechter, G. P.; and Salmon, S. E.: Evidence for the secretion of an osteoclast stimulating factor in myeloma. *New Engl. J. Med.*, 291:1041, 1974.

8. Mundy, G. R.; Shapiro, J. L.; Bandelin, J. G.; Canalis, E. M.; and Raisz, L. G.: Direct stimulation of bone resorption by thyroid hormones. *J. Clin. Invest.*, 1976 (in press).

9. Mundy, G. R.; Shapiro, J. L.; and Raisz, L. G.: Big and little OAF—evidence for the heterogeneity of osteoclast activating factor. *Clin. Res.*, 23:592, 1976.

10. Raisz, L. G.: Bone resorption in tissue culture: Factors influencing the response to parathyroid hormone. *J. Clin. Invest.*, 44:103, 1965.

11. Raisz, L. G.; Trummel, C. L.; Holick, M. F.; and DeLuca, H. F.: 1,25-dihydroxycholecalciferol: A potent stimulator of bone resorption in tissue culture. *Science*, 175:768, 1972.

12. Raisz, L. G.; Luben, R. A.; Mundy, G. R.; Dietrich, J. W.; Horton, J. E.; and Trummel, C. L.: Effect of osteoclast activating factor from human leukocytes on bone metabolism. *J. Clin. Invest.*, 56:408, 1975.

MIDDLE EAR DISEASE RELEASE OF SOLUBLE FACTOR(S) STIMULATING BONE RESORPTION

Joel M. Bernstein, M.D., M.A.
Ernest Hausmann, D.M.D., Ph.D.
John Wright, M.D.

Introduction

The mechanism of bone resorption in chronic otitis media with or without cholesteatoma, is essentially unknown. In the late 50's, Reudi (1958) and Tumarkin (1958) suggested that bone resorption in chronic otitis media was the result of direct pressure on bone from the cholesteatoma mass. Later, Thomsen, et al (1974) suggested that ossicular destruction in middle ear disease resulted from the inflammatory process itself, specifically from the associated hyperemia and release of histiocyte lysosomal enzymes. In support of this hypothesis the authors pointed out the fact that bone resorption in otitis media can occur in the absence of cholesteatoma formation. More recently Sade' and Berco (1974) and Sade' and Halevy (1974) have also suggested inflammation as the major cause of bone destruction although the precise mechanism remains unclarified.

A specific mechanism for osteolysis in middle ear disease has been suggested by the classic work of Abramson (1969) in which middle ear cholesteatomas have been shown to have collagenolytic activity when cultured on native collagen gel. More recently, Abramson, et al, (1975) has proposed that the granulation tissue at the base of the cholesteatoma may be responsible for the bone resorption. Although collagenolytic destruction of bone is suggested as the basic mechanism, it should be pointed out that there are no known diseases in which bone is enzymatically destroyed without antecedent demineralization (Krane, 1975). Thus to date, none of the proposed mechanisms of bone destruction in otitis media are totally convincing.

The purpose of this paper is to present evidence that cholesteatoma or granulation tissue from the middle ear and mastoid are capable of producing a soluble factor(s) which enhances osteoclastic activity, bone mineral matrix resorption and inhibition of bone formation in a bone organ culture system.

Material and Methods

All tissue was obtained from patients undergoing standard middle ear and mastoid surgery for chronic otitis media. Cholesteatomas were exposed, curetted and suctioned; the tissues obtained were immediately placed in warm culture medium containing penicillin and streptomycin. Granulation tissue from chronic otitis media without cholesteatoma was also obtained in the same fashion and transferred to culture medium. The cholesteatoma and granulation tissue was diced into fragments of one to two cubic mm, washed several times in culture medium and placed in tissue culture vessels containing .5 ml modified BJG (Gibco, Grand Island, New York) with 1 mg/ml of bovine serum albumin.

The fetal bone—tissue culture model employed was originally described by Raisz and Niemann (1969). The essential steps of the assay procedure were as follows:

(A) Rats were injected with 45 calcium chloride on the 18th day of gestation.

(B) The rats were sacrificed on the 19th day; the radii and ulnae, including the cartilaginous ends, were isolated and placed in a chemically defined culture medium.

(C) The release of 45 calcium into the culture

medium in the presence of a test agent was compared with the release in bones incubated in control media; the results were then expressed as a ratio. A ratio significantly greater than one strongly suggested initiation of cell mediated bone resorption.

The routine procedure included a 24 hour preculture period in control media followed by a two day culture in the experimental medium. Preculture permitted more precise time control and removal of most of the exchangeable 45 calcium from the bones so that subsequent release of 45 calcium was largely due to active bone resorption. Hematoxylin and eosin stained five micron sections of the cultured bones were examined for the presence of osteoclasts. Necrotic incudes obtained from patients with chronic otitis media, with and without cholesteatoma were also examined histologically.

The ultrafiltrates of two cholesteatomas were prepared using cellulose membranes (UM-2 Amicon with a nominal molecular weight cut off of 1000 daltons) and their effect on 45 calcium release from pre-labeled fetal bone was determined. The concentration of prostaglandins was measured by radioimmunoassay (Levine, et al, 1971).

Results

The effect of cholesteatoma culture medium and corresponding canal skin culture medium on calcium release by embryonic bones during organ culture is tabulated in Table 16. Six of seven cholesteatomas revealed a significant release of 45

TABLE 16

Effect of Ultrafiltrate of Cholesteatoma Culture Medium on ^{45}Ca Release by Embryonic Bones During Organ Culture

	Sample	^{45}Ca Release Ratio (48 hrs.)		
1. a.	Cholesteatoma Culture Medium	4.07 ± 0.19	$p>0.001$	Difference is Significant
b.	U.F.*	2.35 ± 0.17	$p>0.01$	$p>0.001$
2. a.	Cholesteatoma Culture Medium	1.78 ± 0.22	$p>0.02$	Not Significant
b.	U.F.	2.3 ± 0.14	$p>0.001$	

*Ultrafiltrate

^{45}Ca release ratios are mean$\pm$ S.E. for six pairs of cultures in each experiment; 24-hour preculture was used.

calcium from pre-labeled bones when compared with the 45 calcium released from bones incubated in control media. Media from canal skin of three patients tested did not show evidence of significant bone resorption.

Ultrafiltrates of media from two cholesteatomas stimulated bone formation as evidenced by the release of 45 calcium (Table 16) and by an increase of osteoclastic resorption seen histologically (Figs. 59 and 60). In one sample, the

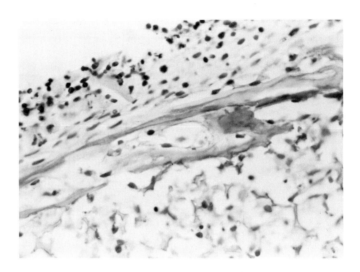

Fig. 59: Fetal bone cortex incubated in control medium. Note the central calcified bone core and thin rim of uncalcified osteoid. Osteoclasts are absent.

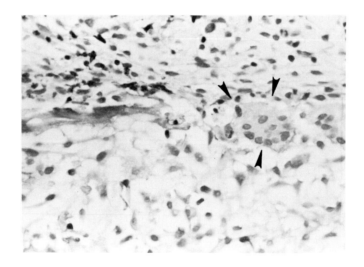

Fig. 60: Fetal bone cortex incubated in cholesteatoma incubation medium. Note the loss of bone cortex associated with the appearance of osteoclasts (arrows). The darkly stained calcified core of residual cortical bone does not have an osteoid covering, and suggests bone formation arrest. Undecalcified hematoxylin and eosin section.

45 calcium release stimulated by cholesteatoma culture fluid was greater than that evidenced by the corresponding ultra filtrate; in another sample, there was no apparent difference between the whole culture medium and the ultrafiltrate in stimulating bone resorption.

The effect of culture fluid from a cholesteatoma on the release of 45 calcium from pre-labeled bones was tested, using fetal bones with viable cells and bones in which the cells had been killed by heat or repeated freezing and thawing. In both instances the media stimulated significant 45 calcium release although the magnitude of stimulating was significantly less in dead bone compared to bone containing viable osteocytes (Table 17).

In addition to studying the effects of otitis extracts in fetal bone in tissue culture, we also had the opportunity to examine incudes surgically removed from ten patients with chronic otitis media. Some of these patients had had identifiable cholesteatomas, others had not. All of the incudes studied showed substantial reduction in the size of the long process and in polarized tissue section these areas revealed an irregular pattern of established lamellar bone admixed with newly formed woven bone. This suggested that considerable remodelling had taken place.

TABLE 17

Effect of Cholesteatoma Culture
Medium on Devitalized Embryonic Bones

	Sample	^{45}Ca Release Ratio		
1. a.	Fetal Bone Cultures	4.07 ± 0.20	$p > 0.01$	Difference is Significant
b.	Heat Killed Fetal Bones	1.58 ± 0.08	$p > 0.001$	$p > 0.001$
2. a.	Normal Fetal Bone Cultures	2.93 ± 0.19	$p > 0.01$	Difference is Significant
b.	Freeze-Thawed Killed Fetal Bone	1.45 ± 0.03	$p > 0.001$	$p > 0.001$

^{45}Ca release ratios are mean $\pm$ S.E. for six pairs of cultures in each experiment; 24-hour preculture was used.

Bones were heated killed by heating in culture media for 5 min. at 70°C and freeze-thaw killed by successively freezing and thawing them 5 times.

One incus (Fig. 61) showed advanced destruction of the long process associated with localized invasion of inflammatory tissue. Irregular scalloped lacunae filled with cellular fibrous tissue strongly suggested recent osteoclastic bone resorption although no actual osteoclasts were, in fact, identified. In addition to these areas of resorption, the core of lamellar bone forming the stump of the eroded long process was irregularly capped by woven bone, thus indicating previous episodes of new bone formation and remodelling. In still other areas a thin rim of osteoid associated with aggregates of osteoblasts represented very recent osteogenesis. Similar evidence of bone resorption and remodelling was totally lacking in the preserved short process portion of the incus.

Table 18 illustrates one middle ear fluid, which was mucoid, which produced significant calcium release from embryonic bones during tissue culture. It can also be noted that mastoid granulation tissue alone, without cholesteatoma, was capable of producing significant calcium resorption.

TABLE 18

Effect of Culture Media from Other Inflammatory Products of the Middle Ear Cleft on Embryonic Bones During Organ Culture

	^{45}Ca Release Ratio	
1. *MEF (Serous)	0.79±0.08	p>0.05
2. MEF (Serous)	0.91±0.01	N.S.
3. MEF (Mucoid)	1.52±0.05	p>0.001
4. Granulation Tissue From Mastoid	1.63±0.18	p>0.02
(No Cholesteatoma)		

*MEF= Middle Ear Fluid
N.S.= Not Significant

Discussion

Bone is an active tissue and in common with all other tissue responds to inflammation with necrosis, removal of necrotic tissue and repair. Nichols (1971) has pointed out that turnover, a phenomenon occurring to some extent in all connective tissues, is uniquely active in bone. Bone resorption requires removal of mineral, breakdown of collagen and the small amounts of mucopolysaccharide which make up the extracellular matrix and perhaps removal of cellular elements. For the formation of new bone, mechanisms for the bio-synthesis of new matrix and for its subsequent mineralization are needed. Recently the cellular basis of metabolic bone disease has been reviewed extensively by Rasmussen and Bordier (1973). They suggest that the sequence of cellular events in a bone remodeling unit on the endosteal bone surface begins initially with the activation of mesenchymal cells which become osteoprogenitor cells and by continued differentiation pro-osteoclasts. The pro-osteoclasts then fuse to become osteoclasts which undergo further modulation to become pre-osteoblasts and after completing their synthetic function become

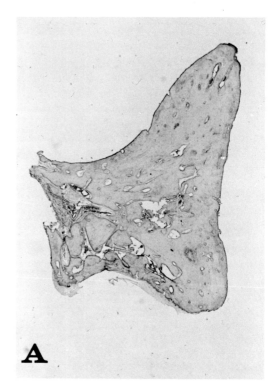

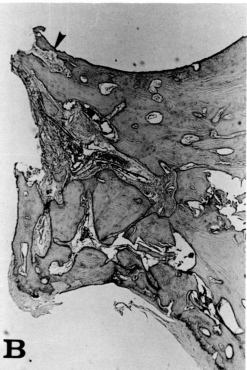

Fig. 61: (A) Incus from a patient with chronic otitis media. The long process has almost completely disappeared. Hematoxylin and eosin. (B) A high power view of the eroded long process reveals an ingrowth of granulation tissue and irregular resorption lacunae (arrow). No recognizable osteoclasts were identified. Hematoxylin and eosin.

osteocytes. In normal bone, net bone loss depends on osteoclast number, size (Rowe and Hausmann, 1975), and function activity (Holtrop, et al, 1974) and net bone formation on the number and activity of the osteoblasts.

Vaes (1969) has reviewed the activity of lysosomes and the cellular physiology of bone resorption. It is his belief that hydrolytic enzymes released from osteoclasts play a critical role in bone resorption not only through an extracellular mechanism which parallels that of mineral solubilizing agents, but also through intracellular digestion within the osteoclast vacuoles. Scott (1967) observed that the lysosome-like granules of the osteoclasts are apparently secreted into the large cytoplasmic vacuoles of the ruffled border of the osteoclasts. Intracellular digestion of materal brought into these vacuoles by pinocytosis could thus be achieved by the lysosomal enzymes as in other·cells. It has also been emphasized that although their quantitative contribution to bone loss seems to be minor (Baylink, et al, 1973), osteocytes may also play a role in bone resorption.

Available evidence today suggests that osteoclasts are actively involved in bone resorption. The border of the osteoclasts adjacent to the resorbed bone surface exhibits a characteristically ruffled appearance ultrastructurally (Holtrop, et al, 1974). A suggested mechanism for osteoclast activity is that it secretes acid such as lactic acid, to dissolve bone mineral and collagenase to hydrolyse bone matrix (Vaes, 1969). This response when initiated by parathyroid hormone elevates bone cell cyclic AMP (Chase and Aurbach, 1970) and results in an influx of calcium into bone cells (Dziak and Stern, 1975). Bone resorption stimulated by osteoclast activating factor is not associated with elevation of bone cell cyclic AMP (Raisz, et al, 1975). The mechanisms for 45 calcium release from pre-labeled fetal bones in tissue culture are primarily metabolic and ion exchange. The magnitude of the ion exchange component can be estimated from the release of 45 calcium from pre-labeled non-viable bones.

The present study suggests that a soluble substance or substances released from cholesteatoma are capable of stimulating osteoclastic resorption in tissue culture and very likely in vivo as well. Stimulation of 45 calcium from pre-labeled dead fetal bones, however, suggests that cholesteatomas also release a factor stimulating mineral release directly, without the mediation of cellular activity. Inasmuch as canal skin alone does not seem to produce this effect, it appears unlikely that the squamous epithelium of cholesteatoma is responsible for bone resorption. It is more likely that the granulation tissue of the subepidermal region is largely responsible for this phenomenon. Possible factors which could be involved include endotoxin (Hausmann, et al, 1972), lipoteichoic acid (Hausmann, et al, 1975), prostaglandins (Klein and Raisz, 1970) and osteoclastic activating factor (OAF) (Horton, et al, 1972), a product of activated lymphocytes (a so-called lymphokine).

Endotoxins are lipopolysaccharides contained in the cell walls of many gram negative organisms and lipoteichoic acids are contained in cell walls of many gram positive organisms. Highly purified endotoxins have been tested on fetal bones in tissue culture and have shown to initiate significant osteoclastic bone resorption (Hausmann, 1974). In 25 of 30 cholesteatomas we have studied, gram negative bacilli containing lipopolysaccharides have been found. The most common organism was pseudomonas aeruginosa; the second most common organism was proteus mirabilis. Occasionally staphlococcus epidermitis or staphlococcus aureus were also found but these may have been contaminants. Furthermore, three of four cholesteatomas examined for endotoxin by the sensitive Limulus assay were found to be positive for endotoxin (Yin, 1975). Thus it is theoretically possible that bone resorption may result from the lipopolysaccharide or lipoteichoic acid present in bacterial cell walls.

Stimulation of bone resorption in organ culture by various purified prostaglandins has been extensively reviewed by Dietrich, et al (1975). The bone resorptive activity in media containing gingival fragments has been shown to result from the release of prostaglandins (Gomes, et al, 1976). The ability of prostaglandin E, F, A, and B to stimulate bone resorption was demonstrated in tissue culture with prostaglandin E being, by far, the most active. We have demonstrated prostaglandin E to be present in the ultrafiltrate of two cholesteatoma supernatants. This cyclic fatty acid was present in quantities which would be capable of bone resorption. This is summarized in Table 19. In one such supernatant, all of the bone resorbing activity was present in the ultrafiltrate suggesting that prostaglandins alone may have been the active agent responsible. On the other hand, in the other cholesteatoma ultrafiltrate, approximately one-half of the calcium resorption activity resided in the ultrafiltrate. The bone resorptive effects of prostaglandins as well as lipopolysaccharide and lipoteichoic acid appears to be mediated by osteoclasts (Hausmann, et al, 1975).

TABLE 19

PGE Levels in Culture Fluids

Sample No.	ng/ml	(mean)
2	2.0* 2.9	(2.5)
4	4.7* 4.3	(4.5)

*Assayed in duplicate; PGB$_1$ equivalent

Finally, Horton, et al (1972) has shown that activated lymphocytes produce a substance which has been called osteoclastic activating factor (OAF). This substance appears to be released by cultured mononuclear leukocytes suggesting that lymphocytes and macrophages associated with chronic inflammatory lesions may have the potential to degrade bone and collagen. Evidence for this is based on the release of 45 calcium in 48 hour treated organ cultures. Increased levels of collagenase in acutely and chronically inflamed tissues in which the connective tissue has been destroyed is demonstrated. This suggests that in an immunologically induced chronic inflammatory lesion where mononuclear leukocytes predominate, antigen stimulated lymphocytes may induce the macrophages to produce collagenase. Although, as yet, there is no evidence to suggest that bone destruction and chronic otitis media, with or without cholesteatoma, represents an immunologically induced condition, more evidence is needed to rule out this possibility.

The results of this study suggest that cholesteatoma is capable of producing calcium resorption which is probably due to osteoclast activation. Using radioactive labelled fetal bones, studies in organ culture suggest that a soluble product from cholesteatoma is capable of producing calcium resorption, osteoclastic activation and inhibition of bone synthesis. The possible factors involved include prostaglandins E, lipopolysaccharides and OAF (Fig. 62).

The incus (see Fig. 61) was very instructive in demonstrating the probable mechanism of in vivo incus destruction in otitis media. The tissue changes strongly suggested that granulation tissue was very closely related to the bone destruction and has been mediated through activation of osteoclasts. The presence of extensive remodelling also suggested that this process had been episodic in nature. One might logically question, however, why this was seen in only one of the incudes examined and why osteoclasts were never actually observed. A partial answer to this may lie in the fact that elective surgery for otitis media and cholesteatoma is invariably preceded by attempts to reduce inflammatory exudate. It is conceivable that the interval between initiation of intensive therapy and surgery is sufficient for the active resorptive phase to be superseded by a reparative one. This is, of course, speculative and additional observations will be necessary to conclusively prove that osteoclastic resorption plays an important role in ossicular destruction in otitis media.

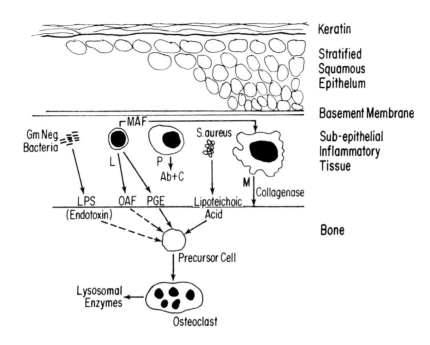

Fig. 62: Potential pathways for bone resorption in COM with or without cholesteatoma.

Summary

Bone resorption occurs in chronic otitis media, with or without cholesteatoma. It may also occur in long standing otitis media with effusion. A specific model of bone resorption has been presented. It is suggested that specific chemical mediators of inflammation are capable of activating osteoclasts which, in turn, initiate bone breakdown as evidenced by calcium resorption in vitro and increased osteoclast formation. There is also some histological evidence to suggest that bone synthesis is inhibited as a result of this soluble factor. Three possible mediators of bone resorption have been discussed. The evidence thus far suggests prostaglandin E as a distinct possibility, but the bacteria present in chronic otitis media may also be responsible through the effect of lipopolysaccharides on osteoclastic activation. There is no evidence yet to support an immunologically induced bone resorption mechanism although it is suggested that osteoclastic activating factor (OAF) from activated lymphocytes may represent such a mechanism. It is noteworthy that the two cells which predominate in the inflammatory exudate of chronic otitis media are the lymphocyte and the macrophage (Bernstein and Fisher, 1976, in press).

References

1. Abramson, M.: Collagenolytic activity in middle ear cholesteatoma. *Ann. Otol. Rhinol. Laryngol,* 78: 112, 1969.

2. Abramson, M.; Asarch, R.; and Litton, W.: Experimental aural cholesteatoma causing bone resorption. *Ann. Otol. Rhinol. Laryngol.,* 84:425, 1975.

3. Baylink, D.; Sipe, J.; Wergedal, J.; and Whittemore, O. J.: Vitamin D-enhanced osteocytic and osteoclastic bone resorption. *Am. J. Physiol.,* 224: 1345, 1973.

4. Bernstein, J. M. and Fisher, J.: The cytology of otitis media with effusion. Manuscript in preparation, 1976.

5. Chase, L. R. and Aurbach, G. D.: The effect of parathyroid hormone on the concentration of adenosine 3^1, 5^1 monophosphate in skeletal tissue in vitro. *J. Biol. Chem.,* 215: 1520, 1970.

6. Dietrich, J.; Goodson, J.; and Raisz, L.: Stimulation of bone resorption by various prostaglandins in organ culture. *Prostaglandins,* 10: 231, 1975.

7. Dziak, R. and Stern, P.: Calcium transport in isolated bone cells. III. Effects of parathyroid hormone and cyclic 3^1, 5^1-AMP. *Endocrinology,* 97: 1281, 1975.

8. Gomes, B. C.; Hausmann, E.; Weinfeld, N.; and DeLuca, C.: Prostaglandins bone resorption stimulating factors released from monkey gingiva. *Calcif. Tiss. Res.,* 19: 285, 1976.

9. Hausmann, E.; Weinfeld, N.; and Miller, W. A.: Effects of lipopolysaccharides on bone resorption in tissue culture. *Calc. Tiss. Res.,* 9: 272, 1972.

10. Hausmann, E.; Luderitz, O.; Knox, K.; and Weinfeld, N.: Structural requirements for bone resorption by endotoxin and lipoteichoic acid. *J. Den. Res.,* 54: (Special Issue B) B94-B99, 1975. J. Den. Res., 54: (Special Issue B) B94-B99, 1975.

11. Hausmann, E.: Potential pathways for bone resorption in human periodontal disease. *J. Periodontol.,* 45: 338, 1974.

12. Holtrop, M. E.; Raisz, L. G.; and Simmons, H. A.: The effects of parathyroid hormone, colchicine and calcitonin on the ultra-structure and the activity of osteoclasts in organ culture. *J. Cell. Biol.,* 60: 346, 1974.

13. Horton, J. E.; Raisz, L.; Simmons, H. A.; Oppenheim, J. J.; and Mergenhagen, S. E.: Bone resorbing activity in supernatant fluid from cultured human peripheral blood leukocytes. *Science,* 177: 793, 1972.

14. Klein, D. and Raisz, L.: Prostaglandins: stimulation of bone resorption in tissue culture. *Endocrinol.,* 86: 1436, 1970.

15. Krane, S.: Skeletal remodeling and metabolic bone disease. In Talmage, R. V.; Owen, M.; and Parsons, J. A.: *Calcium Regulating Hormones.* Amsterdam, Netherlands, Excerpta Medica, 1975, pp. 57-65.

16. Levine, L.; Gutierrez, R. M.; and Van Vunatais, H.: Specificities of prostaglandins B1 and F1a and F2a antigen-antibody reactions. *J. Biol. Chem.,* 246: 6782, 1971.

17. Nichols, G.: Inflammation and bone. In Forcher, B. and Houck, J.: *Immunopathology of Inflammation,* Amsterdam, Netherlands: Excerpta Medica, 1971, pp. 229.

18. Raisz, L. G., and Niemann, I.: Effect of phosphage, calcium and magnesium on bone resorption and hormonal responses in tissue culture, *Endocrinol.,* 85: 446, 1969.

19. Raisz, L. G.; Luben, R. A.; Mundy, A. R.; Dietrick, J. W.; Hoeton, J.; and Trummel, C.: Effect of osteoclast activating factor from human leukocytes on bone metabolism. *J. Clin. Invest.,* 56: 408, 1975.

20. Rasmussen, H. and Bordier, P.: The cellular basis of metabolic bone disease. *New Eng. J. Med.,* 289: 23, 1973.

21. Reudi, L.: Cholesteatosis of the attic. *J. Laryng. Otol.,* 73:593, 1958.

22. Rowe, D. J. and Hausmann, E.: Quantitative and qualitative analysis of osteoclast changes in endotoxin-treated bones. *J. Den. Res.,* 54 (Special Issue A): 149, 1975.

23. Sadé, J. and Halevy, A.: Bone destruction in chronic otitis media. *J. Laryng. Otol.,* 88: 139, 1974.

24. Sadé, J. and Berco, E.: Bone destruction in chronic otitis media. *J. Laryng. Otol.,* 88:413, 1974.

25. Scott, B. L.: The occurrence of specific cytoplasmic granules in the osteoclast. *Ultrastruct. Res.,* 19: 417, 1967.

26. Thomsen, J.; Balslev Jørgensen, M.; Bretlau, P. et al.: Bone resorption in chronic otitis media: a histological and ultrastructural study. I. Ossicular necrosis. *J. Laryng. Otol.,* 88: 975; 1974.

27. Thomsen, J.; Balslev Jørgensen, M.; Bretlau, P. et al.: Bone resorption in chronic otitis media: a histological and ultrastructural study. II. Cholesteatoma. *J. Laryng. Otol.,* 88: 983, 1974.

28. Tumarkin, A.: Attic cholesteatosis. *J. Laryng. Otol.,* 72: 610, 1958.

29. Vaes, G.: Lysosomes and the cellular physiology of bone resorption. In Dingle, J. T. and Fell, H. P.:

(Eds.). *Lysosomes in Biology and Pathology.* North Holland Publishing Company, Amsterdam, Holland, 1969, pp. 217-253, vol. 1.

30. Yin, E. T.: Endotoxin, thrombin and the limulus amebocyte lysate test. *J. Lab. Clin. Med.,* 86:430, 1975.

CHOLESTEATOMA AND BONE RESORPTION

Maxwell Abramson, M.D.
Cheng-Chung Huang, Ph.D.

Only ten years ago, the most popular theory for the effect of cholesteatoma on bone was pressure necrosis. This theory was accepted, although increased pressure has never been demonstrated in cholesteatomas. Since cholesteatomas occur in sacs open laterally, and rarely occur as complete cysts, increased pressure is not likely. Necrosis not only doesn't cause bone resorption, but actually prevents bone resorption as students of archaeology know. Bone destruction requires living tissue involving a specific series of biochemical events which must include the destruction of the principal structural protein, collagen.

Our interest in the interaction of cholesteatoma and bone has moved from the outside in. This research was begun with cholesteatoma specimens collected from the operating rooms at the Massachusetts Eye and Ear Infirmary. We were seeking a specific collagen dissolving enzyme which was demonstrated by lysis of reconstituted collagen gels (Abramson, 1969). Great variations in collagenase activity from one specimen to the other were puzzling until we began to realize that certain surgeons were routinely giving us dead epithelial debris and leaving cholesteatoma matrix in the patient. The collagenase in cholesteatoma did turn out to be quite similar to other collagenase enzymes (Abramson and Gross, 1971), such as the enzyme found in normal human skin (Eisen, et al, 1970) and rheumatoid synovium (Harris and Krane, 1974). Cholesteatoma collagenase is elaborated in vitro by living cells, not stored in the tissue, requires protein synthesis for production, makes a single cut through the collagen molecule, and is inhibited by serum, cysteine, and EDTA (Abramson and Gross, 1971). A single cholesteatoma weighing 100 mg could dissolve as much as 400 micrograms of collagen in four days in vitro—as much collagen as is found in the entire long process of the incus (Abramson, 1969).

Our next question is, what is the source of this enzyme? Is it a product of the epithelium or the connective tissue? Reddick and co-workers (1974) recently localized collagenase in the papillary dermis of skin in the connective tissue stroma of basal cell carcinomas and in fibroblast cell culture. We used a similar immunocytochemical technique with frozen sections of cholesteatoma incubated with a specific antiserum made in rabbits against purified human skin collagenase (Abramson and Huang, 1976). The rabbit antihuman skin enzyme was localized with fluorescein and examined under ultraviolet microscopy. Cholesteatoma tissue incubated with non-immune serum (Fig. 63A) showed epithelial debris, epithelium, and subepithelial connective tissue with no staining.

Cholesteatomas stained with immune serum (Fig. 63B) show bright green fluorescence at the connective tissue, and especially the basement

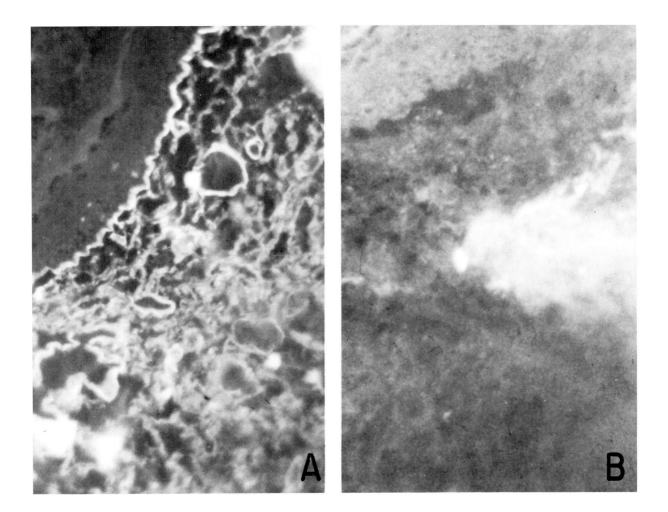

Fig. 63: Fluorescent, dark field photomicrograph of human middle ear cholesteatoma. **(A)** Frozen section stained with antihuman skin collagenase antiserum followed by fluorescein labelled goat antirabbit IgG. Bright staining is seen in the subepithelial connective tissue, particularly around vascular spaces and at the basement membrane. No staining can be seen in the epithelium (middle) layer or the keratinized (upper) layer. **(B)** Section of cholesteatoma incubated with non-immune rabbit serum followed by fluorescent labelled goat antirabbit IgG. No specific staining is present. *(Courtesy of Abramson and Huang, The Laryngoscope, 1977, in press.)*

membrane, but no sign of collagenase in the epithelium or epithelial debris. In looking for the intracellular source of the collagenase, we found the enzyme in typical appearing fibroblasts (Fig. 64). We also found collagenase in certain monocytes (Fig. 65) with characteristic bilobed nuclei and in

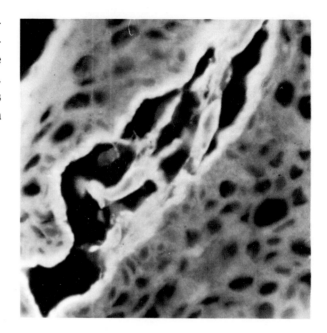

Fig. 64: Fluorescent photomicrograph showing tympanic membrane epithelium above, cholesteatoma epithelium below, separated by a thin layer of connective tissue. Bright staining can be seen in typical appearing fibroblasts as well as in the basement membrane. *(Courtesy of Abramson and Huang, The Laryngoscope, 1977, in press.)*

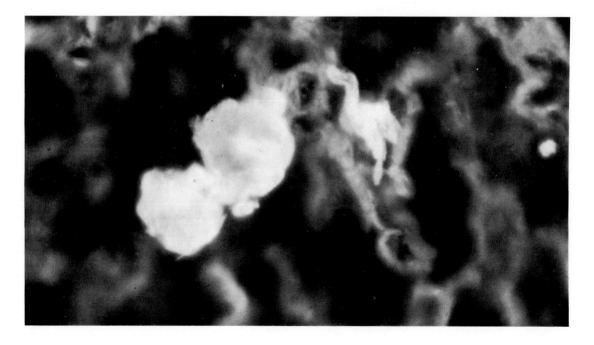

Fig. 65: Collagenase stained fluorescent photomicrograph of the subepithelial connective tissue of a middle ear cholesteatoma showing bright staining within typical appearing monocytes. The characteristic bilobed nucleus can be seen in the upper cell. *(Courtesy of Abramson and Huang, The Laryngoscope, 1977, in press.)*

endothelial cells of capillary buds (Fig. 66). Both capillary buds and monocytes are increased in chronic inflammatory states.

What does the epithelium have to do with bone resorption? Is its function only to maintain the connective tissue in a chronic inflammatory state? We produced fistulas of the cochlea in guinea pigs in a variety of ways using talc granulomas and skin flaps (Abramson, et al, 1975). Bone resorption occurred under epidermal cysts without sepsis, with sepsis and no skin, and even under chronic talc granuloma without sepsis. The bone resorption sites have certain histologic features in common and agree with Thomsen's (1974) and Sade's (1974) findings in human temporal bones. The fistulas are covered by a thin layer of inflammatory connective tissue containing numerous chronic inflammatory cells and capillary buds. Osteoclasts are rarely seen. Bone resorption, therefore, occurs from contact with chronic inflammatory connective tissue regardless of the mechanism of the chronic inflammation. The presence of epithelium, while not crucial, greatly increased the incidence of bone resorption in these animal experiments. Cochlea fistulas occurred in three of eight animals with skin (38%) and three of 47 animals without skin (6%).

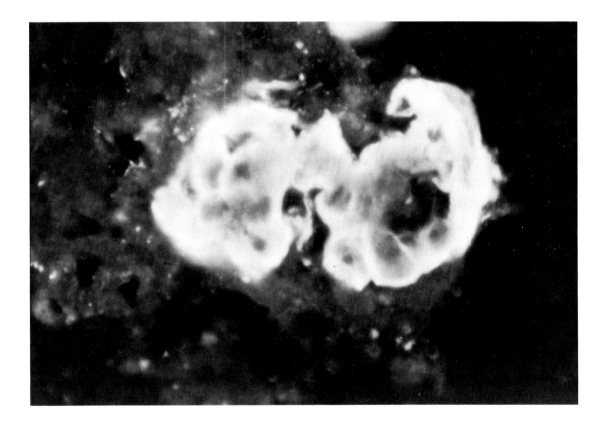

Fig. 66: Collagenase stained fluorescent photomicrograph of middle ear granulation tissue showing bright staining within endothelial cells of two capillary buds. *(Courtesy of Abramson and Huang, The Laryngoscope, 1977, in press.)*

Now, we cannot understand bone resorption by simply studying collagen breakdown. The demineralization process is at least as important and is probably a primary step before collagen breakdown can occur. As we learn more about bone resorption, it begins to appear as a series of cascading events analogous, perhaps, to blood clotting. Otologists interested in chronic otitis media must participate in solving the mechanisms of this complex and essential process.

References

1. Abramson, M.: Collagenolytic activity in middle ear cholesteatoma. *Ann. Otol. Rhinol. Laryngol.*, 78:112, 1969.
2. Abramson, M. and Gross, J.: Further studies on a collagenase in middle ear cholesteatoma. *Ann. Otol. Rhinol. Laryngol.*, 80:177, 1971.
3. Abramson, M.; Asarch, R. G.; and Litton, W. B.: Experimental aural cholesteatoma causing bone resorption. *Ann. Otol.*, 84:425, 1975.
4. Abramson, M. and Huang, C. C.: Localization of collagenase in human middle ear cholesteatoma. *Laryngoscope*, 1976 (in press).
5. Eisen, A. Z.; Bauer, E. A.; and Jeffrey, J. J.: Animal and human collagenases. *J. Invest. Dermatol.*, 55:359, 1970.
6. Harris, E. D. and Krane, S. M.: Collagenases. *New Engl. J. Med.*, 291:557, 605, 652, 1974.
7. Reddick, M. E.; Bauer, E. A. and Eisen, A. Z.: Immunocytochemical localization of collagenase in human skin and fibroblasts in monolayer culture. *J. Invest. Dermatol.*, 63:361, 1974.
8. Sade', J. and Berco, E.: Bone destruction in chronic otitis media: A histopathological study. *J. Laryngol. Otol.*, 88:413, 1974.
9. Thomsen, J.; Bretlau, P.; Balsley, J. M., et al: Bone resorption in chronic otitis media. A histological and ultrastructural study. II. Cholesteatoma. *J. Laryngol. Otol.*, 88:983, 1974.

DECALCIFICATION FACTORS IN GRANULATION TISSUE AND EAR CANAL SKIN

Bruce J. Gantz, M.D.
Constance Clancey, Research Assistant
Maxwell Abramson, M.D.

We are presently studying three questions concerning cholesteatoma disease and its relationship to bone resorption. We wanted to know:

(1) If the tissues that make up the cholesteatoma are capable of resorbing bone?

(2) Is bone resorbing ability limited to a specific histologic type of tissue?

(3) Can a chemical mediator be isolated from these tissues that is responsible for activating bone resorption?

Cholesteatoma consists of keratinizing squamous epithelium overlying chronic inflammatory connective tissue which resembles granulation tissue.

In order to study these tissues separately, granulation tissue was formed in guinea pigs by the subcutaneous injection of carrageenan; skin containing keratinized squamous epithelium and connective tissue was obtained from guinea pig ears and ear canals; and connective tissue was harvested from guinea pig dermis.

An organ culture technique similar to that described by Raisz and Niemann (1969) was used to determine if these tissues had bone resorbing potential. Our technique involves the incubation of individual guinea pig tissues in a bone culture media for 48 hours.

After this period, experimental cell free media from either granulation tissue, skin or connective tissue, or uncultured control media is placed with rat forelimb long bones which have previously been incorporated with radioactive Ca^{45}. After another 48 hour incubation period, an aliquot of the media is analyzed for Ca^{45} activity. Bone resorption is measured as the amount of Ca^{45} released from the rat bones. Our data is expressed as a treated/control ratio, since paired long bones from the same fetus received either experimental or control media.

Table 20 illustrates the results from these initial experiments. Granulation tissue media caused 3.03 times more release of Ca^{45} than controls for a treated/control ratio of 3.03 in fourteen pairs of bones. Skin containing keratinizing squamous epithelium and connective tissue, resulted in a 1.68 treated/control ratio in fourteen pairs of bones. Connective tissue alone resulted in a 1.61 treated/control ratio in nine pairs of bones.

This data suggests that these tissues secreted a substance in culture media that is capable of resorbing bone. Granulation tissue caused almost twice as much release of Ca^{45} than skin or connective tissue. Thirdly, bone resorption was not influenced by the presence of keratinized squamous epithelium, because it appears that bone resorption produced by the skin media was due to its connective tissue component.

The next step was to identify the chemical mediator present in granulation tissue responsible for activating the bone resorption. Prostaglandin was considered because of the inflammatory nature of the disease (Klein and Raisz, 1970). Osteoclast activating factor seemed a less likely mediator because osteoclasts were rarely seen in microscopic sections of the rat bones from the experiments. We did find many mononuclear cells in the bone, however.

In another series of experiments, Indomethacin, an inhibitor of prostaglandin synthesis (Vane, 1971), was cultured with granulation

TABLE 20

The Effect of Tissue Culture Medias on
the Release of Ca[45] from Fetal Rat Bones

Tissue Culture Media	Number of Bone Pairs	48 Hr. CA[45] Release Treated/Control Ratio
Granulation Tissue	14	3.03 ± .19
Skin	14	1.68 ± .08
Connective Tissue	9	1.61 ± .13

tissue. This media was then incubated with radioactive rat bones. Also a radioimmunoassay for prostaglandin was performed òn the granulation tissue culture media and on the granulation tissue culture media plus Indomethacin. In this experiment, the granulation tissue media resulted in a treated/control ratio of 2.7. When this same granulation tissue was incubated with Indomethacin, which inhibits PG activity, the treated/control ratio was reduced from 2.7 to 1.8, which is almost the same level as normal connective tissue. The radioimmunoassay also confirmed the presence of prostaglandins in the granulation tissue culture media.

The radioimmunoassay results are seen in Table 21. Granulation tissue culture media that produced the 2.7 treated/control ratio demonstrated 9.8 ng/ml of prostaglandin E-like material while granulation tissue media with Indomethacin pro-duce only 0.4 ng/ml of PGE-like material.

In summary, these experiments demonstrate that (1) sterile granulation tissue, which is histologically similar to the subepithelial chronic inflammatory tissue found in cholesteatoma, is capable of chemically activating bone resorption in vitro; (2) keratinized squamous epithelium of skin did not influence bone resorption in our system; (3) it appears that prostaglandin, present in chronic inflammatory tissue, is one of the chemical mediators responsible for producing demineralization of bone. Prostaglandin may play an active role in localized bone resorption in chronic middle ear disease.

Acknowledgements
The authors wish to thank Dr. Jacob Sade´ and Dr. C. C. Huang for their advice and criticism.

TABLE 21

E-Like Prostaglandin Level in Granulation Tissue

Tissue Media	Prostaglandin E-Like Activity Ng/Ml
Granulation Tissue	9.8
Granulation Tissue + Indomethacin	0.4

References

1. Klein, D. C. and Raisz, L.: Prostaglandins: Stimulation of bone resorption in tissue culture. *Endocrinology*, 86:1436, 1970.
2. Raisz, L. G. and Niemann, I.: Effect of phosphate, calcium, and magnesium on bone resorption and hormonal responses in tissue culture. *Endocrinology*, 85:446, 1969.
3. Vane, J. R.: Inhibition of prostaglandin synthesis as a mechanism of action for aspirin-like drugs. *Nature New Biology*, 231:323, 1971.

QUESTIONS AND ANSWERS

Dr. Austin: I was rather disturbed by the first two papers in that they both came to a similar conclusion, which was, to paraphrase, skin is not important to bone destruction. At the risk of intruding my clinical self on your alter ego, I have made some counts in this regard in terms of studying incus destruction. As you probably are all aware, incus destruction occurs in approximately one-half of our cases if we lump all chronic ear disease together. In studying these cases of incus destruction with a much lower powered microscope, by the way, because sometimes the power magnification kind of interferes with seeing what is happening, I find the following little statistics: (1) If we looked at the intrusion of skin in my low-powered microscopic view of the middle ear upon the incus, that is when the skin, to my eye, is attached to the incus, the necrosis took place in 95%. (2) If, on the other hand, we just studied those cases in which there was collapse and retraction of the drum head onto the incus, again we found necrosis in 95%. It seems to me that if the presence of skin is not essential in this condition, then perhaps we are dealing with the wrong experimental model or animal. There may well be granulation tissue or whatever between the skin and the incus that is destroyed. However, to get the skin off I have to use a knife. When the skin is not attached to the incus, it is not likely that necrosis takes place.

Dr. Laurence: When epidermis grows right on bone, it is surprising that necrosis does not occur more often. The epidermis is an avascular organ and it has got to have its blood supply from somewhere, and it is usually from the dermis. It is the skeleton of the dermis which molds the shape of the epidermis. So Dr. Toller was surprised that you didn't get rete pegs. The rete pegs are a function of the skeleton of the dermis and the blood vessels run in. After hyperplasia, you didn't get any more rete pegs. You just got them longer. If you have scar tissue over a fibrin mass, which is flattened and no columnar skeleton, you get a flat epidermis. So I wasn't surprised that you didn't get epidermis lying right adjacent to bone unless it was a necrotic bone where there are a lot of nutrative materials, just as a plaque growing up the side of teeth.

Not only is it avascular, but lymphatics do not grow through it. I was reminded of Dr. Toller's concept of pressure due to implanted tumors. Now if anybody has worked on implanted tumors, you implant them under the skin and when you get them out to take little pieces to reimplant, you put your scalpel in and the next thing that happens it is all over your face. You have a tremendous amount of pressure inside the tumor. How that develops, I don't know except there is a lot of necrotic tissue there. It is well vascularized that I think it has a lymphatic system because it can metastasize and metastasis is usually via the lymphatics.

The other point I have to make is the epidermis is a very stable structure in the adult. All the vitamin A studies for metaplasia are done on the chick. I have been looking up the literature and I couldn't find any metaplasia in adult tissues. There seems to be one example if I am to believe Dr. Sadé because he has an example of metaplasia in an adult. It must be the only one. I know that occurs in rats. Therefore QED, I have to challenge his theory and I think it is about time some of the basic scientists did a bit of challenging, so I will lead off.

Dr. Benda: This lack of epithelium invading bone is contrary to the collection of Professor Ruedi that he has shown us in a span of several generations. I wonder who is going to throw away Professor Ruedi's work.

Dr. Abramson: This concept of pure epithelium or epidermis in isolation is an artificial situation and something that only occurs in experimental conditions or in the mind of the researcher. Epithelium does not exist without its connective tissue. When we talk about a cholesteatoma we talk about a structure that has within it a subepithelial inflammatory connective tissue. Perhaps we are talking about something where the epithelium in migrating maintains this connective tissue in a primitive and inflammatory state.

Dr. Khan: Dr. Schuknecht, may I ask two questions? First, when you remove the cholesteatoma, do you do a tympanoplasty—I mean do you remove the cholesteatoma and do the tympanoplasty at the same time? Second, when you find the ossicular chain completely missing, the footplate and the round windows being all that is left, do you do type III or type IV reconstruction?

Dr. Schuknecht: I always remove the matrix, as we used to call it anyway, the squamous epithelium, even if there is a fistula, peel it out of the mastoid and get rid of the entire squamous epithelial lining. I have only failed to do that once and that was when I got cold feet about six months ago, when I was doing it on an only-hearing ear. As I started to peel the squamous epithelium off the fistula I could see the perilymphatic space open up a little bit. So, I laid it back down. In an only-hearing ear, I think that is good judgment. Other than that I see no virtue in leaving this lining if you are practicing modern otology, in which the objective is to either eliminate the mastoid entirely by leaving the canal wall up or minimizing its size by obliterating it.

The type IV is the one I do if all of the ossicles are destroyed except for the footplate and the drum is also destroyed. If there is a half of a drum or more and some ossicle left, then I think given other advantages of, let's say an ear that is not too seriously involved in cholesteatoma and so on, I would suggest an operation in which an attempt is made to create a tympanic space. In other words, an intact canal wall technique and possibly even a two-stage procedure if it is a child or the opposite

ear is involved, etc. I am sure that these are principles that are used by most of you here today.

Dr. Sadé: I feel compelled to answer Dr. Laurence in respect to metaplasia in adults. This is not a question of theory. If you will consult your local pathologist, he sees it daily in adults in chronic inflammation of mucosa, bronchitis, bronchiectasis, genitourinary infection and sinusitis. This is a daily occurrence.

Dr. Laurence: Let's have a good argument. Yes, I think this is perfectly true, but this is surely from the mucous metaplasia going to a keratinized one. You get it in bladder, trachea, bronchus, and so on. But do you get metaplasia from squamous epithelium to a mucous type?

Dr. Sadé: I don't really know. The only one which goes from squamous into mucous was cited. I cite the only information that I have is of patches of epithelium left in the ear which disappeared later. I cited five surgeons and the sixth one volunteered. I don't have any other information besides that in this direction.

Dr. Laurence: This is interesting because if so, this is a case of squamous epithelium going to mucous. I couldn't find any other one in the literature at all. I was interested because I got interested in vitamin A, and so I have been looking it up.

Dr. Plester: Ladies and gentlemen, we nearly got the impression this afternoon that cholesteatoma is not necessary for destruction of middle ear and temporal bone, but rather granulation tissue. This was demonstrated by Sadé, for instance, by showing that the amount of destruction of the ear ossicle in chronic otitis media is not nearly as great as in cholesteatoma. I got the same feeling. We must keep in mind that what is true for the ear ossicles is not necessarily true for labyrinth bone and the other bone of the temporal bone because we rarely see destruction of the bone of the otic capsule itself. We never see a fistula (nearly) without a cholesteatoma.

Dr. Bellucci: We must differentiate the pattern of advancement of cholesteatoma in two ways. Granulation tissue causes the destruction and the advancement of the cholesteatoma over it. This is proved by some men this afternoon that endotoxins are liberated by some organisms and these are very common organisms in the cholesteatoma, such as proteus, and pseudomonas. These are the ones that have this endotoxin. It makes sense to me to see that the granulation of subepithelial layer is the active layer being worked upon by the organisms which are normally present in a cholesteatoma. Instead of looking at it as the epithelium advancing, you ought to think about it as the epithelial structures following the subepithelial structures in its advancement in response to infection. At surgery we must consider the control of infection, if we are ever going to cure this disease permanently.

Dr. Friedberg: We have heard some very nice explanations of how squamous epithelium gets to the site of disease, if I can use that term. I think all the mechanisms described at one time or another probably do obtain. We can all give very concrete examples of this. Probably no one fits at all times. We have also seen some very dramatic work demonstrating the effect of various mesenchymal factors and unquestionably many of these things are important in bone destruction and collagenase activity and all the rest.

With all this sophisticated information the surgeon goes in with a knife and fork and carries out an extremely gross procedure, at least in terms of the things we have seen today, and he scrapes out some skin, some bone, some granulation tissue and lo and behold the wonder of it all is not that there is a recurrence or persistence of disease, but that very often the disease is cured. I mean that in its absolute sense the disease is cured. Well, what has he done? Very often he has left "matrix" and there is no difference between that and the stuff he scraped out. It is still cholesteatoma. He has left granulation tissue. He has gotten some of it out, but we have heard that it isn't necessary to get all the granulation tissue out. He hasn't changed the genetics or the basic biochemistry of this tissue. He has left various raw areas which subsequently re-epithelialized with skin, if I may use the term, and the patient is cured. What in fact has he done? The only thing I can see is that he has taken an ear that, for some reason, has epithelium that has lost its capacity to migrate and we know that epithelium does migrate, and has converted it back to an ear that can migrate. Subsequently he has aborted all these other things that are very real, but which subsequently cause all this destruction we are worried about. The only thing the surgeon has done is enable it to migrate normally and stopped everything else.

Dr. Lim: Concerning whether the epidermis erodes the bone or not, perhaps we've been looking at the problem from the wrong angle. It has been proven that a cholesteatoma destroys bone. Perhaps we have been talking too much about osteoclasts and bone destruction, and have overlooked bone remodeling in terms of bone regeneration as a result of inflammation.

I would also like to comment on Dr. Thomsen's data that he failed to see osteoclasts. Also, he alluded to the study done in the otosclerotic stapes where they failed to see osteoclasts. I haven't seen one single specimen where osteoclasts kept eating up the bone and there is finally a collapsed temporal bone. It doesn't happen. You always see new bone formation right next to osteoclasts. I think the osteoclast may be the time-honored sequence of events when it destroys the bone the same time it is being regenerated.

Dr. Bernstein: When we perform surgery for chronic ear disease, we almost always see resorption of the lenticular process and long process of the incus. Nothing has been mentioned about blood flow to the ossicles. Why is it that the head of the malleus seems to be so hardy and very often the entire malleus, even when it is surrounded by cholesteatoma, is not resorbed? Very often the short process of the incus surrounded by cholesteatoma is not resorbed. Could anybody make a comment on the frequency of why the long process and lenticular process seem to be so often the first bone that does, followed, I think, by the superstructure of the stapes? Could it possibly be related to obstruction of blood flow, rather than the mechanisms that we mentioned today? These are questions that need answers.

Section II

Etiological Aspects

Chapter 3

Pathogenesis

CHOLESTEATOMA PATHOGENESIS: EVIDENCE FOR THE MIGRATION THEORY

Maxwell Abramson, M.D.
Bruce J. Gantz, M.D.
Richard G. Asarch, M.D.
Ward B. Litton, M.D.

Most otologists today believe that migration explains the pathogenesis of middle ear cholesteatoma—that canal wall skin grows medially into the middle ear to form an epidermal sac. We will discuss this theory on the available evidence to see if this is justified and to apply it to the various forms of cholesteatoma. We again need to define cholesteatoma and to delineate its diverse forms, since migration may not apply equally to all its forms. Cholesteatoma is a three dimensional epidermal and connective tissue structure, usually in the form of a sac, and frequently conforming to the architecture of various spaces of the middle ear, attic, and mastoid. This structure has the capacity for progressive and independent growth at the expense of underlying bone and has a tendency to recur after removal.

Cholesteatomas present themselves in three clinical forms. They occur behind intact tympanic membranes and often are called "primary" or "congenital" cholesteatomas. They appear as diverticula of the pars flaccida, are of limited size, occur in patients with middle ear atelectasis or secretory otitis media, and have little or no history of otorrhea. This form of the disease is often called "primary acquired" cholesteatoma. Finally, cholesteatomas appear with posterosuperior perforations containing granulation tissue polyps and considerable foul smelling otorrhea; a disease process filling the antrum, mastoid, and frequently attic and middle ear as well. This type is often called "secondary acquired" cholesteatoma. Yet, all cholesteatomas are secondary though it is not clear what the primary processes are. Unfortunately, cholesteatomas occur beyond our view; and they are painless.

What evidence is there that migration of epithelium plays a role in the pathogenesis of cholesteatoma? If we are asking whether migration is necessary for epidermal sac formation, the answer is "yes". The formation of a sac requires both cell migration and cell division. There is considerable evidence from studies in organogenesis (Grobstein, 1967 and Slavkin, et al, 1968) and in epithelialization of wounds (Ordman and Gillman, 1966; Christophers, 1972; and Krawczyk, 1972) that migration of existing cells is a primary process and can proceed to a variable, but significant extent in the absence of cell division. However, if the cholesteatomas arise from the outside in, rather than from the inside out, the answer is not obvious. What evidence there is on this question, may not apply to all forms of the disease. The medial or lateral pathogenesis question is of great importance; a question we must consider in determining the appropriate surgical treatment for the various forms of cholesteatoma. We must study the reasons for our surgical failures, especially in differentiating persistent from recurrent cholesteatomas.

Now, the study of fundamental processes of skin will not tell us exactly how cholesteatoma is formed in the middle ear, but it will tell us the factors that influence epithelial behavior in other situations that bear similarity to cholesteatoma. Skin is well suited for its primary role of covering and protection by its ability to migrate. This capacity is held in check under conditions of stability and is released under a variety of injurious and inflammatory conditions (Christophers, 1972). Epithelial cells lose attachments to basement membranes and move with cell processes by way of temporary attachments to adjacent cells activated through contractile intracellular microfilaments (Krawczyk, 1972). What controls the direction of this movement? It is clear that epithelial orientation and direction is not a property inherent in the epithelium itself. It is derived from tactile clues from the epithelial substratum, or connective tissue (Weiss, 1959-60).

The flimsiness of the subepithelial connective tissue of the tympanic membrane, especially the pars flaccida, the susceptibility of connective tissue fiber reorientation due to middle ear pressure changes, as well as inflammatory induced connective tissue contraction of attic mesenteries, have made the migration theory both logical and popular. In fact, it seems reasonable to ask not whether the skin migrates into the middle ear, but why doesn't epithelial migration occur in all cases of otitis media? What keeps the skin out of the middle ear? In central perforations, it seems that the dense connective tissue of the middle layer of the tympanic membrane acts as a barrier to epithelial migration. Of course, at the pars flaccida and at the marginal perforation of the posterosuperior quadrant of the tympanic membrane, there is no connective tissue barrier, no annulus tympanicus. While wound healing has been an attractive model for cholesteatoma pathogenesis, it is well to point out some shortcomings of the analogy. Wounds typically are temporary processes. The epithelial migration stops, the mitotic rate falls, hyperplasia subsides, and the connective tissue matures after the defect has been covered (Christophers, 1972 and Krawczyk, 1972). In cholesteatomas, we are dealing with a non-healing, non-maturing, usually progressive process.

None of this general schema is of particularly recent discovery. In fact, the mechanisms and rationale for the migration theory of cholesteatoma pathogenesis have been described over 80 years ago. Habermann (1888) discussed the question of whether cholesteatomas grow from inside out or from inside in, just as we do today. At that time, the metaplasia theory espoused by Von Troltsch and Wendt was popular. Habermann based his conclusions on migration from the autopsy findings of one patient and followed it with case histories of three similar cases. The patient he described died of a cerebellar abscess associated with chronic otitis media. He traced a strip of epidermis from a defect in the cerebellar dura through the posterior canal wall, connecting to the edge of the posterosuperior perforation. He based his view of lateral versus medial growth on the presence of normal mucosa surrounding the epidermal strip throughout its course. He contended that canal wall skin migrated into the middle ear to "heal".

Soon after that, Bezold (1892) described his views of cholesteatoma genesis. He was impressed by the occurrence of cholesteatoma in previously atelectatic ears and believed that intermittent mild eustachian tube obstruction caused retraction of pars flaccida against the malleus neck, with inflammation causing microscopic ruptures. The presence of skin in the middle ear led to inflammation that stimulated further epithelial growth. He based his view of medial migration of canal skin on a case in which he observed progressive growth of skin from an attic perforation to line the middle ear and attic. He observed this through a large posterior canal wall defect.

The senior author (M. A.) first became interested in the pathogenesis of middle ear cholesteatoma during his residency at the Massachusetts Eye and Ear Infirmary in studying its temporal bone collection. Most of the cases were too extensive to determine the pathogenesis. In early lesions and retractions (Fig. 67), the inflammatory process extends medially and the tympanic membrane epithelium appears to have no respect for the basement membrane or tympanic membrane connective tissue. There are certain advantages in studying cholesteatomas with human temporal bone histology. The authentic disease can be studied in situ, and tissue types can be determined with certainty, as opposed to some guesswork in observations made in the operating room. Histology by itself, however, has certain deficiencies in determining the mechanisms of a process. There are problems associated with sampling error. Each bone represents a single instantaneous observation of a chronic disease having a natural history measured in years. More important, the observation is usually made many years after the development of the disease. For example, the mean age of cholesteatoma patients coming for treatment at the University of Iowa in 1974 was 25 years, and most of these patients had a past history dating several years before that.

Animal Model Studies

The need to study cholesteatoma pathogenesis through systematic observations at various stages led many investigators to study cholesteatomas in animal models. Most of this work was based on a presumed inductive effect of inflammatory connective tissue on epithelial migration and consisted of injecting irritating agents through the tympanic membrane. This was begun by Berberich (1927), who used hot tar. Among the pioneers in this field are Friedmann (1955), who developed an animal model of otitis media with pathogenic bacteria, and showed that a certain percentage of these animals developed skin in the middle ear. Fernandez and Lindsay (1960) injected quinine into the bulla of guinea pigs inducing epithelial migration in three of 30 animals. They found no tympanic membrane perforation in one of these three animals. The experimental finding of epithelial migration without tympanic membrane perforation was also demonstrated by Ruedi (1959).

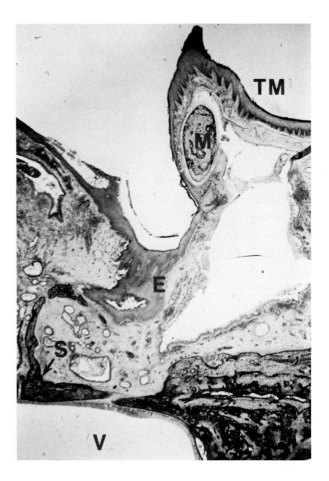

Fig. 67: Human temporal bone showing epithelium (E) of a retraction pocket extending medially against the stapes (S) which is undergoing resorption. The tympanic membrane (TM) malleus handle (M) and vestibule (V) are also shown.

Our interest in animal models of middle ear cholesteatoma was stimulated by concern with factors which enhance epithelial migration, plus a need to develop a model of middle ear bone resorption. Epidermal cysts at the cochlea were induced in a variety of ways (Abramson et al, 1975), using skin as free grafts and flaps. The addition of talc increased our yield of cysts. We could induce a 33% incidence of epidermal cyst with a flap of skin alone placed under the mucosa of the bulla (Fig. 68). Epidermal cysts could not be induced with free skin grafts without talc, or with talc alone. These

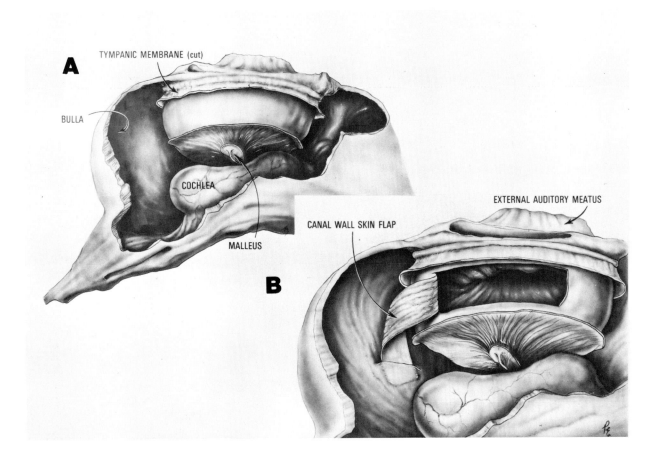

Fig. 68: Operative approach used to produce middle ear epidermal cysts in guinea pigs showing the left ear from a ventral approach. In (**A**), the bulla wall and tympanic membrane have been removed. The method producing a three in ten incidence of epidermal cysts is shown in (**B**) as a flap of canal wall skin inserted into a mucosal pocket. *(Courtesy of Ann. Otol. Rhinol. Laryngol., 84: 426, 1975.)*

cysts ranged from small (Fig. 69) to large (Fig. 70), and, in fact, resembled human middle ear cholesteatomas. The incidence of epidermal cysts at the cochlea was 15%, or eight of 55 animals.

We attempted to increase the incidence of epithelial migration by using a chemical irritant placed into the bulla followed by a marginal perforation at the dorsal portion of the tympanic membrane. In a series of twelve animals in which perforations followed oxalic acid inflammation (Table 22), followed from three days to six months, epithelial migration into the middle ear was noted

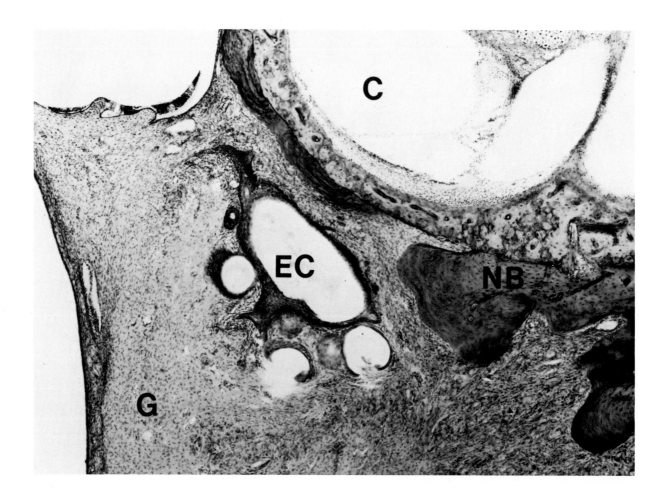

Fig. 69: Guinea pig temporal bone shown three months after a free graft of canal wall skin and talc were placed on the cochlea (C). A small epidermal cyst (EC) is seen within granulation tissue (G) adjacent to the cochlea (C) which contains new bone (NB). *(Courtesy of Ann. Otol. Rhinol. Laryngol., 84: 426, 1975.)*

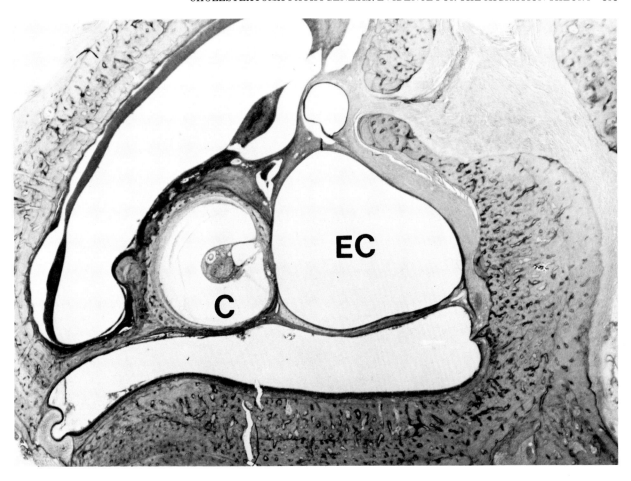

Fig. 70: Temporal bone from group of guinea pigs having canal skin flap inserted under bulla mucosa as shown in Figure 68B. A large epidermal cyst (EC) lies against the cochlea (C) causing a cochlea fistula. *(Courtesy of Ann. Otol. Rhinol. Laryngol., 84: 426, 1975.)*

TABLE 22

Epithelial Migration after Oxalic Acid and Perforation of Tympanic Membrane in Guinea Pigs

Time after Perf. (weeks)	No. of Animals	Skin into Middle Ear	TM Healing
.5	1	0	0
1	2	2	0
2	2	2	0
3	1	0	0
4	3	3	0
25	3	2	0
Total:	12	9 (75%)	

in nine, for an incidence of 75%. The middle ear was lined by skin as early as two weeks after perforation (Fig. 71). Skin with epithelial hyperplasia was found four weeks after perforation (Fig. 72). In six animals having tympanic membrane perforations without pretreatment with irritants, the tympanic membranes appeared healed at four weeks after injury but did not show epithelial hyperplasia or cones of epithelium extending into the middle ear.

In summary, animal experiments show clearly that canal wall skin can be induced to migrate into the middle ear and even form a cyst under a variety of inflammatory influences, and that tympanic membrane perforation is not necessary in epithelial migration into the middle ear as long as persistent inflammation is present.

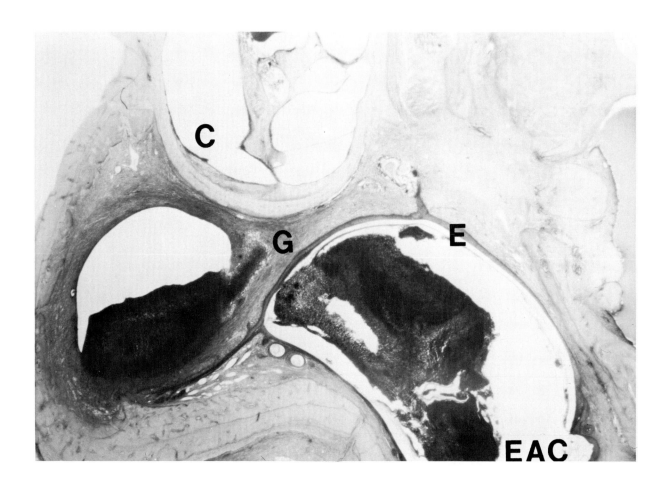

Fig. 71: Guinea pig temporal bone shown four weeks after oxalic acid instillation and two weeks after a marginal tympanic membrane perforation. Epithelium fills the middle ear lying on granulation tissue (G) covering the cochlea (C). A cone of epithelium at (E) extends into the attic. The external auditory canal (EAC) is below.

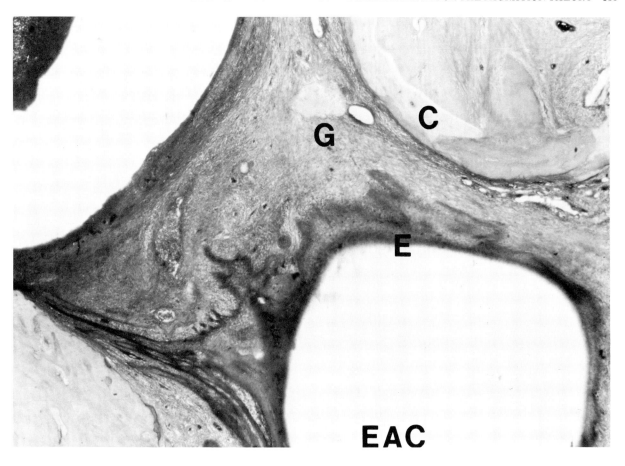

Fig. 72: Guinea pig temporal bone shown six weeks after oxalic acid instillation and four weeks after tympanic membrane perforation. Granulation tissue (G) covered by invasive appearing squamous epithelium (E) overlies the cochlea (C). The external auditory canal (EAC) is below.

Clinical Study

All animal model experiments, of course, suffer from varying degrees of dissimilarity from conditions found in human disease. In order to understand the pathogenesis of cholesteatoma, it is necessary to study the disease in humans at a time when the process is taking place. We studied the records of all patients undergoing surgical treatment for cholesteatoma at the University of Iowa in 1974. The history, physical findings, clinical course, and operative findings were reviewed in attempt to find information on the following questions: Can cholesteatomas be divided into three distinct clinical types? If cholesteatoma grows from outside in, can this process be observed? We paid particular attention to recurrent cholesteatoma in attempting to answer this. And finally, if cholesteatoma develops through migration of canal wall or tympanic membrane epithelium, operative findings should document the presence of epidermal sacs attached laterally, but separated from medial structures by normal mucosa. In 1974, 95 patients underwent 103 operations for cholesteatoma in our clinic. Cholesteatomas were divided into small and large, based on site of occurrence. Cholesteatomas present only in the middle ear or attic were considered small, while cholesteatomas present in the aditus, antrum, or mastoid were considered large cholesteatomas. All cholesteatomas involving the aditus, antrum, or mastoid were extensive, having some connection to the middle ear or attic. Our patients ranged in age from five to 72 years, with a mean of 22.2 for small cholesteatomas and 28.2 for large, with 25.3 for the total population. Patients with small and large cholesteatomas, therefore, did not differ significantly in age.

Of the 95 patients treated in 1974, 72 were treated for cholesteatomas in that ear for the first time, while 23 patients had previous treatment or recurrence during 1974.

The cholesteatomas in our series were almost equally divided into 51 small lesions, treated with exploratory tympanotomy, or atticotomies, and 52 large lesions, or mastoid cholesteatomas, treated by modified radical mastoidectomy, facial recess middle ear approach with mastoidectomy, or a complete mastoidectomy by itself (Table 23).

Could the presenting history and physical findings help differentiate these cholesteatomas into types? Seventeen patients (Table 24) presented with intact tympanic membranes. Of the 11 patients undergoing exploratory tympanotomy, ten had persistent cholesteatoma from previous surgery. The remaining six patients with intact tympanic membranes had a history of otorrhea in childhood and could have had subsequent healing of tympanic membrane sealing off the migrating process from the outside. Of course, otorrhea is so common that there are few individuals who can completely deny its past history. The large and small cholesteatoma patients did present somewhat different histories. They had so much overlap, however, that differentiation was difficult until the extent was determined at exploration. The small cholesteatomas tended to have a history of secretory otitis media with tube insertion, little drainage, and middle ears showing some atelectasis, while the large cholesteatomas had a history of otorrhea frequently occurring after swimming rather than after upper respiratory infections. This finding suggests that many of these large cholesteatomas began as small retractions and got infected from the outside. The large cholesteatomas were more likely to have posterosuperior perforation with granulation tissue rather than dry attic retractions. Are these cholesteatomas separate and distinct types, or can sepsis convert one form into the other? The only evidence we

TABLE 23

Surgical Treatment of Patients with Cholesteatoma 1974

Expl. Tympanotomy	20
Atticotomy	31
Modified Radical	44
Facial Recess	7
Complete Mastoid	1
Total:	103

TABLE 24

Physical Findings in Patients with Cholesteatoma

	Intact TM	Retr. Pocket with Ext.	Perf. or Retr.	Total
Exp. Tymp.	11	0	9	20
Atticot.	4	3	24	31
Mod. Rad.	2	7	35	44
Canal Up	0	0	7	7
Comp. Mast.	0	0	1	1

have on this question comes from recurrent cholesteatomas. Eight of our 23 recurrent cholesteatomas converted from small to large after initial surgery. However, this could be due either to growth and migration, or represent persistent antral or mastoid disease that was missed at the primary operation.

Evidence for a developing, migrating epithelial process could be determined in ten patients in our series. This was based on more than one observation in which a retraction, whose depths could be felt or seen, was noted to have extended on a subsequent visit. Of the seven patients, in the category undergoing modified radical mastoidectomy, four had previous atticotomies with the development of a retraction pocket extending gradually out of sight.

In review of the operative records of small cholesteatomas, we were not able to obtain evidence of retraction pockets surrounded medially by normal mucosa. Epidermal sacs were attached laterally, but had replaced mucosa medially, showing that skin and mucosa do not coexist in apposition. We determined the position of cholesteatoma sacs in the 31 atticotomies, finding the skin lateral to the incus body and/or malleus head in 16, inferior in four, and medial in 11. The lateral, or inferior position of the sac would tend to support a lateral to medial progression of the disease, rather than the reverse.

Summary

The evidence in favor of migration in cholesteatoma pathogenesis can be summarized as follows: (1) Epidermis is well suited for its role for protection and cover by its capacity for migration under conditions of injury and inflammation; (2) animal experiments have clearly shown that canal wall skin can be induced to migrate into the middle ear under inflammatory conditions likely to occur there, and will form bone resorbing epidermal cysts; (3) middle ear and attic cholesteatomas as well as large recurrent cholesteatomas appear to develop as retraction pocket diverticula and grow from lateral to medial; (4) the mechanism of pathogenesis of large previously untreated mastoid and antral cholesteatomas is not clear, but epithelial migration must play a role in the morphogenesis of the epidermal structure; and (5) the development of human cholesteatomas occur asymptomatically and, in most cases, beyond our view.

It seems then that the pathogenesis of cholesteatoma requires an inflammatory process and probably eustachian tube dysfunction. These combine to injure the middle ear mucosa, change the orientation of the attic mesenteries and pars flaccida connective tissue, and stimulate both migration and growth of canal wall and tympanic membrane epidermis. Basically, we are restating the conclusion of Habermann and Bezold. In order to go beyond the classical descriptions of 75 years ago, we will need to determine the precise relationships of these processes in the ear.

Acknowledgement

This investigation was supported by PHS grant NS 10608 from the National Institute of Neurological Diseases and Stroke and the Deafness Research Foundation.

References

1. Abramson, M.; Asarch, R. G.; and Litton, W. B.: Experimental aural cholesteatoma causing bone resorption. *Ann. Otol. Rhinol. Laryngol.*, 84:425, 1975.

2. Berberich, J.: Das experimentalle mittelohrcholesteatoma. *Z Hals-Nas-Ohrenheilk*, 10:881, 1927.

3. Bezold, F.: Cholesteatoma, perforation of Shrapnell's membrane, and occlusion of the tubes—an etiological study. *Arch. Oto.*, 21:232, 1892.

4. Christophers, E.: The kinetic aspects of epidermal healing. In Malbach, H. I. and Rovee, D. T.: (Eds). *Epidermal Wound Healing.* Year Book Medical Publishers, Inc., Chicago, Illinois, 1972, pp. 52.

5. Fernandez, C. and Lindsay, J. R.: Aural cholesteatoma. Experimental observations. *Laryngoscope*, 70:1119, 1960.

6. Friedmann, I.: The comparative pathology of otitis media. Experimental and human. II. The histopathology of experimental otitis of the guinea pig with particular reference to experimental cholesteatoma. *J. Laryngol. Otol.*, 69:588, 1955.

7. Grobstein, C.: Mechanisms of organogenetic tissue interaction. *Nat'l. Cancer Inst. Monograph*, 26:279, 1967.

8. Habermann, J.: Zur entstehung des cholesteatoms des mittelohrs (cysten in der schleimhaut der paukenhohle, atrophie der nerven in der schnecke). *Arch. Ohrenheilk.*, 27:42, 1888.

9. Krawczyk, W. S.: Some ultrastructural aspects of epidermal repair in two model wound healing systems. In Malbach, H. I. and Rovee, D. T.: (Eds.). *Epidermal Wound Healing.* Year Book Medical Publishers, Inc., Chicago, Illinois, 1972, pp. 123.

10. Ordman, L. J. and Gillman, T.: Studies in the healing of cutaneous wounds. I. The healing of incisions through the skin of pigs. *Arch. Surg.*, 93:857, 1966.

11. Ruedi, L.: Cholesteatoma formation in the middle ear in animal experiments. *Acta Otolaryngol.*, 50:233, 1959.

12. Slavkin, H. C.; Beierle, J.; and Bavetta, L. A.: Odontogenesis cell-cell interactions in vitro. *Nature*, 217:269, 1968.

13. Weiss, P.: The biologic foundations of wound repair. *Harvey Lecture Series*, 55:13, 1959-60.

EVIDENCE FOR THE MIGRATION THEORY: ULTRASTRUCTURAL CELL TYPES IN THE EPITHELIAL LAYER OF CHOLESTEATOMA

Georges Bremond, M.D.
Jacques Magnan, M.D.

The electron microscopic study of the epithelial layer of cholesteatoma shows the existence of keratinocytes. The morphology of these keratinocytes is the same as that of the skin, and their potential evolution is similar. They result in the formation of keratin scales.

There are also two other, very particular, types of cells: Langerhans' cells and Merkel's cells. These two cells were first described in the skin. The ultrastructural aspect of the skin in the bony portion of the acoustic meatus appears to be exactly the same as that of cholesteatoma.

Cholesteatoma is a lesion of the inflammatory pseudotumor type. Its histological appearance is always identical: cholesteatoma is keratinizing stratified squamous epithelium on a layer of connective tissue. This combination of epithelial and subepithelial tissue together is called the "matrix."

With ultrastructural observations, one can determine precisely the fine structure of cholesteatoma, and distinguish the presence of particular cell types in the epithelial layer.

Material and Methods

Our observations are based on smears removed during surgery, from 35 patients who have chronic cholesteatomatous otitis. These smears were immediately fixed in 2% glutaraldehyde, buffered with sodium cacodylate at PH $7._2$ for one hour at 4° C.

The fragments, subsequently cut into little squares 1 mm in diameter, were rinsed for 12 hours in the same buffer, and post-fixation in osmium tetraoxyde for one hour. Next, the smears were dehydrated with serial concentration of acetone, and then they were embedded in EPON 812 mixture. Semi-fine cuts were contrasted with uranyl-acetate for 30 minutes, then with lead citrate for two minutes. Afterwards, they were observed through a Hitashi H S 7 S or a Philips 300 electron microscope.

Results

Malpighian epithelium (Fig. 73). It is made up of four or five cell layers that convey basal cell differentiation towards the surface. The ultrastructural characteristics of the different cell layers are no different from those found in the epidermis.

The cells (keratinocytes) are joined together by desmosomes and in their cytoplasm they have tonofibrils that are inserted on the desmosomes and are condensed to thick bunches at the stratum spinosum. Dense masses appear in the cytoplasm of the stratum granulosum; they are formed by condensation of fibrillar structures and correspond to keratohyalin. In the stratum corneum these granules meet and fill the cytoplasm, while the pycnotic nucleus disappears. These keratinized cells, matured fully, degenerate and become squamous. The keratin scales, especially important for cholesteatoma, have an electron-dense and homogenous structure.

With electron microscopy one can examine two particular cell types in cholesteatoma. They are also found in skin, but are rarely described in cholesteatoma.

Langerhan's cells (Fig. 74). These are observed in the stratum spinosum between keratinocytes. These cells are not joined up with the keratinocytes, but are separated from them by a clear

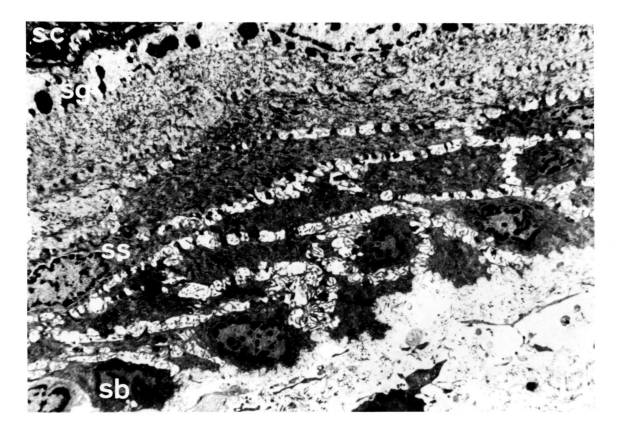

Fig. 73: The ultrastructural characteristics of cholesteatoma's different cell layers are similar from those found in the epidermis. The basal stratum (SB) formed of a unicellular layer. The stratum spinosum (SS) where the keratinocyte's maturation is accompanied by two characteristic phenomena: (1) the flattening of the cells and (2) the grouping of tonofilaments. The stratum granulosum (SG) characterized by keratohyalin grains aligned parallel to the surface. The stratum corneum (SC), the cell becomes a dead shell filled with keratin fibers that are electron dense.

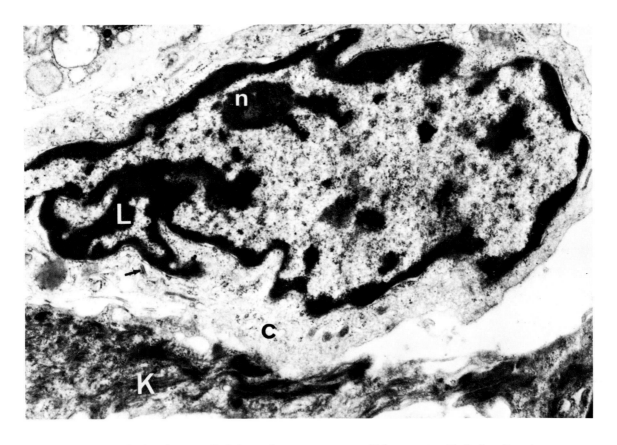

Fig. 74: The Langherans cell (L) has a clearer appearance which contrasts with the keratinocytes (K) darker aspect. The nucleus (N) is irregular and the cytoplasm (C) has no tonofilaments.

space. Their appearance is clear, their irregular nucleus is hollowed by multiple notches. The cytoplasm has no tonofilaments, but contains voluminous mitochondria and, especially, a characteristic cellular element that appears as a small vesicle prolonged by a stick-like shape, 400A in diameter and 0.1 to 0.3 in length, (Fig. 75).

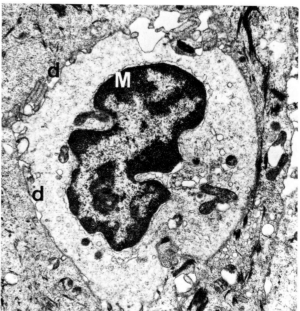

Fig. 76: The Merkel cell (M) looks globular; it has a large nucleus and clear cytoplasm. It is joined to neighboring keratinocytes by desmosomes (D).

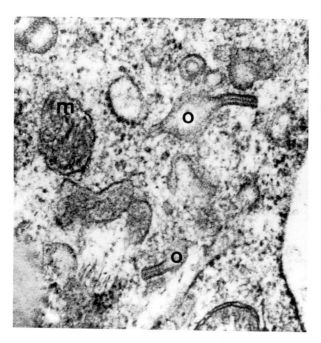

Fig. 75: The Langherans cell contains voluminous mitochondria (M) in its cytoplasm and a characteristic cellular element (O) that looks like a small vesicle with a stick-like prolongation.

Merkel's cells (Fig. 76). These clear cells are located in the stratum germinativum and are connected to neighboring keratinocytes by desmosomes. Their large, lobular, distorted nucleus looks like the Langerhans' cell nucleus, but these Merkel cells are smaller, more globular in shape and have no stick-like cellular elements.

Their clear cytoplasm contains numerous mitochondria and, especially, small, dense, rounded, osmiophilic granules, (Fig. 77).

No melanocytes type cells were observed in the cholesteatoma.

Basal membrane

It is attached to basal cells by hemidesmosomes and to the connective tissue by reticulinic fibrils. It has no particularities. The idea is now accepted that the origin of the basal membrane comes from epithelial cells that it supports, rather than from the connective tissue. In fact, the epithelial cells have the same antigenic properties and the same staining as the basal membrane.

Subepithelial layer

In the connective tissue there are a number of non-specific alterations, analogous to those found in all types of chronic inflammations.

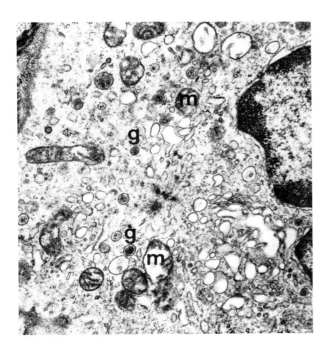

Fig. 77: The Merkel cell contains numerous mitochondria (M) and especially small, dense, rounded, very osmiophilic granules (G) in its cytoplasm.

Discussion

The discovery of two particular cell types in cholesteatoma needs some comment.

The presence of Langerhans' cells is well-known in the skin, the thymus and the stroma of certain tumors. It has already been observed in cholesteatoma (Ikeda, 1968; Bodelet and Wayoff, 1972; Lim and Saunders, 1972; Magnan, 1972; Bremond et al, 1975). Their mesenchymatous origin from histiocytic cells has been accepted (Winkelmann, 1969).

Merkel cells are sensory. They are usually found in certain cutaneous zones (finger pulp), as well as in nasal and buccal mucosa (Zelickson, 1967), but up till now they have never been described in cholesteatoma.

Since these cells do not normally exist in the middle ear mucosa (Lim et al, 1967; Lim and Hussl, 1969; Lim and Klainer, 1972; Kawabata and Paparella, 1969; Hentzer, 1970 and 1972; Coquin, 1970; Bremond and Coquin, 1972; and Hilding and Heywood, 1971). Their presence in cholesteatoma seems to provide a good argument in favor of the migratory theory in this lesion.

Metaplasia of middle ear mucosa can give epidermoid squamous epithelium, but not keratinizing squamous epithelium.

Furthermore, it is hard to believe that this metaplasia results in the formation of such particular cells as Langerhans' and Merkel cells, usually not found in the mucosa lining.

Thus far, ultrastructural descriptions of epithelial metaplasia into a stratified squamous type, especially in the ear (Bodelet and Wayoff, 1972) and bronchial mucosa (Gould et al, 1971), do not mention the presence of these two cell types.

On the contrary, the skin at the bottom of the external auditory meatus has the same histological and ultrastructural appearance as cholesteatoma.

References

1. Bodelet, B. and Wayoff, M.: Notes préliminaires sur l'ultrastructure du cholestéatome. *Ann. Otolaryngol. Chir, Cervicofac.*, 87: 449, 1970.

2. Bodelet, B. and Wayoff, M.: Métaplasie et cholestéatome. *Ann. Otalaryngol. Chir. Cervicofac.*, 89: 411, 1972.

3. Bremond, G. and Coquin, A.: Ultrastructure of normal and pathological middle ear mucosa. *J. Laryngol. Otol.*, 86: 457, 1972.

4. Bremond, G.; Magnan, J.; and De Micco, C.: Aspects microscopiques du cholestéatome. *Cahiers d'Oto Rhinolaryngologie*, 10: 303, 1975.

5. Coquin, A.: *Ultrastructure de la muqueuse normale et pathologie de l'oreille moyenne.* Thése Méd. Marseille Universite d'Aix, 1970.

6. Gould, V. E.; Wenk, R.; and Sommers, S. C.: Ultrastructural observations on bronchial epithelial hyperplasia and squamous metaplasia. *Cander*, 28: 426, 1971.

7. Hentzer, E.: Ultrastructure of the normal mucosa in the human middle ear, mastoid cavities, and eustachian tube. *Ann. Otol. Rhinol. Laryngol.*, 79: 1143, 1970.

8. Hentzer, E.: Ultrastructure of the middle ear mucosa in chronic suppurative otitis media. *J. Laryngol. Otol.*, 86: 447, 1972.

9. Hilding, D. A. and Heywood, P.: Ultrastructure of middle ear mucosa and organization of ciliary matrix. *Ann. Otol., Rhinol. Laryngol:* 80: 306, 1971.

10. Ikeda, M.: Electron microscopic studies of the fine structures of cholesteatoma epidermis. *J. Otolaryngol. Jpn.*, 71: 84-91, 1968.

11. Kawabata, I. and Paparella, M.: Ultrastructure of normal human middle ear mucosa. Preliminary report. *Ann. Otol. Rhinol. Laryngol.*, 78: 125, 1969.

12. Lim, D.; Paparella, M.; and Kimura, R. S.: Ultrastructure of the eustachian tube and middle ear mucosa in the guinea pig. *Acta-otolaryngol. (Stockh)*, 63: 425, 1967.

13. Lim, D. J. and Hussl, B.: Human middle ear epithelium—an ulstrastructural and cytochemical study. *Arch. Otolaryngol.*, 89: 835, 1969.

14. Lim, D. J. and Saunders, W. H.: Acquired cholesteatoma: light and electron microscopic observations. *Ann. Otol. Rhinol. Laryngol.*, 81:1, 1972.

15. Lim, D. J. and Klainer, A.: Cellular reactions in acute otitis media—scanning and transmission electron microscopy. *Laryngoscope*, 81: 1772, 1972.

16. Magnan, J.: *Le cholestéatoma (notions actuelles)* Thése Méd. Marseille Universite d'Aix, 1972.

17. Winkelmann, R. K.: The skin in histiocytosis X. *Mayo Clin. Proc.:* 44-535, 1969.

18. Zelickson, A. S.: *Ultrastructure of normal and abnormal skin.* Lea and Febiger, Philadelphia, Pennsylvania, 1967.

CHOLESTEATOMA OF THE MIDDLE EAR: PATHOGENESIS AND SURGICAL INDICATION

George T. Nager, M.D.

Pathogenesis

The first description of a cholesteatoma was given by Cruveilhier in the early part of the nineteenth century (1829). He referred to it as tumeur perleé or pearly tumor. Pathologically, the lesion represents an epidermal inclusion cyst. The term cholesteatoma—a misnomer—will be retained here because of its long-established place in the otological literature. The characteristic feature of a cholesteatoma is the presence of keratinizing stratified squamous epithelium within the middle ear cleft. This epithelial lining forms the matrix, which desquamates keratohyalin lamellae continually in a radial concentric direction. The layers of exfoliative keratin accumulate in an onion-skin-like fashion and form the bulk of the cholesteatoma. Because of the thin matrix, the capsule of the cholesteatoma is very delicate. The concentric lamellar structure of the cyst and the resultant interference of incident light gives the surface its characteristic mother-of-pearl sheen.

The cholesteatoma or epidermal inclusion cyst arises, with few exceptions from the skin lining, the deep portion of the external auditory canal, and the outer surface of the tympanic membrane. This area of skin is special in that it is thin, lacks the papillary and reticular layer of the dermis, and rests directly on the periosteum of the canal and on the middle layer of the tympanic membrane. The majority of cholesteatomas arise either from retraction of certain areas of the pars flaccida or pars tensa of the tympanic membrane, or from papillary downgrowth and migration of the squamous epithelium into the epi- or mesotympanic space (Figs. 78 and 79).

Dependent upon the site of origin, cholesteato-

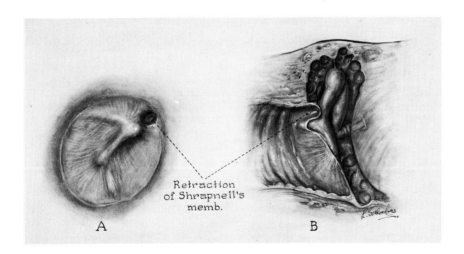

Fig. 78: (A) Illustrates the most frequent site of a retraction pocket in Shrapnell's membrane. (B) This pocket extends medially into the superior recess of the tympanic cavity or Prussack's space. Prussack's space is bounded laterally by the pars flaccida and medially by the neck of the malleus. The floor of this recess is formed by the lateral process of the malleus.

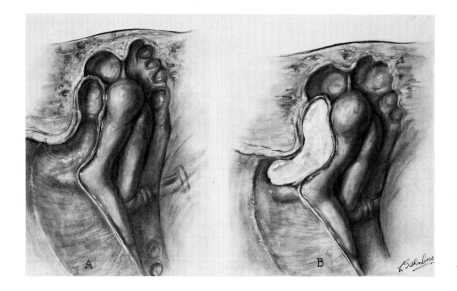

Fig. 79: **(A)** Illustrates the empty, skin-lined retraction pocket in Shrapnell's membrane which has become adherent to the walls of Prussack's space. **(B)** The accumulation of keratin within that pocket leads to the development of the attic retraction cholesteatoma.

mas may be divided into: (1) pars flaccida or Shrapnell-cholesteatomas and (2) pars tensa cholesteatomas.

The two basic mechanisms involved in the pathogenesis of the attic or Shrapnell's cholesteatoma are: (1) retraction of Shrapnell's membrane (attic retraction), and (2) active epithelial immigration, each with the propensity of forming an attic cholesteatoma.

The conditions that may predispose to the formation of an attic retraction cholesteatoma include: (1) a hereditary disposition; (2) hypocellular pneumatization; (3) a decrease in intratympanic pressure and (4) the presence of persistent embryonic, or newly formed connective tissue.

The threat of a cholesteatoma arises only once the retraction pocket begins to accumulate keratin and once it becomes superinfected. Accumulation in turn is enhanced by piling-up of epithelial debris in a small hollow space or cavity and difficulty or inability of evacuation of the aggregated material to the outside (Figs. 80 and 81).

The other, probably more frequent mechanism involved in the development of an attic cholesteatoma is active papillary proliferation and migration of the epidermis into the underlying connective tissue of the middle ear.

The predisposing factor for this mechanism are: (1) the inherent growth potential of the basal cells in the epidermis of Shrapnell's membrane

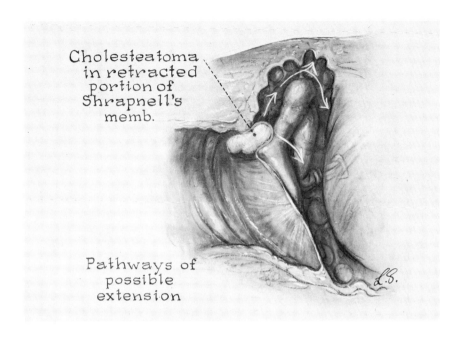

Fig. 80: Illustrates, in a coronal section, the directions in which the attic retraction cholesteatoma may expand within the anterior and superior region of the epitympanic recess.

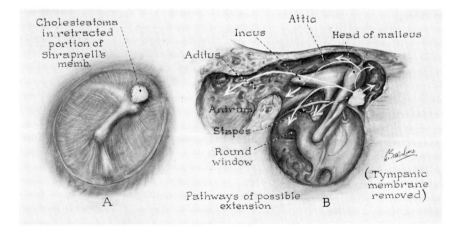

Fig. 81: Illustrates, in a lateral view, the directions in which the attic retraction cholesteatoma generally develops, and the routes by which it reaches the aditus, antrum, and the mesotympanum.

and in a circumscribed area of the meatal skin; (2) the submucosal connective tissue layer in the middle ear space, and (3) a hypocellular pneumatization.

The causative factor is an inflammatory stimulus associated with recurrent acute or chronic otitis media in childhood. The further development and local behavior is identical for the two forms of cholesteatomas. The majority of attic cholesteatomas present with a small perforation and an extension already to or beyond the mastoid antrum at the time of clinical recognition (Fig. 82).

It is conceivable that there is some overlapping in the mechanisms of the two types of attic cholesteatomas and that inflammation is not the only stimulus that can incite epithelial migration (Nager, 1976).

The pathogenesis of the pars tensa cholesteatoma is practically identical with the one of the cholesteatoma originating from the pars flaccida or Shrapnell's membrane. It arises in general either from retraction or from a typical papillary downgrowth of the squamous epithelium in certain predilective areas of the tympanic membrane. Ac-

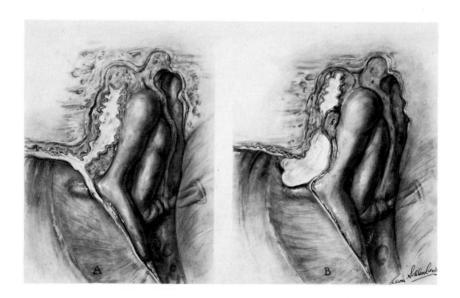

Fig. 82: (A) Illustrates an attic papillary cholesteatoma which evolves from papillary downgrowth of the keratinizing squamous epithelium lining Shrapnell's membrane, and the migration into the lateral recess of the attic. **(B)** It is conceivable that the two mechanisms (attic retraction and papillary downgrowth) may co–exist, in a rare instance, in the development of an attic cholesteatoma.

cordingly, a central and posterosuperior pars tensa retraction pocket and a central and posterosuperior near marginal pars tensa papillary cholesteatoma may be distinguished.

Central pars tensa retraction pockets have long been observed. Wittmaack (1918) and Steurer (1929) first mentioned their existence. They are frequently associated with ipsi- or contralateral attic retraction pockets. (Beichert 1957 and Schwarz 1966). Epithelial proliferation, accumulation of keratin, and to some extent an inflammatory irritation of the middle ear mucosa, are significant contributory factors. The pars tensa retraction pocket cholesteatoma results from chronic tubotympanic disease and its associated decrease in intratympanic pressure. Perforation of the cholesteatoma sac leads to superinfection and enhances the conversion of an initially "dry" to a "moist" cholesteatoma with otorrhea. Although the pathogenesis of the attic and pars tensa cholesteatoma is identical, the latter occurs much less frequently. (Fig. 83).

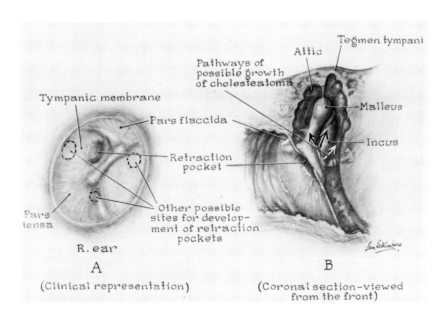

Fig. 83: (A) Illustrates the possible locations for the development of retraction pockets in the pars tensa. Progressive retraction of the posterosuperior quadrant of the drum may lead to invagination anterior and/or posterior to the long crus of the incus into the adjacent compartments of the epitympanic recess. (B) Arrows indicate the directions in which a pars tensa retraction pocket cholesteatoma may expand.

The posterosuperior pars tensa retraction pocket cholesteatoma differs from the central form in its location, mode of development, sequels and frequency. Its relation to adjacent bony structures, like in the attic retraction cholesteatoma, predisposes from the beginning to a development into and enlargement within the tympanic cavity; the narrow and unyielding opening into the external ear canal. Thus, plays a significant role in its initial and subsequent evolution. The retraction of the pars tensa leads in sequence to atrophy, apposition and adherence to the long crus of the incus. Further retraction may proceed in two directions, anterior and posterior to the long crus of the incus into the respective portion of the posteroinferior epitympanic recess. Occasionally, two retraction pockets may develop, one anterior, the other, posterior to the incus. Cholesteatomas arising in these retraction pockets have long been recognized otologically (Schwarz, 1966). Progressive enlargement of the cholesteatoma may lead to necrosis of the matrix, inflammation, periosteitis and osteitis with erosion of the annulus and adjacent bone. Increasing erosion of the tympanic bone may eventually result in a spontaneous radical cavity created by nature. On the other hand, a posterosuperior marginal pars tensa perforation, as pointed out by Ruedi (1958, 1959) may result in many instances from outward perforation of an epitympanic cholesteatoma (Fig. 84). The further development of the cholesteatoma is in the direction of least resistance either lateral

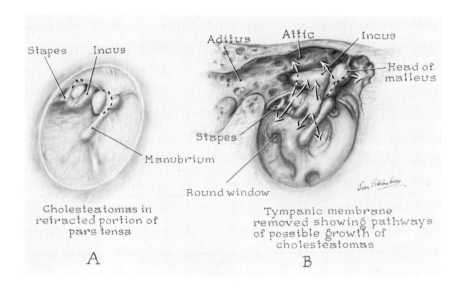

Fig. 84: (A) Illustrates one of the most frequent locations of a retraction pocket cholesteatoma in the pars tensa of the tympanic membrane. (B) Arrows indicate the routes by which posterosuperior pars tensa retraction pocket cholesteatomas generally reach the aditus, antrum, and other areas of the tympanum.

or medial to the ossicular chain or towards the hy-potympanum and tubal orifice. Progressive erosion of the ossicular chain and enlargement of the perforation leads to characteristic defects. The incus is either totally or partially destroyed, and the cholesteatoma at the time of clinical diagnosis usually extends to or beyond the antrum in about 80% of instances.

It was Kupper, who in 1876 first recognized the existence of the central pars tensa papillary cholesteatoma, and Habermann, who in 1889 initially described the developmental mechanism. Originally developing within the pars tensa, the cyst may perforate into the outer ear canal. The central perforation, therefore, is the result rather than the cause for the origin of the cholesteatoma.

Epidermal papillae normally are either very small or non-existent (Fig.85). However, in the presence of a chronic inflammatory process, the squamous epithelium begins to proliferate and form papillae. The papilla has a tendency to grow towards and into inflammatory granulation tissue. Such granulation tissue may develop within the tympanic membrane, following local necrosis of the fibrous layer of the eardrum, or exist on its undersurface as an inflammatory altered, embryonic, or newly formed connective tissue. The further finger-like penetration of a papilla into

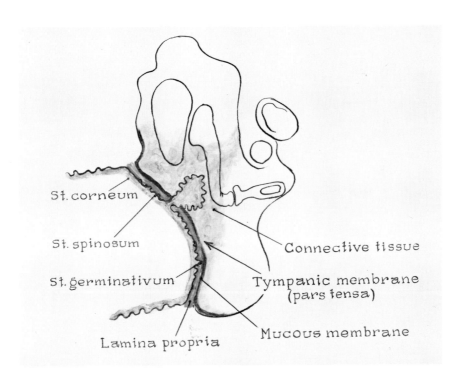

Fig. 85: Illustrates the development of papillary cholesteatoma of the pars tensa. A papilla from the epidermis, lining the outer surface of the tympanic membrane, protrudes through the drum into the underlying connective tissue to form an epidermoid inclusion cyst which subsequently may perforate into the outer ear canal.

the middle ear depends to a great extend upon this granulation tissue, with the epidermoid cyst developing in the center of the deeply penetrating papilla. Early rupture of the cholesteatoma within the middle ear may lead to a carpet-like spread of the matrix along the undersurface of the drum, already observed by Bezold in 1890 (Fig. 86).

Although the central papillary cholesteatoma may develop anywhere in the pars tensa, the posterosuperior quadrant is a predilective site. Progressive colliquation necrosis of the tympanic membrane, annulus and tympanic bone may lead to a marginal perforation. The further development is very similar to the one of the central pars

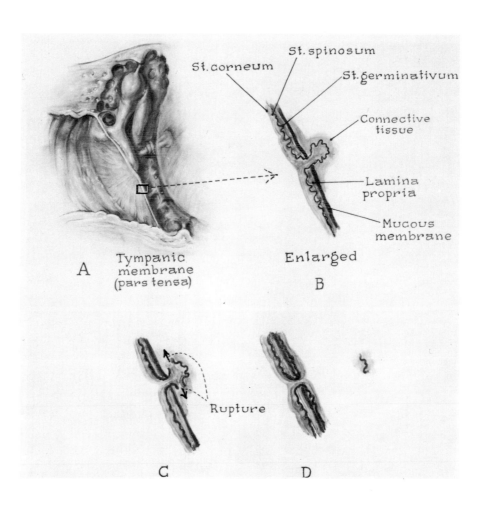

Fig. 86: A papillary pars tensa cholesteatoma may remain intact and gradually expand within the middle ear, or rupture early in its development, and give rise to a carpet-like spread of the cholesteatoma matrix over the undersurface of the tympanic membrane.

tensa retraction pocket cholesteatoma. Loss of hearing develops early and often reaches a considerable degree.

The posterosuperior pars tensa cholesteatoma which develops adjacent to the annulus is characterized in general by its deep location in the aditus or antrum, by its spherical form and by its long, slender, occasionally no longer recognizable connection to the tympanic membrane. It is recognized for its tendency to stimulate polypoid granulation tissue and the preservation of the ossicular chain in about 50% of instances (Schwarz, 1966).

The retraction pocket cholesteatoma develops on the basis of a chronic tubo-tympanic disease and is therefore associated with manifestations of decreased tympanic pressure and with initially transient, recurrent, but subsequently permanent decrease in hearing. Since this cholesteatoma in its initial stage is "dry", the inflammatory components are lacking, and it is the hearing impairment rather than the otorrhea which prompts the patient to see an otolaryngologist. The otoscopic examination often reveals a retraction of the pars flaccida, as well as of the pars tensa, or an adhesive process, bilaterally. Hypocellular pneumatization is the rule. The reaction of the middle ear mucosa remains restricted. By nature of its spherical form and clear demarcation, the cholesteatoma can be removed with ease, and the prognosis to achieve a dry and healed operative cavity is promising.

In the papillary cholesteatoma the circumstances are different. The stimulus and prerequisite for active epithelial immigration is a productive inflammatory process of the middle ear mucosa in the presence of embryonic or acquired connective tissue. The presence of this connective tissue is obvious. Varying in extent and location, it may obliterate the epi-, meso-, and hypotympanic space. The inflammatory component, its tendency to polypoid degeneration and its association with hypocellular pneumatization are striking. A papillary cholesteatoma in the majority of instances affects one ear only.

To differentiate between a cholesteatoma that has developed on the basis of retraction of a certain area of the tympanic membrane and one that has arisen from papillary downgrowth and epithelial immigration, may be difficult, and in a more advanced stage can only be assumed on clinical grounds. The distinction becomes easier and more reliable histologically when reviewing a cholesteatoma in serial sections of the temporal bones.

Surgical Indication

The decision between conservative and surgical management depends upon the nature of the disease process. The cholesteatoma of the middle ear is characterized, in general, by its chronic progressive course and lack of spontaneous healing. The complications are considerable and their nature and significance are well recognized. Conservative management, therefore, has little to offer, and is justified only in exceptional cases. A hesitant attitude, by loss of valuable time, increases the surgical difficulties and risks and reduces the chances for preservation of hearing and permanent eradication of the disease. For these reasons, early operation has long become the generally accepted treatment of choice. Thus, the indication does not depend upon the developmental stage or the hearing level, rather upon the responsibility to eradicate the pathological process, to avoid complications, and to preserve cochlear and vestibular function.

Early surgical management depends on accurate assessment of a cholesteatoma in good time and on a clear understanding of the pathogenesis of its different forms, its predisposing factors, biology and regional behavior. The influential factors—heredity, pneumatization, tubal anatomy and physiology, persistence of embryonic—(or development of new reactive connective tissue), the role of a local or adjacent inflammatory process, and the host response must all be thoroughly understood. The mechanisms which lead to the involvement of adjacent structures, bone, facial nerve, membranous cochlea and vestibular labyrinth, blood vessels, endocranium, etc. have to be perceived. To this must be added the surgical experience of others and one's own which has long taught us that the majority of cholesteatomas by the time of their clinical recognition already extend to or beyond the mastoid antrum, and that there are forms of cholesteatomas that are clearly more treacherous than others. Whereas, the papillary cholesteatoma by nature of its pathogenesis has no chance to be arrested in its evolution, the beginning retraction pocket cholesteatoma can be controlled by meticulous cleaning and elimination of the stimulus responsible for the epithelial proliferation. Finally, there are situations in which a cholesteatoma should be managed conservatively and can indeed be controlled without further loss of sensory function or additional risks for the patient. We share the concept that not every cholesteatoma has to be managed surgically. Thus, the decision when, and at what stage to advocate an operation, and the selection of the appropriate approach and technique requires a thorough understanding of the pathogenesis of the middle ear cholesteatoma in addition to surgical expertise.

Summary

The majority of middle ear cholesteatomas arise either from retraction of certain areas of the pars flaccida or pars tensa of the tympanic membrane or from papillary proliferation and immigration of the squamous epithelium lining the outer surface of the drum into the epi-, or mesotympanic compartment, of the middle ear.

Dependent upon the site of origin, pars flaccida (Shrapnell) cholesteatomas, and pars tensa cholesteatomas may be distinguished. According to the pathogenesis a retraction pocket cholesteatoma may be differentiated from a papillary cholesteatoma.

The predisposing factors for retraction of the tympanic membrane include: (1) a genetic disposition; (2) hypocellular pneumatization; (3) decrease in intratympanic pressure; and (4) presence of persistent embryonic or newly formed, reactive connective tissue in the middle ear.

The threat of a cholesteatoma arises only once the retraction pocket begins to accumulate keratin and once it becomes superinfected.

The predisposing factors for papillary proliferation and immigration of squamous epithelium into the middle ear comprise: (1) an inherent growth potential of the basal cell layer of the epidermis covering the outer surface of the drum; (2) the submucosal connective tissue in the middle ear, and (3) hypocellular pneumatization. The provocative impulse for active epithelial proliferation and immigration is an inflammatory process, generally in the middle ear.

The two mechanisms involved in the pathogenesis of these cholesteatomas in all likelihood overlap in some instances, and inflammation may not be the only stimulus that can incite epithelial proliferation.

The majority of attic cholesteatomas present with a small perforation, and most attic and middle ear cholesteatomas extend already to or beyond the mastoid antrum at the time of clinical recognition.

Since the middle ear cholesteatoma is characterized, in general, by a chronic progressive course, conservative management has little to offer, and is justified only in exceptional instances. The otologist's responsibility is to permanently eradicate the disease to avoid possible serious complications, and to preserve cochlear and vestibular function.

The prerequisites of competent management are: (1) a clear concept of the pathogenesis, nature, and regional behavior of the middle ear cholesteatoma, and (2) surgical expertise.

Acknowledgement

Mr. Leon Schlossberg, Assistant Professor, Department of Art as Applied to Medicine, provided the illustrations.

Mr. Chester F. Reather, RBP, Director of the Photomicrography Laboratory, Department of Otolaryngology, provided the photographs.

References

1. Beickert, P.: Hernienartige entstehung und entwicklung von cholesteatomen. *Zschr. Laryng.*, 36:154, 1957.

2. Bezold, F.: Cholesteatom, perforation der membrana flaccida Shrpanelli und tubernverschluss, eine atiologische studie. *Zschr. Ohr. hk.*, 20:5, 1890.

3. Cruveilhier, L. J. B.: *Anatomie Pathologique du Corpus Humani.* Vol. 1, Book 2, J. B. Bailliere, Paris, France, 1829.

4. Habermann, J.: Entstehung des cholesteatoms des mittelohres. *Arch. Ohr. Nas. Kehlk. hk.*, 27:42, 1889.

5. Kupper: Cholesteatom des trommelfells. *Arch. Ohr. Nas. Kehlk. hk.*, 11:6, 1876.

6. Nager, G. T.: Theories on the origin of attic retraction cholesteatomas. In Shambaugh: *Fifth International Workshop on Middle Ear Microsurgery and Fluctuat Hearing Loss.* Northwestern University Medical School, Chicago, February 29-Mar. 5, 1976.

7. Ruedi, L.: Cholesteatosis of the attic. *J. Laryngol. Otol.*, 72:593, 1958.

8. Ruedi, L.: Cholesteatomformation in the middle ear in animal experiments. *Acta Otolaryng.*, 50:233, 1959.

9. Schwarz, M.: *Das cholesteatom in Gerhorgang und im mittelohr. Zwangslose Abhandlungen aus dem Gebiete der Hals-Nasen-Ohrenheilkunde, Heft 8.* Georg Thieme, Stuttgart, Germany, 1966.

10. Steurer, O.: Zur pathogenese der mittelohrcholesteatome. *Zschr. Hals-Ohr. hk.*, 24:402, 1929.

11. Whittmaack, K.: Die cholesteatomeiterung und die falsche cholesteatombildung. In Henke, F. und Lubarsch, O.: *Handbuch der Speziellen Pathologischen Anatomie und Histologie, Bd. XII. Gehororgan,* Julius Springer, Berlin, Germany, 1962.

HYPOTHESIS BASED ON ANATOMICAL ABERRATION AND CERTAIN CONDITIONS RESPONSIBLE FOR CHOLESTEATOMA FORMATION

Cyrus S. Amiri, M.D.

Among the theories for the establishment of acquired cholesteatoma, invasion via marginal perforation seems to be the most acceptable.

Acquired cholesteatoma usually arises either from Shrapnell's area or posterosuperior marginal perforations. Why is it that we seldom see small marginal perforations elsewhere on the tympanic frame? To answer this question, one must carefully examine the anatomical peculiarities of these areas.

The annular ligament and fibrous layer of the tympanic membrane act as a supporting structure over which squamous epithelium can grow. The presence of an intact annular ligament makes the formation of a small marginal pars tensa perforation impossible. We know from experience that in persistent cases of serous otitis media prior to the days of drainage tubes, one was never able to keep a small artificial perforation open for drainage unless part of the annular ligament was removed.

Even with large anteroinferior or posteroinferior marginal perforations, cholesteatoma formation is not often found, because the squamous epithelium with its subepithelial layer from the lateral surface of the drum membrane and the cuboidal epithelium from the medial surface of the drum membrane meet and prevent further migration of the squamous epithelium; however, in certain cases of necrotizing otitis media, where a large pars tensa perforation occurs, the cuboidal epithelium on the medial surface of the tympanic membrane and even on the medial tympanic wall is damaged. This allows the squamous epithelium to migrate into the middle ear and onto the medial wall, forming an exteriorized cholesteatoma. This would explain the finding in patients such as some

of those reported by Goodhill (1960).

Why then are marginal perforations of the posterosuperior pars tensa or pars flaccida perforations or retractions potentially dangerous? The answer to this lies in the anatomical variations which may occur in these areas and their relationship to the neighboring tympanic frame.

The annular ligment normally resides in its sulcus which extends about the entire periphery of the tympanic frame except for the notch of Rivinus.

(1) In certain individuals, the annular ligament does not extend all the way to the posterior spine of the Rivinian notch but instead, narrows and disappears before reaching the posterior spine. This can be observed in some individuals undergoing stapedial surgery (Fig. 87).

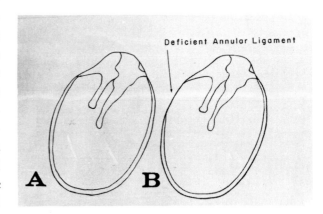

Fig. 87: (A) Normal relationship of fibrous annulus in posterosuperior canal wall. (B) Deficient fibrous annulus in posterosuperior quadrant.

(2) In some individuals, the posterosuperior portion of the annular ligament does not reside in its sulcus, but is instead located posterolateral to the sulcus, allowing a shelf of bone to exist anteromedially to the posterosuperior portion of the annular ligament (Fig. 88).

(3) In some instances, the chorda tympani will be found entering the middle ear from the posterosuperior bony canal wall. In these ears, very often a bony shelf exists medial to the posterosuperior annular margin (Fig. 89).

(4) In some individuals, a shelf of bone is found extending medially from the notch of Rivinus. A pouch-like invagination of Shrapnell's membrane in response to a negative middle ear pressure will come in contact with the medially extending shelf of bone in these individuals (Fig. 90).

Retraction of Shrapnell's membrane alone cannot cause cholesteatoma unless certain conditions

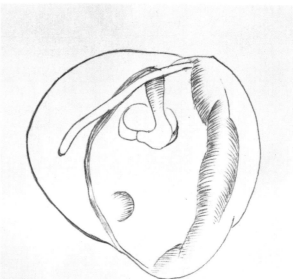

Fig. 89: Bony shelf medial to posterosuperior annular margin.

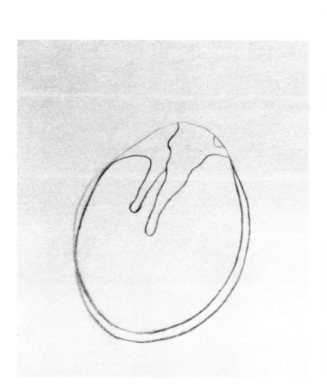

Fig. 88: Shelf of bone anteromedially to the posterosuperior portion of annular ligament.

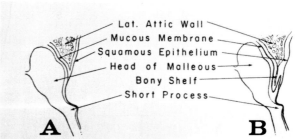

Fig. 90: (A) Normal relationship of mucous membrane and squamous covering of the lateral attic wall. (B) Extension of bony shelf from lower margin of lateral attic wall.

are added to it such as external inflammation with the presence of moisture, granulation, trauma, or otitis media to cause perforation.

Frequently, we see adhesion or close relation of chorda tympani nerve to the eardrum (Fig. 91).

In severe retraction of eardrum (T.M.) in case of serous otitis media, or, adhesive otitis media, there is a good possibility of having the membrane plastered against the incus or neck of malleus. Under this condition, pars flaccida and even pars tensa perforation allows direct contact of squamous epithelium from the external auditory canal with medially extended shelf of unprotected bone or structures previously mentioned, (Fig. 92). If any of the anatomical variations or conditions described above exist, the anterior margin of such a perforation will not have a good contact with posterior margin. Such a perforation cannot heal since the squamous epithelial margins of the perforation are not directed toward each other. A study of the above anatomical relationship will show that these potential cholesteatoma patients are the victims of a slight anatomical variation. Were it not for this, a marginal posterosuperior perforation would heal as benignly as other tympanic membrane perforations do (Amiri, 1966).

Summary

Lack or displacement of annular ligament, bone and structures situated under the edge of perforation act as a guide line for migration of squamous epithelium into the middle ear and is thought to be an underlying factor for establishment of acquired cholesteatoma.

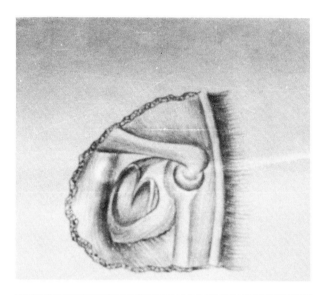

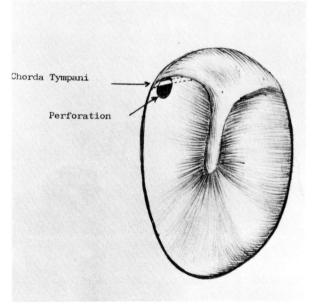

Fig. 91: Adhesion or close relation of chorda tympani nerve to eardrum.

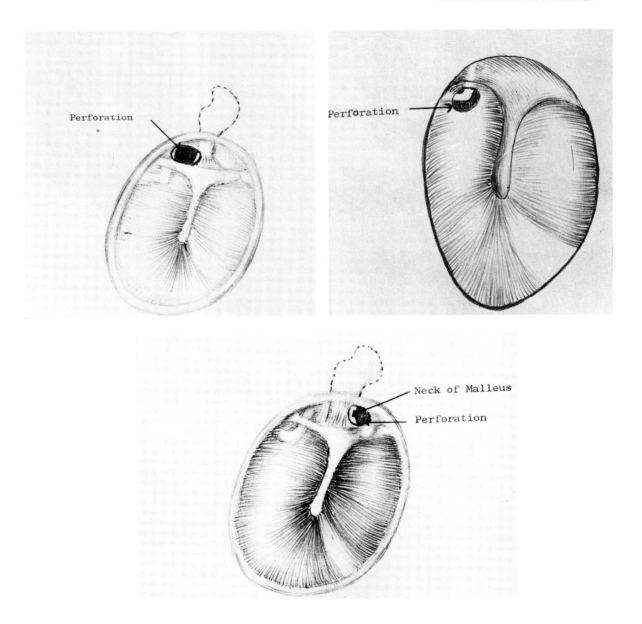

Fig. 92: Edges of incus and neck of malleus are seen through the perforation.

References

1. Amiri, C.: Anatomical observations relating to the
   etiology of cholesteatoma. *Laryngol.*, 76:1662,
   1966.

2. Goodhill, V.: The lurking latent cholesteatoma.
   Ann. Otol. Rhinol. Laryngol., 69:119, 1960.

ETIOLOGICAL ASPECTS IN CONGENITAL CHOLESTEATOMA

Eugene L. Derlacki, M.D.

In 1965, at a meeting of the American Otological Society, Dr. Jack D. Clemis and I presented our concept of the genesis, the pathology and classification of cholesteatoma in general, and congenital cholesteatoma more specifically in our article "Congenital Cholesteatoma of the Middle Ear and Mastoid". In our experiences, including those in 1976, we have found no reason to amend that detailed exposition. This writing recapitulates concepts previously expressed in four of my previous papers (Derlacki and Clemis, 1965; Derlacki et al, 1968; Derlacki, 1973 and 1976).

Since our 1965 presentation, Schechter (1969) has published an extensive review of cholesteatoma pathology from which he developed a schematic representation of the pathogenesis of cholesteatoma. In his concept, the process begins with upper respiratory pathology which ultimately results in eustachian tube obstruction producing mechanical ventilation problems. With this tubal condition as a substratum, it is the timing of the inflammatory component that determines the mechanism by which migration and proliferation of squamous epithelium results in cholesteatoma. In any case, the tympanic membrane is involved in the pathologic process, either by collapse and disruption, or by actual chronic perforation.

Schechter's schema, of course, does not provide a mechanism for the genesis of a tympanic or attic cholesteatoma early in childhood, and, for the most part, behind a normal intact tympanic membrane and without a history of middle ear infections. Clemis and I emphasized the following points in defining congenital cholesteatoma of the tympanum and mastoid: (1) development behind an intact tympanic membrane, (2) without previous history of aural infections, (3) arising from embryonal inclusion of squamous epithelium or from undifferentiated tissue which changes to squamous epithelium in the developing temporal bone.

Our interest in congenital cholesteatoma was stimulated by hearing and subsequently reading Cawthorne's (1961 and 1963) two papers on so-called primary or congenital cholesteatoma of the temporal bone.

The second paper carried a description of one patient with a cholesteatoma visualized through an intact tympanic membrane "in brilliant mint condition", and readily extracted by turning a tympanomeatal flap. This case led Cawthorne to postulate that cholesteatoma, certainly when it starts in the petrous bone and possibly when it starts in the attic, can be independent of external agencies such as an in-drawing of the pars flaccida or the spreading inward of epithelium through a perforation.

Cruveilhier (1829) introduced the term "tumeurs perleés" in describing three intracranial masses "looking like a great pearl in its setting of reddish brain tissue making a most beautiful picture." One of these was his own case, while the other two had been previously reported in 1807 by Le Prestre (in article by Bailey, 1920) and Dupuytren (in article by Cushing, 1922). After discovering cholestrin crystals in the interior of these tumors, Müller (1838) described three more and may forever be held accountable for the misnomer "cholesteatoma" which he applied to these masses. Afterwards, Virchow (1854) described four additional cases, and although he returned to the term "pearly tumor", accuracy had yielded to tradition and the term cholesteatoma has persisted as accepted nomenclature. For some time thereafter, an academic battle ensued over their epithelial or endothelial derivation. Today there is fairly general agreement with von Remak (1928) who first postulated in 1854 that these growths are due to the development of congenital epithelial cell rests.

The historical development of the etiology of aural cholesteatomas is fascinating. Körner(1964), who had analyzed these reports of intracranial cholesteatoma, compared them with aural cholesteatoma and hypothesized their derivation from congenital cysts in 1830, thus establishing the tumor theory. Because cholesteatomata of the ear associated with chronic infections were as common as pearly tumors were rare, a great deal of dispute arose concerning the congenital origin of the aural type. This led Nager (1925) to remark that primary cholesteatoma of the ear is "such a rarity as to lose all practical importance for diagnosis or therapy". Juers (1965) states ". . . . all cholesteatoma lesions which I have observed at surgery have, without any doubt in my mind, been the result of retraction or migration of epithelium through a perforation from the external meatus or tympanic membranes".

In 1873, Wendt proposed that the middle ear mucosa was stimulated to squamous metaplasia by inflammatory changes. His theory fell into disfavor, then was revived and modified by Tumarkin in 1938, and presently has little following. However, Bendek in 1963, reported that a significantly high percentage of biopsy samples taken from the promontory lining in 40 cases of serous otitis media and 35 cases of chronic suppurative otitis media revealed squamous epithelium. Each of these ears had been subject to inflammatory stimulation, be it from infection or allergy, and although cholesteatomas were not found, the presence of squamous epithelium implies either squamous metaplasia or congenital squamous cell rests, supporting either the tumor or metaplasia theories.

Since these two theories were not at all satisfactory, Habermann (1888) and Bezold (1908) focused attention on the probability of invasion of the middle ear and attic space by canal skin. It was known that epithelium could migrate through a marginal type of perforation and pave the middle ear space only to desquamate and produce a secondary acquired cholesteatoma as described by Shambaugh (1959). Bezold (1908) suggested that with eustachian tube obstruction the resulting negative middle ear pressure leads to retraction of Shrapnell's membrane and desquamation from the epithelial surface producing a plug of epithelial debris. Wittmaack (1933) expanded the theory and today it is widely accepted in the etiology of primary acquired cholesteatoma.

Ruedi in 1957, in 1959, and again in 1963, suggested that in response to inflammatory stimulation, basal cells of the posterosuperior canal skin proliferate. The resulting finger-like invaginations with central cornifications enter the posterior attic establishing a cholesteatoma without a tympanic membrane perforation. By progressive growth and/or infection, Shrapnell's membrane or the drum head may perforate secondarily. Contemporary acceptance favors the immigration theories, each of which is initiated by one or two of three prerequisites, i.e., marginal perforation, inflammation and negative intratympanic pressure. Cholesteatomas have been produced in laboratory animals, corroborating the immigration theories, (Table 25).

TABLE 25

Classification of Cholesteatoma Genesis

Tumor theory—Korner, 1830

Metaplasia theory—Wendt, 1873

Immigration theory

    Direct extention via marginal perforation
    (Secondary acquired cholesteatoma)

    Attic retraction theory—Bezold, 1888
    (Primary acquired cholesteatoma)

    Proliferation of basal cells of canal skin, 1957
    (Primary acquired cholesteatoma)

Pathology

Cholesteatomas are epidermoid cysts which, when uncomplicated by infection, are typically opaque white and glistening, startlingly resembling mother of pearl, both in tint and lustre, and assume the shape of the cavity housing them. They are usually easily pealed from their surroundings, are void of blood vessels and the cut surface reveals a crumbly mass of white dry flakes. The matrix is composed of stratified squamous epithelial cells overlying a connective tissue stroma with encapsulated concentric layers of desquamated epithelial cells, cholestrin crystals and fat globules. The matrix of dermal cysts or dermoids, on the other hand, is composed of epidermis plus dermis and dermal elements, while the cyst contents in addition to squamous and cholestrin contain hair and sebaceous material. Although epidermoid cysts are common in the temporal bone, dermoids are unreported in this location, and they are rarely found within the cranium. Finally, one must consider the subject of implantation cysts which may be of either dermal or epidermal type, depending on the nature of the tissue implanted. Since cholesteatomas have been reported in an otherwise normal ear some time after head injury or myringotomy, one must postulate the possibility of a congenital cholesteatoma existing prior to the trauma in addition to considering the more obvious, acquired implantation epidermoid cyst.

Classification of Cholesteatoma

To avoid confusion with the other adjectives used in the literature such as true, primary, silent, latent, genuine or cholesteatoma verum, which are sometimes used with totally different meaning, we shall employ the term "congenital cholesteatoma". Congenital cholesteatoma auris implies a cholesteatoma which develops behind an intact tympanic membrane in a patient without previous history of aural infections, and presumably arises from embryonal inclusion of squamous epithelium or undifferentiated tissue which changes to squamous epithelium in the developing temporal bone.

Although much has been postulated about congenital cholesteatoma, few well documented case studies have been reported. Our search of the literature reveals a division by location into three sites within the temporal bone; the petrous pyramid, the mastoid, and the middle ear cleft. Hence our classification of cholesteatoma of the temporal bone has evolved into a simple one as shown in Table 26.

TABLE 26

Classification of Cholesteatoma

Primary acquired cholesteatoma

Secondary acquired cholesteatoma

Congenital cholesteatoma

   Petrous pyramid type

   Mastoid type

   Tympanic type

Discussion

After reviewing our previous papers in preparation for the "First International Conference on Cholesteatoma", I hoped to find that the conference would answer certain questions. What causes the difference in biological activity of congenital epithelial cell rests? One 3 year old child may grow an isolated pearly tumor whose exact site of origin is difficult to detect during the easy surgical delivery, whereas another child of three years may have developed a cholesteatoma matrix whose extensive migration has lined the middle ear space, attic, antrum, and even the mastoid cavity with a broad attachment to underlying mucosa. These large epidermoid cysts assume the shape of the cavities housing them, and may have unattached satellite plaques or lobules most often found in the hypotympanum and the anterior middle ear space.

When one discovers an epidermoid cyst which fulfills our criteria for a congenital cholesteatoma, except for the age of discovery and less frequently in adulthood, has there been a different etiogenesis consistent with the metaplastic theory? It may well be that the conference will create more questions than answers. Should this be the case, future conferences and workshops on cholesteatoma will be justified.

References

1. Bailey, P.: Cruveilhier's "tumeurs perlées". *Surg. Gynec. Obstet.*, 31:390, 1920.

2. Bendek, G. A.: Histopathology of transudatory-secretory otitis media. *Arch. Otolaryngol.*, 78:33, 1963.

3. Bezold, F. and Siebenmann, F.: *Textbook of Otology.* E. H. Colgrove, Chicago, Illinois, 1908, p. 189.

4. Cawthorne, T.: Congenital cholesteatoma. *Arch. Otolaryngol.*, 78: 248, 1963.

5. Cawthorne, T. and Griffith, A.: Primary cholesteatoma of the temporal bone. *Arch. Otolaryngol.*, 73: 252, 1961.

6. Cruveilhier, J.: *Anatomie pathologique du corps humain.* J-B. Balliere, Paris, France, Vol. 1 and 2, 1829, p. 341.

7. Cushing, H.: A large epidermal cholesteatoma of the parieto (temporal) region deforming the left hemisphere without cerebral symptoms. *Surg., Gynec. Obstet.*, 34:557, 1922.

8. Derlacki, E. L.: Congenital cholesteatoma of the middle ear and mastoid: a third report. *Arch. Otolaryngol.*, 97:177, 1973.

9. Derlacki, E. L.: Congenital cholesteatoma of the middle ear and mastoid: a fourth report. Shambaugh Fifth International Workshop on Middle Ear Microsurgery and Fluctuant Hearing Loss, March, 1976.

10. Derlacki, E. L. and Clemis, J. D.: Congenital cholesteatoma of the middle ear and mastoid. *Ann. Otol.*, 74:706, 1965.

11. Derlacki, E. L.; Harrison, W. H.; and Clemis, J. D.: Congenital cholesteatoma of the middle ear and mastoid: a second report presenting seven additional cases. *Laryngoscope*, 78:1050, 1968.

12. Habermann, J.: Zur Entstehung des Cholesteatoms des Mittelhors. *Arch f Ohrenh*, 27:42, 1888.

13. Juers, A. L.: Cholesteatoma genesis. *Arch. Otolaryngol.*, 81:5, 1965.

14. Körner, cited by Portmann, G.; Portmann, M.; and Claverie, G.: *The Surgery of Deafness.* Valetta - Malta: Progress Press, 1964.

15. Müller, J.: *Über den Feinern Bau und die Formen der krankhaften Geschwülste.* G. Reimer, Berlin, Germany, 1838, p. 50.

16. Nager, F. R.: The cholesteatoma of the middle ear. Its etiology, pathogenesis, diagnosis and therapy. *Ann. Otol. Rhinol. Laryngol.*, 34:1249, 1925.

17. Ruedi, L.: Pathogenesis and treatment of cholesteatoma in chronic suppuration of the temporal bone. *Ann. Otol. Rhinol. Laryngol.*, 66:283, 1957.

18. Ruedi, L.: Cholesteatoma formation in the middle ear in animal experiments. *Acta Otolaryngol.*, 50:233, 1959.

19. Ruedi, L.: Acquired cholesteatoma. *Arch Otolaryngol.*, 78:252, 1963.

20. Schechter, G.: A review of cholesteatoma pathology. *Laryngoscope*, 79:1907, 1969.

21. Shambaugh, G. E., Jr.: *Surgery of the Ear.* W. B. Saunders, Philadelphia, Pennsylvania, 1959, p. 178.

22. Tumarkin, A.: A contribution to the study of middle-ear suppuration with special reference to the pathogeny and treatment of cholesteatoma. *J. Laryngol. Otol.*, 53:685, 1938.

23. Virchow, R.: Über Perlgeschwulste. *Arch f path Anat Berlin*, 8:371, 1854.

24. von Remak, cited by Critchley, M. and Ferguson, F.: The cerebrospinal epidermoids (cholesteatomata). *Brain*, 51:334, 1928.

25. Wendt, H.: Desquamative entzündung des mittelhors ("Cholesteatom des Felsen beins" der Autoren). *Arch f Heilk, Leipz*, 14:428, 1873.

26. Wittmaack, K.: Wie entsteht ein genuines cholesteatom? Arch f Ohren-, Nasen-u. Kehlkopfh, 137:306, 1933.

PATHOGENESIS OF ATTIC CHOLESTEATOMA: THE METAPLASIA THEORY

Jacob Sadé, M.D.

Stratified squamous epithelium (S.S.E.) in the middle ear indicates a cholesteatoma. Yet, S.S.E. is found in the middle ear under several different clinical situations which are pathogenetically and clinically different.

(A) Metaplastic islands of mucosa in the middle ear cleft are often found to be transformed into S.S. epithelium (Sade, 1973; Karma, 1972; and Palva, et al, 1968) (Fig. 93). Usually this is in the presence of a perforation (whether it be central or marginal) accompanied by some degree of chronic inflammatory ear disease. Ear polyps which are associated with either type of perforation are also often covered by S.S.E. Such metaplasia occurs under inflammatory conditions in most mucosas of the body and is seen in nasal turbinates and nasal polyps, chronic sinusitis, bronchitis, cervicitis, urinary tract infections, etc. The principles governing this in situ process are today better understood in light of advances in molecular biology and have been extensively discussed elsewhere (Sadé and Weisman, 1977; Nevo, et al, 1975; and Willis, 1962).

(B) In advanced state of atelectasis (grade IV or adhesive otitis media), the remaining drum (Sadé and Berco, 1976) is found receding and at times adherent to the medial middle ear wall. In this situation an S.S.E. lined pocket is formed which usually has a broad aperture (Fig. 94). This is referred to as a retraction pocket and is usually self-cleansing. The nature of the pocket is today partially understood through the collapse of a drum whose "backbone," i.e., the collagenous middle layer, was previously destroyed by a chronically infected process. While such a pocket may be found near the facial nerve or even the lateral semicircular canal or even higher, it has not been demonstrated and documented that it does in effect "retract" to form a narrow necked epidermoid cyst behind the ossicular chain (or into the mastoid region). Many otologists who know that many cholesteatomas are associated with such pockets do however "feel" that they have "seen" this happen. It is indeed possible that the same background and factors ("eustachian tube dysfunction" and underaeration) responsible for the emergence of attic cholesteatoma are also responsible for the formation of such pockets. On the other hand, only two out of 72 such atelectatic pockets were found by us to be associated with attic cholesteatoma. Partial surgical atticotomies with time may show a similar "retraction"—the graft, or tympano-meatal flap, collapsing into what was left from the attic—through the defect created by the surgically removed scutum! This latter situation is less commonly self-cleansing especially when a deep recess is thus created with a narrower opening or "neck." Infection of such

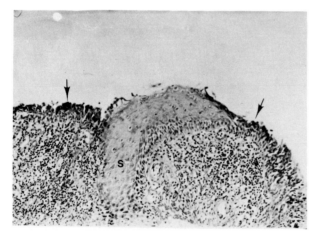

Fig. 93: An island of metaplastic stratified squamous epithelium (s) surrounded by respiratory epithelium (arrows).

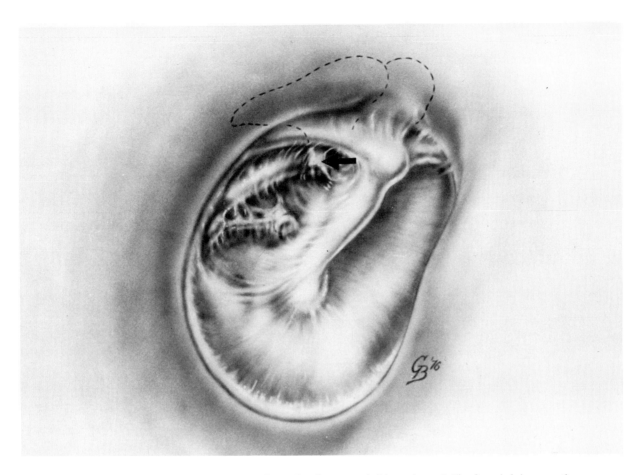

Fig. 94: Atelectasis of the posterosuperior quadrant showing an eroded incus (arrow). The drum is lying over the promontorium, stapes, and facial nerve.

cul-de-sacs are therefore not uncommon. Also in the occasional postoperative posterior tympanotomy which shows posterior wall bone absorption (Weinberg and Sadé, 1971)—S.S.E. will be seen to invaginate into the mastoid through this defect. Some degree of mesenchymal interaction with epithelial migration and especially a slight negative pressure (1.7 -5 mm H_2O) should be seen as operative in these entities (Buckingham and Ferrer, 1973 and Sadé, et al, 1976).

(C) The third and most complex entity is found in the form of epidermoid cysts which are mostly seen in the attic antrum and mastoid. These are usually connected (fistulizing) with the external ear canal—often through a rather narrow neck and/or perforation and are called "attic cholesteatomas". As is well known this fistulization usually takes place through a marginal or Shrapnell perforation and often involves scutum destruction to a lesser or greater extent. The big discussion, as to the origin of "cholesteatoma", centers on this particular attic entity. Indeed, some—including myself—consider that only this form should be termed a true cholesteatoma.

Many otologists (Nager, 1925; Ojala and Saxen, 1952; Fernandez and Lindsay, 1960; McGuckin, 1961; Buckingham, 1968; and Lim and Saunders, 1972) believe that attic cholesteatomas originate in the external canal skin invading (or invaginating) the attic through a pre-existing perforation, or are extensions of the retraction pockets mentioned above. This is a simple, uncomplicated, and on the face of it a logical explanation; however, others (Virchow, 1855; Wingrawe, 1910; Cushing, 1922; Holmes, 1938; McKenzie, 1931; Tumarkin, 1938; Diamant, 1948 and 1952; and Cawthorne, 1963) look upon this explanation as over-simplified.

One of the typical features of attic cholesteatoma is that we encounter it when it is already well-developed. Their average diameter measured by me in autopsies was 6 mm—a size corresponding to the cholesteatomas encountered by us at surgery. Of special interest are those ears which come without any previous history, presenting a pin-point Shrapnell's perforation leading into a sizable epidermoid cyst (cholesteatoma) in the attic suggesting a previously rather long and unnoted history. Others have a longer though insidious clinical history—altogether the average time for patients who have had their symptomatology (usually running, itching ear) before presenting themselves for surgery was found by us to be ten years (Sadé and Halevy, 1976). The initial steps of attic cholesteatoma have so far not been documented and are therefore only speculated. Time sequential clinico-pathological follow-up or suitable experimental models are not yet available. It is therefore possible that no direct evidence for attic cholesteatoma genesis will be at hand for some time and we will have to content ourselves with circumstantial evidence. Circumstantial evidence is seldom conclusive, and thus the opinions on this issue are quite divergent.

Trying to understand this puzzle led me to study attic cholesteatomas in situ and in toto. The material I was able to examine comprised histological sections of 22* such temporal bones, 19 of which communicated with the external canal. In 17 (80%) of the 22, the epidermal sac was mainly situated medially to the ossicular chain (Figs. 95, 96 and 97). In the other four, the ossicles were destroyed to such a degree as to make the distinction of lateral or medial impossible. Seldom is it explicitly appreciated that attic cholesteatomas are in effect situated so often as deeply as that. Any study of cholesteatoma pathogenesis should include an explanation of how such an epidermoid cyst had access into such an inaccessible topographic location. Seven of these sectioned ears showed in addition a small separate epidermoid cyst lateral to the malleus (communicating with the external ear canal) (Figs. 98 and 99) corresponding to a frequently clinically observed supramalleus dimple—also termed by many "retraction pocket". Yet, when such a depression is larger, it is referred to as "nature's atticotomy".

Attic cholesteatoma could be defined as epidermoid cysts situated deep in the attic, making "self-cleansing" difficult and improbable. The lack of self-cleansing and the accumulation of debris will be the prime cause of the secondary infection of these cysts—being responsible for most of the bone resorption that occures thereafter (Grippaudu, 1958; Harris, 1962; Sadé and Berco, 1974; and Thomsen, et al, 1974). Indeed the gram-negative bacteria so often found in infected cholesteatomas are typically secondary invaders. It is of course the origin of these epidermoid cysts in the attic which we are trying to find and which is so difficult to prove.

What is the evidence that attic cholesteatoma originates from the external ear canal epithelium? Proponents of the external origin look upon S.S.E. bridging the external ear canal (where S.S.E. is naturally found) and the cholesteatomatous sac in the attic as evident proof that skin from the external ear invades the middle ear. This seems a logical conclusion especially considering that the nor-

*Dr. M. Paparella, Dr. F. Nager, Dr. D. Lim, Dr. J. Lindsay, and Dr. B. McCabe kindly made available to me their histological material.

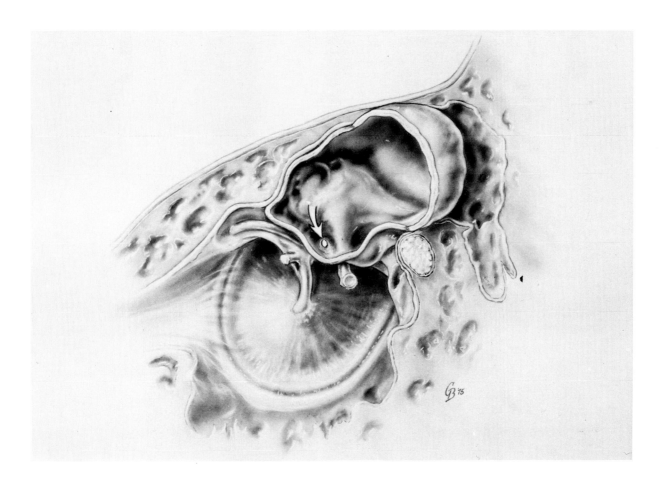

Fig. 95: Cholesteatoma sac situated medial to the ossicular chain—viewed from within. Shrapnell's perforation is seen between malleus and incus (arrow).

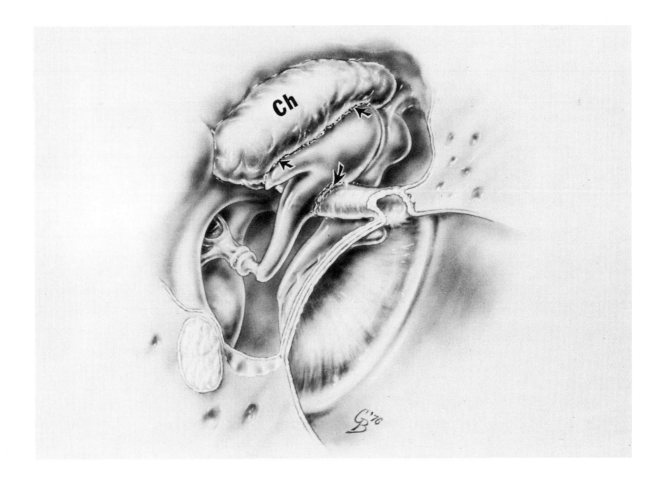

Fig. 96: Cholesteatoma sac situated medial to the ossicular chain. Its connecting neck is seen to pass between the incus and malleus—ending in a Shrapnell perforation. Contacts with bone (arrows).

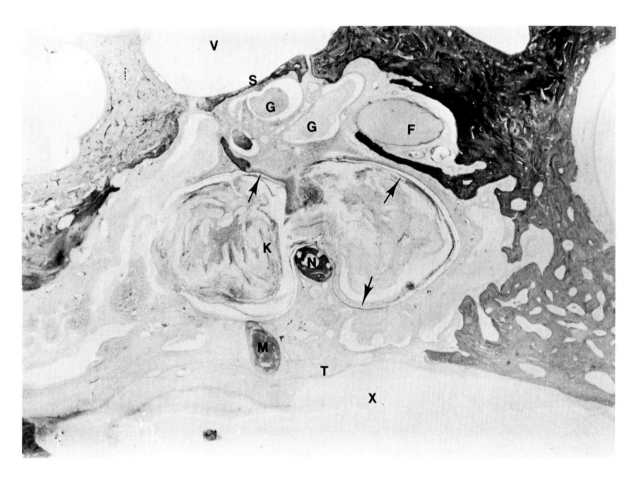

Fig. 97: Histological section showing a kidney shape cholesteatous sac filling the attic medial to the ossicular chain (m and n). Keratin (k). Lining of sac (arrows). Facial nerve (f). Glands in attic (g). Tympanic membrane (t). External canal (x). Malleus (m). Incus (n). Stapes (s). Vestibule (v). Note: The S.S.E. is directly related to both in the incus and malleus— with no other epithelium in between the two.

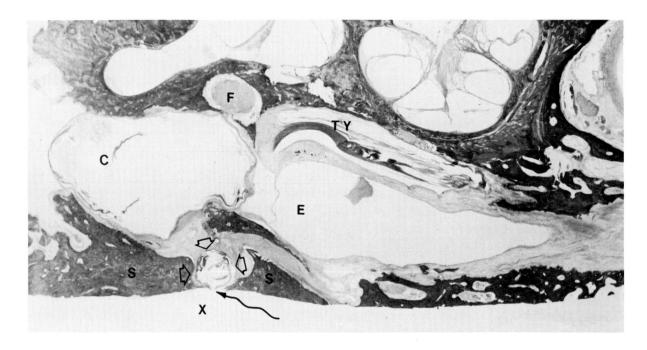

Fig. 98: Cross section of a middle ear showing a small epidermoid cyst lateral to the ossicular chain (hollow arrows)—communicating (waving arrows) with the external ear canal (x). Lateral to the ossicular chain there is another cholesteatous sac (c). Scutum (s). Eustachian tube (e). Tensor tympany (ty). Facial nerve (f).

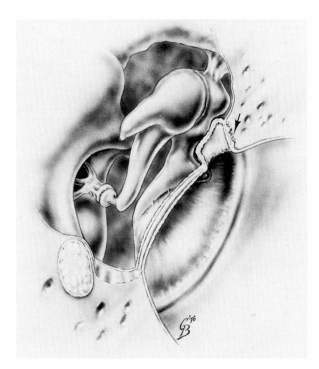

Fig. 99: Schematic drawing corresponding to the histological picture in Figure 98 showing a "cut" through a "Shrapnell dimple"—Which in actuality represents a small epidermoid cyst lateral to the ossicular chain and often referred to as a "retraction pocket". Part of the scutum is eroded by the process (arrow).

mal attic is not lined with S.S.E. However would the origin of this cyst take place for some unforeseen reason in the attic and break secondarily through into the external canal—(i.e., fistulization), epithelialization of the connecting tract, will also ensue. Therefore, this particular evidence may work both ways and cannot really be accepted as valid.

The migratory proponents view S.S.E. as an aggressive agent which invades the middle ear. To do so that epithelium has often to find its way through the Shrapnell membrane or part of the scutum (Fig. 100) (destroy it?) then infiltrate medial to the ossicles and finally expand (up!) into the attic and form a cyst? Another theoretical possibility, often entertained, would be a pre-existing marginal and/or scutum perforation through which the external canal skin invades the attic (again upwards!).

Epithelial migration is not known to be an aggressive phenomenon, killing other cells in order to advance and occupy their place. Epithelium migrates to fill epithelial loss over denuded surfaces as happens in wound healing. In effect, an

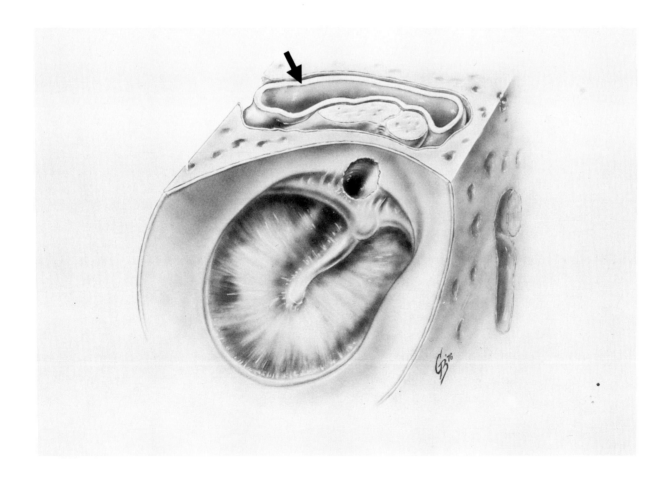

Fig. 100: Schematic representation of a perforation through the Shrapnell membrane and adjacent scutum. A view from the top shows the incus and malleus head (cut) while medial to them is a cholesteatoma sac (arrow).

epithelium which migrates naturally when "unopposed" promptly stops when it encounters another epithelium. This is a well-established basic biological phenomenon termed contact inhibition and is routinely seen when two identical epithelium migrate one towards the other in tissue culture. The only exception to this biological rule is seen in malignant cells. There the migrating cells do not stop! Interestingly enough S.S.E. on "meeting" mucosal cells also shows contact inhibition as demonstrated by Nevo, et al (1975) in our laboratory in tissue cultures (Fig. 101). Suitable examples of a similar contact inhibition in the middle ear

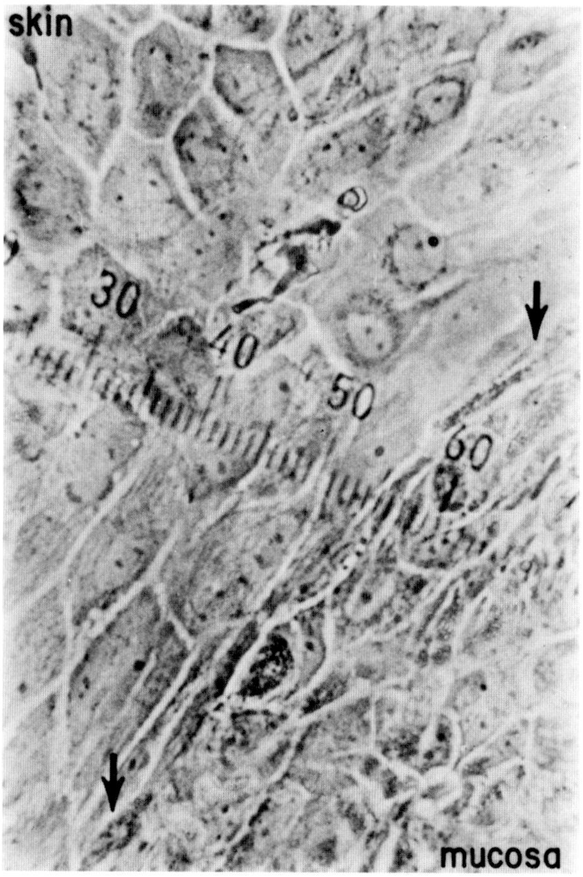

Fig. 101: Tissue culture of stratified squamous epithelium and mucosa both being arrested when they meet. Seam line (arrows).

are abundantly found in central perforation which demonstrates well how the skin usually stops at or near the margin (Fig. 102)—when it encounters another epithelium, i.e., the middle ear mucosa. In effect, central perforations which are three times more common than marginal lead into a cholesteatomatous sac only exceptionally.

What about a pre-existing perforation through which S.S.E. may invade the middle ear, i.e., Shrapnell and marginal perforations? The actual formation of such perforations have not been observed (nor documented) under any condition— certainly not as a result of acute otitis media. I have never seen a marginal or Shrapnell perforation precede an attic cholesteatoma, nor have I seen a necrotizing otitis media which is supposed to result in a perforation suitable for intratympanic epithelial migration. All of the hundreds of cholesteatomas observed by me had already a perforation the moment an attic cyst was present, whether this cyst was large or small. In these observations I join others such as McKenzie (1931) and Diamant (1948). Occasionally I have seen a posterior perforation in simple chronic otitis media without leading into an attic cholesteatoma which did touch the annulus but I have not seen it progress towards an attic cholesteatoma. Furthermore, such marginal perforations were indeed also created experimentally (Rogers and Snow, 1968), but they always closed, leaving no cholesteatoma behind.

Those who recognize these facts postulate a hypothetical negative pressure in the middle ear which is supposed to suck the external canal skin into the attic. This negative pressure is postulated to be secondary to eustachian tube obstruction; however, the only negative middle ear pressures directly measured in ears relevant to this disease were shown to be on the average of -1.7 or -5 centimeters of water. Such small pressures (almost near normal) are rather unlikely to bring about such gross pathological changes, i.e., pulling the canal skin through the drum (at times through scutum) between the ossicles, to end up in the roof of the attic. Furthermore, the eustachian tube has

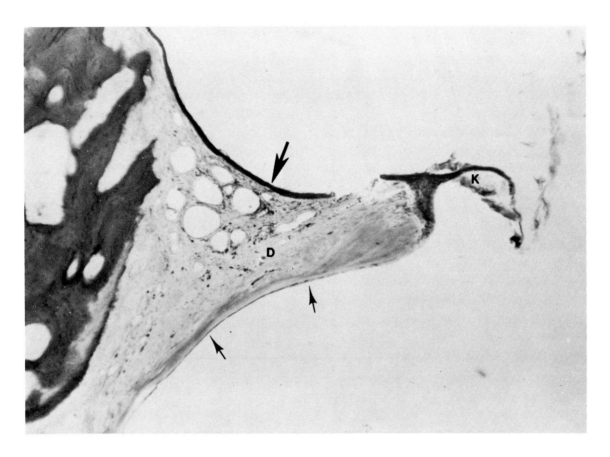

Fig. 102: Edge of tympanic membrane perforation showing "contact inhibition". Rest of tympanic membrane (d). Stratified squamous epithelium (large arrow). Mucosa (small arrows). Keratin (k).

really never been shown to be obstructed in these cases (this does not mean that the eustachian tube functions properly). Likewise the progression of an atelectatic ear or shallow supra-Shrapnell dimple (see Figs. 94, 98 and 99) (at the scutum area) into an attic cholesteatoma, though often taken for granted, has never been documented, and I personally have never seen it happen.

Examining histologically 39 ossicles removed from cholesteatoma ears, or larger cholesteatoma surgical specimens as well as the present series of 22 temporal bones (Fig. 103), I found all of the ossicles to be lined only by one type of epithelium; either S.S.E. or middle ear mucosa. The epithelium (whether mucosa or S.S.E.) was separated from the ossicles only by connective tissue. No mucosa was found between the ossicles and the S.S.E. Actually if the invagination theory were correct one would expect to find, at least occasionally, three such epithelial layers: (1) S.S.E. originating from the external ear canal, (2) the adjacent middle ear mucosa, and (3) the mucosal enveloping ossicles.

The other factor which should be considered is

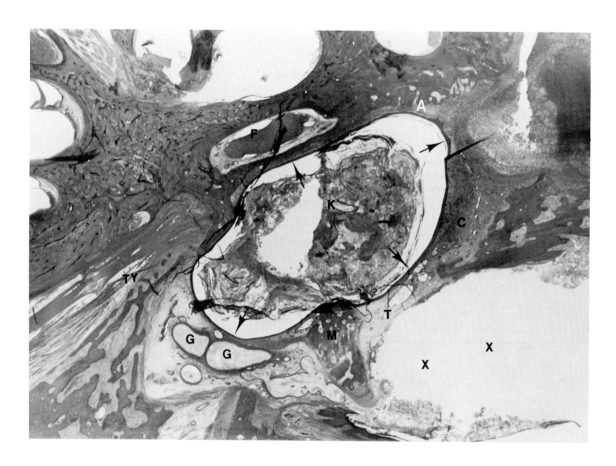

Fig. 103: Cross section of attic which is completely filled by a keratin containing cholesteatoma glands and mesenchymal tissue. Mesenchyma (a). Keratin (k). S.S.E. (arrows). Glands (g). Malleus (m). Facial nerve (f). Upper part of tympanic membrane (t). External ear canal (x). Tensor tympany (ty). Note: The S.S.E. is directly related to the malleus—with no other epithelium in between them.

the migration pattern and direction of external ear epithelium. The migratory invagination theory is obviously based on the concept of epithelium migrating inwards (medial direction) toward the attic (Simmons, 1961). This will be a "backwards" migration as the external ear canal epithelium usually clears itself laterally—towards the concha.

However, when I placed India ink dots at the margins of atelectatic depression of the pars tensa, or attic "retractions", as well as cholesteatoma perforation, migration of all the India ink dots followed swiftly (0.1 mm per day) the physiological pattern, i.e., laterally (Fig. 104) as described in the normal by Alberti (1964) and Litton (1968).

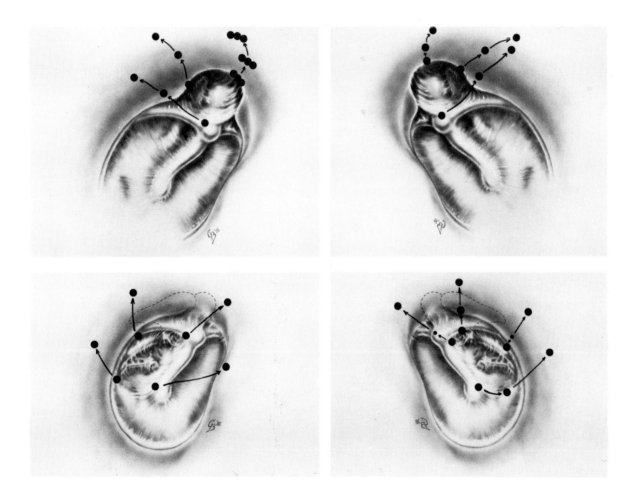

Fig. 104: India ink cleared from the edges of "retraction pocket". Their traveling direction is towards the external meatus away from the "retraction"—their speed averaging 1 mm per day.

However, ink dots, blood or epithelial debris at the bottom of such pockets were found to migrate out very slowly.

All these facts make me doubt the possibility that external canal skin invades the attic and can primarily form a deep-seated retro-ossicular epidermal cyst in the attic, and prompted me to look—at least by exclusion, for the origin of this epidermal cyst in the only alternative site, i.e., the attic itself. Indeed, I have often seen on histological slides the cholesteatoma sac molding itself in the attic in the shape of a kidney with its epithelium being flattened (see Figs. 97 and 107). This speaks of a centrifugal growth with pressure from its inside on its walls—at least at one time during its development. Such a situation is likely to develop in a closed expanding cyst.

Virchow (1855), Cushing (1922), Holmes (1938), McKenzie (1931), Diamant (1948 and 1952) and Cawthorne (1963) also looked for the origin of cholesteatoma in the attic. Some of them postulated an awakening of ectodermal embryonic rests—i.e., this is the so-called "congenital theory" (Alberti, 1964). The theory is that some or all attic cholesteatomas are in effect epidermoid cysts arising from embryonic rests, eventually bursting out into the external canal. They leaned on the presence of such intact cysts (the so-called congenital cholesteatomas) which are occasionally found in the attic. While attic cholesteatomas unconnected to the external ear are indeed periodically described and termed congenital cholesteatomas, the embryonic rests (Peron and Schuknecht, 1975) which are supposed to be their forerunners were never demonstrated. The basic reason for this "embryonic rest" theory is the need to explain the presence of S.S.E. ectoderm in an endodermal region—the attic. We know today however that any dividing cell of the middle ear lining can transform itself into various cell types including keratinizing cells, a process called metaplasia and described in detail elsewhere. Metaplasia into S.S.E. is very common in the middle ear and is seen to some degree in about 60-100% of all chronic ears (Sade and Weinberg, 1969). The inducer or trigger which is responsible for changing metaplasia into S.S.E. is not known to us today but having made progress in understanding such chemical mediators in mucus metaplasia (Sade, et al, 1975) we might in the future find the same for the induction of S.S.E. The inherent capability of the middle ear lining to transform itself into S.S.E. does not yet explain the formation of S.S.E. cysts in the attic.

However three of the previously mentioned 21 serially sectioned ears containing cholesteatoma had no connection with the external canal—and would ordinarily be termed as "congenital cholesteatomas." One of these cholesteatomas did partly replace the middle ear mucosa (Fig. 105); its abundantly keratin forming S.S.E. is bordered on all sides by respiratory mucosa. Of the other two, one developed as an S.S.E. cyst in the middle of middle ear connective tissue, and the other was too large to determine how it started. Furthermore, when observing cholesteatomatous sacs which did have a connection with the external ear canal, seven out of 19, i.e., 38%, showed the epidermoid cyst to be only partly lined by S.S.E.—islands of typical respiratory epithelium-forming mucus (and not keratin) were found in various places (Fig. 106). Of the 19 cases, two showed total S.S.E. involvement of the promontorium and hypotympanum (i.e., beyond the extension of the cholesteatomatous sac)—the other 17 showed metaplastic S.S.E. islands studied in various points of their mucosa. These observations show that attic epidermoid cysts, whether they do or do not communicate with the external ear canal, have a lining which often is mixed—partly S.S.E. and partly respiratory epithelium producing mucus. The inescapable conclusion is that at least in part the process is metaplastic.

Epithelium spreading on a surface behaves differently than when it is buried in tissue, for in the latter it tends to form a cyst which can be considered a primitive organ. Thus, mucus cells will form glands when deep below the surface and S.S.E. will form under these epidermoid cysts. Clinical experience points to this (surgical epider-

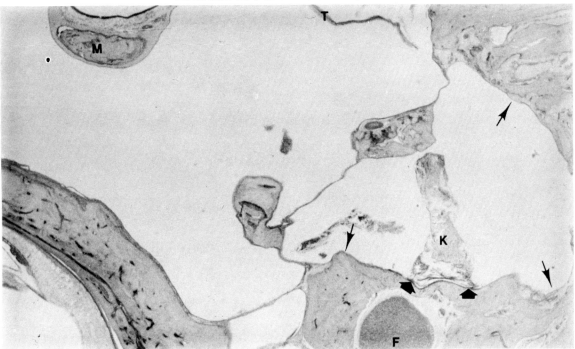

Fig. 105: Histological section through middle ear showing stratified squamous epithelium (between the two fat arrows), producing keratin (k). This metaplastic area is surrounded by mucosa (thin arrows). Facial nerve (f). Tympanic membrane (t). Malleus handle (m).

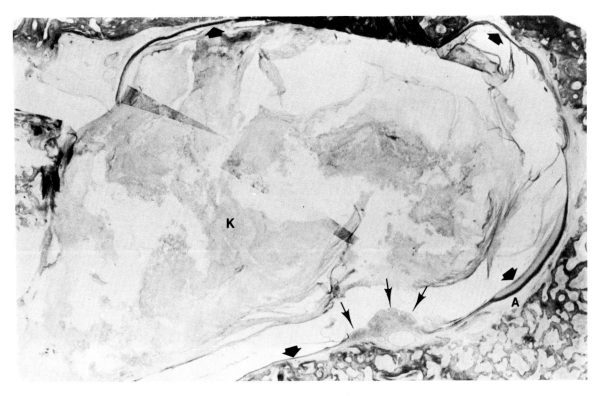

Fig. 106: Cross section of a cholesteatoma sac filled with keratin (k). Stratified squamous epithelium lining of the sac (big arrows). Part of the cholesteatomatous sac shows island of respiratory mucosa (thin arrows).

mal inclusion cysts) and Abramson (1975) has reproduced epidermoid cysts in such a manner experimentally.

Mucus producing cysts are extremely common in the midst of attic connective tissue in ears which are or have been inflamed. Could we not have, by the same token, epidermoid cysts develop in the same place? As epithelial cells which line the attic can be triggered to develop into keratin producing cells—just as well as they can into mucus producing cells even during adult life. If these cells were buried in connective tissue, they would then form epidermoid cysts or mucus cysts (glands) respectively. At times I did indeed encounter islands or tongues of S.S.E. in the midst of attic connective tissue (Fig. 107). Scanning many serial sections I also encounter occasionally the actual budding from the middle ear lining of such epithelial cells and cords (Fig. 108) infiltrating and embedding themselves in the midst of the attic connective tissue. These embedded epithelial cords and cells could be viewed as precursors of

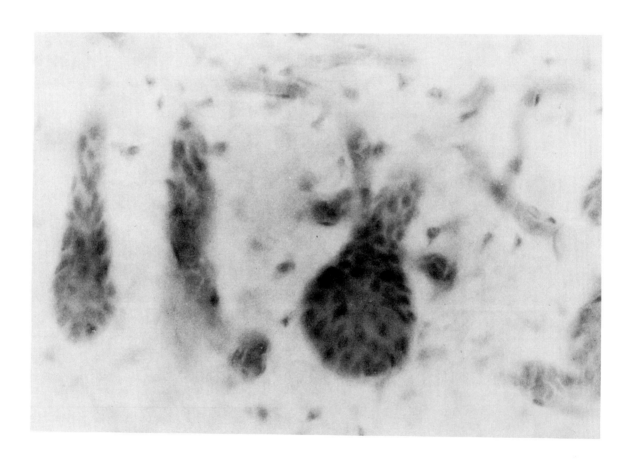

Fig. 107: Stratified squamous epithelium islands in attic mesenchyma.

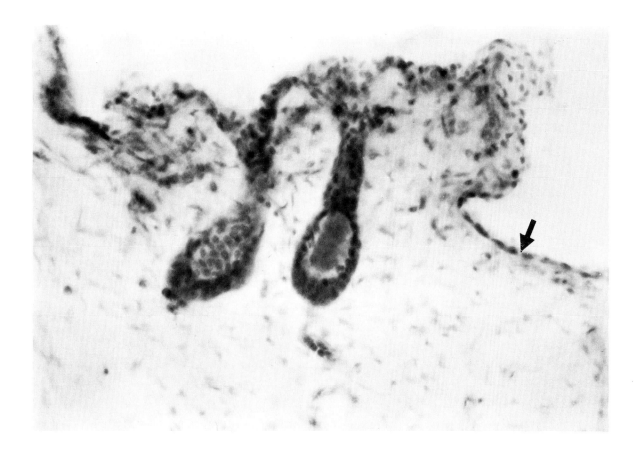

Fig. 108: Epithelial buds invaginating attic mesenchyma. Their origin is seen to be the epithelial lining (arrow).

epidermal cysts.

Attic cholesteatomas could therefore be viewed as epidermoid cysts originating primarily in the attic probably through a metaplastic process and developing secondarily a fistulous tract into the external canal. At times one can find such a cyst in connection with the external ear canal without (histologically) an epithelial layer lining connecting the two—which can be interposed as a tract prior (the fistula) to its epithelialization (Fig. 109). Epithelialization of such a tract can indeed be considered as a process which is governed by epithelial migration—both from the external canal as well as from the attic epidermal cyst. The

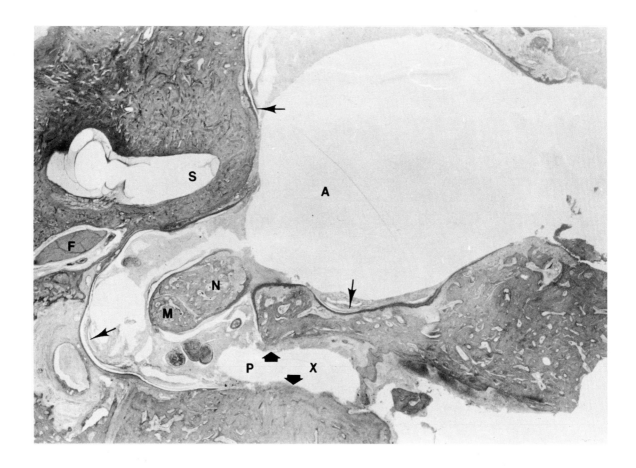

Fig. 109: Attic cholesteatoma "bursting" (p) into external ear canal (x). Antrum (a). Malleus (m). Incus (h). S.S.E. (thin arrows). Semicircular canal (s). Facial nerve (f). Note: the tract, or fistula, connecting the middle ear with the external ear canal is lined only by an inflammatory exudate (thick arrows) with no epithelial cells being as yet present.

slow self-cleansing ability of such deeply buried sacs could account for them becoming secondarily infected. These medial epidermoids are different from those which are in the lateral part of the ossicular chain and which, due to their closeness to the surface, are self-cleansing: the latter are the small "nature's micro-atticotomies" (Fig. 110). It seems plausible that the large "nature's radicals" are medial cholesteatomas which due to a low grade of infection and exceptional self-cleansing capabilities, have reached that particular condition unnoticed. Between the medial situated sac and the lateral one, one can indeed find all the spectrum of transitions of one into the other as

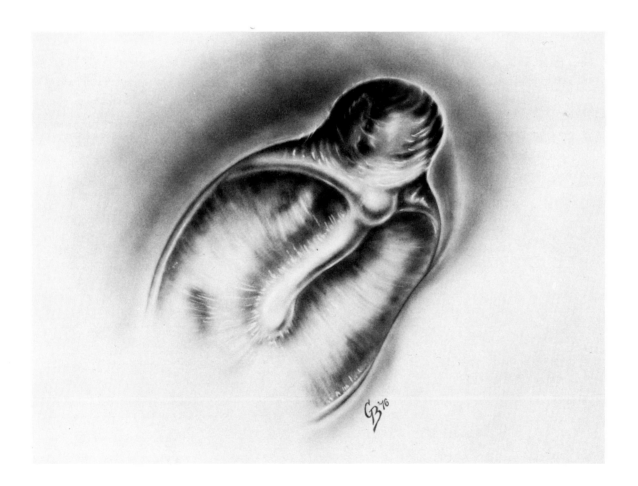

Fig. 110: Nature's atticotomy—no attic "retraction pocket" which in effect is an epidermoid cyst which is due to being lateral to the ossicular chain turned—after exteriorizing itself—into a benign self-cleansing pocket.

well as all imaginable extensions anteriorly and especially posteriorly.

The mechanism by which these epidermal cysts "find their way" into the external ear canal has to do with two different phenomena: (1) direction, and (2) penetration. The mechanism of direction finding eludes us completely. However, the penetration is probably due to pressure and the local inflammatory reaction—the latter which is probably a reaction to the cholesteatomatous sac—as was discussed elsewhere (Abramson, et al, 1975).

Among the wide spectra of possibilities of the final communication of the attic mastoid cholesteatoma with the external canal there are two principle ways. The one in front of the incus (behind or in front of the malleus)—when a Shrapnell perforation will be formed (see Fig. 96)—the other behind the incus when a posterosuperior perforation will be mostly formed. In the latter case the accompanying slow infection will often damage the drum which thereafter may show either a large posterosuperior perforation of the "membrana tensa" or its collapse forming a secondary local atelectasis.

Why do epidermal cysts reside mostly in the attic and mastoids? Thought should be given to the possibility that the flat attic epithelium in distinction from the mucociliary epithelium found in the meso— and hypotympanum, has a predisposition or special commitment towards metaplasia into S.S.E. Its relative clearance deficiency due to paucity of cilia there (Sade, 1966) may be a factor as well. The other local specific factor is the ease with which the attic shuts off from the middle ear. This is due to the relatively small communicating apertures from the attic to the tympanic cavity. Even moderate swelling seen in inflammatory processes will close these apertures. Beaumont (1966) demonstrated experimentally that air spaces will fill themselves with mesenchymal tissue after being isolated from the air, forming among others cholesterol granuloma like lesions. Indeed such swollen mucosa will at times fill the attic (see Figs. 97 and 103), almost completely

creating an environment wherein a S.S.E. cell might find it suitable to progress into a cyst—just as when it is buried in mesenchyme. The high incidence of cholesteatoma among secretory otitis media population, as reviewed by Kokko (1974), may stem from the clustering of the attic in these ears, by a swollen inflammatory mucosa (Sade, 1966) for a long period of time. Bluestone (1976) and Severeid (1976) showed eustachian tube dysfunction as an accompanying parameter in cholesteatomas. Severeid's high incidence (about 9%!) of cholesteatomas in a cleft palate population is by itself indicative, as this is a group excessively prone to secretory otitis media. The association with total or partial collapse of the tympanic membrane becomes therefore a very logical combination and the postulated, undocumented genesis of cholesteatoma from such retraction pockets becomes unnecessary. However, how eustachian tube malfunction predisposes cholesteatoma genesis remains a mystery.

Summary

Stratified squamous epithelium (S.S.E.) is presented in the middle ear in several clinical entities—such as metaplastic islands of the mucosa or atelectatic drum. However, only an epidermoid cyst, commonly found in the attic, is herewith defined as attic cholesteatoma. Histological examination of 19 temporal bones with attic cholesteatomas show them to reside mainly medial to the ossicular chain. This explains the difficulty of their self-cleansing as well as the ensuing secondary infection. When a similar process occurs lateral to the ossicles a small self-cleansing dimple is formed, the so-called "upper" retraction pocket. It is difficult to entertain invasion of external canal skin into the upper medial attic (often through the scutum), especially in the face of such evidence as epithelial contact inhibition, or the invariable outward migration of S.S.E. from edges of "retraction pockets" or cholesteatoma perforations. Also, large cholesteatomas are usually found simultaneously with their perforations and no documentation of the evolving process from a pre-existing perforation exists. The possibility of such attic cholesteatomas arising primarily in the attic is thus supported. The frequency with which cholesteatoma sacs (including the "congenital" type) show mucosal cells as part of their lining, suggests a metaplastic phenomena. This is (in this case) the inherent ability of mucosal stem cells to form also keratinizing S.S.E. The formation of epidermoid cysts from S.S.E. is discussed in analogy with the frequent glandular formation in the attic. Such "organ" formations may arise when their respective cells (forming mucus or keratin) grow in the midst of connective tissue rather than on its surface. Histologic evidence for the latter is brought forth.

References

1. Abramson, M.; Asarch, G. C.; and Litton, W. B.: Experimental aural cholesteatoma causing bone resorption. *Ann. Otol. Rhinol. Laryngol.*, 84:425, 1975.
2. Abramson, M.: Personal communication, 1976.
3. Alberti, P. W.: Epithelial migration on the tympanic membrane. *J. Laryngol. Otol.*, 78:808, 1964.
4. Beaumont, D. G.: The effects of exclusion of air from pneumatized bones. *J. Laryngol. Otol.*, 80:236, 1966.
5. Bluestone, C.: Functional eustachian tube obstruction in acquired cholesteatoma and related conditions. Proc. First International Conference on Cholesteatoma, May 26-29, 1976, Iowa City, Iowa.
6. Buckingham, R. A.: Etiology of middle ear cholesteatoma. *Ann. Otol. Rhinol. Laryngol.*, 77:1054, 1968.
7. Buckingham, R. A. and Ferrer, J. L.: Middle ear pressure in eustachian tube malfunction: manometric studies. *Laryngoscope*, 83:1585, 1973.
8. Cawthorne, I.: Congenital cholesteatoma. *Arch. Otolaryngol.*, 78:248, 1963.
9. Cushing, J.: Large epidermal cholesteatoma of the parieto-occipital region. *Surg. Gynecol. Obstet.*, 34:557, 1922.
10. Derlacki, E. L. and Clemis, J. D.: Congenital cholesteatoma of the middle ear and mastoid. *Ann. Otol. Rhinol. Laryngol.*, 74:706, 1965.
11. Diamant, M: *Chronic Otitis: A Critical Analysis.* S. Karger, New York, New York, 1952.
12. Diamant, M.: Cholesteatoma and chronic otitis. *Arch. Otolaryngol.*, 38:581, 1948.
13. Fernandez, C. and Lindsay, J.: Aural cholesteatoma. Experimental observations. *Laryngoscope*, 70:1119, 1960.
14. Grippaudu, M.. Histopathological studies of the ossicles in chronic otitis media. *J. Laryngol. Otol.*, 72:177, 1958.
15. Harris, A. J.: Cholesteatosis and chronic otitis media. *Laryngoscope*, 72:954, 1962.
16. Holmes, A.: A review of 303 cases of cholesteatoma. *Ann. Otol. Rhinol. Laryngol.*, 47:135, 1938.
17. Karma, P.: Middle ear epithelium and chronic ear disease. *Acta Otolaryngol.* (Supp) (Stockh), 307:1, 1972.
18. Kokko, E.: Chronic secretory otitis media in children. A clinical study. *Acta Otolaryngol.* (Supp) (Stockh) 327:1, 1974.
19. Lim, D. F. and Saunders, W. H.: Acquired cholesteatoma. *Ann. Otol. Rhinol. Laryngol.*, 81:2, 1972.
20. Litton, W. B.: Epidermal migration in the ear: the location and characteristics of the generation center revealed by utilizing a radioactive desoxyribose nucleic acid precursor, *Acta Otolaryngol.* (Supp) (Stockh), 240:5, 1968.
21. McGuckin, F.: Concerning the pathogenesis of destructive ear disease. *J. Laryngol. Otol.*, 75:949, 1961.
22. McKenzie, D.: The pathogeny of aural cholesteatoma. *J. Laryngol. Otol.*, 46:163, 1931.
23. Nager, F. R.: The cholesteatoma of the middle ear. *Ann. Otol. Rhinol. Laryngol.*, 34:1249, 1925.
24. Nevo, A. C.; Weisman, Z.; and Sadé, J.: Cell proliferation and cell differentiation in tissue cultures of adult mucociliary epithelia. *Differentiation*, 3:79, 1975.
25. Nevo, A.; Weisman, Z.; and Sadé, J.: Contact inhibition of epithelia of different structures. To be published.
26. Ojala, L. and Saxen, A.: Pathogenesis of middle ear

cholesteatoma arising from Shrapnell's membrane. *Acta Otolaryngol* (Supp) (Stockh), 33:5, 1952.

27. Palva, T.; and Palva, A.; and Dammaret, J.: Middle ear mucosa and middle ear disease. *Arch. Otolaryngol.*, 87:21, 1968.

28. Peron, D. L. and Schuknecht, H. F.: Congenital cholesteatoma with other anomalies. *Arch. Otolaryngol.*, 102:498, 1975.

29. Rogers, A. K. and Snow, B. J.: Closure of experimental tympanic membrane perforations. *Ann. Otol. Rhinol. Laryngol.*, 77:66, 1968.

30. Sadé, J.: Middle ear mucosa. *Arch. Otolaryngol.*, 84:137, 1966.

31. Sadé, J.: Pathology and pathogenesis of secretory otitis media. *Arch. Otolaryngol.*, 84:297, 1966.

32. Sadé, J.: Cellular differentiation of the middle ear lining. *Ann. Otol. Rhinol. Laryngol.*, 80:376, 1971.

33. Sadé, J.: The biopathology of secretory otitis media. *Ann. Otol. Rhinol. Laryngol.* (supp), 83:59, 1973.

34. Sadé, J. and Weinberg, J.: Mucus production in the chronically infected middle ear. *Ann. Otol. Rhinol. Laryngol.*, 87:148, 1969.

35. Sadé, J. and Berco, E.: Bone resorption in chronic otitis media. *J. Laryngol. Otol.*, 88:413, 1974.

36. Sadé, J.; Weisman, Z.; Nevo, A. C.; and Drucker, I.: Effects of environmental factors on respiratory epithelia. Proc. International Symposium on Respiratory Diseases and Air Pollution. OHALO Symposium, 1975.

37. Sadé, J. and Berco, E.: Atelectasis and secretory otitis media. *Ann. Otol. Rhinol. Laryngol.* (Supp 25), 85:66, 1976.

38. Sadé, J. and Halevy, A.: The natural history of chronic otitis media. *J. Laryngol. Otol.*, 1976. In press.

39. Sadé, J.; Halevy, A.; and Hadas, E.: Clearance of middle ear effusions and middle ear pressures. *Ann. Otol. Rhinol. Laryngol.* (Supp 25), 85:58, 1976.

40. Sadé, J. and Weisman, Z.: The phenotypic expression of middle ear mucosa. *Ann. Otol. Rhinol. Laryngol.* (Supp), 1977. In press.

41. Severeid, L.: Development of cholesteatoma in children with cleft palates. Proc. First International Conference on Cholesteatoma, May 26-29, 1976, Iowa City, Iowa.

42. Simmons, B. F.: Epithelial migration in central type tympanic perforations. *Arch. Otolaryngol.*, 74:435, 1961.

43. Thomsen, J.; Jørgensen, M. B.; Bretlau, P.; and Kristensen, H. K.: Bone resorption in chronic otitis media. A histological and ultrastructural study. *J. Laryngol. Otol.*, 88:875, 1974.

44. Tumarkin, A.: A contribution to the study of middle ear suppuration with special reference to the pathogeny and treatment of cholesteatoma. *J. Laryngol. Otol.*, 53:685, 1938.

45. Virchow, R.: Uber Perlgeschwulste. *Archiv fur Pathologische Anatomie and Physiologie und Klinische Medizin (Berlin)*, 8:371, 1855.

46. Weinberg, J. and Sadé, J.: Postoperative cholesteatoma occurrence through the posterior wall. *J. Laryngol. Otol.*, 85:1189, 1971.

47. Willis, R. A.: *The Borderland of Embryology and Pathology*. Butterworths, London, England, 2nd Ed., 1962, pp. 319.

48. Wingrawe, W. V. H.: Notes on the pathogeny of cholesteatoma. *Proc. R. Soc. Med.*, 3:63, 1910.

AURAL CHOLESTEATOMA AND EPIDERMIZATION: A FINE MORPHOLOGICAL STUDY

David J. Lim, M.D.
Herbert G. Birck, M.D.
William H. Saunders, M.D.

Introduction

Despite extensive histological studies on aural cholesteatoma (Eggston and Wolff, 1947; Ojala and Saxen, 1951; Friedmann, 1955; Harris, 1962; Ruedi, 1963; Schwarz, 1966; Maeda, et al, 1967; Ikeda, 1968; and Schuknecht, 1974) and experimental investigation, (Friedmann, 1959; Ruedi, 1959; and Fernandez and Lindsay, 1960) many questions regarding the basic aspects of this condition remain unanswered. The pathogenesis of acquired cholesteatoma also remains controversial, although the immigration theory appears to have supportive evidence from clinical observation, temporal bone histology (Ruedi, 1963) and animal experiments. Congenital cholesteatoma has been supported mainly by clinical observation and is considered rare (Derlacki and Clemis, 1965). In recent years, the metaplasia theory has also been revived and has gained some circumstantial evidence from clinical observation as well as from histopathological findings (Sade, 1974 and Nager, 1976).

This report is an attempt to clarify the fine morphology of cholesteatoma and keratinizing squamous epithelium (epidermization) in the middle ear in order to answer the following questions: what are their morphological characteristics? How are they formed and how do they migrate? How do they interact with the perimatrix or mucosal epithelium?

Material and Methods

A total of 75 aural cholesteatoma specimens obtained from surgery was prepared for ultrastructural study by the procedure described in our earlier paper (Lim and Saunders, 1972). Three serial-sectioned human temporal bones with cholesteatoma are also included in this study. A total of 17 mucosal biopsy specimens which showed epithelial squamous metaplasia out of 180 biopsies obtained from the promontories of children with otitis media with effusion (serous or mucous otitis media) is also included in this study. The specimens were processed as reported earlier (Lim and Birck, 1971). Plastic embedded tissues were examined, using either a phase contrast microscope with 1 μ sections or a transmission electron microscope (Philips 300) with thin sections.

Results and Discussion

General fine morphology: The matrix of the cholesteatoma, or epidermization, showed a typical epidermal structure identical to that in the tympanic membranes described earlier (Lim, 1968 and Matoltsy and Parekkal, 1967). It is formed by the stratum basale, stratum spinosum, stratum granulosum, and stratum corneum. The combined stratum basale and stratum spinosum form the stratum Malpighii. These cells are firmly attached together by numerous desmosomes (Fig. 111).

Large numbers of Langerhans' cells were frequently observed in some specimens and rarely in others. These cells are characterized by dendritic cell processes and Langerhans' granules and often have a clear cell body which lacks desmosomal contact with squamous cells. The paucity of melanocytes in the cholesteatoma matrix is striking in contrast to the previous report by Ikeda (1968) and the possibility that there might be more

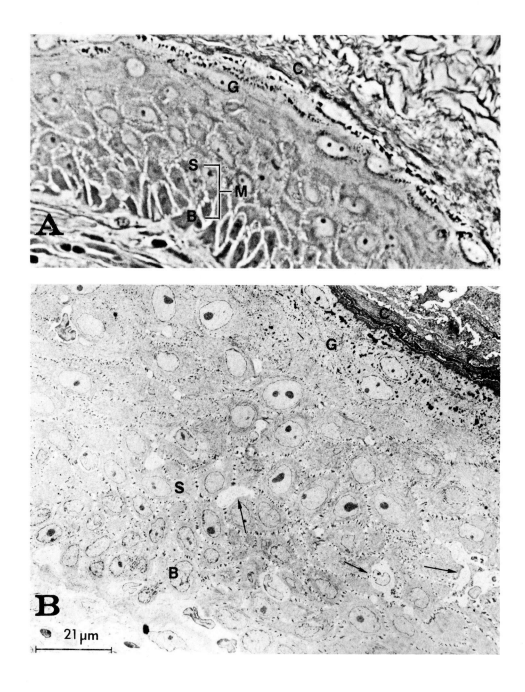

Fig. 111: (A) A phase contrast micrograph shows cholesteatoma matrix which is made up of basal (b), spinous (s), granular, and cornified (c) layers. Malpighian layer (m). **(B)** An EM photograph of the cholesteatoma matrix shows cellular details. Arrows indicate numerous dendritic Langerhans' cells.

amelanotic melanocytes than we are able to recognize cannot be ruled out. Having the Langerhans' cells and melanocytes in the cholesteatoma matrix may further suggest an epidermal origin, from canal skin or tympanic membrane which also possess these cell elements.

The thickness of the cholesteatoma matrix (epidermis) varied considerably among cases: measurements ranged from 3 μ to 20 μ. When the matrices were thin, they often lacked the stratum spinosum (Fig. 112).

There is a well-developed basal lamina at the

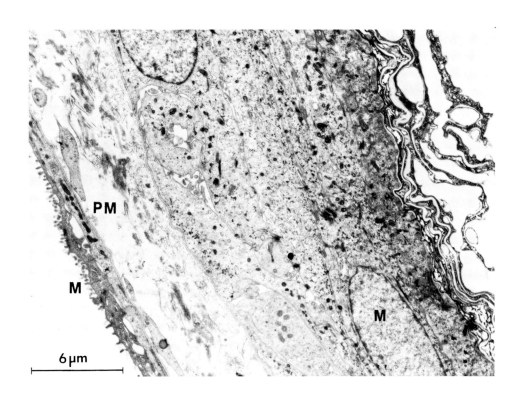

Fig. 112: A thin wall of pearly cholesteatoma shows matrix (m) and perimatrix (pm), and mucous membrane (m) on the outside. The perimatrix is formed by scanty connective tissue.

dermal-epidermal junction, and this membrane is adhered to the basal cells by hemidesmosomes and partly anchored to the dermis by fine reticular fibers (Fig. 113). The basal lamina is made up of collagen and presumably serves as a molecular filter. When basal cells are either damaged or migrate upward as a natural process of keratinization, the basal lamina remains intact and

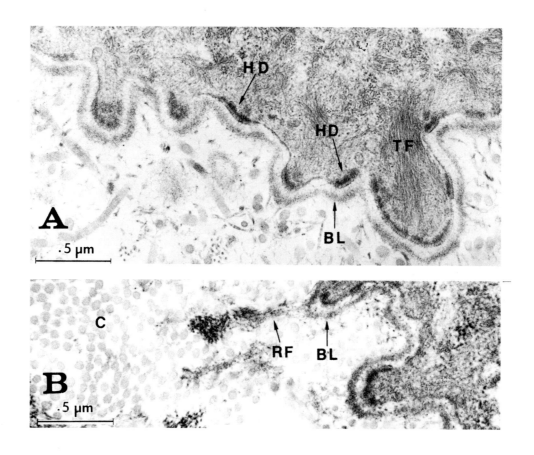

Fig. 113: (A) Basal portion of the cholesteatoma basal cell is adhered to the basal lamina (bl) with hemidesmosomes (hd) which are closely related to the tonofilaments (tf). (B) Basal lamina (bl) of the basal cell is often attached to the fine reticular fibrils (rf). Collagen fibers (c).

serves as a guide for the new epithelial cells that migrate to the empty spaces (Fig. 114). On the other hand, owing to this arrangement, if there should be a localized inflammatory reaction in the dermis near the basal lamina, physical distortion of the basal lamina will occur and the orderly migratory behavior will be disrupted, as will be shown below.

The perimatrix (or lamina propria) also showed great variability. Some were extremely thin (5-10 μ), while others were very thick (30-40 μ). Thick perimatrix usually contained a few too many fibrocytes, collagen fibers, reticular fibers, and capillaries. In places, localized round cell or PMN leukocytic infiltration was observed. Rarely, some mast cells were also noted.

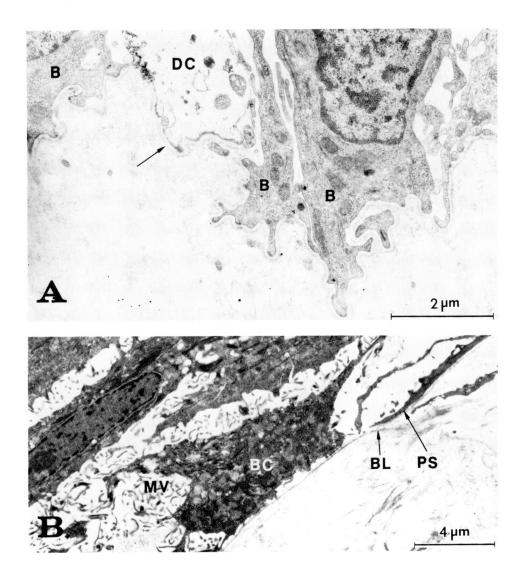

Fig. 114: (A) One of the basal cells (b) of the cholesteatoma has degenerated (dc), but its basal lamina (arrow) is still intact. Note lack of desmosomes. (B) Basal cells (bc) apparently migrate by pseudopod (ps) along the old basal lamina (bl), which is partly disrupted. Numerous microvilli (mv) are observed in these basal cells.

Abundant keratohyalin granules—a prerequisite for the keratinization process—were positively identified in close association with tonofilaments in all confirmed cholesteatoma (Fig. 115A). Numerous membrane coating granules (or Odland's bodies) were also observed in the granular layer (Fig. 115B). Although the exact function of these bodies is not known, they are thought to contribute to the bioprocess of keratinization by being expelled into the extracellular space (Matoltsy and Parekkal, 1967). When keratinization is complete, there are always unmistakable cornified keratin flakes in an orderly arrangement, which show positive birefringence under

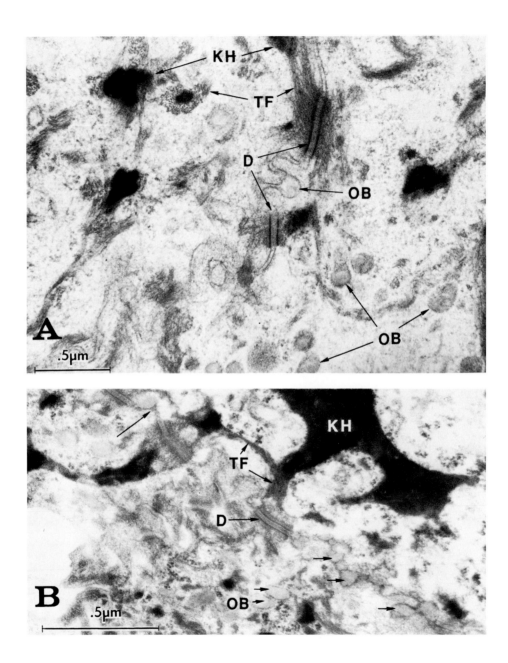

Fig. 115: (A) Granular cell of the cholesteatoma shows numerous tonofilaments that are attached to desmosomes (d). Keratohyalin granules (kh) are closely associated with tonofilaments (tf). Numerous Odland's bodies are seen. (B) Odland's bodies (ob) are apparently expelled into the intercellular space (arrows). Tonofilaments (tf) are associated with keratohyalin granules (kh).

polarized light.

Keratin formation did not appear to be directly proportional to the thickness of the epidermis, since even thin epidermis produced large quantities of keratin flakes. Rather, the thick matrix appeared to be the result of the inflammatory response in the area (Fig. 116A). It appears that the matrix with large quantities of keratohyalin granules actively produces keratin. However, keratinization also appeared well advanced even when the keratin granules were only scanty in the stratum granulosum.

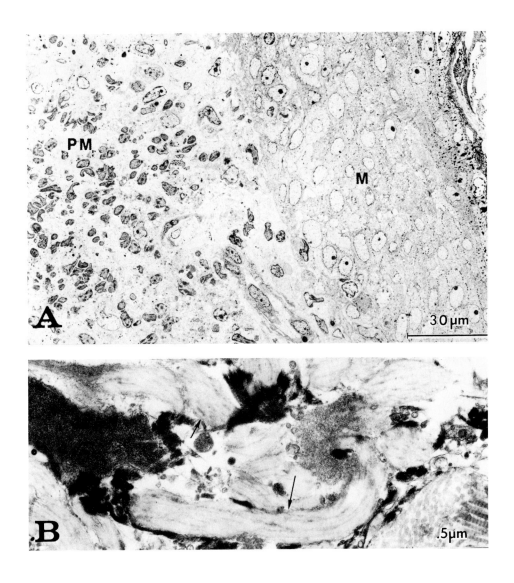

Fig. 116: (A) A thick cholesteatoma matrix (m) and perimatrix (pm) that are infiltrated with numerous inflammatory cells. (B) A close-up view of elastic fibers (arrows) in the perimatrix of cholesteatoma.

Morphologically speaking, there are no differences between the cholesteatoma matrix and epidermization, or between the cholesteatoma matrix and the epidermis of the tympanic membrane. However, there are a few exceptional cases where true keratinization did not occur. These cases are found among the epidermization cases and will be discussed below under metaplasia.

The outer surface of shiny pearl formation is made up of mucosal epithelium. These cells can be simple squamous, cuboidal, or even tall columnar cells with goblet and ciliated cells, as already described by the authors (Lim and Saunders, 1972).

Advancing Front and Cyst or Pearl Formation

A majority of the cholesteatomas we examined had a cystic form, but a few of them were in a typical pearl form. The former type of cholesteatoma appears to be the result either of the ingrowth of epidermis from the tympanic membrane perforation, mainly from Shrapnell's membrane, or of total perforation of the whole drum. Some of them appear to originate from an indrawn tympanic membrane (retraction pocket), of which the mucous layer has adhered to the middle ear connective tissue by inflammation. If the pars flaccida is retracted, the perimatrix contains elastic fibers (Fig. 116B). The elastic fibers are not found in middle ear connective tissue. Therefore, we can assume that the elastic fibers found in the perimatrix came from the pars flaccida. We have not yet seen cases where the cholesteatoma is formed from retracted pars tensa unless its lamina propria, which is made up primarily of square reticular fibers, is severely compromised. The pars tensa fibers are morphologically distinct from collagen fibers and are not seen in the cholesteatoma perimatrix.

When the cholesteatoma maintains a clean pearl formation, the matrix and perimatrix are usually very thin due to the distension of the sac by the collection of keratin matter in it. However, when the cholesteatoma is in a cystic form in direct contact with inflamed mucosal tissue such as granulation tissue and glandular formation of the mucosa, invariably there are thickened matrices with heavy infiltration of inflammatory cells in the perimatrix. Importantly, where the localized inflammatory reaction takes place, the papillary projection of the dermis is evident. In some instances, the cholesteatoma matrix with or without a papillary projection may form a pearl (Fig. 117A) similar in mechanism to that of Ruedi's (1959) experimental cholesteatoma.

It appears that an important prerequisite for cholesteatoma invasion or pearl or cyst formation of acquired cholesteatoma is an inflammatory reaction. The most successful experimental results in producing cholesteatoma were obtained from middle ear infection or chemical stimulation of the tympanic membrane (Abramson, et al, 1975). These stimuli induce intense inflammatory reaction, which in turn provides: (1) stimulation of the basal cells to divide and proliferate, or (2) fibrin clotting and fibrillar formation as a result of inflammatory response, causing the adhesion of the basal lamina or the migration of basal cell processes (pseudopods) to orient themselves to move toward the middle ear cavity (Fig. 117B). The present material also frequently showed irregularity or destruction of the basal lamina, presumably by physical disruption by local inflammation or the action of hydrolytic enzymes released by inflammatory cells.

A similar phenomenon is also observed in fresh wound healing, where migrating basal cells leave their basal laminae and their leading cell processes make contact with fibrin nets and use them as a guide (Martinez, 1972). Earlier Paul Weiss (1959) proposed an important concept known as the "contact guidance" system, which operates in cell orientation and locomotion. This means there is a certain guiding system which makes the cells orient themselves in a certain direction and move by this guiding mechanism. In his classic study of cell culture using connective tissue, Weiss demonstrated that the orientation and locomotion of cells largely depends on their microenvironment,

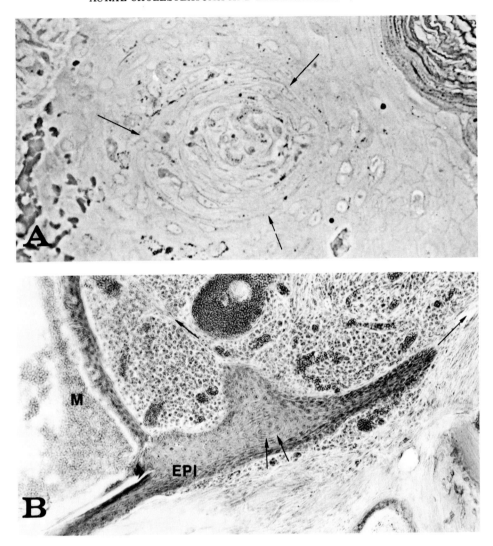

Fig. 117: (A) A whorl formation of the cholesteatoma matrix is indicated by arrows. This may be an early stage of pearl formation. (B) A papillary formation of the advancing front of epidermis (epi) Two-prong advancement is clearly associated with fiber orientations (arrows). Observe localized inflammatory cell infiltration under the mucous membrane (m) and closely associated with the advancing front. A double arrow points to a whorl formation in the epidermis.

specifically plasma fibrin meshwork. In tissue culture, cells orient themselves along the lines of tension which are created by plasma clotting. Centripetal migration of the epidermal cells in wound healing can be explained by the initial swelling of the wound by oozing plasma and the subsequent contraction of the wound by plasma clotting attached to the basal lamina which will orient fibrils toward the center of the wound (Giacometti and Parekkal, 1969).

When the advancing front of the epidermis is examined, almost without exception there are localized inflammatory reactions at the junction, generally in the connective tissue of the mucosal end. More important, there are numerous fine fibrils attached to the basal cells serving as a guide (Fig. 118). Examples of several different modes of epidermal advancement can be found in temporal bone sections where varying advancing fronts can be studied in a serial manner. Depending on the direction of the guiding fibrils, the advancing epidermal basal cell projection is oriented either to undermine the mucosal epithelium or to form a papillary projection (see Fig. 117B). When there are already well-formed fibrillar nets, the epidermis appears to migrate following the fibrillar orientation. Electron microscopic findings of such advancing fronts confirm the light microscopic observations and further show that the basal lamina is disrupted and the pseudopodial

extension of the migrating cells can be observed in contact with the fine fibrils (Fig. 119). Migrating or newly migrated epidermal cells lack desmosomes—structures binding cells together, perhaps, limiting their mobility (see Fig. 114).

These findings are particularly important for both theoretical and practical consideration. This finding would imply that the behavior of the migrating epidermis is dictated by the fibril formation and subsequent shrinkage as a result of local inflammation, not as a result of a presumed invasive nature of the epidermal cells in the cholesteatoma, as suggested earlier. It can be hypothesized that the extent of invasive behavior may be determined by the microchemical environment, particularly the contraction of plasma, surrounding the migrating front. This concept is also in line with the common clinical experience that a quiescent cholesteatoma can suddenly become active with aural infection.

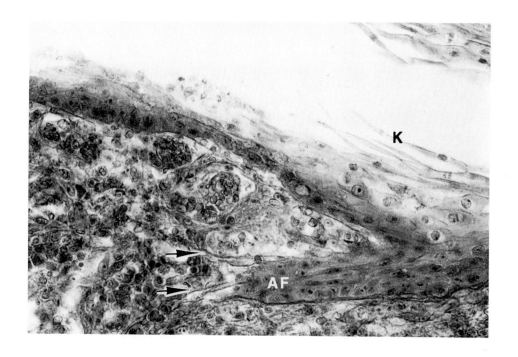

Fig. 118: An advancing front (af) of epidermization shows its attachment with fine fibrils (arrows) that are oriented in the same direction as the advancement. Also observe round cell infiltration in the perimatrix of the advancing front. Keratin (k).

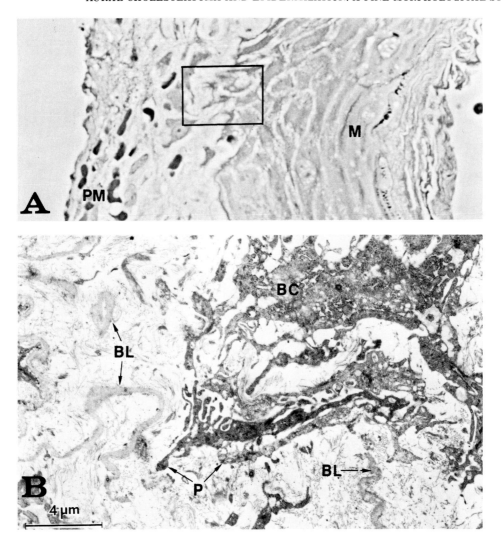

Fig. 119: (A) A phase contrast micrograph shows an early stage of basal cell disruption which may lead to the formation of an advancing front. **(B)** An EM photograph of the rectangle above shows the disrupted basal lamina (bl) and cell process (p) of basal cells (bc), indicating their active migration.

A still unanswered question is the nature of the underlying inflammation: how this localized inflammatory reaction at the advancing front comes about in the absence of generalized infection in the middle ear. It is possible that the inflammatory reaction can be induced at the advancing front by keratin, which may serve as an irritant, or micro-organisms may gain access to the lamina propria through a gap in the epidermal-mucosal junction. The other possibility is that there might be some immunological tissue reaction. Further ultrastructural and immunochemical study is needed to clarify this question.

Cyst formation by implanted skin was noted by

Christophers (1972). When a piece of guinea pig ear skin is cut out and implanted intradermally in the ear tissue pocket, a cyst is formed by the implanted skin regardless of the orientation of the implanted skin—whether it is facing the ear epidermis or against it. Keratin is always shed into this cystic cavity. He reasoned that this cyst formation is due to an early connection between the dermal tissues of the host and the implants, the outgrowing epidermal cells being moved along the roof of the host pocket, which was heavily infiltrated by inflammatory cells. This cyst formation in the implant can be explained by the contact guidance system of the wound formation. On the other hand, when ear skin is explanted in semiliquid medium, the explant forms an epiboly and not a cyst. Abramson (1975) also observed similar findings when epidermis was transposed to the bulla. These experiments would again suggest that the cyst-forming nature of the skin implants does not reside in the epidermis itself but in the environment surrounding the implants.

Weiss (1959) suggested that when a mass among aggregated fibrins expands, the direction of the surrounding fibrins runs parallel to the surface of the sphere. This is analogous to the pearl formation of cholesteatoma, where the epidermal cells are programmed to migrate along the surface by their spherically oriented guiding system (Lim and Saunders, 1972). When this guiding system is disrupted by local inflammatory reaction, distortion of the basal lamina will occur as a result of the shrinkage of reticular fibrils or fibrins attached to the basal lamina and the subsequent attachment and pulling of the pseudopods from the basal cells. This would cause an outward (centrifugal) movement of the dermis to form a papillary advancing front. Once such a direction is set by the fibrils present in the perimatrix, the epidermis (or matrix) will migrate along this fibrillar orientation. This phenomenon is analogous to the railroad track by which a train is guided. When the inflammatory reaction ceases, the advancing front becomes blunted and forms a pearl. Once the pearl is formed, the accumulation of keratin in the sac will keep expanding. The pearl- or cyst-forming nature of the cholesteatoma does not lie in the inherent nature of the matrix; rather it lies in the connective tissue of the inflamed middle ear. This concept was already expressed by Walsh et al (1951).

Metaplasia

Squamous metaplasia of the middle ear mucosal membrane was observed in 17 biopsies out of 180 cases of children with otitis media with effusion (serous or mucous otitis media). Only three cases had typical keratinizing squamous epithelial cells (Fig. 120). That none of them had had a prior myringotomy strongly suggests that they had true

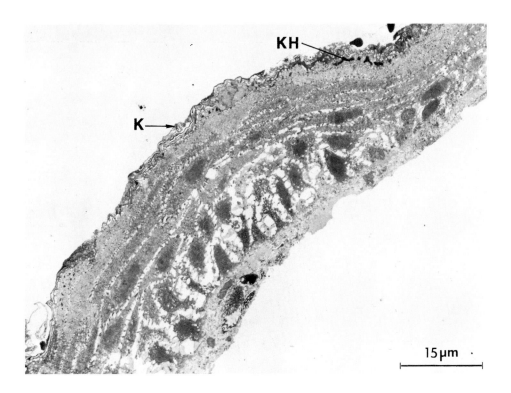

Fig. 120: A mucosal biopsy from a child suffering from otitis media with effusion (serous otitis media) shows a typical keratinizing epithelium (k). The patient had an intact tympanic membrane at the time of the myringotomy. Keratohyalin granules (hg).

metaplasia. About 10 cases showed signs of squamous metaplasia but lacked signs of true keratinization, such as the absence of keratohyalin granules or horny layer (Fig. 121). However, they showed well-developed tonofilaments. The superficial squamous epithelial cells showed some microvilli. This type of metaplastic epithelium somewhat resembles non-keratinizing epithelium

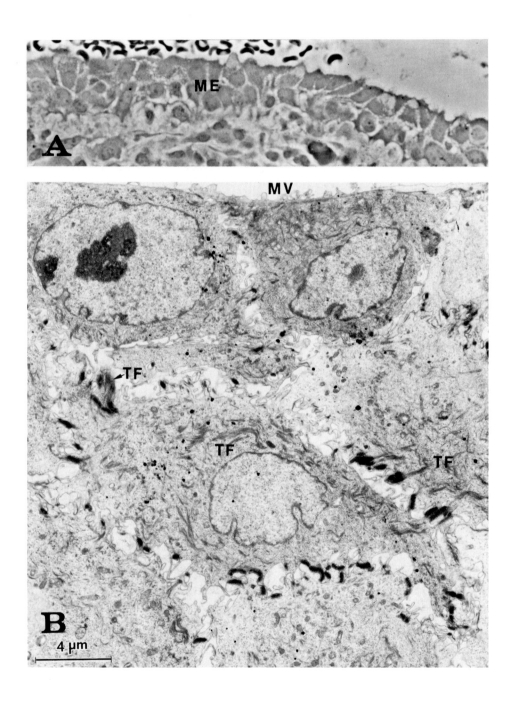

Fig. 121: (A) A phase contrast micrograph of a mucosal biopsy from a child with serous otitis media shows metaplastic transitional epithelium (me). (B) An EM photograph of the above shows stratified cuboidal epithelium with numerous tonofilaments, but without keratohyalin granules. Surface cells are covered with microvilli (mv).

of the human esophagus (Bloom and Fawcett, 1975). Whether this type of metaplastic epithelium is a distinct class of non-keratinizing squamous epithelium or is in a transitional form to eventually become a keratinizing epithelium could not be determined.

The remainder of the cases showed only keratin-like flakes in the absence of true epidermis. In these cases, without exception, there were numerous micro-organisms, giving evidence of infection (Fig. 122). Pseudokeratin (or keratin-like flakes) may be formed by degenerating epithelial cells and foreign body giant cells that are somehow packed together to become dehydrated, resem-

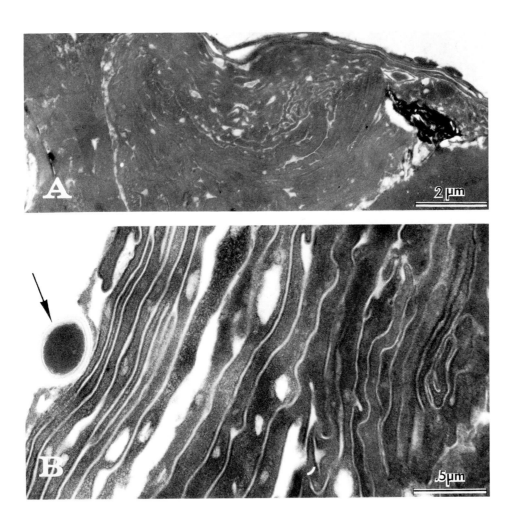

Fig. 122: (A) A mucosal biopsy of a child with otitis media with effusion shows keratin-like substances. (B) A close-up view of the keratin-like substance from the above specimen shows a micro-organism (arrow).

bling keratinized epithelium (Fig. 123). It is also possible that they are infected keratin and that there is cholesteatomatous epidermal tissue in the middle ear somewhere, but dermis is missing from the biopsy.

These new biopsy findings bring out the possibility of metaplasia of the middle ear mucosa, and it is worthwhile to discuss the laboratory evidence to support or dispute such a notion. It is known that respiratory mucosa can transform into keratinizing epithelium in the trachea for certain stimuli such as tobacco tar (Greenberg and Hallman, 1964). Recently, Greenberg et al (1973) showed that middle ear mucosa also can be transformed into keratinizing epithelium by the application of tobacco tar. This experiment undoubt-

edly enhances the possibility of mucosal metaplasia as a mode of cholesteatoma formation, although critical evidence is still lacking that such metaplastic epithelium will remain as epidermis and eventually develop into cholesteatoma.

The multipotentiality of the epithelial cells is well known to biologists (Montagna, 1962). An entire family of epithelial cells, which includes the keratinizing appendages and numerous glands, all derive from the ectoderm of the embryo. The development of glands capable of secreting mucin or lipids is a characteristic of dermis and shares the same genetic message stored in the germinal cells. Phylogenetically speaking, the mucus protection system of an animal's skin surface is developed earlier than the keratin protection system

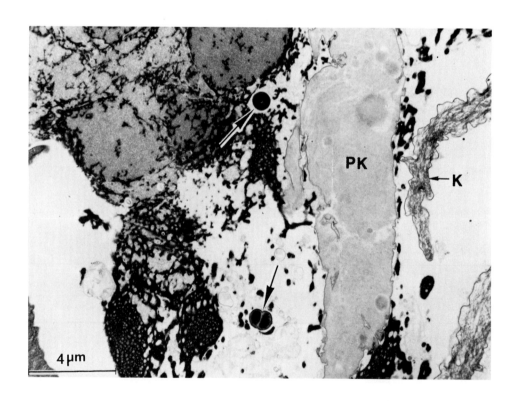

Fig. 123: Mucosal biopsy from a child with otitis media with effusion shows numerous keratin-like (k) materials, which may have come from an exfoliated cell or degenerating giant cells. Pseudokeratin (pk)? Arrows point to the micro-organisms.

(Mercer, 1961). It has been shown that the determination to become either mucus-secreting or keratin-forming cells is not irrevocable and that the cells of the germinal layer itself remain effectively multipotential even in freely differentiated epithelium (Billingham and Silvers, 1968). This evidence was often cited as a favorable theoretical ground for the metaplasia hypothesis of cholesteatoma (Sade, 1971).

It is known that the modulation between mucus-secreting cells and keratin forming cells is dependent on sex hormones in vaginal epithelia. However, experiments with high doses of estrogen failed to produce metaplasia of middle ear mucosa even though vaginal epithelium showed keratinization (Friedmann, 1959).

In epithelial cell culture, O_2-CO_2 levels have proven to be a critical factor for keratogenesis. Illuminating experimental data were presented by Moscona (1964) who showed that high O_2 serves as an initiating factor for keratogenesis of chorioallantoic epithelial cells. When 5% CO_2 was added to 95% O_2, the keratinization was completely prevented. At relatively high CO_2 levels, keratogenesis is suppressed and the cells function as respiratory epithelia, producing mucus. Sadé (1974) postulated, and later proved, (Sadé, 1976) that the high CO_2 gas level in the middle ear of the secretory otitis patient is the underlying reason for the increased mucus production by the mucosa; conversely, he postulated that high O_2 gas may produce keratin secreting cells. So far, his organ culture experiment has not shown positive evidence of keratinizing metaplasia from mucus membrane. Even if we subscribe to high O_2 as a keratogenetic factor in the middle ear, it is hard to explain how keratinization occurs in ears that suffer from secretory chronic otitis media, which presumably have high middle ear CO_2 levels due to poor tubal function (Ingelstedt, et al, 1975). The high CO_2 environment would not be suitable for producing keratinizing epithelium. In fact, none of 81 squirrel monkeys developed squamous metaplasia of the middle ear mucosa following chronic tubal obstruction of up to six months in our experi-

ment, although many of them developed serous otitis media (unpublished experiment conducted jointly with Dr. Michael Paparella).

It is also well proven that certain factors can influence the irreversible differentiation of the epithelial embryogenesis. Fell and Mellanby (1953) established that the presence of vitamin A in the culture medium in which chick embryo ectoderm was growing prevented keratin formation but initiated mucin-secreting and cilia-bearing cells. When vitamin A is not added to the medium, the ectoderm produces keratinizing epithelium. The same phenomenon was observed using human embryonal skin (Lansnitzki, 1956). However, there is no evidence so far to suggest that vitamin A is involved in cholesteatoma formation.

There is ample experimental evidence provided by grafting to suggest that the factors responsible for localized specialization arise in the underlying mesoderm. For example, using the embryonic chick, by grafting mesoderm from a presumptive foot bud beneath wing ectoderm, one can cause the formation of a claw instead of wing feathers (Cairns and Saunders, 1954). This phenomenon is known as epithelial-mesenchymal interaction. In the first place, the external environment imposes a class of differentiation on epithelial cells and, second, the mesodermal (mesenchymal) organization further limits differentiation and gives rise to site-characteristic development. Numerous experiments (Zwilling, 1956; Waddington, 1956; and McLoughlin, 1968) have shown that the underlying mesenchymal tissue induces and maintains the epidermal differentiations. If this concept is directly applicable in keratogenesis in the middle ear, we have to assume that the mesenchymal cells in the perimatrix are responsible for such metaplasia. But critical evidence to confirm this notion in cholesteatoma is still lacking. In fact, our own unpublished experiment (conducted jointly with Dr. Daniel Jackson), with implanted skin in the cat's bulla, showed that a large area of the epidermis was regressed and replaced by mucous membrane and formed epiboly. This finding would indicate that the mesenchymal tissue obtained from skin failed to maintain epidermis in the bulla but successfully supported mucosal epithelium. Therefore, it can be suggested that, at least in fully developed skin, connective tissue does not have any unique genetic characteristics in determining mucosal epithelium or keratinizing epithelium.

Another difficulty of the metaplasia hypothesis lies in the lack of temporal bone documentation to prove that such metaplasia is common in patients with chronic otitis media (Schuknecht, 1974). Only one convincing example which may support the middle ear metaplasia or congenital origin was recently reported by Dr. George Nager (1976) at the last Shambaugh Workshop. He showed a small island of keratinizing epithelium in the promontory of a presumably normal ear.

Contrary to the lack of supportive evidence from temporal bone findings, a high incidence of metaplasia has been reported from biopsy materials. Sadé (1969) found that 60% of the mucosal biopsies obtained from chronic otitis media showed evidence of squamous cell metaplasia, and 42% showed keratinization. Bernstein et al (1972) also reported that 11% of the biopsies obtained from promontories of patients suffering from secretory otitis media showed stratified squamous metaplasia and 8% showed keratiniza-

tion. These big discrepancies in the incidence of keratinization of the middle ear mucosa cannot be explained, but they may perhaps be due to the differences in patient population, size of biopsy, and chronicity of the disease. But it also could be due to the dynamic (or modulating) nature of the pathology. However, it also could be that they have more of the congenital type of cholesteatoma, which is known to be a rare occurrence, in their series, or the pathology may be rapidly changing during the course of the disease. The squamous metaplastic changes may revert back to the mucus-secreting cells following the cure of the middle ear disease.

With the given evidence, we can only tentatively suggest that such metaplasia (true keratinizing epithelium) can occur in the middle ear in a few cases. But this evidence should be considered only circumstantial. No definitive conclusion regarding true metaplasia can be drawn in the absence of definitive evidence and critical experimental data.

Acknowledgement

The authors wish to thank Ilija Karanfilov, Joan Osborne, Jonathan Darby, Nancy Sally, and Katherine Abramson for their valuable technical assistance.

References

1. Abramson, M.; Asarch, R. G.; and Litton, W. B.: Experimental aural cholesteatoma causing bone resorption. *Trans. Am. Otolol.* Soc., 63:80, 1975.
2. Bernstein, M. M.; Hayes, E. R.; Ishikawa, T. et al: Secretory otitis media; A histopathologic and immunochemical report. *Trans. Am. Acad. Ophthalmol. Otolaryngol.*, 76:1305, 1972.
3. Billingham, R. E. and Silvers, W. K.: Dermoepidermal interactions and epithelial specificity. In Fleischmajer, R. and Billingham, R. E.: (Eds.). *Epithelial-Mesenchymal Interactions. 18th Haber-*

mann Symposium. Williams and Wilkins Company, Baltimore, Maryland, 1968, p. 252.
4. Bloom, W. and Fawcett, D. W.: *A Textbook of Histology.* W. E. Saunders Company, Philadelphia, Pennsylvania, 1975, p. 639.
5. Cairns, J. M. and Saunders, J. W.: The influence of embryonic mesoderm on the regional specification of epidermal derivatives in the chick. *J. Exp. Zool.*, 127:221, 1954.
6. Christophers, E.: Kinetic aspects of epidermal healing. In Maibach, H. I., and Rovee, D. T.: (Eds.).

Epidermal Wound Healing. Year Book Medical Publishers, Chicago, Illinois, 1972, p. 53.

7. Derlacki, E. and Clemis, J. D.: Congenital cholesteatoma of the middle ear and mastoid. *Ann. Otol. Rhinol. Laryngol.*, 74:706, 1965.

8. Eggston, A. and Wolff, D.: *Histopathology of the Ear, Nose and Throat.* Williams and Wilkins Company, Baltimore, Maryland, 1947.

9. Fell, H. B. and Mellanby, E.: Metaplasia produced in cultures of chick ectoderm by high vitamin A. *J. Physiol.*, 119:470, 1953.

10. Fernandez, D. and Lindsay, J.: Aural cholesteatoma. Experimental observations. *Laryngoscope,* 70:1119, 1960.

11. Friedmann, I.: The comparative pathology of otitis media. Experimental histopathology of experimental otitis of guinea pig with particular reference to experimental cholesteatoma. Part II. *J. Laryngol. Otol.*, 69:588, 1955.

12. Friedmann, I.: Epidermoid cholesteatoma and cholesterol granuloma. *Ann. Otol. Rhinol. Laryngol.*, 68:57, 1959.

13. Giacometti, L. and Parekkal, P.: Skin transplantation: Orientation of epithelial cells by the basement membrane. *Nature*, 223:514, 1969.

14. Greenberg, S. D.; Dickey, J. R.; and Neely, J. G.: Effects of tobacco on the ear. *Ann. Otol. Rhinol. Laryngol.*, 82:311, 1973.

15. Greenberg, S. D. and Hallman, G. L.: Changes in respiratory epithelium induced by single large application of tobacco tar: An experimental study in dogs. *South. Med. J.*, 57:417, 1964.

16. Harris, A. J.: Cholesteatosis and chronic otitis media. The histopathology of osseous and soft tissues. *Laryngoscope*, 72:954, 1962.

17. Ikeda, M.: Electron microscopic study of fine structures of cholesteatoma epidermis. *Nichi Jibigingo (Japan)*, 71:84, 1968.

18. Ingelstedt, S.; Jonson, B.; and Rundcrantz, H.: Gas tension and pH in middle ear effusion. *Ann. Otol. Rhinol. Laryngol.*, 84:198, 1975.

19. Lansnitzki, I.: The effect of 3-4 Benzpyrene on human foetal lung grown in vitro. *Brit. J. Cancer,* 10:510, 1956.

20. Lim, D. J.: Tympanic membrane: Electron microscopic observation. Part I: Pars tensa. *Acta Otolaryngol (Stockh).*, 66:181, 1968.

21. Lim, D. J.: Human tympanic membrane: An ultrastructural observation. *Acta Otolaryngol. (Stockh.)*, 70:176, 1970.

22. Lim, D. J. and Birck, H.: Ultrastructural pathology of the middle ear mucosa in serous otitis media. *Ann. Otol. Rhinol. Laryngol.*, 80:838, 1971.

23. Lim, D. J. and Saunders, W. H.: Acquired cholesteatoma: Light and electron microscopic observations. *Ann. Otol. Rhinol. Laryngol.*, 81:2, 1972.

24. McLoughlin, C. B.: Interaction of epidermis with various types of foreign mesenchyme. In Fleischmajer, R. and Billingham, R. E.: (Eds.). *Epithelial-Mesenchymal Interactions. 18th Habermann Symposium.* Williams and Wilkins Company, Baltimore, Maryland, 1968, p. 244.

25. Maeda, M.; Tabata, T.; Shimada, T.; and Ikeda, M.: Histological and histochemical studies on cholesteatoma epidermis. *Ann. Otol. Rhinol. Laryngol.*, 76:1043, 1967.

26. Martinez, I. R., Jr.: Fine structural studies of migrating epithelial cells following incision wounds. In Maiback, H. I. and Rovee, D. T.: (Eds.). *Epidermal Wound Healing.* Year Book Medical Publishers, Chicago, Illinois, 1972, p. 323.

27. Matoltsy, A. G. and Parekkal, R. F.: Keratinization. In Zelickson, A. S.: (Ed.). *Ultrastructure of Normal and Abnormal Skin.* Lea and Febiger, Philadelphia, Pennsylvania, 1967, p. 76.

28. Mercer, E. H.: *Keratin and Keratinization: An Essay in Molecular Biology.* Pergamon Press, London, England, 1961.

29. Montagna, W.: *The Structure and Function of Skin.* Academic Press, New York, New York, 1962.

30. Moscona, A. A.: Studies on stability of phenotypic traits in embryonic integumental tissue and cells. In Montagna, W. and Lobitz, W. C.: (Eds.). *The Epidermis.* Academic Press, New York, New York, 1964, p. 83.

31. Nager, G.: Theories on attic retraction pocket cholesteatoma. Paper presented at The Shambaugh Fifth International Workshop on Middle Ear Microsurgery and Fluctuant Hearing Loss, February 29-March 5, 1976, Chicago, Illinois, in press.

32. Ojala, L. and Saxen, A.: Pathogenesis of middle ear cholesteatoma arising from Shrapnell's membrane (attic cholesteatoma). *Acta Otolaryngol. (Stockh.).,* Suppl. 100:33, 1951.

33. Ruedi, L.: Cholesteatoma formation in the middle ear in animal experiments. *Acta Otolaryngol. (Stockh.).,* 50:233, 1959.

34. Ruedi, L.; Acquired cholesteatoma. *Arch. Otolaryngol.*, 78:252, 1963.

35. Sadé, J.: Cellular differentiation of the middle ear lining. *Ann. Otol. Rhinol. Laryngol.*, 80:376, 1971.

36. Sadé, J.: The biopathology of secretory otitis media. *Ann. Otol. Rhinol. Laryngol.*, Suppl 11, 83:59, 1974.

37. Sadé, J.: Middle ear mucosa and secretory otitis media. Paper presented at The Shambaugh Fifth International Workshop on Middle Ear Microsurgery and Fluctuant Hearing Loss, February 29-March 5, 1976, Chicago, Illinois, in press.

38. Sadé, J. and Weinberg, J.: Mucus production in the chronically infected middle ear: A histological and histochemical study. *Ann. Otol. Rhinol. Laryngol.*, 78:148, 1969.

39. Schuknecht, H. F.: *Pathology of the Ear.* Harvard

University Press, Cambridge, Massachusetts, 1974.

40. Schwarz, M.: *Das Cholesteatom im Gehorgang und im Mittelohr: Pathogenese-Diagnose-Therapie.* George Thieme Verlag, Stuttgart, Germany, 1966.

41. Waddington, C. H.: *Principles of Embryology.* George Allen and Unwin Ltd., London, England, 1956.

42. Walsh,T. E.; Covell, W. P.; and Ogura, J. H.: The effect of cholesteatosis on bone. *Ann. Otol. Rhinol. Laryngol.,* 60:1100, 1951.

43. Weiss, P.: Cellular dynamics. In Oncley, J., et al: (Ed.). *Biophysical Science - A Study Program.* John Wiley and Sons, New York, New York, 1959, p. 17.

44. Zwilling, E.: Interaction between limb-bud ectoderm and mesoderm in the chick embryo. IV. Experiments with a wingless mutant. *J. Exp. Zool.,* 132:241, 1956.

IMPLANT CHOLESTEATOMA IN THE MASTOID

Edward C. Brandow, Jr., M.D.

The high incidence of residual or recurrent cholesteatoma following operation is a problem to the otologic surgeon, particularly with the intact canal wall technique. Failures are distressing, to the patients and surgeons, and in this condition, this complication occurs in from 2% to 30% of cases, and in children, sometimes as high as 50%. DeGuine has reported that at revision operation in 140 patients, there was a 54% incidence of epidermoid cysts or pearls in the mastoid. It is not always the intact canal wall technique that gives rise to residual or recurrent cholesteatoma. Open cavity procedures are also followed by failures; here the rate is not as high, but the problems become significant if followed long enough. Gristwood reported, after eight years of follow-up an incidence of 17% recurrence after the modified radical operation. Even with meticulous care, recurrence has been too high in my own series. The reappearance of cholesteatoma may occur after ten or more years because of the insidious slow growth, especially in non-infected patients. Since some patients are eventually lost to follow-up, a true incidence of recurrence is difficult to determine.

We believe that the most common cause for the reappearance of cholesteatoma is from bits of residual disease being left behind. In 1962, Guilford suggested that the use of a drill for exposure of cholesteatoma caused fragmentation of the matrix with dissemination of epithelial cells throughout the operative field. Some of these cells, he claimed, have the potential to take as a graft in the mastoid and give rise to recurrent cholesteatoma. The purpose of this paper is to elaborate on this hypothesis, to re-emphasize its importance, and to suggest that this factor may help explain the high incidence of recurrent cholesteatoma.

It is well known that skin, particularly a thin split-thickness graft, takes well in the mastoid cavity and for a time, back in the 1950's, it was extensively used. The raw bony surface of the cavity provides a good bed for implantation of epithelial cells or small broken-off fragments of the matrix. Dissection and removal of cholesteatoma is often difficult and the sac usually cannot be kept intact. During surgery, at one time or another, it is pushed around and crushed. It is torn apart, shredded, and when drilled down upon with cutting burrs, innumerable cells are disseminated throughout the operative field. Although most of these cells are washed with irrigating solution, a few may remain, together with tiny fragments of the matrix. Microscopic bits of epithelium get caught up in the sticky serum or blood clots that collect in the cavity. This blood provides a media for the support of an implant. It is also suggested that irrigation might force some epithelial cells down into the depths of the cellular system and possibly into opened haversian canals in the bone. These tiny bits of epithelium that implant, grow as tiny grafts and give rise to small pearly tumors, eventually forming a new cholesteatoma.

This theory was derived from observations during the "second look procedure" following the intact canal wall operation. A planned second stage exploration following most cholesteatoma operations is mandatory because of the anticipated high incidence of regrowth. In retrospect, I believe that recurrence represents implanted epithelial fragments, "seeding" of the mastoid cavity. When reopened, many were found to have multiple, separate pearls in the mastoid cavity—some in open areas which had been under direct vision in the cavity and where there had been no question of exposure. The operative notes indicated that the sac had been completely dissected from the mastoid with careful microsurgical technique. No difficulty had been experienced and there had been no anticipated residual disease or recurrence.

In one patient, eight months after the initial surgery, reoperation disclosed three separate pearls (Fig. 124), one on the mastoid tip, a second in the sino-dural angle and the third, 5 mm in diameter was found on the exposed surface of the lateral semi-circular canal directly beneath the microscope in the center of the field. It is unlikely that this was from a remnant of the matrix left behind. In another ear, (Fig. 125) a pearl was found in an area of the mastoid where previously the sac had not extended. This case also does not represent residual disease.

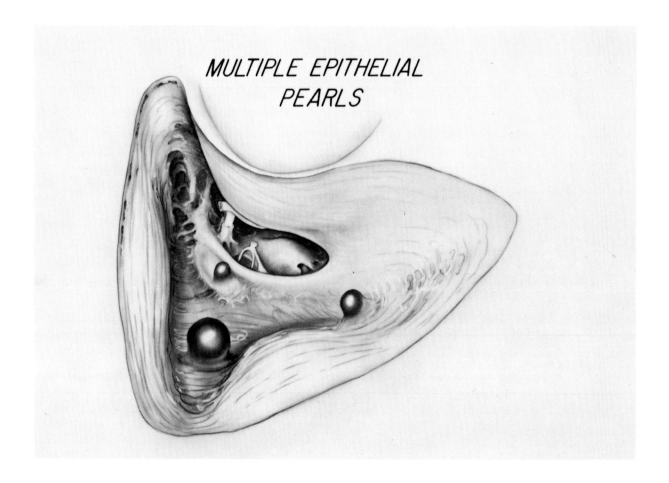

Fig. 124: Multiple recurrent epithelial pearls with a discrete cyst on the semicircular canal under direct microscopic view.

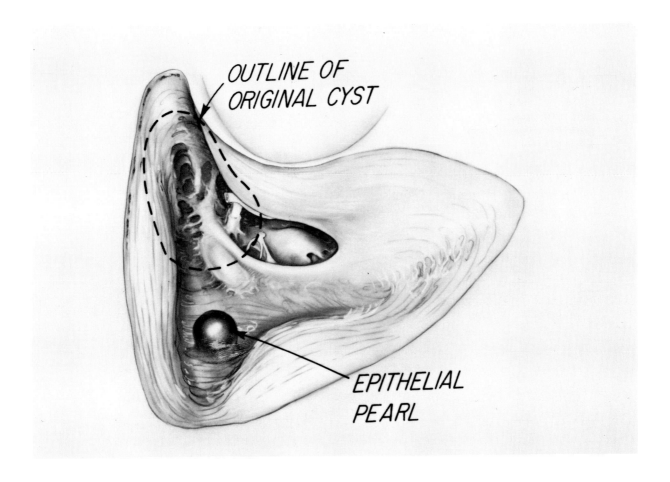

Fig. 125: Recurrent epithelial pearl in an area of the mastoid separate from the original cyst.

Implants would not be expected to be common in the middle ear as mucous membrane does not make a suitable site for implantation. Middle ear pearls or cysts more likely represent evidence of residual disease that was left behind.

The time lapse before staged reoperation is important and is best done within nine to twelve months. One must wait until the reaction from surgery of the ear and mastoid has subsided, and yet allow adequate elapse of time for the cyst to reform, if they will. Exact timing is difficult because of the number of years that it may take for the recurrence to develop. However, if too much time elapses, the pearls will collapse and form one large mass filling the mastoid cavity.

Smyth, Glasscock, Austin, Sheehy, and others have all reported staged operations and found no evidence of the residual cholesteatoma when it had, for one reason or another, not been removed. Sade' believes in the ability of the middle ear or mastoid epithelium to undergo metaplasia and change its characteristics. Certain unknown factors or mechanisms control epithelial differentiation in the ear and can switch squamous cells to mucous producing cells. Squamous epithelium can also lose its ability to form keratin, and when it becomes non-keratinizing, it is harmless.

Certainly, not all remaining fragments of epithelium develop pearls or the mastoid would be filled with an unlimited number of tiny cysts. However, some cells undoubtedly do implant and must be responsible for recurrent cholesteatoma.

In summary, the concept of epithelial implants has been presented as a possible explanation for the high incidence of reappearing cholesteatoma pearls in the mastoid. The question postulated is whether these multiple cysts represent residual disease left behind at the original operation or whether they arise from the implantation of cells or seeding of the mastoid. This transplant concept is theoretical and is unfortunately only derived from clinical observations, but it does offer a logical explanation. If this hypothesis is accepted, we otological surgeons can feel relieved to know our surgical skills are not always to blame for the residual or recurrent cholesteatoma.

QUESTIONS AND ANSWERS

Dr. Friedmann: I fully agree with Dr. Abramson on his excellent exposition of the migration theory. My interpretation of the material that has been presented would be that this squamous epithelium has ingrown or migrated into the middle ear from the outside and not from the inside out. I can't accept that when you have an epidermoid lining it is metaplasia. If it were metaplasia, the columnar epithelium would have been replaced by squamous epithelium. We have plenty of examples of this. When you see columnar epithelium beneath an epidermoid cyst, it couldn't be metaplasia because the columnar epithelium would have been replaced by the epidermoid tissue. Instead, it is undermining the middle ear mucosa. I am convinced that the metaplasia and congenital theories are operative in some cases of cholesteatoma, but I second Dr. Abramson.

Dr. Lim: This concerns Dr. Abramson in that we were quite interested in the dermal and mucosal interaction. We were impressed by the fact that nine out of 10 cases where mucosa meets skin we always seem to have localized inflammation at this junction. This is quite impressive. I think this is where the balances are tipped so that the migration of one epithelium will take over the other. I would like to point out again, even if Jacob today showed that the cholesteatoma may form behind Shrapnell's membrane, you cannot completely rule out the possibility that somewhere a stimulation behind the drum invited the migration of the basal cells to form cholesteatoma. It is not warranted to conclude that it necessarily be metaplasia.

Dr. Palva: Thank you, Dr. Lim. Dr. Ruben?

Dr. Ruben: To Dr. Abramson, in the experimental work in the guinea pig, two questions: One, did you have a control where you just used oxalic acid and what happened? Second, it seems that you are getting into the same logic trap that Dr. Sadé suggested, that you can't really prove the skin has come in from the external auditory canal. Perhaps experiments either with tritiated thymidine or something primitive like India ink marking would be a way to do that.

A question to Dr. Sadé. He speaks of the patients which we have all seen with retraction pockets and states that nobody has seen a cholesteatoma formed from one of these. I wonder if he is not looking at a biased sample because these are the patients who come to us that we're able to clean out once a month, twice a year, etc.

Dr. Plester: Dr. Sadé, do we have any idea why these epidermal cysts are usually formed in the majority of the cases just behind the pars flaccida and why are they always formed in the close vicinity of this retraction pocket? There is so much mucous membrane lining all over the ear and so much opportunity to form metaplasia, that I am wondering why it is going in this particular place?

Dr. Sheehy: In relationship to what Dr. Sadé said in terms of not having seen one of these posterior atelectases go on to cholesteatoma under your own eyes where there was not cholesteatoma before, certainly I have. I am sure my associates have. In fact this presents one of the problems in terms of whether you operate prior to the time there is an active cholesteatoma in order to prevent the problem of ossicular destruction. So certainly we have seen that. I also wanted to make one plea. We saw this morning two of the three speakers using an either/or between recurrence and residual cholesteatoma. I would hope the speakers will differentiate disease left behind from recurrent disease. I don't care if they use the terms we do, but at least differentiate them.

Dr. Khan: Dr. Derlacki, I have three questions. First, what do we understand by the term cholesteatoma? Second, what is the classification of cholesteatoma, and how long did you observe the patients before you operated and found an epidermoid cyst? Third, is it not possible that there was a serous otitis media in childhood with a small perforation and epithelium migrated in and then the perforation healed? And, in due time a cholesteatoma or cyst developed, which you operated upon?

Dr. Delvillar: In Spain many years ago, Rodriguez Aldratas advanced the theory that the so-called congenital cholesteatoma could be due to the fact that in the last days or hours of fetal life, the fetus can absorb through the eustachian tube amniotic liquid charged with epithelial cells. The cells could be included in the attic portion of the middle ear of the fetus and remain there as an inclusion. Eventually there forms a cholesteatoma of the attic without the presence of a retraction pocket or perforation. The diagnosis is made 25 or 35 years after, when the growth of the pearl reaches a size capable of interfering with hearing.

Dr. Ekvall: Dr. Sadé said that no one believing in the retraction theory had ever measured the actual middle ear pressure. We have tried to do it in some cases. In our experiments, pressure recordings obtained from the middle ear of the patient by way of ventilating tube demonstrate that a forceful nasal inhalation or sleep may produce a considerable pressure reduction in the middle ear. Actually this pressure reduction, which we have recorded in several patients, is equivalent to a sudden descent from about 1,000 feet in less than one-fifth of a second. This is possible, of course, if the tube is sufficiently patent. One of our patients had a life-long history of sniffing, which she did several hundred times a day. Her middle ear showed bilateral attic retraction pockets with cholesteatoma. In our clinic we have last year found an increasing number of patients with a classic history of patulous tube, but these classic signs were previously disregarded because of chronic otitis. These patients all have been sniffers and the wider their tubes, the more often and the more forcefully they try to close their tubes by sniffing. We think it is reasonable to assume that this might

be one cause of cholesteatoma formation of the retraction type and maybe it is inability to close the tube in many cases.

Dr. Austin: May I speak briefly on the problem of congenital cholesteatoma? The conference has been unable to reach any agreement in definition of cholesteatoma. I think we are deluding ourselves using the term congenital cholesteatoma. Dr. Pulec yesterday afternoon referred to the fact that our definition left out the congenital cholesteatomas which occur in the petrous apex, the cerebellopontine angle or the squamous portion of the temporal bone. I would suggest that we would simply call these what they are and that is epidermoid cysts, no more, no less. Let's not play games with the mythical term cholesteatoma. They have no relation to classic cholesteatoma in terms of the disease process. The treatment is totally different.

Dr. Redfield: May I comment on Dr. Sadé's photograph or diagram with the cholesteatoma having its external connection inferior to the junction of the malleus head and the incus. Speaking from my own experience, I don't see this except in very rare instances. I do see the great majority of my cholesteatomas with epithelial debris accumulating and protruding from this space going lateral to the malleus head and medial to the scutum.

Dr. Ruben: A question to Dr. Sadé. It was shown that India ink would move away from the retraction pocket. This was actually used as an argument that the migration is to the periphery and not to the center. To me it seems just the opposite. The action is at the center of the sac and not in the periphery. It could be not imagined that an infection at the center of the sac would speed up production of cysts. Actually it leads to an increased growth of a cul-de-sac actually forming a cholesteatoma. This seems to be crucial.

Second, to Dr. Abramson. If you put talcum on top of the remaining squamous epithelium, could you always expect cysts which could be easily removed with surgery?

Dr. Abramson: In reply to Bob Ruben's question about the oxalic acid, we did use it by itself and we were not able to produce cholesteatomas with it alone. This is in contradistinction to Dr. Lindsay, who was able to produce them with oxalic acid itself.

The question as to whether the experimental cholesteatoma occurred from outside in or inside out is a very difficult thing to prove. Looking at the time sequence of our cases, it would seem that we have smaller amounts of migration in shorter periods of time after injury and larger amounts of migration in longer times. That doesn't clinch the argument. It would be better to do a triated thymidine experiment, however life is short and we choose those few experiments that we can do in our time.

I comment on David Lim's slides. We did an experiment where we took little bits of skin, isolated them, and put them in a cul-de-sac in between bullar mucosa and bullar bone. In about five days we got beautiful cysts. We thought here we were going to produce great cholesteatomas. After five days they were about 20 microns and grew up to 50 microns. They never got any larger; in fact they regressed! I wonder if that is not what happens to a lot of these bits of metaplastic epithelial patches that occur. If you don't have a ready source of squamous epithelium, you don't have this very independent process that we are talking about of continual and progressive growth. The metaplasia theory implies that there is an inflammatory irritant process that not only causes the metaplasia, but it causes it to go to a sac as large as that which we see and yet never shows any evidence of breaking through the tympanic membrane until the sac gets there.

Dr. Derlacki: In our written text, we state we consider a cholesteatoma an epidermoid cyst whether it is a congenital or acquired. All cholesteatoma we consider epidermoid cysts. I don't see what difference it makes when I am faced with its surgical removal whether it is from the petrous bone or from the middle ear cleft. The term congenital cholesteatoma is more or less inherited. We used it to define that particular entity that has been described in the old nomenclature when we

had the three types, primary acquired, secondary acquired and congenital.

How long would we observe? Well, I think this is surgical philosophy. When I identify a cholesteatoma behind an intact tympanic membrane, I consider this a surgical entity and the sooner that ear is operated upon, the better. I am not going to run an experiment at the cost of a three year old child to find out how long it is going to take for it to perforate. I have already had several patients referred to me with intact tympanic membranes with cholesteatomas visualized, and by the time they reached me they had perforated. Some were infected, making it a much tougher problem. So the minute it is identified, I treat. I will not sit here and be a scientist. I am a surgeon.

As far as the question of preceding otitis media with a healed perforation which then forms a cholesteatoma behind the intact tympanic membrane, I made the point that the majority of our cases have had acute otitis media at some time, so I can't really answer that question.

I am a little surprised that Dick Buckingham didn't get up and answer Dr. Sadé when he had asked me of proof of the posterosuperior retraction pocket becoming a secondary acquired cholesteatoma. Buckingham has a magnificient series of slides in which he has depicted exactly this sequence and the reversal of that sequence by the insertion of ventilating tubes. I think everybody has seen this and as far as attic retraction pockets are concerned, I think anyone with much experience with cholesteatomas has watched attic retraction pockets develop into cholesteatomas in the attic and in my experience most of them are lateral to the ossicles, not medial to them.

Dr. Sadé: I have quite a few questions to answer. A few months ago we had the good fortune of having Nelson Kiang here. The Department of Otolaryngology here quite often has visiting professors and Nelson Kiang is, of course, one of the brightest we could have. Somebody asked him about his interest in ear research. He said, "I am not in the ears at all". We asked, "What are you interested in"? He said, "Actually, my central interest is in how to know that something is true".

The ear is just a model. We do not really realize how difficult it is to find if something is so or not. An example is we have projected since yesterday about 5,000 slides from maybe 500 specimens each of which could be interpreted one way or the other and each could be looked upon for half an hour and somebody will say one thing and somebody another.

A comment about animal experiments. Animal experiments are very much in vogue. People take them a bit too seriously. The analogy is not always fitting. I will give you an example. One of them was by Jim Snow. He performed operations which should produce cholesteatomas, but didn't.

As far as the mucosa is concerned, if there is a cholesteatoma behind an ossicle (and I was also surprised to find that most of them are behind) and if you look at a section in the appropriate plane you see stratified squamous epithelium medially and mucosa laterally here exactly like Imre showed us. If you would take it in a different plane, you will never find mucosa in between. Time is too short now to go into this extensively.

David Lim is right. I do not have final proof. I did not really want to say that I have final proof that what we have is a metaplastic process. I wanted to say, really, that it is very difficult for me to accept this invasive theory. I tend to think that it arises from within, and it makes sense to me and it has a theoretical basis. There is some circumstantial evidence that it might be a metaplastic process. This is as far as I can go.

Now as to the retraction pockets, I did not say—if I said it, I take it back—that it never happens that a posterosuperior retraction pocket will form a cholesteatoma. What I said is that I have never seen it. I have looked for it for 16 or 17 years, under the operating microscope, and I have never seen it. I would challenge you at the next Cholesteatoma Congress to bring such a case that you have followed up proving it, and going all the way to the attic. Is it really a retraction pocket and a year later here it is behind the ossicles? Maybe it can happen. I have not seen it.

Why in the attic exclusively, Dr. Plester? This is a crucial question. I don't have an answer. I can tell you two things that I can think of. One of them, we know that the middle ear mucosa is not the same lining everywhere. The attic mucosa is relatively flat in comparison with mesotympanic mucosa and there is a possibility that the cells in the attic, which are flat, are really squamous and not stratified squamous, might have a different inclination towards metaplasia than in the mesotympanum. This is a possibility, they might have a different behavior once they are entrapped. The second is even more interesting and again I don't have proof. I have, and I am not the only one, the feeling that we see more cholesteatomas today than ever before. As a matter of fact when I compared my figures to Bezold's, and Bezold is an otologist who counted, it seemed to me that I see tenfold the cholesteatomas as they had at that time.

It is possible that this might be really a complication of secretory otitis media (in the sense that secretory otitis media is really a complication of acute otitis media which was treated with antibiotics and not drained). Again, it is possible. I know of no direct evidence.

As far as pressure is concerned, which Dr. Ekvall of Sweden mentioned, he did measure pressure. Dr. Buckingham, found, in a similar group, pressures of an average of 5 mm. of water. I found 1.7 mm. This, in my opinion, does not explain what is happening. I don't really know what a patulous tube is. I am a little flabbergasted with that.

It is true that I said we have cholesteatomas which are behind the ossicular chain and we have those ones which are in front or lateral to them? These are self-cleansing and these are the cholesteatomas which we are dealing with. This is an oversimplified way of looking at it. You have a whole spectrum of combinations among them.

To Dr. Friedmann, I have never seen a perforation with a cholesteatoma behind it close. It might occur, but, I haven't seen it.

Dr. Abramson: I wanted to say a word about the

pearl formation. We've had this in several forms and in several discussions. I think it is a piece of squamous epithelium that is left in the ear or is implanted, as Dr. Brandow says, on a flat surface. I think the process that results is as follows. The loss of contact inhibition occurs, the epithelium will migrate beyond its mitotic rate and will thereby form a cystic structure. As it forms this cystic structure, it exceeds its blood supply and kills itself. The pearl we see is dead epithelium. It's not a progressive process. If it's left there it's not going to change. Now, on the other hand, if you have an inflammatory event, perhaps infection, it may change the inhibiting factors and allow for increased mitosis. If this is a place in a crevice, so that as it begins to form itself into a cyst it is able to obtain blood supply from two surfaces, it may in fact become a progressive process. I think that these pearls we often see when we go back in the middle ear, if we didn't do anything, nothing would happen.

Dr. Sadé: The comment that I would like to make is that I think Dr. Brandow's paper was of extreme importance because it really describes a phenomenon for which we don't have an explanation. I accept your observation at full value. I accept that you removed everything up to the bone with a microscope and in those places which were absolutely exposed as far as bone is concerned, you came later on and found pearls. This is very important and I don't think we now know how it happens. I have some doubts that it is seeding. I have some doubts, also, that what my friend, Dr. Abramson, just explained is the mechanism for that. According to the information I have, if you have epithelium, I absolutely accept that you remove the epithelium. If you would have left some epithelium, then it would have migrated. In order to have a cyst we probably have to have an epithelium below an epithelial surface. In your experiments, you were able to form actual cysts only when you buried them. When you didn't bury them you couldn't form them. I just want to emphasize that what you pointed out does happen, and needs clarification. It is absolutely true that many of

them die, but maybe not all of them die.

Dr. Abramson: I think that once it's white, it's dead. If it's pink, it might be alive. The experience that I've had was based on those times years ago as a resident when I would take middle ear material and I would look for collagenase. Whenever it was a pearl, there was no living cell on histology. That's very different from the sac or the cholesteatoma we're talking about.

Dr. Brandow: Well, I appreciate the comments and I certainly don't know. But, I will tell you that we did cut a histological section from one of these pearls which did show living cells and it did appear as though this was a new little cholesteatoma.

Dr. Harker: It's been my experience that some of the pearls that form will enlarge and continue to enlarge until they are marsupialized or removed. The second thing is that the mastoid cavity, of course, does in all probability fill with blood and if there is an epithelial remnant which is left implanted or whatever, it will be covered by something and then would quite easily be able to encyst itself.

Dr. Sadé: This is really how the whole conference started, discussions between Max, Lee and myself. It went on for an entire year like that.

As to the proof of dead or alive, I doubt that whether you find collagenase or do not, or rather if you do not find it, this is proof of death of a cyst. The histology is not proof at all of dead or alive. There are actually three proofs of a tissue being dead or alive. One of them is vital stains. Another is to measure oxygen consumption. It is very difficult, nobody did it on those pearls. The third is to do tissue culture which is not that easy. I only wanted to point out that it is not that easy to clinch.

Dr. Abramson: What you say only refers to the presence of cells, to determine whether a cell is dead or alive. If you have no cells then this question is not relevant. You have to have cells in order to have life.

Dr. Lim: One comment which I would like to make about the electron microscopic findings that Professor Bremond's group presented is an interesting one. In the cholesteatoma epidermis they saw in cases a large number of Langerhans' cells which we have reported. Also from Japan this was reported some years ago. They also found pigment cells, which occur in the skin elsewhere. This was a rather interesting finding but I didn't quite know what to make of it. If it is proven that it never occurs in the metaplastic epithelium, then this is absolutely crucial: it is our proof that this skin is migratory and not metaplastic.

Chapter 4

Microbiological Considerations

THE BACTERIOLOGY OF CHOLESTEATOMA

L. A. Harker, M.D.
Franklin P. Koontz, Ph.D.

The purpose of this study was to assess the total bacteriologic flora of a number of cholesteatomas cultured at surgery taking special precautions to look for anaerobic bacteria. It seemed likely that anaerobic organisms might be present not only because of the reduced aeration and cellular development of many of these ears, but also because anaerobes have recently been isolated in over half of the surgical specimens from chronic suppurative sinusitis, (Frederick and Braude). Furthermore, brain abscess, a sequelae to both suppurative ear and sinus disease is often caused by anaerobic organisms.

While the departmental staff was aware of the study, treatment decisions were uninfluenced by it; results of the cultures were not made available to the staff. Because of this, the usual and customary treatment prevailed. Half of the patients received preoperative antibiotics—in all but one (who received pre-op ampicillin) this consisted of two or three 250 mg oral dose of erythromycin the day preceding surgery. No patient received intraoperative antibiotics. One-third had received combination antibiotic otic drops in the days preceding the operation.

Specimens were collected from 32 cholesteatoma ears between June 1975 and February 1976. Attempts were made to culture all cholesteatomas surgically exposed at atticotomy or mastoidectomy whether "dry" or "infected". Reasons for not culturing a given cholesteatoma were failure of the collection team to get to the operating room before the surgeon had removed the cholesteatoma, or breakdown of the specialized anaerobic equipment, which occurred twice during the study period.

All cultures were taken from the surgical field and not from the external auditory canal to avoid external contamination. Only cholesteatoma matrix was cultured, usually in at least a 2 x 4 mm sheet, rather than a dry swab of the area. The preferred sites of culture were the antrum, followed by the attic, and then the middle ear. Specimens were collected as soon after surgical exposure of the disease as was feasible, usually within 15 minutes.

The thioglycollate broth culture medium had been boiled for 10 minutes no more than one hour before its use to ensure total reduction of the medium (anaerobiosis) by driving off the oxygen absorbed during media storage. The broth was then cooled, transported to the operating room where the cholesteatoma sample was immersed into it, and hand carried back to the laboratory for processing. These steps took from one-half to two hours at the maximum.

In the laboratory, the specimens were immediately placed in the total anaerobic environment available in the Anaerobic Chamber (glove box), a large flexible, heavy duty, polyethylene structure filled with anaerobic gases (85% nitrogen, 10% hydrogen, and 5% carbon dioxide). Culture media are stored and used in this chamber and everything in it is rendered totally anaerobic (including the pencils) making possible the identification of even the most fastidious anaerobes.

Handling the specimens in this fashion markedly decreases the possibility of isolating the obligate aerobes, organisms which must have oxygen to survive and flourish. Practically, this applies only to Bacillus anthracis; and there shouldn't be too many "anthraxed ears" around.

The aerobic and anaerobic bacterial isolates obtained by this method were purified and identified by standard procedures involving the use of accepted enzyme determinations, sugar reactions, amino acid utilization, and appearance on inhibitory media. In addition, a "primary guide" to the anaerobes was obtained by gas-liquid chromatographic separation of their volatile acid by-products. The actual differentiation (speciation) criteria were those devised or endorsed by the Center for Disease Control of the United States Public Health Service, (Lennette, et al, 1974 and Dowell and Hawkins, 1972).

This study only sought to identify what organisms were present, not the relative importance of each organism in relation to the other organisms or the clinical picture.

Results

Two patients were excluded from the study because the material cultured was not cholesteatoma matrix; thus, 30 patients were studied. Their age distribution is shown in Table 27. The peak incidence is in the second decade of life, which is representative of the clinical material at this institution. In four of the patients, no organisms were cultured (Table 28). However, in 17, or 57%, more than one organism was identified. If we look at these multiple isolates (Table 29), it is evident that frequently very many different organisms are present in the same cholesteatoma matrix.

TABLE 27

Age Distribution

Age in Years	No. of Patients
0-10	7
11-20	11
21-30	3
31-40	2
41-50	0
51-60	4
61-70	2
71-80	1
	N = 30

TABLE 28

Number of Organisms per Patient

Organisms	No. of Patients	Percent
None	4	13
One	9	30
Multiple	17	57

TABLE 29

Multiple Isolates

No. of Organisms	No. of Patients
2	4
3	4
4	1
5	5
7	1
8	1
10	1
11	1

The average number of organisms identified was slightly over three and there were nine ears where five or more different bacterial species were identified.

In two-thirds of the patients, anaerobic organisms were present (Table 30). In 70%, aerobic organisms were present, and in half of the ears, both anaerobes and aerobes were identified.

TABLE 30

Culture Results

	Number	Percent
No Growth	4	13
Anaerobes Present	20	67
Aerobes Present	21	70
Both Present	15	50

The aerobic organisms which were seen are shown in Table 31. Pseudomonas aeruginosa was the most frequent aerobic organism identified and pseudomosa fluorescens was also seen. The rest of the aerobes represent a very mixed flora of enteric organisms, and numerous others.

TABLE 32

Anaerobes

Bacteroides	13
Peptococcus-Peptostreptococcus	11
Propionibacterium Acnes	8
Fusobacterium	4
Bifidobacterium	3
Clostridium	3
Eubacterium	2

TABLE 31

Aerobes

Pseudomonas Aeruginosa	11
Pseudomonas Fluorescens	2
Proteus Species	4
Escherichia Coli	4
Klebsiella-Enterobacter-Serratia	4
Streptococcus	
β Hemolytic	2
α or μ Hemolytic	5
Faecalis	1
Alcaligenes-Achromobacter	3
Staphylococcus Aureus	1
Staphylococcus Epidermidis	2
CDC Group F	2

When only aerobic organisms were identified, most frequently only a single organism was present (Table 33), and most commonly, a pseudomonas. As previously mentioned, when anaerobes alone were isolated, they were commonly a pure culture of propionibacterium acnes (Table 34).

TABLE 33

Aerobes Only

No. of Patients	
1	Staph Aureus
3	Pseudomonas
1	Pseudomonas + Achromobacter
1	β Hemolytic Strep + Serratia + Klebisiella

TABLE 34

Anaerobes Only

No. of Patients	
4	Propionobacterium Acnes
1	Peptostreptococcus + Bacteroides Melanogenicus

The anaerobic organisms identified are shown in Table 32. Bacteroides was most frequently encountered with varieties of the anaerobic staphylococcus or streptococcus next most frequent. It was characteristic of the latter group of organisms to have several (up to nine or ten) morphologically different colony types of the same organism. When this was present, it was counted only as one organism for the data. The propionibacterium acnes group is interesting because, frequently, these were a single isolate with no other organism present and they were frequently seen in older patients. By and large, the anaerobic organisms identified mirror the aerobic ones, in the fact that most of the organisms identified are known aggressive pathogens.

When a foul smell to the drainage was noted preoperatively, in all but one case, multiple organisms were identified (Table 35), the exception, only the pseudomonas aeruginosa was isolated. In all of the other cases, there were anaerobes as well as aerobes present. From what is known of anaerobic infections elsewhere in the body, it is likely that anaerobic organisms were also present but not identified in the patient who had the pure culture of pseudomonas with foul drainage. Pure cultures of pseudomonas in the laboratory do not have a foul smell and anaerobic infections characteristically do. The other six patients with foul drainage illustrate this well.

Conclusions

(1) Aerobic and anaerobic cultures of the cholesteatoma matrix will identify the bacterial population present in the ear at that time.

(2) The majority of these ears harbor a number of bacteria within the cholesteatoma matrix.

(3) Half of these bacteria are anaerobic and the other half aerobic organisms.

(4) A foul odor in ear drainage from cholesteatoma usually indicates that many organisms, both aerobic and anaerobic, are present.

(5) When a patient has a suspected septic complication of cholesteatoma, as sigmoid sinus thrombophlebitis, or epidural or brain abscess, the anaerobic and aerobic organisms present in the ear should be identified.

TABLE 35

Foul Smell Pre-op

No. of Organisms	No. of Patients
1	1
5	3
7	1
10	1
11	1

References

1. Dowell, V. R. and Hawkins, T. M.: *Laboratory Methods in Anaerobic Bacteriology—CDC Laboratory Manual.* Center for Disease Control, Atlanta, Georgia, 1972.
2. Frederick, J. and Braude, A. I.: Anaerobic infections of the paranasal sinuses. *New England Journal of Medicine,* 290:135.
3. Lennette, E. H.; Spaulding, E. H.; and Truant, J. P.: *Manual of Clinical Microbiology.* (Ed. 2). American Society for Microbiology, Washington, D. C., 1974.

MICROBIOLOGICAL IMPLICATIONS OF KERATINIZATION

Bryan Larsen, Ph.D.

It has been well stated by others at this conference that the essence of cholesteatoma might be partly understood by studying other tissues, and this is also true for its bacteriology.

My own research has involved the bacteriology of the rat vaginal tract. As seen in Figure 126, the total number of bacteria in the vaginal tract changes significantly and cyclically with the estrous cycle and the greater number of bacteria are present during the estrogen dominated phase.

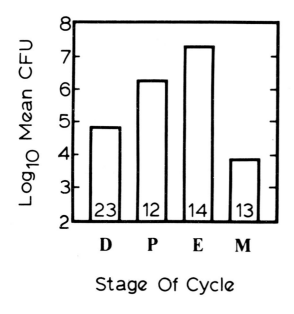

Fig. 126: The bacterial content of the rat vaginal tract is related to the stage of the estrous cycle. The histogram shows bacterial counts expressed as colony forming units per rat (CFU). Stage of the cycle is indicated by the boldface letters; (p) proestrus; (e) estrous; (m) metestrus; (d) diestrus. The number of observations is enclosed in each bar.

At the ultrastructural level in the non-estrogen stimulated rat, virtually no bacteria are found in the vaginal epithelium. This is illustrated in the scanning electron micrograph (Fig. 127). This is in contrast to the scanning electron micrograph (Fig. 128) which shows the change that occurs in tissue architecture and in bacterial colonization in the estrogen stimulated rat. Notably, after estrogen treatment, cells are thin and sheet-like and bacteria associated with the tissue are numerous.

In thin sections of vaginal tissue from non-estrogen treated rats, an epithelium free of bacteria and possessing a microvillous-like border is seen. This is illustrated in Figure 129. If a sprayed animal is treated with estrogen, changes are seen in the vaginal epithelium which are consistent with keratinization. Cells become flattened, layered and filled with electron-dense granulofilamentous material as illustrated by Figure 130. Although bacteria are associated with this surface, they are more abundantly associated with cells which have become detached and exfoliated into the vaginal folds. Squamous cells which have detached from the epithelial substratum and have collected in the vaginal folds are represented by the material seen in Figure 131. In addition to the striking abundance of bacterial forms, note also that the exfoliated cells appear more electron lucent than the underlying tissue suggesting the loss of some or all of the intracellular keratin. It may be possible that release of the keratin or some derivative of the keratin into the environment promotes bacterial growth, an hypothesis which is still under study. Regardless of the mechanism, the similarity between this tissue and the cholesteatoma keratin, seen in Figure 132, is obvious.

Bacteriologists have examined a variety of keratinizing epithelia from human and animal

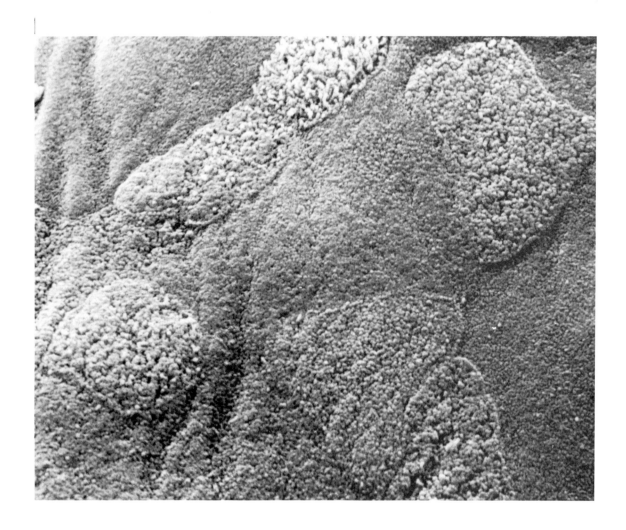

Fig. 127: Scanning electron micrograph of rat vaginal epithelium during diestrus; note the absence of bacteria and the microvillous appearance of cellular surface.

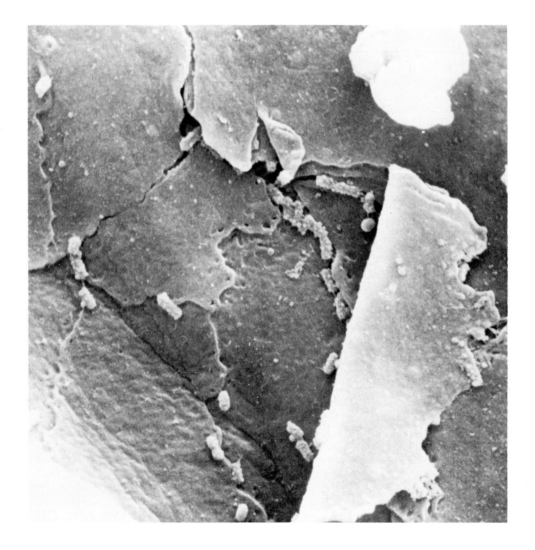

Fig. 128: Scanning electron micrograph of estrogen stimulated rat vaginal epithelium. Bacteria are abundant and cellular surface is obviously cornified.

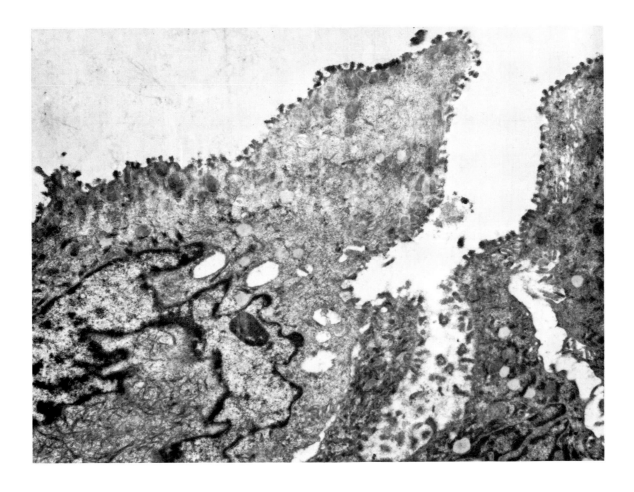

Fig. 129: Electron micrograph of thin sectioned tissue from estrogen non-stimulated rat vagina. Note the appearance of the cellular surface which is consistent with the microvillous surface seen in Figure 127.

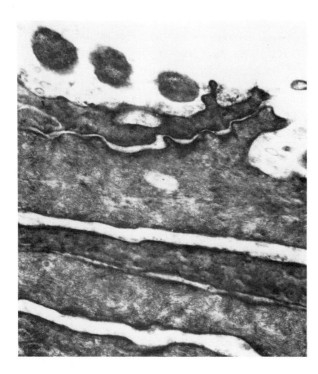

Fig. 130: Electron micrograph showing the appearance of estrogen stimulated epithelium. Bacteria are present and the epithelial cells are flattened and lack intracellular organization characteristic of living cells. The intracellular space is composed of electron dense granulofilamentous material keratin.

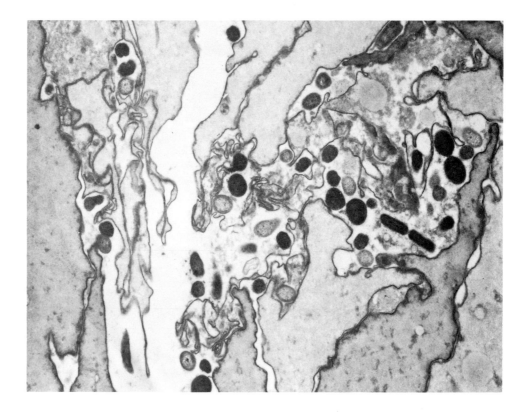

Fig. 131: Electron micrograph of exofiliated keratinized cells. The abundance of bacteria is notable.

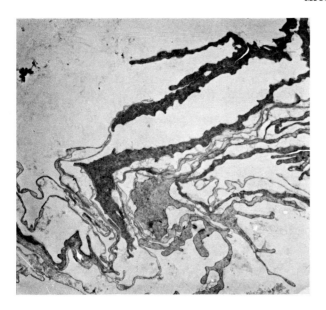

Fig. 132: Cholesteatoma keratin. Note the similarity between this tissue and that in Figure 131.

sources including skin, buccal mucosa, esophagus of certain animals and the stomach of rodents and the vagina as just presented. It appears likely that keratinized epithelia exposed to the environment may normally become colonized. Could it be that the bacteria associated with the cholesteatoma reflect this more generalized phenomenon of bacterial colonization of keratinized epithelia?

As long as cholesteatoma is with us it seems a worthwhile venture to ask if cholesteatoma is a possibly normal microbial habitant and examine both the ultrastructural relationship between bacterial and host structures and physico-chemical interactions between host and microbial community. Such information may provide new insights into one of the complications of cholesteatoma encountered in clinical practice.

QUESTIONS AND ANSWERS

Dr. Palva: If I may start the discussion, I would like to ask how many of those ears were dry ears.

Dr. Harker: Some were clinically dry at the time and it was very surprising to have one of the dry ears with multiple organisms, one had eight or nine. The note at surgery was that there was no free pus in the antrum and that it was a dry cholesteatoma at that point. I should add that this study sought only to identify the organisms which were present. It did not seek to determine which are most prominent where there was a heavy growth vs. a light growth. The clinical significance of the organisms individually we did not determine.

Dr. Bellucci: We emphasize the type of organism as important in determining whether there is activity from the eustachian tube. The saprophytes are usually associated with the cholesteatoma. They can be present and are not as virulent as those that arrive from the eustachian tube, such as strep, staph, etc. I think this is a good indication of eustachian tube contamination and I think that cultures in ears that cannot be controlled medically are important before doing tympanoplasty surgery.

Dr. Mangat: I have two questions. First, do you have any indications how these might compare with the preoperative cultures? Second, how difficult would it be to get preoperative anaerobic cultures, say if you just used pre-reduced thyoglycolate broth without the anaerobic chambers?

Dr. Harker: We did not compare preoperative cultures with the intraoperative. That would have been desirable. We talked about it, but the laboratory facilities and the fact that we would be comparing a swab of discharge vs. a piece of tissue led us to not do that. It should be entirely possible to have well reduced media with thyoglycolate there and to take either granulation tissue or cholesteatoma debris present and available in the external canal, or even discharge, and identify an anaerobic organism. In general the number of anaerobic organisms found in the body mirrors how hard people are looking for them.

Section III

Clinical Aspects

Chapter 5

Epidermiology

CHOLESTEATOMA: EPIDEMIOLOGICAL AND QUANTITATIVE ASPECTS

Ronald Hinchcliffe, M.D.

When one considers how prevalent cholesteatoma is and that its existence has now been recognized for nearly a century and a half, it is surprising that so little information is available on its epidemiology. Indeed, epidemiological studies have been conspicuous by their absence. Thus, what I have to say here is not so much to review the previous studies on the subject, but to make a plea for future work.

For convenience, I shall divide the paper into six parts, i.e. First, a consideration of ethnogeographic factors, secondly, of socio-economic factors, thirdly, of climatological factors, fourthly, of longitudinal studies, fifthly, of the influence of antibiotics, and, finally, of what conclusions might be drawn, including pointers to future endeavor.

Ethnic and Geographic Factors

In a consideration of the operation of broad ethnic factors, we have the experience of otologists whose work covers, or has covered, patients from more than one ethnic group. Although much of this evidence is on an anecdotal level, it should be considered when viewing the picture as a whole.

During a recent study visit to Japan, I discussed the problem with otologists who had worked in North America and Europe. Dr. Taguchi of Shinshu University, considers cholesteatoma to be much more common in Canada than in Japan. Another otologist has found cholesteatoma to be more common in Germany than in Japan. However, the general observation is that chronic suppurative otitis media is much more extensive in Japan than in Germany. The observations of Prasansuk and Sekorarith in Thailand are that cholesteatoma is a very common occurrence in their patients, especially in young children. Martin, who has worked in Uganda for many years, has observed that cholesteatoma is much less frequent in the indigenous people there than it is in British patients either there or in the United Kingdom.

In the North American continent, both Johnson (1967) and Jaffe (1969) have studied ear disease in the Navajo Indian. In Johnson's series of Navajo school children, 6.4% had chronic otitis media, and in Jaffe's series of Navajo school children, 4.8% had chronic otitis media, associated almost exclusively with a central perforation. Cholesteatoma was infrequent, but when present, it was associated with total perforation of the pars tensa.

Jaffe reported that no cholesteatoma was seen in over 200 tympanoplasties for central perforations in the Navajos, even though careful examination of the middle ear was performed routinely.

Among urban Alaskan Eskimo school children, Beal (1972) found that 19% suffered from active chronic suppurative otitis media and, of these, 13% had cholesteatoma. However, in a study of 3,770 Baffin Zone Eskimos of all ages, Baxter and Ling (1974) found that only 99 cases suffered from chronic suppurative otitis media. Only two of these cases showed cholesteatoma.

As he organized an otological health service for the people of North Newfoundland and Labrador, Ratnesar (1976) was able to study ear disease in three ethnic groups (Eskimos, Algonkian Indians, and Caucasians) living under the same broad environmental conditions. Ratnesar observed no case of cholesteatoma among the 17 Eskimos with chronic suppurative otitis media, two cases among the 15 Algonkian Indians with chronic suppurative otitis media, and 23 cases among the 50

Caucasians with chronic suppurative otitis media.

The American Indian, Eskimo and Japanese are all members of the xanthodermi so that it would appear that this racial group is less likely to develop cholesteatoma than the leucodermi. However, in view of observations made on the Thais and the Alaskan Eskimos, the Southern Mongoloids and the Eskimos of the Pacific littoral may be exceptions to this statement. Similarly, the melandodermi may also be less likely to develop cholesteatoma than the leucodermi. As Cody (1976) and Coman and McCafferty (1976) indicate, this apparent relative racially-based immunity to cholesteatoma may be secondary to the "protective" effect of central perforations.

In a narrower ethnic context, Sadé and his colleagues (1974) have analyzed the prevalence of cholesteatoma in relation to the ethnic group of patients attending a hospital in Israel. The ethnic distribution of bilateral cholesteatomatous perforations was significantly different from that of other types of aural pathology. To what extent this difference is due to geogens and not genes has yet to be determined.

Socio-Economic Factors

There is no direct evidence as regards the influence of socio-economic factors on the prevalence or development of cholesteatoma. However, since this lesion is intimately connected with chronic otitis media, socio-economic influences on the latter condition may well be reflected in the epidemiological parameters of cholesteatoma.

Socio-economic factors have been incriminated in the pathogenesis of chronic otitis media (Tumarkin, 1959 and Jain 1966). Cambon and his colleagues (1965) surveyed middle ear disease in the American Indians of the Mount Currie Reservation (100 miles north of Vancouver, British Columbia). The prevalence of middle ear disease was six times greater in the Indians given a socio-economic rating of "bad" than it was in those given a rating of "good". Pal, et al (1974) pre-

sented the results of an otological survey of an urban community in Lucknow. The screening took the form of a direct examination of 4,528 persons of 835 families living in the area served by an urban Health Centre. Information was also obtained on the socio-economic status of the subjects examined. Inter alia, the prevalence of chronic otitis media was found to be related to family income. A power function describes the curve of best fit for the data presented by Pal, et al, i.e.

$$P = 63.2 \, I^{-0.376}$$

P = prevalence of chronic otitis media per 1,000 population

and I = per capita family income in Rs per month.

On the basis of this equation, Table 36 shows the predicted number of cases and the actual number of cases of chronic otitis media noted in this survey.

TABLE 36

Lucknow Survey
(Pal, et al, 1974)
Chronic Otitis Media

Social	Cases in Samples	
Class	Actual	Predicted
I	5	
II	9	9
III	17	18
IV	23	20
V	32	34

In a previous paper on epidemiology of otitis media, and viewing the prevalence in global terms, the author indicated that the prevalence of chronic otitis media in children is also an inverse power function of the per capita GMP of the country concerned (Hinchcliffe, 1972).

If chronic otitis media is a poverty related disease, can its prevalence be reduced by elevating the socio-economic level of the involved population? Beal (1972) reports that, following the discovery of oil near one Alaskan village, there was "a much improved standard of living and chronic otitis media all but disappeared". But, would this effect be applicable to cholesteatoma?

Related to socio-economic status is the person's pattern of life in the broadest sense. Baxter and Ling's studies of the Eskimos in Baffin Zone, showed that, after the age of ten, the prevalence of chronic suppurative otitis media declined with age, being non-existent in Eskimos older than about 30 years. This trend is also evident in Ratnesar's data. Baxter and Ling hypothesized that acute and secretory otitis media may not so readily have progressed to a chronic form 25-30 years ago. At that time the whole mode of Eskimo life was completely different. They were fewer in number, lived an isolated, nomadic life, and subsisted on a high protein diet. In contrast, the modern Eskimo lives in an over-crowded, over-heated prefabricated house in settlements which are not isolated and where sanitation is not always ideal. In the majority of settlements, dietary patterns are also inferior. This supports the hypothesis that contact with civilization is associated with a high prevalence of chronic otitis media. An alternative hypothesis is that the lower prevalence of otitis media in the older age groups is simply due to a spontaneous healing of perforations with the passage of time.

It is of note that the prevalence of chronic suppurative otitis media varied appreciably (up to a factor of ten) from one Eskimo settlement to another. In Igloolik (northeast of the Melville Peninsula) the prevalence of chronic suppurative otitis media was six per 1,000 of population; in Frobisher Bay (in southeast Baffin Island) the prevalence was 64 per 1,000 population. Hildes and Schaefer (1973) have interpreted changes in the health of Eskimos with increase of urbanisation and Schaefer (1971) has specifically referred to the detrimental effect of bottle feeding in respect of the incidence of otitis media in children.

Climatological Factors

Schuknecht (1974) points out that, if the epithelialized pocket of cholesteatoma is dry, the rate of exfoliation is slow and the keratin mass may accumulate slowly for years without creating complications; however, in the presence of infection, the cholesteatoma may develop rapidly. It is conceivable that, although this may not contribute to the pathogenesis of either cholesteatoma or otitis media, climatic, or microclimatic conditions might predispose to the frequency and severity of superadded infection, thus accelerating the growth of the lesion and enhancing the severity of the disease process.

Longitudinal Studies

Sadé (1976) suggested that the prevalence of cholesteatoma has increased since the time of Bezold, which increase may have been associated with an increase in the prevalence of secretory otitis media.

Baxter and Ling's studies on the Baffin Zone Eskimos indicate that many ears heal spontaneously. Examination of the Cape Dorset (south Baffin Island) Eskimos in 1972, showed that one-third of the patients whom Ling and his colleagues found to have discharging ears in 1968, subsequently developed imperforate (but scarred) tympanic membranes and hearing within normal limits. While this may apply to chronic middle ear infection in the absence of cholesteatoma, it almost certainly does apply to ears with cholesteatoma. Spontaneous healing of central perforations might explain the rising cholesteatoma/otitis media that Tschopp (1976) reports.

In ears operated on for cholesteatoma, the question is not whether cholesteatoma occurs, but in what percentage of operated ears it occurs, and at what rate. Gristwood and Venables (1976) have collected and analyzed detailed information relating to both the recurrence rate and the growth rate of cholesteatoma, which recurred in a group of 141 ears that had been treated surgically for chronic otitis media in association with cholesteatoma. This study should provide a model for future work on this problem. The minimal cumulative percentage of detected recurrences (Fig. 133) increased in proportion to the logarithm of time, i.e.

$$P = 16 \log_{10}t - 14.7$$

where P = minimal cumulative % age of detected cholesteatoma recurrences

and t = time in months after operation.

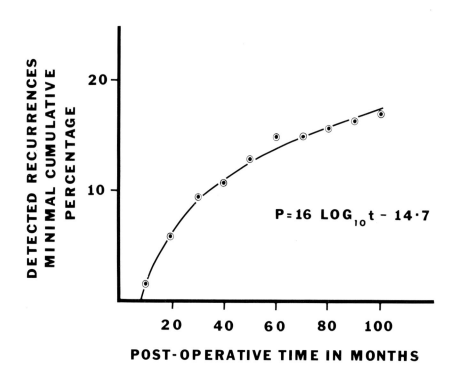

Fig. 133: Minimal cumulative percentage of detected recurrences of cholesteatoma as a function of time in months following operation. (After Gristwood and Venables, 1976.)

These values are minimal in the sense that they do not take into account (a) that an increasingly smaller proportion of cases were of a greater postoperative age (Fig. 134) and also (b) that, with increasing lapse of time following operation, the chance of retrieval for follow-up diminishes. The data showed that case retrieval fell off exponentially with time according to the equation:

$$N = 97e^{-0.0534t}$$

where N = % age of cases retrieved for follow-up at time

and t = time lapse in years after surgery

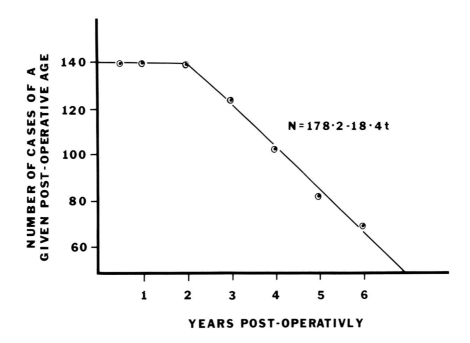

$$N = 178 \cdot 2 - 18 \cdot 4\,t$$

Fig. 134: Composition (re-postoperative age) of cases in whom the recurrence rate of cholesteatoma was studied. (After Gristwood and Venables, 1976.)

As indicated in Table 37, this equation is a satisfactory predictor of actual cases retrieved. Decreasing case retrieval as a function of lapsed time bedevils many prospective hospital-based epidemiological studies. It will be of interest to know to what extent other series of cases show the same, or similar, change. Can one assume that the characteristics, especially, in this case, of disease recurrence, are similar in the unretrieved group and '" retrieved group? Or are cases retrieved for . .ow-up simply because there has been a recurrence of the disease? If the unretrieved cases are similar to the retrieved cases, then correcting the "minimal" recurrence data for this bias, together with that for the smaller number of postoperatively older cases, might be held to indi-

TABLE 37

Case Retrieval as Function of Time

Time After Surgery	Sample Size	Cases Retrieved	
		Actual	Predicted
0.5	141	133	133
1	141	129	130
2	141	119	123
3	125	103	103
4	104	80	81
5	83	65	62
6	70	49	49

cate that recurrences will occur in all patients with the passage of a sufficient length of time (Fig. 135). Incidentally, values predicted from this figure are not excessive; they are not unrepresentative of other data quoted at this conference.

Gristwood's and Venables' data is also unique in providing information on the actual growth rates of cholesteatoma. When follow-up detected the recurrence of an epidermoid cyst, the cyst diameter was measured and the post-operative lapsed time noted. The data for the epitympanic recess, mastoid and mesotympanum were reported separately. Although these authors fitted exponential equations to their data, a Gompertz function might be considered to be a more appropriate fit. A Gompertz function is defined by the equation:

$$Y = Vg^{h^X}$$

where both g and h are constants and V is a limiting value of Y. Thus, a Gompertz function can accomodate the limits of growth which are observed in cholesteatoma. Figures 136, 137, and 138 show Gristwood's and Venables' epitympanic recess, mastoid and mesotympanic data fitted to Gom-

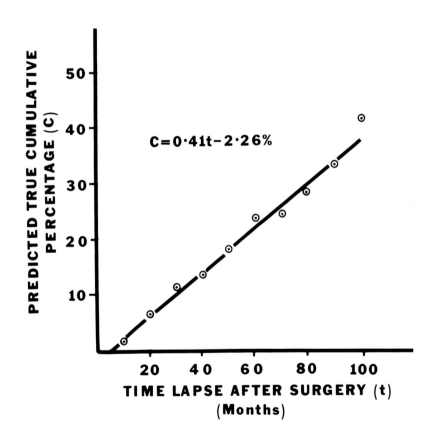

Fig. 135: Predicted cumulative percentage of detected recurrences of cholesteatoma as a function of time in months following operation.

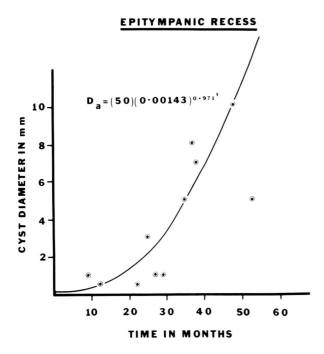

Fig. 136: Growth of recurring epitympanic recess cholesteatomata. Data with the Gompertz function. (After Gristwood and Venables, 1976.)

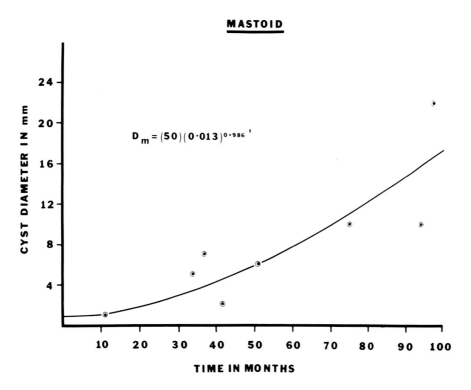

Fig. 137: Growth of recurring mastoid cholesteatomata. Data fitted with a Gompertz function. (After Gristwood and Venables, 1976.)

MESOTYMPANUM

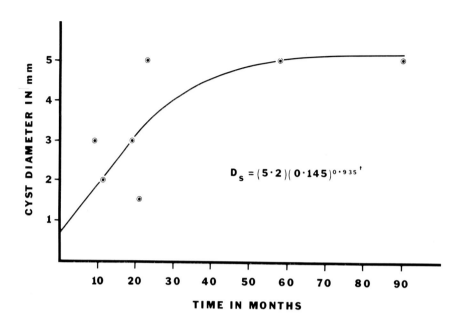

$$D_s = (5\cdot2)(0\cdot145)^{0\cdot935^t}$$

Fig. 138: Growth of recurring mesotympanic cholesteatomata. Data fitted with a Gompertz function. (After Gristwood and Venables, 1976.)

pertz functions, such that:

$$D_a = (50)(0.00143)^{0.971^t}$$
$$D_m = (50)(0.013)^{0.986^t}$$
$$\text{and } D_s = (5.2)(0.145)^{0.935^t}$$

where D_a = diameter of epitympanic recess cyst in mm

D_m = diameter of mastoid cyst in mm

D_s = diameter of mesotympanic cyst in mm

and t = postoperative elapsed time in months

Influence of Antibiotics

I could find no dependable data on this point. However, Rambo's (1972) experience is perhaps representative of that of others in this respect: "In a series of 50 cases of suppurative chronic mastoiditis in children referred to me for surgery, I found cholesteatoma in 73%. . . . . Practically all these children were treated extensively with antibiotics, and it was a frequent comment by their parents that they could not understand what had happened, that they had always taken the child to the doctor and had done everything they were told". The indications then are that the course of cholesteatoma is unaltered by antibiotics.

During the eight years that data has been available on the frequency of cholesteatoma at the Royal National Throat, Nose and Ear Hospital, London, there has been no discernable trend. The proportion of chronic suppurative otitis media cases with this lesion has remained at a 6% level over that period of time.

Conclusions and Proposals for Future Work

Clearly, the epidemiology of cholesteatoma is not synonymous with that of chronic otitis media. Different factors may be involved in each case, not only in respect of determining the causation, but also the course of the condition. Nevertheless, because of the intimate association of cholesteatoma with middle ear infection and ventilation, future epidemiological studies must provide a broad otoscopic picture. The minimal otoscopic data should be as set out in the schema put forward by Naunton's (1972) working group at the National Conference on Otitis Media in 1970. Measures should be made available on known or suspected etiological factors such as: geographic location and climatic profile, ethnic group, socioeconomic status, family and medical history and duration of breast feeding (for children), together with indices of structural integrity or of function: radiological (for degree of pneumatization and evidence for bone destruction), audiometric and tympanometric (in respect of the imperforate tympanic membranes) examinations. Correlation matrices should be obtained for the data and multivariate analyses should be conducted to extract the principal factors influencing the conditions.

As well as point prevalence studies, prospective longitudinal studies should be conducted to determine not only the natural course of cholesteatoma but also, from studies in children, which ears are likely to develop this lesion. Severeid's (1976) study provides an example of how some of these studies should be conducted.

Perhaps the first overriding requirement is to determine the intra- and inter-observer variation in respect of reporting cholesteatoma and, associated with this, the criteria that are adopted for such judgements. It is, of course, particularly important that the epidemiological studies which are to be conducted should be controlled for observer variation in judging cholesteatoma.

If these basic suggestions are borne in mind, we should hope to see an epidemiological contribution to the knowledge and causation and pathogenesis of cholesteatoma in the foreseeable future.

References

1. Baxter, J. D. and Ling, D.: Ear disease and hearing loss among the Eskimo population of the Baffin zone. *Canad. J. Otolaryngol.*, 3: 110, 1974.
2. Beal, D. D.: Prevention of Otitis Media in the Alaskan Native. In Glorig, A. and Gerwin, K. S.: (Ed.). *Otitis Media: Proceedings of the National Conference, Callier Hearing and Speech Center, Dallas.* Charles C Thomas, Springfield, Illinois, 1972, p. 158.
3. Cambon, K.; Galbraith, J. D.; and Kong, G.: Middle-ear disease in Indians of the Mount Currie Reservation, British Columbia. *Canad. Med. Assoc. J.*, 93: 1301, 1965.
4. Cody, D. T.: The definition of cholesteatoma. In McCabe, B. F.: (Ed.). *First International Conference on Cholesteatoma*, May 26-30, Aesculapius Publishing Company, Birmingham, Alabama, 1977.
5. Coman, W. B. and McCafferty, G. J.: Cholesteatoma in Australian Aboriginal children. In McCabe, B. F.: (Ed.). *First International Conference on Cholesteatoma*, May 26-30. Aesculapius Publishing Company, Birmingham, Alabama, 1977.
6. Gristwood, R. E. and Venables, W.: Growth rate and recurrence of residual epidermoid cholesteatoma. *Clinical Otolaryngol.*, 1:164, 1976.
7. Hildes, J. A. and Schaefer, O.: Health of Igloolik Eskimos and changes with urbanization. *J. Human Evolution*, 2: 241, 1973.
8. Hinchcliffe, R.: Epidemiological aspects of otitis media. In Glorig, A. and Gerwin, K. S.: (Eds.). *Otitis Media: Proceedings of the National Conference. Callier Hearing and Speech Center, Dallas.* Charles C Thomas, Springfield, Illinois, 1972, p. 36.
9. Jaffe, B. F.: The incidence of ear diseases in the

Navaho Indians. *Laryngoscope,* 79: 2126, 1969.

10. Jain, S. N.: Studies in Kakinada. In *Proceedings of II All-India Workshop on Speech and Hearing Problems in India.* Deafness Research Project, Christian Medical College, Vellore, India, 1967, p. 59.

11. Johnson, R. L.: Chronic otitis media in school age Navajo Indians. *Laryngoscope,* 77: 1990, 1967.

12. Ling, D.; McCoy, R. H.; and Levinson, E. D.: The incidence of middle ear disease and its educational complications among Baffin Island Eskimo children. *Canad. J. Public Health,* 60: 385, 1969.

13. Martin, J. A. M.: Personal communication, 1976.

14. Naunton, R. F.: Epidemiology. In Glorig, A. and Gerwin, K. S.: (Eds.). *Otitis Media: Proceeding of the National Conference. Callier Hearing and Speech Center, Dallas.* Charles C Thomas, Springfield, Illinois, 1972, p. 275.

15. Pal, J.; Bhatia, M. L.; Prasad, B. G. et al: Deafness among the urgan community—an epidemiological survey at Lucknow (U.P.). *Indian J. Med. Res.,* 62(6): 857, 1974.

16. Prasansuk, S. and Sekorarith, C.: Unpublished data.

17. Rambo, J. H. T.: Surgical Treatment of Chronic Otitis. In Glorig, A. and Gerwin, K. S.: (Eds.) *Otitis Media: Proceeding of the National Conference. Callier Hearing and Speech Center, Dallas.* Charles C Thomas, Springfield, Illinois, 1972, p. 207.

18. Ratnesar, P.: Chronic ear disease along the coasts of Labrador and northern Newfoundland. *The J. Otolaryngol.,* 5(2): 121, 1976.

19. Sadé, J.; Konak, S.; and Hinchcliffe, R.: Ethnic factors in the pathogenesis of chronic otitis media in Israel. A preliminary investigation. *J. Laryngol. Otol.,* 85: 349, 1971.

20. Sadé, J.: Pathogenesis of Attic cholesteatoma—The metaplastic theory. In McCabe, B. F.: (Ed.). *First International Conference on Cholesteatoma.* May 26-30. Aesculapius Publishing Company, Birmingham, Alabama, 1977.

21. Schaefer, O.: Otitis media and bottle-feeding. An epidemiological study of infant feeding habits and incidence of recurrent and chronic middle ear disease in Canadian Eskimos. *Canad. J. Public Health,* 62: 478, 1971.

22. Schuknecht, H. F.: *The Pathology of the Ear.* Harvard University Press, Boston, Massachusetts, 1974.

23. Severeid, L. C.: Development of cholesteatoma in children with cleft palate: A longitudinal study. In McCabe, B. F.: (Ed.). *First International Conference on Cholesteatoma.* May 26-30. Aesculapius Publishing Company, Birmingham, Alabama, 1977.

24. Taguchi, T.: Personal communication, 1976.

25. Tschopp, C. F.: Chronic otitis media and cholesteatoma in Alaskan native children. In McCabe, B. F.: (Ed.). *First International Conference on Cholesteatoma.* May 26-30. Aesculapius Publishing Company, Birmingham, Alabama, 1977.

26. Tumarkin, A.: On the nature and significance of hypocellularity of the mastoid. *J. Laryngol.,* 73: 34, 1959.

DEVELOPMENT OF CHOLESTEATOMA IN CHILDREN WITH CLEFT PALATE: A LONGITUDINAL STUDY

Larry R. Severeid, M.D.

The establishment of cleft palate clinics has afforded a unique opportunity to follow patients with predictable ear disease from birth to adulthood. It is well appreciated that the incidence of ear disease and eustachian tube dysfunction are high in the cleft palate population.

The medical records of 191 patients with cleft palate were reviewed. All of these patients have been enrolled in the University of Iowa Cleft Palate Clinic since infancy and have been followed at regular intervals, usually every six months or more often. One hundred and sixty of these patients had eustachian tube dysfunction with impairment of middle ear ventilation. The age range of these patients is shown in Table 38. The mean age of this group is 16 years.

Findings

Thirty-one of the cleft palate patients never demonstrated eustachian tube dysfunction, either by clinical examination or audiometric studies. These 31 patients (16% of the series) are free of middle ear disease.

The remaining 160 cleft palate patients all had at some time eustachian tube dysfunction. However, the eustachian tube dysfunction decreased with advancing age. I had reviewed this same patient population five years ago. Table 39 shows the percent of patients in each age group who had not yet established normal tubal function. This is important to appreciate, that in the cleft palate population, tubal dysfunction is self-limiting; however, it is protracted. The otologist's goal

TABLE 38

Age Distribution of Patients and Number in Each Group

Age in Years	Number of Patients
10-13	88
14-16	24
17-22	34
23-27	10
28-32	4

TABLE 39

Percent of Subjects with Eustachian Tube Dysfunction Classified According to Age Groups

Age in Years	Percent with Tubal Dysfunction
5-8	66%
9-12	29%
13-17	17%
18-22	10%
23-27	0%

is to properly manage these patients until that critical time of established tubal function occurs.

Incidence of Cholesteatoma

At the time of this study 7.1% of the 160 patients who had data, there have been 15 operative procedures for cholesteatoma.

All of these patients had long standing eustachian tube dysfunction, manifest by secretory or serous otitis media and conductive hearing loss. All of these patients had had multiple ventilating tube insertions in an attempt to maintain middle ear ventilation. One patient had had ventilating tubes inserted on 12 different occasions. Temporary middle ear ventilation was the rule because of extrusion of the tubes. No patient was noted to develop a cholesteatoma while the ventilating tubes were in place, nor can any cholesteatoma formation be attributed to myringotomies. Retraction pockets were not noted in the myringotomy sites, which were in the antero-inferior quadrants of the tympanic membranes.

Origin of the Cholesteatomas

All of the cholesteatomas, with the exception of one, were noted to originate from progression of tympanic membrane retraction pockets. All patients were noted to have retraction pockets on previous visits, however, in many cases, either the degree of retraction was not appreciated, or there

was significant progression of the disease. Table 40 shows the location of the retraction pockets. Four cholesteatomas developed from retraction pockets of the pars flaccida. Eleven originated from retraction pockets of the pars tensa in the posterosuperior quadrant and one was a residual cholesteatoma cyst discovered at the time of a staged ossicular reconstruction following an atticotomy procedure.

There was no clinical difference in the histories between those patients who developed in "primary acquired" (pars tensa) and the "secondary acquired" (pars flaccida) cholesteatoma. The only difference was in the location of the retraction pocket in the tympanic membrane.

TABLE 41

Types of Surgical Procedures Performed and the Number of Cases of Each

Procedure	No. of Cases
Radical Mastoidectomy	4
Modified Radical Mastoidectomy	2
Canal Up Mastoidectomy	2
Endaural Atticotomy	5
Tympanotomy	2

TABLE 40

Location of the Cholesteatoma Source and the Number of Cases

Location	No. of Cases
Primary Acquired (Pars Flaccida)	4
Secondary Acquired (Pars Tensa)	11
Cholesteatoma Cyst (Residual)	1

One patient had two distinct cholesteatoma sacs, one from the pars tensa and one from the pars flaccida.

Surgical Procedures

The surgical approach employed usually depended on the clinical extent of the disease. The type of surgical procedures and the number of cases are shown on Table 41.

The relatively large number of endaural atticotomy and canal-up procedures performed can be attributed to early detection as well as changes in concepts of management of cholesteatoma. In spite of the fact that surgical intervention was done early in the course of the cholesteatoma progression, five of these seven patients already had ossicular erosion with discontinuity at the time of surgery.

Radical mastoidectomies were performed in four patients. Three patients were noted to have cholesteatoma in the middle ear cleft which could not be, to the surgeon's satisfaction, adequately removed, i.e., skin in round window niche, sinus tympani or auditory tube orifice. All three of these cholesteatomas originated from pars tensa retraction pockets. The fourth was a pars flaccida cholesteatoma with minimal middle ear involvement but there was extensive tympanosclerosis of the middle ear lining and ossicles.

Age at the Time of Surgery

All of the patients had surgery before or during their teens. The age distribution at the time of surgery is shown on Table 42. It appears that critical time for the development of the cholesteatoma occurs during the period of prolonged tubal dysfunction. If this function is restored prior to significant retraction pocket formation, the likelihood of a cholesteatoma developing is nil. Such a statement remains speculative, since it must be remembered that the mean age of this patient population is 16 years and much can still happen.

Summary

Cholesteatoma occurred only in cleft palate patients who had long standing persistent auditory tube dysfunction. The most frequent source of the cholesteatoma was the pars tensa retraction which also accounted for the highest incidence of ossicular erosion and extensive middle ear involvement requiring radical mastoidectomies. In spite of a significant number of atticotomies and canal-up procedures, to-date, residual cholesteatoma has been found in only one ear. The less radical procedures were possible because of early detection of the disease.

I am sure that if this patient population is reviewed again in five years, the incidence of cholesteatoma will be even higher. That is, unless new approaches for the prevention and/or management of this disease are discovered.

TABLE 42

The Age Distribution and the Number of Operations
in Each Age Group

Age In Years	No. of Operations
0-5	0
6-10	6
11-15	8
16-20	1
21-25	0
26-30	0

CHRONIC OTITIS MEDIA AND CHOLESTEATOMA IN ALASKAN NATIVE CHILDREN

Charles F. Tschopp, M.D.

Chronic otitis media in Alaska is a disease of this century. This is confirmed by studies of the Canadian Eskimo by Baxter (1976) who reports relatively little ear pathology present in Eskimos born before 1950. A review (Fortuine, 1971) of the written literature concerning the health of the Eskimo between 1576 and 1884 does not mention the most common sign of chronic otitis media, otorrhea. Specific EENT problems were noted however, such as epistaxis and corneal clouding. This would infer the absence of chronic suppurative ear disease.

Those physicians practicing in Alaska after World War II were very aware of the high incidence of otorrhea among native children. The distinct odor of suppuration, related to numerous draining ears was often noted by physicians visiting school rooms in the villages. Documentation of the high incidence of ear disease came in 1957 in an article in Northwest Medicine by Hayman and Kester. They estimated 739 Eskimos needed mastoidectomies and 2,785 needed tonsillectomies (Hayman and Kester, 1957).

In 1969, Maynard, in a study of villages in the Bethel area, found that otitis media, with its chronic sequelae, was one of the most important causes of morbidity among Eskimo children. The onset of their ear disease was often before the age of two. There was no sex, or seasonal predilection in occurence.

Relatively little is mentioned in the literature about complications of chronic otitis media in the Alaskan natives. However, as a young medical officer in Anchorage in 1960, I knew of three patients who were admitted to the Alaska Native Medical Center with otitis meningitis. All were operated on shortly after admission and one died several days after surgery. All had large cholesteatomas.

Surgery for chronic otitis media was begun in the late 1950's. The first operations were mainly radical mastoidectomies, and later Rambo's. Many of the Rambo's were subsequently revised because of cholesteatomas. Fortunately, there were no central complications. Most of this type of cholesteatoma presented as soft tissue swelling, or draining postauricular fistulas.

In July 1968, in an attempt to initiate action, a multi-disciplinary conference was held concerning the problem of chronic otitis media in school children. The Otitis Media Project was begun in 1969 and funded by Congress in 1970 through the help of various native groups. The objects of the Otitis Media Project were:

(1) Reduce the number of newly occurring cases of chronic otitis media in pre-school children to 3% or less.

(2) To examine the entire school population and in the following order of priority:

(A) Find and provide prompt surgery for all cholesteatomas.

(B) Provide restorative surgery for all bilateral disease.

(C) Provide restorative surgery for all unilateral disease.

(D) Continue surveillance of this population and continue evaluation of surgical results.

(E) Provide hearing aids or other amplification where degree of disability indicates.

To achieve these objects, an educational, medical, and surgical program was initiated.

Early in the project (Beal, et al, 1971), 75% of all the school children in the western and northern parts of Alaska were surveyed audiologically and/or otologically. Otologic findings in 4,193 children showed 1,274 had perforated tympanic membranes and of these, 144 or 11% had cholesteatoma. The date from the computer as of February, 1976, indicating the prevalence of chronic otitis media and cholesteatoma is presented in the following graphs (Figs. 139 and 140).

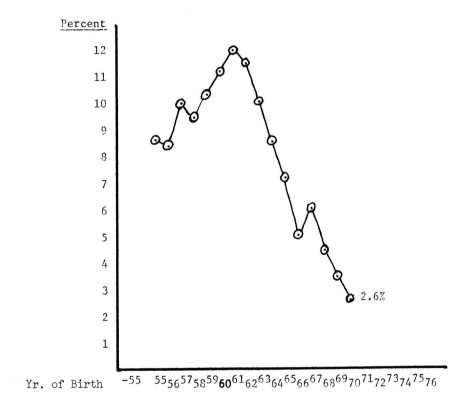

Fig. 139: The prevalence rates for chronic otitis media shows a decline from a high for the children born in 1961 of 12% to a low of 2.6% for those born in 1970. That the incidence of chronic otitis media has truly been reduced, has been verified by recent surveys in the villages.

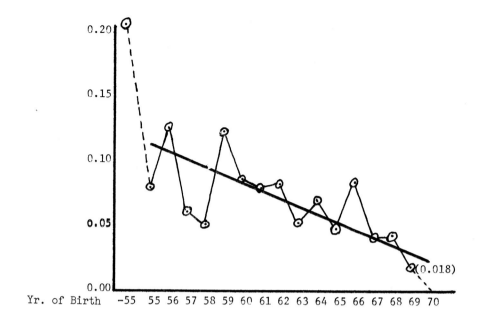

Fig. 140: This illustrates a decline in the ratio of cholesteatoma to chronic otitis media by decreasing age. It can also be interpreted as indicating an increase in the ratio with increasing age. However, with control of chronic otitis media, I believe that the children born in 1970 will never have as much problem with cholesteatoma, as those born in 1960. Time and continued surveillance will tell. One point of concern is whether the children who have had their perforations closed will go on to develop retraction pockets and attic cholesteatomas. At present, almost all cholesteatomas we see in children are secondary acquired cholesteatomas. It may well be that the high incidence of chronic otitis media indicates basic eustachian tube dysfunction. While we have not seen much serous otitis media in children after tympanoplasty, preliminary results of tympanometry in head start children in the Bethel area have shown a high incidence of abnormal tympanograms. Chronic otitis media in Alaskan native children has been reduced by early and appropriate medical care of acute otitis media. This in turn has reduced the number of cholesteatomas. No central complications have occurred from chronic otitis media for over ten years. Whether primary acquired cholesteatomas as seen in more medically advanced areas will be a problem in the future remains to be seen.

References

1. Baxter, J. D.: *Ear Disease Among the Population of the Baffin Zone. Procedures of the Third International Symposium on Circumpolar Health.* Shephard and Itoh (Ed.) University of Toronto Press, Toronto, Canada, 1976, pg. 382.
2. Beal, D.; Stewart, K.; and Fleishman, J.: The surgical program to reduce the morbidity of chronic otitis media in Alaska. Unpublished data, 1971.
3. Fortuine, R.: The health of the Eskimo, as portrayed in the earliest written accounts. *Bulletin History of Medicine,* 45:97, March-April, 1971.
4. Hayman, C. and Kester, F.: Eye, ear, nose and throat infections in natives of Alaska. *Northwest Medicine,* 56:423, 1957.
5. Maynard, J.: Otitis media in Alaskan Eskimo children, an epidermiological review with observations on control. *Alaska Medicine,* Sept.: 93, 1969.

CHOLESTEATOMA IN AUSTRALIAN ABORIGINAL CHILDREN

Gerard J. McCafferty, F.R.A.C.S.
William B. Coman, F.R.A.C.S.
Elizabeth Shaw, B. Sp. Thy.
Neil Lewis, M.A.

For many years the factors responsible for the development of cholesteatoma have been under close scrutiny by otologists interested in chronic otitis media. Recently, we have carried out extensive otological studies of Australian Aboriginal Communities, mainly school children. Our observations have revealed a high prevalence of chronic otitis media but a low incidence of cholesteatoma. This paper presents the method, results and clinical impressions of our studies.

Not much is known about the health status of Aboriginal Australians before the coming of European colonists. It is reasonable to assume, however, that the rigors of a harsh environment would have produced a hardy race of people and that low population density and a nomadic way of life would have discouraged the spread of infective diseases.

Medical anthropologists, indeed, attribute many of the health problems of present day Aboriginals to immunological and cultural differences that prohibit rapid adaptation to the settled community life style now favoured by the dominant European culture. Certainly, the adaptation process has been costly for the Aboriginal people. An abundant literature attests to the inordinately high prevalence of many diseases, including respiratory tract infections (Maxwell, 1972); intestinal parasite infestations (Jose, Self and Stallman, 1969); malnutrition and growth retardation (Jose and Welch, 1970); episodic bowel infections (Gracey and Bower, 1973) and middle ear disease (Stuart, Lewis and Barry, 1973).

Concern with the high prevalence of ear disorders among Aboriginal children led the present authors to initiate a Hearing Conservation and Aural Treatment Program for Aboriginal Communities living in remote areas of the State of Queensland. The target populations are scattered over vast distances. (Fig. 141). Climatic conditions throughout the state range from sub-tropical in the south to tropical in the north. There is considerable diversity of sociological structure from one community to another although heavy governmental expenditure in recent years has done much to improve living standards, housing, educational amenities and health care on all communities. Traditional activities and customs have disappeared among southern communities and are rapidly dying out in the north. Comparatively few people of pure aboriginal descent remain in the southern half of the state but, in the extreme north, there has been much less inter-racial dilution.

The communities served by the Hearing Conservation and Aural Treatment Program contain approximately one-third of Queensland's Aboriginal and Torres Strait Island population estimated by the Australian Census of 1971 to comprise 32,000 inhabitants.

Methods and Materials

The population. As already stated, the Aboriginal communities involved in the program are located for the most part in remote areas of the state inadequately served by established otological facilities. The major thrust of the program has been directed towards children attending schools and pre-schools although parents have been encouraged to have younger children

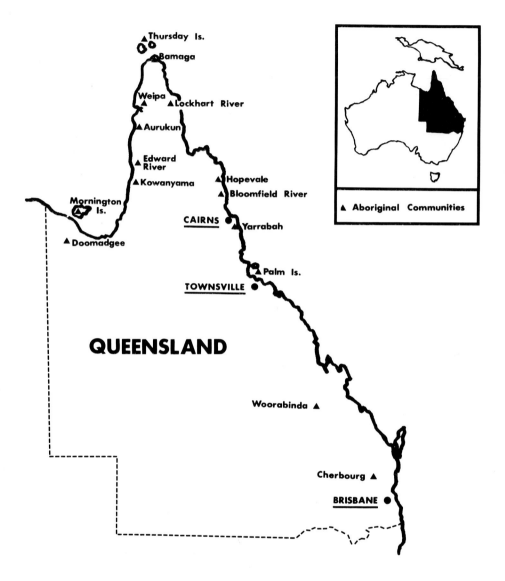

Fig. 141: Map of Queensland showing location of Aboriginal communities in relation to major urban centers.

examined and to undergo examination themselves. The program has an on-going commitment to visit each of 16 different communities annually. The figures currently reported relate, however, only to the 1975 survey which encompassed a total of 3663 individuals in the age range of 0-14 years.

Survey Strategy. To identify individuals in need of otological treatment, a visiting team of audiologists and audiometricians examined all available school children and others in each community. Evaluations included pure tone audiometry, tympanometry and acoustic reflex registrations. As part of the identification process, otoscopic examination was carried out either by a medical officer or a trained nursing sister.

All cases who failed the screening battery were then referred to an out-patient clinic conducted by visiting otologists. On the basis of the audiological findings and a comprehensive E.N.T. examination, the otologist decided whether to treat each case conservatively, to assign it to an operating list for immediate surgery, or to refer it to the E.N.T. Department of a major regional hospital.

Audiometric evaluation. All tests of hearing sensitivity were performed by trained audiometrists using portable, battery operated audiometers (Angus and Coote Type PD1) calibrated to Australian Standard Reference zero-Z43, Part II, 1970. Air conduction thresholds were determined for each ear at four frequencies 500, 1000, 2000 and 4000 Hz, the results being expressed as an average hearing level in terms of the National Acoustic Laboratories four frequency averaging formula.* Experience has shown that although the average hearing level criteria are less sensitive to minor impairments than are single frequency criteria advocated by the American Speech and Hearing Association, they are substantially less prone to measurement error when tests are being conducted under field survey conditions. Three categories were used to describe the audiometric findings.

Category 1: NORMAL HEARING—an average hearing level not exceeding 25 dB

Category 2: MILD HEARING LOSS—an average hearing level of 26-40 dB

Category 3: MODERATE TO SEVERE HEARING LOSS—an average hearing level of 41 dB or more.

Tympanometric evaluation. For each ear, measurements were made of middle ear pressure, static compliance and pressure/compliance function. The characteristics of the pressure/compliance function were then classified into Tympanogram Types A, B or C in accordance with Jerger's (1970) nomenclature. In all cases the instrumentation used for this purpose was a Peter's Model AP 61 Electro-Acoustic Bridge.

Otoscopy. Examination of the ears, nose and throat was accomplished with the aid of a full range of E.N.T. instruments. Adequate electric suction apparatus and a portable operating microscope were available. Complete assessment of difficult ears has been carried out under general anaesthesia. More recently, using an adapted fiber-light nasopharyngoscope, we have attempted photographic documentation of ears. We have recorded our observations and subsequently collated them to facilitate description of the otological state of each ear in standard terminology (See Table 44).

Results

(a) Otoscopy: A total of 7326 ears was examined.

Table 43 shows the percentage of ears in each of several otoscopic categories. Most of the classifications are self explanatory but the "abnormal intact" category requires further definition. Into this category we have cast all ears in which there was evidence of resolving or resolved

---

* National Acoustic Laboratory: Average Hearing Level (C.A.L. Hearing Impairment Tables, 1958)

Ave. H/L = $\frac{1}{6}$ [H/L 500 Hz + (2 × H/L 1000 Hz) + (2 × H/L 2000 Hz) + H/L 4000 Hz]

TABLE 43

Otoscopic Findings in Aboriginal Children

Otoscopic Findings	Percentage of Ears
Normal	29.0
Abnormal Intact	43.25
Retraction (Attic or Posterosuperior Quandrant)	0.2
Sero-mucinous Otitis Media	15.7
Chronic Otitis Media	11.7
Atelectatic T.M.	0.1
Cholesteatoma	0.05

TABLE 44

Percentage Distribution of Average Hearing Levels

Hearing Category	Number of Ears	Percentage of Ears
1. (Ave. H/L 0-25 dB)	2895	59.7
2. (Ave. H/L 26-40 dB)	1806	37.4
3. (Ave. H/L 41 dB or more)	145	2.9

disease, but in which there appeared to be no significant activity at the time of the examination. This included ears which still had a satisfactory middle ear space despite scarring or general retraction of the tympanic membrane. It also included ears in which the tympanic membrane was "lack lustre", showed tympanosclerosis, or vascular changes without discernible fluid in the middle ear.

Approximately 40% of the population surveyed show evidence of resolving or resolved inflammatory ear disease and in a minimum of 27% active ear disease is present. The rarity of cholesteatoma in this population is striking.

Figure 142 shows the age distribution of ears suffering chronic otitis media. The peak incidence of this condition seems to occur in children under the age of five years.

(b) Audiometry:

Pure tone audiograms were obtained on 4846 ears. Table 44 shows the percentage of ears in this sample that were assigned to each of the hearing categories described earlier. Some 40% of ears suffered hearing impairment, but most of the losses were of mild degree.

(c) Tympanometry:

Tympanometric findings for 5317 ears are shown in Table 45. The results have been broken down further into age categories in Figure 143. No attempt was made to obtain tympanograms from ears that were actively discharging or from ears that were obviously perforated. Tympanometric abnormalities were significantly more prevalent in the younger children.

TABLE 45

Percentage Distribution of Tympanometric Types

Tympanogram	Number of Ears	Percentage of Ears
Type A	2142	52.6
Type B	377	7.1
Type C	2802	40.3

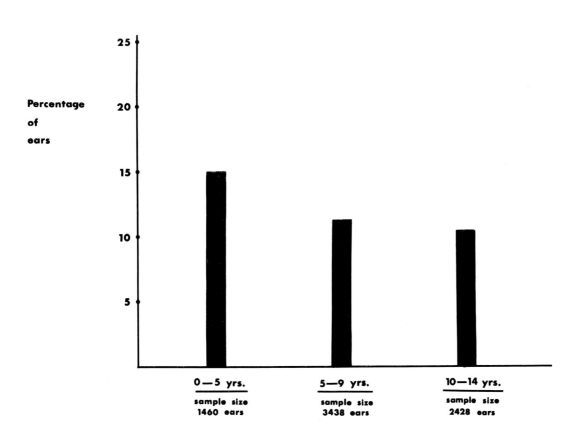

Fig. 142: Age distribution of ears suffering chronic otitis media.

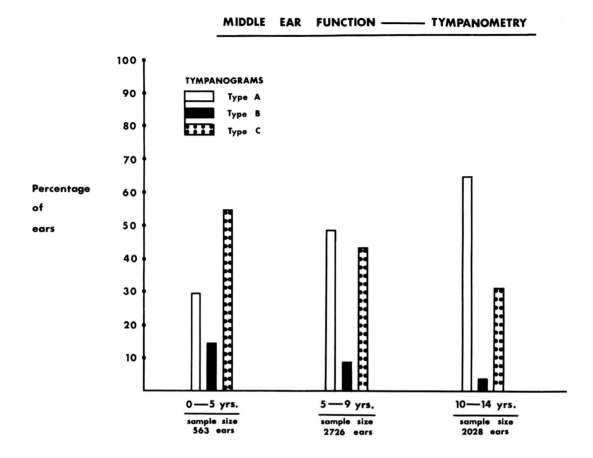

Fig. 143: Age distribution of tympanometric types.

Discussion

An extensive otological and audiological survey of Aboriginal children in Queensland suggests that large numbers either have middle ear disease or are liable to develop it. Chronic otitis media was quite common, as, indeed, was sero-mucinous otitis media. Atelectatic ears were rare, however, and cholesteatoma was found to be exceedingly uncommon. From the data obtained, we believe that the progression of ear disease in this population follows the course depicted in Figure 144.

In early life, Aboriginal children develop an upper respiratory tract infection either bacterial or viral in origin. Biopsies of nasal mucosa indicate that in approximately forty percent of cases there is an allergic component as evidenced by eosinophile infiltration of the nasal mucosa. Associated with this upper respiratory tract infection, seromucinous otitis media occurs. Otitis media in this environment is rarely acute but rather of an indolent type which does not appear

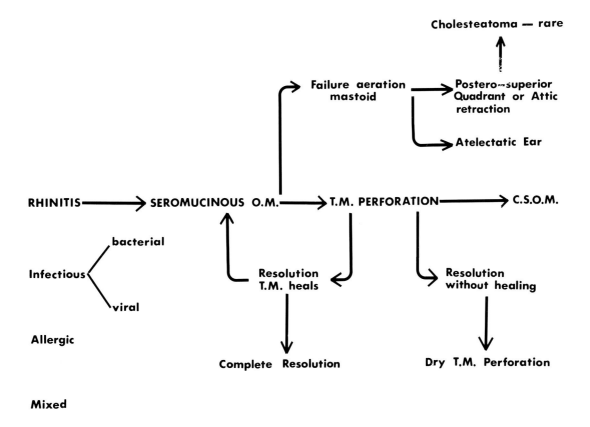

Fig. 144: Flow diagram depicting probable course of ear disease in Aboriginal children.

to cause severe pain or discomfort to those affected. If secondary infection of this sero-mucinous otitis media is virulent, tympanic membrane perforation results. Again this does not appear to be of the acute necrotising type, as initially, perforations are small and often heal spontaneously with recurrence of sero-mucinous otitis media. Large perforations appear to result from repeated episodes of perforation and the fact that children swim in polluted water while their ears are actively discharging. Swimming also causes reinfection in ears which have previously perforated. In other cases, sero-mucinous otitis media persists without perforation, with resultant failure of mastoid aeration and possible development of a retraction pocket, an atelectatic ear or cholesteatoma.

We wish to stress that the situation, as we see it, is extremely fluid. The state in a particular individual will vary from time to time but if atelectasis, postero-superior quadrant retraction, attic retraction or cholesteatoma develop the change does not appear to be spontaneously reversible.

In such a situation it is surprising to find such a low incidence of atelectatic ears and cholesteatoma. Congenital cholesteatoma as described by Cawthorne (1963) has not been detected. However, we have not conducted mass radiological surveys. Metaplasia of middle ear mucosa to keratinizing squamous epithelium has not been observed. Migration of keratinizing squamous epithelium through a perforation also has not been seen. The cholesteatoma we have noted appear to result from an indrawing of the tympanic membrane either above or below the chorda tympani with "pocketing" of keratinizing squames. The exfoliated cells accumulate remorselessly in the recess with gradual expansion and erosion of neighbouring structures. In the attic, the membrana flaccida is lax and readily indrawn by negative intratympanic pressure. When retraction occurs in the postero-superior quadrant below the chorda tympani, the collagenous layer of the membrana tensa has been destroyed by previous inflammation. We have noted that if the opening of the retraction is large, or its edges not acute, clearance of desquamated epithelium continues without significant accumulation of debris.

We have given considerable thought as to why, in a virtual morass of aural pathology, cholesteatoma should be so infrequent. Our deliberations have raised the following questions.

(1) Bezold (1879) stated, "I have not seen a perforation form in Shrapnell's membrane in the course of a genuine or secondary acute suppuration of the middle ear". Marcus Diamant (1948) also made the pertinent comment that "Marginal perforation has never yet been observed by anybody to occur in close association with acute otitis". Could it be that the low incidence of cholesteatoma results from the high prevalence of central membrana tensa perforation? Specifically, are central membrana tensa perforations allowing middle ear aeration with resultant prevention of cholesteatoma?

(2) Could the Aboriginal tympanic membrane be more resistant to negative intratympanic pressure than the Caucasian? We do not know but electron microscopy studies of Aboriginal skin by a dermatologist at the University of Queensland reveal that the collagen layer in the dermis shows less degeneration with age than that of the Caucasian. (Mitchell, 1968).

(3) Could there be a genetically determined characteristic of the meatal epidermis which decreases the propensity of the basal cells to penetrate into the submucous connective tissue of the middle ear in response to negative intratympanic pressure and inflammation?

None of these questions can be answered now. We intend to continue our observations and with the assistance of other disciplines, further investigations and more detailed analysis of our findings, and we hope that we might uncover preventative principles that could be applied to other populations.

Acknowledgement

The authors gratefully acknowledge the support of the Department of Aboriginal and Islanders Advancement, Queensland and the Department of Aboriginal Affairs, Canberra, Australia.

References

1. Bezold and Seibenmann: *Textbook of Otology.* Lecture XXI. In Jordan, R. E.: Secretory otitis media in etiology of cholesteatoma. *Arch. Otolaryng.,* 78:261, 1879.
2. Cawthorne, T.: Congenital cholesteatoma. *Arch. Otolaryng.,* 78:248, 1963.
3. Diamant, M.: Cholesteatoma and chronic otitis. *Arch. Otolaryng.,* 47:581, 1948.
4. Gracey, M. and Bower, G.: Fatal diarrhoeal disease in Australian Aboriginal children. *Aust. N. Z. J. Med.,* 3:255, 1973.
5. Jerger, J.: Suggested nomenclature for impedance

audiometry. *Arch. Otolaryng.*, 96:1, 1972.

6. Jose, D. G.; Self, M. H. R.; and Stallman, N. D.: A survey of children and adolescents on Queensland Aboriginal settlements. *Aust. Ped. J.*, 5:71, 1969.

7. Jose, D. G. and Welch, J. S.: Growth retardation, anaemia, and infection, with malabsorption and infestation of the bowel: The syndrome of protein-calorie malnutrition in Australian Aboriginal children. *Med. J. Aust.*, 1:349, 1970.

8. Juers, A. L.: Cholesteatoma genesis. *Arch. Otolaryng.*, 81:5, 1965.

9. Maxwell, G. M.: Chronic respiratory disease in Aboriginal children. Report of the First Australian Ross Conference. Ross Laboratories.

10. Mitchell, R. E.: The skin of the Australian Aborigine; a light and electronmicroscopical study. *Aust. J. Derma.*, 9:314, 1968.

11. Reudi, L.: Acquired cholesteatoma. *Arch. Otolaryng.*, 3:252, 1963.

12. Stuart, J. E.; Lewis, A. N.; and Barry, M.: Hearing and ear disease in primary school children on three Queensland Aboriginal settlements. *Aust. Ped. J.*, 9:164, 1973.

AERATION—A FACTOR IN THE SEQUELAE OF CHRONIC EAR DISEASE ALONG THE LABRADOR AND NORTHERN NEWFOUNDLAND COAST

P. Ratnesar, F.R.C.S.

The high incidence of ear disease and deafness prevalent among the three ethnic groups, namely the Eskimos, Algonkian Indians and Caucasians living along the Labrador and Northern Newfoundland Coast is presented. A similar finding has been reported by Baxter and Ling 1974 when they reported their survey in the Eastern Arctic in the Baffin Zone. Brodozsky and others 1974 also reported the high incidence of ear disease and deafness in the Keewatian Eskimos.

Though the Eskimos and Indians were both mongoloids, they were ethnically and culturally different. The Caucasians were mostly settlers from the British Isles and France, though there is some mixture present now (Fig. 145).

The role of socio-economic factor in the incidence and sequelae of ear disease in this population was similar to the other studies among the natives of Alaska, Canada, and Greenland. Cambon (et al, 1965), Schaefer (1971). The variation of ear disease in the different ethnic groups showed a definite relation to aeration of the middle ear cleft.

Method

The air cell system of the mastoid antrum was determined by X-rays and confirmed when surgical exploration was undertaken to clear disease with or without tympanoplastic procedures.

The patency of the eustachian tube was assessed clinically and by the use of impedance audiometer. The patency was confirmed and mean diameter assessed by the use of ureteric catheters when the patients had an anesthetic for (Fig. 146):

(1) Examination of the ear with microscope for suction clearance or myringotomy and possible insertion of grommets.

(2) Exploration of the mastoid with or without tympanoplastic procedure.

(3) Gross assessment of the post-nasal space including the making of moulds of the postnasal space in five patients, aged fifteen in each ethnic group (Fig. 147).

Findings

This study is based on material collected in the three year period 1973-1975. The various types of ear disease were grouped into the following categories:

(1) Serous otitis media (includes "glue" ears).

(2) Chronic otitis media (C.O.M.).

(3) C.O.M. with cholesteatoma.

(4) Tympanosclerosis (Table 46).

Though C.O.M. was common among the three ethnic groups, the incidence of cholesteatoma was almost completely in the Caucasians. When the most frequent type of ear disease was compared to the size of the eustachian tube as assessed by ureteric catheters it was found that Eskimos invariably showed the incidence of C.O.M. with or without tympanosclerosis and had large eustachian tubes, whereas Caucasians invariably showed evidence of chronic suppurative otitis media with cholesteatoma, and had very small eustachian tubes (Table 47).

The Eskimos had a larger nasopharynx than the Caucasians especially in breadth, thus enhancing the aeration of the middle ear cleft.

Discussion and Conclusion

For a long time the development of cholesteatoma was associated with poor aeration. If a nega-

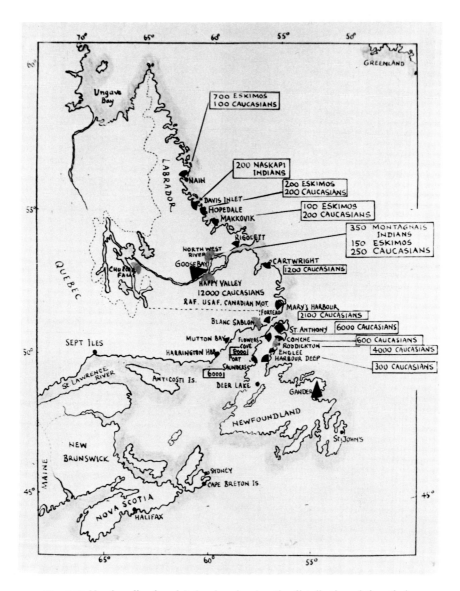

Fig. 145: Newfoundland and Labrador showing the distribution of the ethnic
groups.

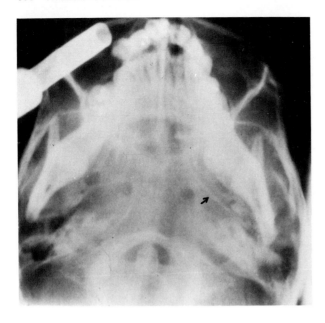

Fig. 146: Submento vertical view x-ray of the base of the skull showing ureteric catheter in the eustachian tube.

tive pressure is created in the middle ear due to eustachian tube malfunction, this must surely produce a lowering of O_2 tension. Buckingham and Ferrer 1969, and Buckingham 1971, have highlighted the negative pressure caused by tube malfunction to be a factor in the aetiology of cholesteatoma.

Baxter and Ling 1974 in a survey of the Eskimos of all ages in the Baffin Zone of Eastern arctic noted normal tympanic membranes in adults and a high prevalence of perforated drums and suppurative otitis media in the children. They concluded that C.O.M. with drum perforation is more common now than formerly. Still, the incidence of cholesteatoma among Eskimos was rare.

Prevalence of aural disease was related to poor social conditions, poor nutrition and presence of nasal discharge. This similar observation has been made by Hildes and Schaefer 1973 and Baxter and Ling 1974 in their surveys.

The observations along this coast confirms that

of other authors that C.O.M. rates high as a cause of morbidity in this population, but this also shows that the absence of cholesteatoma in Eskimos is related to the adequate aeration of the middle ear cleft (Ratnesar 1976).

Tympanosclerosis was more marked in patients with good air cell system of the middle ear cleft as seen more often in Eskimos.

Thus aeration is an important factor in the sequalae of chronic ear disease and especially the incidence of cholesteatoma.

Acknowledgements

I am grateful to the International Grenfell Association, Department of Otolaryngology Toronto and the Hearing and Research Group at Guy's Hospital for helping me with this work for the last four years.

My thanks also to Mr. Leng of the Medical Photographic Department and Miss Evelyn Tunney for helping me with the manuscript.

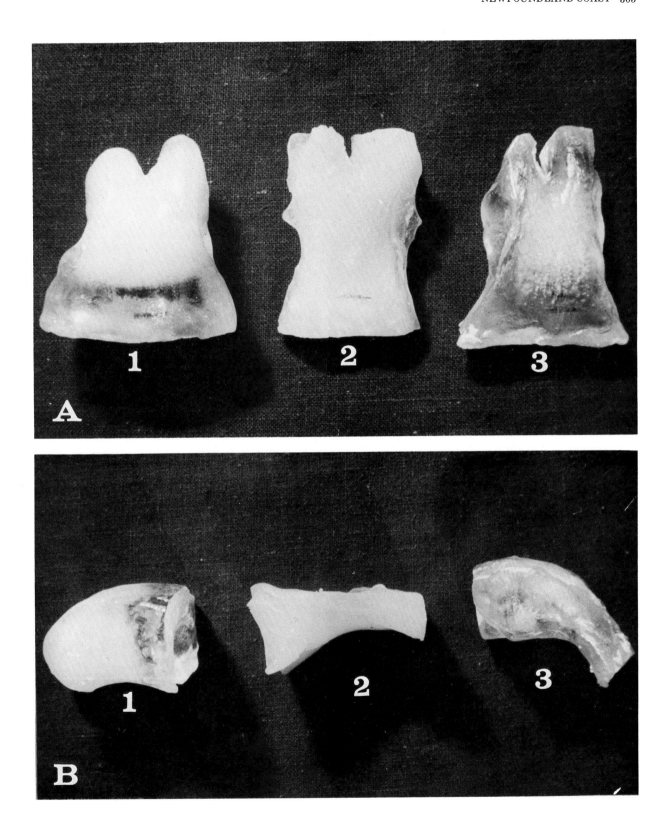

Fig. 147: Moulds of the post nasal space in the three ethnic groups: (1) Eskimo and Naskapi; (2) Caucasian; and (3) Montagnais Indians.

TABLE 46

	0 - 10			11 - 20			21 - 40			41 and over			Total	
	E	I	C	E	I	C	E	I	C	E	I	C		
Serous Otitis Media	5	2	12			13							32	7:25
Chronic Otitis Media	10	4	14	6	7	17	1	2	6				67	30:37
Cholesteatoma		1	4		1	10			8			1	25	2:23
Tympanosclerosis	1		7	6	1	6	1	1	3				26	10:16
	60			67			22			1			150	Ratio
	23 : 37			21 : 46			5 : 17			0 : 1			Eskimo & Indian To Caucasian	
	49 : 101													

TABLE 47

Ethnic groups	Most frequent Ear Disease	Average size of Eustachian tube using Ureteric catheter	Total Population	% Incidence of Ear Disease
ESKIMO Inuits	Chronic otitis media Tympanosclerosis	4-6FG 1.33-2.00 m.m.	1075	2.8
INDIAN	C.S.O.M.	4-6FG	550	3.5
CAUCASIAN	Cholesteatoma Tympanosclerosis	3FG 1.00 m.m.	46565	0.2

References

1. Baxter, J. D. and Ling, D.: Ear disease and hearing loss among the Eskimo population of the Baffin zone. *Canad. J. Otolaryng.*, 3:110, 1974.

2. Brodozsky, D.; Woolf, C.; Hedd, L. M.; and Hildes, J. A.: Proceeding of the Circumpolar Health Conference, July, 1974, In press.

3. Camben, K.; Galbraith, J. D.; and Kong, G.: Middle ear disease in Indians of the Mount Currie Reservation, British Columbia. *Canad. Med. Assoc. J.*, 93:1301, 1965.

4. Schaefer, O.: Otitis media and bottle feeding. *Canad. J. Pub. Health.*, 62:478, 1971.

5. Hildes, J. A. and Schaefer, O.: Health of Igloolik Eskimos and changes with urbanization. *J. Human Evol.*, 2:241, 1973.

6. Ratnesar, P.: Chronic ear disease along the Labrador and Newfoundland coast. *Canad. J. Otolaryng.*, Vol. 5, No. 2, April 1976.

CHOLESTEATOMA: AN INCIDENCE STUDY

L. A. Harker, M.D.

The present study was undertaken to attempt to determine the incidence of cholesteatoma in Iowa. From the epidemiologic standpoint, incidence is defined as the number of new cases of a disease occurring during a given period of time, often one year. It is expressed as a ratio with the numerator being the number of new cases of the disease in question and the denominator being the entire population at risk for being a case. Incidence differs from prevalence which measures all cases of a disease, whether old or new. One way to determine the prevalence and incidence of cholesteatoma in Iowa would be to examine all Iowans on a given day and count the number of cholesteatomas—this would be the prevalence. Then, if all these cases were surgically eradicated and one year later all Iowans were again examined and all new cases of cholesteatoma were tallied, the new figure would represent the incidence of cholesteatoma for that year. However, this method seemed impractical and a simpler one was sought.

Iowans tend to seek their specialized health care needs regionally rather than traveling to far away places, and in this part of the country only otolaryngologists treat cholesteatoma surgically. If all the otolaryngologists who perform cholesteatoma surgery on Iowans reported all their cases, and if they operated on the great majority of new cases that they saw, an incidence figure could be obtained. This is what was attempted.

All otolaryngologists listed in the Directory of the American Academy of Otolaryngology as practicing in Iowa were contacted by letter (and usually by phone as well) as were representatives of the Mayo and Gundersen Clinics in Rochester, Minnesota and LaCrosse, Wisconsin; the University of Nebraska Medical School in Omaha; and practitioners in Sioux Falls, South Dakota, and Rock Island and Moline, Illinois. Many had excluded surgical otology from their practice and referred cholesteatoma patients to other otolaryngologists. Of the twenty-five in Iowa known to operate for this disease, responses were received from twenty-two. Responses were also received from four of the five surrounding communities.

Results

In the six month period between September 1, 1975 and February 29, 1976, eighty-six surgically verified cholesteatomas occurring in Iowa residents were reported (Table 48). Since the population of Iowa is slightly over 2.8 million people, this gives an annual incidence of 60 per 1,000,000 or 6 per 100,000. Incidence figures were calculated for each decade of life by similarly relating number of cholesteatomas to population at risk (Table 49). Not surprisingly, these show the peak incidence to be during the second and third decades of life.

Discussion

The overall incidence of 6/100,000 seems low. But if there were actually twice as many cholesteatomas removed outside the University Hospitals and the Iowa City Veterans Hospital as were reported, the incidence would still be only 10/100,000 or 0.01%. Iowa's population is almost exclusively Caucasian and predominantly socioeconomically middle class. There are no ghettos and no large segment of the population without medical care. Most figures available for comparison represent either prevalence data rather than incidence of the disease, or represent a different population. While the present figure is low, it is felt to represent a realistic incidence of cholesteatoma in this population.

TABLE 48

Cholesteatoma Incidence

No. of cases in 6 months	86
Total Iowa population	2,824,376 (1970)
Total annual incidence	6.01/100,000

TABLE 49

Cholesteatoma Incidence by Age

Age in Years	No. of Cases	Population*	Incidence/100,000
0-9	12	256,656	4.68
10-19	26	283,457	9.17
20-29	15	185,598	8.08
30-39	7	144,602	4.84
40-49	11	156,540	7.03
50-59	7	146,637	4.78
60-69	7	117,400	5.96
70-79	2	82,481	1.21

*Population is halved to relate the number of cases reported in the six month study prior to an annual incidence.

References

1. Austin, D. E. and Werner, S. B.: *Epidemiology for the Health Sciences.* Charles C Thomas, Springfield, Illinois, 1974.

QUESTIONS AND ANSWERS

Dr. Paparella: I really did enjoy these presentations because, for the first time at least in meetings, I don't recall any better discussion relating to population, genetic factors, and epidemiological factors, which really gets at the underlying cause of the problem of cholesteatoma. I do have a few brief comments to make which will be really questions which I will pose to the presenters. As I listened to these discussions it seemed to me there were three main conclusions. The first is the role of genetics versus environment and natural pathogenesis of cholesteatoma. I simply am going to ask every one of these presenters to speculate briefly on that question, the relative role of genetics, be it individual genetics or population genetics, and the effect of environmental or extrinsic factors. The second important message I got out of the presentations is that it clearly is impossible to separate cholesteatoma out as a specific entity without considering its relevance and how it relates to other entities, other diseases, all under the overall title of otitis media. We have heard some of the presentations describe how middle ear effusions lead to chronic otitis media of which cholesteatoma is a part. So, cholesteatoma becomes a specific example of chronic otitis media which may indeed evolve from these very early examples of inflammation of the middle ear, the middle ear effusions, and again, I would like each presenter to comment briefly on that. The third comment really relates to that, and that is again the overall significance of otitis media. I combine those two remarks.

First, for Dr. Larry Severeid, who discussed ear diseases in cleft palate children, I think that does provide another interesting group to study. Please comment as we ask the general question, why did some of these children go from serous otitis media to cholesteatoma and some not? Again, you commented upon tubal function as being of significance in this group, and the question is, have you considered other factors? I am certain that you must agree that there must be other factors aside from tubal function, immunological factors, etc. For Dr. Tschopp, who discussed cholesteatoma in Alaskan natives, and especially in Alaskan children, I am especially interested in this from an epidemiological and a genetic point of view. I like his observations on the genetic importance of cholesteatoma in Alaskans. He incidentally did seem to give us about the highest percentage of cholesteatomas in chronic otitis media. As I understood him, it was about 11%. The other reports this morning indicated a much lower percentage. Perhaps he could comment upon that. The next presentation was by Dr. Harker, and I think he did give us a good sampling from a midwestern state, composed largely of Caucasians of middle class, indicating a very low incidence of cholesteatoma. The question is, does he know of other studies done in any comparable state? I think this is an interesting approach. To Drs. Coman and McCafferty: again, the same question, genetics versus environment. Dr. Ratnesar looked at three comparative groups, Caucasians, Eskimos, and Indians. He indicated that the Caucasian had an extremely low incidence of cholesteatoma, 2.8% for Eskimos, and 3.5% for Indians. Dr. Hinchcliffe finalized the presentations this morning and commented upon the importance of longitudinal studies and epidemiological studies.

Dr. Harker: With regard to the question of genetics versus environment, we have seen that cholesteatomas do exist. My feeling is that in all probability the environment may be more important than genetics. We have seen changes in the general health of populations and changes in disease patterns. We have not seen acute necrotizing otitis medias as was so common in the earlier part of this century. There is certainly a great change in the incidence of acute coalescent mastoiditis, which may reflect the introduction of antibiotics, but there are many cases of acute suppurative otitis media, and still the incidence of acute coalescent mastoiditis seems quite low. I think that the population we are dealing with changes, and certainly one of the things which is different in the population now compared to before in times past, is housing. Another is socio-economic status, and another diet. These things reflect the general health of the individual, and in all probability, their susceptibility to this disease.

Dr. Paparella: Dr. Tschopp, 11% in your study of those who had otitis media or chronic otitis media had cholesteatomas. That is the highest yield we heard of today. Comment please.

Dr. Tschopp: If you are cooped up in small houses, and there are many people in the house, there is a higher incidence of recurrent respiratory infections. We believe that with recurrent acute otitis media, you develop chronic otitis media. The story I related of the Eskimo lady who brought her child to the clinic because it was the only one of her 12 children that did not have draining ears was true. One of the ways we tried to solve the problem was to educate the families and village health aids in proper care of acute otitis media.

Dr. Severeid: The cleft palate patient is one who does not respect socio-economic lines. It is an hereditary disease affecting most races, some more predominantly than others. The one underlying problem is the eustachian tube which is related to the cleft. I think the important point in this 191 patients is that the cleft or the cholesteatoma is just a small part of the overall disease entity. Perforations are common. Granulation tissue polyps are common. Atelectasis is common. Dr. Hinchcliffe commented on patients with perforations. If left alone, the incidence of cholesteatoma decreases. This is certainly our experience. I think there is a need for longitudinal observation. You cannot examine one group once, make your obser-

vations, and make rational conclusions. I want everybody to know that I could probably juggle that incidence any way I wanted to. Ironically, I looked at it from the 160 patients who had eustachian tube problems. In other words, if I would have considered the whole 191, it would have been less. I would imagine if I wanted to look at posterior-superior retraction pockets that did not have squamous debris I could make it much higher. It probably represents any group that is carefully followed, because prolonged eustachian tube problems are so common.

Dr. Coman: With respect to genetics, one of the few areas that we can look at and say a genetic change has occurred in a race occurs with the separation of Tasmania from the mainland of Australia. This occurred ten to twenty thousand years ago, and yet that race of Tasmanian aborigines who are now extinct were studied by anthropologists and found to be quite different from their mainland brothers. So, if you are considering how long it takes a genetic trait to occur that is measurable, there is a definite period of time. With respect to diet and nutrition, we measured serum immunoglobulins in the ears and in the nasopharynx. We measured all parameters and we strongly believe that it is a nutritional factor rather than a genetic factor that predisposes them to the ear problems.

Dr. Ratnesar: The natives in Ceylon are related to the aborigines of Australia, and the incidence of cholesteatoma in both is very low. However, many of the patients had perforations with discharge from their ears. Yet, I did not see a retraction pocket, and the natives had good eustachian tube function. I was never able to measure it. When I treated the perforations and discharging ears with general hygiene, some of the small perforations healed spontaneously. Also, I agree with Dr. Tschopp and others that nutrition and hygiene play an important role in the incidence of chronic ear disease.

Dr. Austin: My comment is relative to the study with cleft palate patients, and in opposition to

Jim, I was struck by the very high incidence of cholesteatoma reported in this series. For example we have a series in Chicago in which over 100 patients who had had cleft palates repaired disappeared from medical care for a period of 10 to 15 years and had no medical attention. They were called back and examined. The incidence of chronic ear disease in this group was very, very low. As you implied, their ears did return to health, or the fluid left the ears as they grew older, but the incidence of cholesteatoma was in the 1 to 2% range. My question is, is it not possible that therapy during the young years led to your 6 to 7% incidence of complication?

Dr. Bellucci: I wish to know from Dr. Tschopp whether you ever see an entire family with seven or eight children all with ear disease, and if you have does it correlate with a general hypodevelopment of the nasopharynx?

Dr. Severeid: In response to Dr. Austin's question, yes, I think that it is very possible. It would be interesting to know at what age your patients were lost to follow-up. I think it would be important to compare the two. All of these patients had ventilating tubes. I think that you have to look at your patient population whenever you talk about statistics, because the patients that I am discussing have been followed intimately. That makes for a very broad sample, compared to just a small group whose ears were seen at any one time.

Dr. Tschopp: I don't believe that there is a familial difference as far as the shape of the skull is concerned. I really don't have many facts at all. It is just my impression that the shape of the skull isn't that much different in the Alaskan native to warrant a conjecture that this relates to chronic otitis media.

Dr. Ratnesar: There is a specific difference in the structure in the three ethnic groups as I showed you. There was a broader nasopharynx and also the Eskimos had a deeper lateral recess. Those that had the recess had a greater tendency for a chronic discharge, as opposed to the others.

Chapter 6

Hereditary and Congenital Factors

HEREDITARY FACTORS IN CHRONIC OTITIS MEDIA IN GENERAL AND CHOLESTEATOMA IN PARTICULAR

Dietrich Plester, M.D.

The pneumatization of the retrotympanic spaces shows a considerable variation in extent. Chronic suppurative otitis media and cholesteatoma in its primary and secondary forms are regularly associated with reduced or absent pneumatization. Obviously, the degree of pneumatization of the middle ear will give an important clue in the diagnosis and prognosis of chronic middle ear disease.

Several factors have been suspected of interfering with the development of pneumatization of the middle ear. Wittmaack (1937), who first described the close relationship between cholesteatoma formation and lack of pneumatization, pointed out that it could be due to infections of the middle ear during early childhood. He thought that otitis media of the infant produced a chronic hyperplastic or hypoplastic middle ear mucosa.

Irreversible alterations of the mucosa due to repeated infections reduce the capacity of the mucosa to create pneumatic cells in the spongy bone of the mastoid. This he considered an active process of the middle ear mucosa.

My predecessors in the ENT Department in Tübingen, Albrecht (1925) and Schwarz (1944), concentrated their scientific interest on hereditary or genetic factors influencing the degree and form of pneumatization of the middle ear. Wittmaack later admitted that hereditary factors might play some role but mainly in the reaction to environmental influences. These influences subsequently act on the middle ear mucosa which possibly determines the size of the cellular system and generates a somewhat greater susceptibility to chronic ear disease.

In order to evaluate genetic factors as far as mastoid pneumatization is concerned, Albrecht investigated monozygotic and dizygotic twins. The monozygotic twins offer the greatest opportunity of proving hereditary influences, if physical characteristics are similar. Differences in monozygotic twins result from environmental factors, whereas differences in dizygotic twins are due to genetic and environmental influences. For these reasons investigations on monozygotic or dizygotic twins seem to yield the most valuable information about different influences on human body characteristics.

Albrecht's early investigations were completed by Schwarz (1929) on 56 monozygotic and 35 dizygotic twins. The study was based mainly on clinical material of the Tübingen University. Therefore, the zygotic standard of our twins could be proved in most cases by amnion studies after birth. Detailed studies of these twins were conducted by Weitz (1929) and von Verschuer (1929).

The high degree of corresponding extent of mastoid pneumatization in acellular mastoids is demonstrated in Figure 148. It is not the frequency of reduced pneumatization itself which is remarkable, but rather the degree of conformity of pneumatization in monozygotic twins.

The conformity of pneumatization, even the bony structure with its regularities and irregularities, and the anatomical relations of the sigmoid sinus are highly significant in monozygotic twins. This demonstrates the important role of hereditary factors for its development. Dahlberg and Diamant (1945) later fully confirmed these findings of Albrecht and Schwarz. Besides investigating twins, they extended the research to families, measuring the size of the mastoid cells by planimetric means. A close relationship between mastoid pneumatization of the

	Number of temporal bones	Number of acellular mastoid processes	Corresponding extend of pneumatisation	percentage
monozygotic twins (N 59)	236	60 (25,5 %)	10 = 40 mastoid processes	66,6
dizygotic twins (N 35)	140	17 (12,1 %)	1 = 4 mastoid processes	-

Fig. 148: Sixty out of 236 temporal bones in monozygotic twins were found to be acellular or nearly acellular. Two-thirds of these belonged to monozygotic brothers or sisters (Schwarz, 1929).

parents and children was demonstrated, again underlining the importance of hereditary factors. The genealogical tree of a family, carefully investigated by Schwarz, shows highly reduced pneumatization of all members of the family (Fig. 149), obviously introduced by the father. He him-

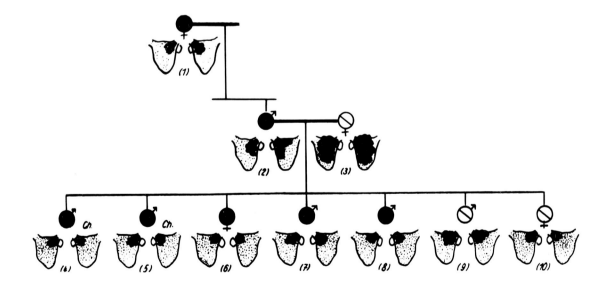

Fig. 149: Genealogical tree of the family G. Demonstration of mastoid pneumatization. The pneumatized part of the ear is blackened. (Schwartz, 1940) ●-epitympanic retraction. ch-cholesteatoma formation.

self inherited this characteristic from his mother.

Two brothers, whom I had previously treated for mucoserotympanonitis, developed at the age of 10 and 12 years, attic cholesteatoma in the left ear; the father of these children also had undergone cholesteatoma surgery eight years previously on the left ear. Similar observations have been reported by Virchow (1966) as early as 1856, and later by Rüedi (1958), Walb (1966), and Schwarz (1940).

Chronic otitis media and a reduced pneumatization are often associated. On one hand, a reduced infection or cholesteatoma; on the other hand, not every ear with reduced pneumatization reveals signs of this disease.

Diamant's investigations showed that the size of the cellular system has an important bearing on susceptibility to chronic otitis. In Dahlberg's terminology, chronic otitis media might have a constellational character, affecting only a part of the population. In this case it would be provoked by a combination of hereditary and environmental factors.

Until now there has been no scientific proof whether the middle ear mucosa is unable to produce or form an extended or "normal" pneumatization or whether susceptibility of the mucosa to chronic ear disease and lack of pneumatization are due to a "silent gene" affecting both.

Clinical observations have revealed an astonishing change in cholesteatoma formation. Cholesteatoma with a large marginal perforation or an almost completely destroyed ear drum has become rare. The so-called secondary cholesteatoma originates from necrotizing otitis media following scarlet fever, measles or influenza, predominantly in childhood. Thanks to antibiotic treatment, we rarely find these complications today.

Most of the cholesteatoma we find nowadays follows invagination of the pars flaccida, which is provoked by chronic irritation, as demonstrated by Rüedi, or is due to chronic tubal dysfunction.

Chronic otitis media or cholesteatoma forma-

tion is unknown in the animal and even in the anthropomorphous ape. The human middle ear seems to be predisposed to this disease. Anatomical investigations demonstrate the development of the clivus angle (Fig. 150) of the skull is associated with the upright position in man, which shortens the base of the skull.

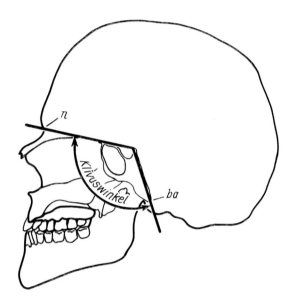

Fig. 150: Clivus angle and base of the skull (Oltersdorf).

The upright position and the enlargement of the skull in man during the development of the human race have altered the base of the skull. This has had important consequences for the osteogenesis of the temporal bone. It is evident that the curvature of the skull of the ape when compared with the same line in man, (Fig. 151) that the shortening of the base of the skull affects the middle ear, mainly the eustachian tube.

In animals, the muscles of the nape of the neck are well developed to hold the head, whereas in man the muscles of the anterior part of the neck are comparatively stronger. The mastoid process has evolved in man as a consequence of the upright position and the formation of the clivus angle.

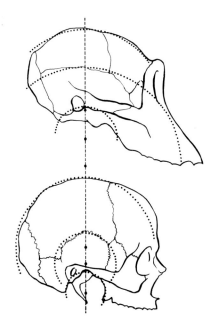

Fig. 151: Comparison of the curvature of the skull (Krummungskreis) in ape and man (Oltersdorf).

The tympanic bone, which forms the base of the outer ear canal and of the eustachian tube, is still in a horizontal position in the ape: it is fixed at the base of the temporal bone. In man, on the other hand, the tympanic bone is placed nearly at the vertex of the clivus angle. Due to this intrusion of space, the tympanic bone has a nearly vertical position in human beings.

The observations of Oltersdorf (1962) of the ENT Department in Tübingen have shown a close and statistically significant relationship between the clivus angle and the extent of pneumatization. The eustachian tube, which is round and wide in animals, becomes oval and often narrow in man, sometimes even forming an angle between the osseous and cartilaginous part near the isthmus of the tube. In deforming the tube, the base of the human skull might influence the aeration of the middle ear and the pneumatization as well.

Insufficient pneumatization contributes to the development of chronic ear disease and the configuration of the skull in man favors this condition. The result of the upright position and pronounced enlargement of the skull of the human is a predisposition to chronic ear disease.

References

1. Albrecht, W.: Die Bedeutung der Konstitution bei den Erkrankungen des Ohres und der Luftwege. *Z. Laryng. Rhinol. Otol.*, 14:1, 1925.
2. Dahlberg, G. and Diamant, M.: Hereditary character in the cellular system in the mastoid process. *Acta. Otolaryng.*, 33:378, 1945.
3. Okasaki, M.: Röntgenologische Studien über die Bedeutung der Ebfaktoren bei der Pneumatisation der Warzenfortsatze. *Zbl. HNO-Heilk.*, 29:217, 1938.
4. Oltersdorf, U.: Pneumatisation des Warzenfortsatzes und Schädelform. *Arch. Ohr-, Nas.-*

Editor's note: This interesting anthropological note does not take into account the fact that quadrupeds hold their head in just the same position relative to the horizon as bipeds.

Kehlk.-Heilk., 180:602, 1962.

5. Rüedi, L.: Cholesteatosis of the attic. *J. Laryng. Otol.*, 72:593, 1958.

6. Schwarz, M.: Die Bedeutung der hereditären Anlage für die Pneumatisation der Warzenfortsatze und der NNH. *Arch. Ohr.-, Nas.-, Kehlk,-Heilk.*, 123:161, 1929.

7. Schwarz, M.: Familiare Schrapnell-Einsenkung. *Erbbl. f. d. HNO-Arzt*, 31:11, 1940.

8. Schwarz, M.: Zur Erblichkeit der Schrapnelleinsenkung. *Arch. Ohr-, Nas.-, Kehlk.-Heilk*, 154:165, 1944.

9. Schwarz, M.: *Das Cholesteatom im Gehörgang und im Mittelohr.* G. Thieme Verlag, Stuttgart, Germany, 1966.

10. von Verschuer: zit. n. Schwarz, M., 1929.

11. Virchow, R.: Über Perlgeschwulste. zit. n. Schwarz, 1966.

12. Walb: zit n. Schwarz, 1966.

13. Weitz: zit n. Schwarz, 1929.

14. Wittmaack, K.: Über die Entstehung der Schleimhautkonstitution des Mittelohres. *Acta Otolaryng.*, 25:414, 1937.

THE MASTOID AIR CELLS

Herman Diamant, M.D.
Marcus Diamant, M.D.

I. The varying sizes of the mastoid air cell system.

Early in otology a clinical correlation was observed between the size of the mastoic air cell system and the occurrence of middle ear otitis. This combination can be classified as follows:

(1) Acute otitis media with a "large" cell system.

(2) "Chronic otitis media" with a "small" cell system.

It must be stressed that the knowledge in those days of the variation in size of the mastoid air cell system in the population was defective partly because the selection factor limited the survey to be comprised only of patients attending ear departments. Furthermore, the estimation of size was still made according to visual inspection, even when roentgenograms were available as a basis for determining the size. Thus, Schwartz classified five main groups, and the Schwartz-Barth classification has been accepted in many quarters. Briefly, it is as follows:

Group I: Temporal bones with an unusually extensive air cell system.

Group II: Temporal bones with an air cell system still large and extending not only into the mastoid process but also into the squama temporalis and arcus zygomaticus regions.

Group III: Temporal bones with air cells throughout, or in most of the mastoid process, but without pneumatization of the other regions mentioned under Group II.

Group IV: Temporal bones with an air cell system only in the antral portion of the mastoid bone and, perhaps, in the aditus ad antrum. In this group, accordingly, marked inhibition or retardation of the pneumatization process is already present.

Group V: Temporal bones without air cell development.

Marcus Diamant's systematic examination of his first normative material was of patients infected with scarlet fever, then always treated in an epidemic hospital (1940). He presumed that scarlet fever could hardly be expected to infect only people with a special size of the mastoid pneumatization, even if some sizes of air cell systems can be combined with certain frequencies of otitis in the total size variation in the population. The measurements were made on X-ray pictures taken on a special skull-table allowing an exact position at its exposition and also of stereopictures. A planimeter-measuring technique was used also allowing exact determination of the methodical sources of error. In a normal group of about 350 individuals a variation of size between 0 − 30 cm^2 and a frequency distribution according to the probability curve for biological variation was established. The frequency distribution within the normal material was later shown in a three times greater sample and again in the representative population. When correlating the measures on the lateral X-ray exposition with those of the frontal ones, the correlation coefficient was computed to be 0.86. It was performed on 900 individuals representing a normal material as well as on an additional group of monozygotic and dizygotic pairs of twins. Dahlberg and Diamant (1945) could show in the latter that hereditary factors definitely play the greatest role for the growth of size of the air cell system and that the factors play a much lesser role. These environmental factors may in fact not be pathological at all. Birthweight differences may for instance depend on the fact that the umbilical cords have given more nourishment to one of the twins than to the other.

However, the finding in a normal material as such may not be taken as definite proof for a biological variation of the size in the air cell system, since conclusions cannot be deduced from statistical calculations.

Moreover, other authors have later shown a corresponding range of variation and frequency distribution, both at planimetric and volumetric studies (Flisberg and Zsigmond, 1965).

A corresponding distribution could also be shown to exist for the right and left ears in the same individual when asymmetrical. The standard deviation was significantly less which, is to be expected, as a correlation between the two ears in the same person is greater than between all ears in different individuals.

Both the inter—and intraindividual normal distribution can be expected when environmental factors influencing the growth are non-pathological, though of course it still cannot be maintained to prove non-pathogenicity. Thus, pre—and postnatal infections or presence of meconium in the middle ear at birth can still hypothetically be looked upon as pneumatization-inhibiting, but even such a hypothesis must be shown at least to be probable, when maintaining that these factors are causing a pathologic hampering of the pneumatization or a total pathologic lack of air cells. Wittmaack's so-called pneumatization theory is totally based on histopathological studies of the mucous membrane (1918). Above all, it may be stressed that Wittmaack himself denies any correlation to the size of the air cell system (1937). His studies are furthermore carried out on a small post-mortum material and are quite unscientific from the point of view of the selection factors. In addition Alexander (1927) could show that all the three mucous membrane types described by Wittmaack could be found in the same histopathological preparation.

The pneumatization studies made by Opheim (1944) and Ojala (1950) show that there are great difficulties in checking the development of the air spaces in the humeri in the chicken. Only after total destruction of punctum pneumaticum could a non-pneumatization be achieved. Besides, their finding cannot be used for judging conditions in the human middle ear. There are no such destructive influences without visible symptoms in man, either during the pre-natal life, or later on. Finally, their conclusions are contradictory to their own finding, a point very obvious when comparing their own statements in the separate parts of their studies.

Acute otitis media with or without complications in an adult presumably producing a diminishing air cell system already developed to some degree, could not within reason occur except as developing in a biologically varying normal sample except step by step, from the periphery to the center, as illustrated by M. Diamant (Fig. 152).

Clinical findings of such a reduction of previously existing large size has not been evidenced. On the other hand, it may be conceived that biological forces for the growth of the mastoid air cell system may be stopped pre-natally at different degrees and that thereby size differences may be caused. This should, however, not produce the actual frequency distribution of the normal material. It seems improper to attribute the relevent influencing power to the pre-natal meconium occurring in the middle ear which cannot be attributed to the clinically observed acute media otitis in children. It has furthermore not been shown that the so-called "chronic" otitis causes a disturbance of the growth of the air cell system with a variation ranging from 1 cm^2 to 10 cm^2 in cases with a marginal ear drum perforation. Finally, Diamant's and Lilja's (1948) X-ray studies of so-called chronic mastoiditis did not show any diminishing of the air cell system in the X-ray film, despite their protracted observation and that histopathological postoperative examinations showed reactive and reparative processes in the walls of the individual air cells.

Friedmann's (1955) experiments must be mentioned. He has shown sclerosing changes in the bulla of guinea-pigs. The bulla in guinea-pigs can-

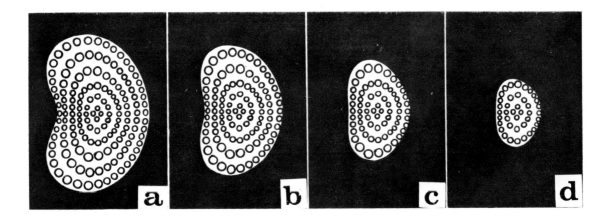

Fig. 152: Acute otitis media with diminishing air cell system.

not give information as to the mastoid cells in man. The sclerosing of the bulla by new bone formation has not been shown to eliminate the tracing of its original borders on the roentgenogram.

Concerning Tumarkin (1957), it is realized that his groups from the slums of Liverpool differed somewhat from the population in general as to size of the mastoid air cell system. From his pneumatization examination it is possible to conclude that there is a smaller average of size in the slum as compared with that of the normal material. This difference may be due to hereditary factors and to the risk of infection from overcrowding and poor hygiene. It cannot be concluded that elimination of poverty will eliminate all ear disease as every otologist has wealthy patients who have sustained any and all various middle ear diseases.

II. The size of the air cell system and otitis media—acute and "chronic".

Marcus Diamant also examined a more differentiated material based on otitis media (1952). With his strict demands for the exactness of measurement of relevant size as well as of selection factors he could assess the varying size distribution as correlated to healthy and diseased ears.

In his research, M. Diamant has shown that there is a strong "affinity" between the size of the air cell system and the origin of different types of otitis if these are divided into three groups, acute otitis media, central ear drum perforation and marginal ear drum perforation. However, Diamant emphasizes that the size of the air cell system itself has not been shown to cause this "affinity". Thus, the patient's resistance as well as the different grade of affinity to different ear diseases can be related to the size of the air cell system as an indicator of the biological factors which command both the growth in size and resistance. The size for the various kinds of ear disease can be seen in Figure 153. This resemblance and "affinity" concerns the single ear of the individual. Thus, it is not tied to the individual as a whole. If size of the air cell system of one ear exceeds 25 cm^2 and the other reaches below this size, otitis media may not occur at all in the "larger" ear, but may occur in the "smaller" one. Of course, otitis media never should occur in any ear, even when there is no mastoid pneumatization at all.

This possibility to make prognostic conclusions is unique. This medical information is thus valid for each ear. M. Diamant has described a case of primary cancer in the middle ear where the size of

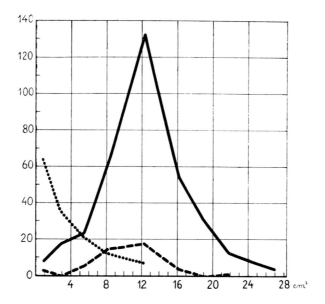

Fig. 153: Normal material (solid curve), chronic otitis (dotted curve) and acute otitis (broken curve) at the ages of 10-30 years, grouped according to the size of the cellular system.

the air cell system led to the right diagnosis, since it was statistically possible to exclude a central or marginal perforation as the cause of an affection giving a swelling of the meatus that made inspection impossible. It may be added that the very frequent secretory otitis has been shown to attack ears having a size distribution in accordance with acute otitis media. This must not however be taken as a base for the conclusion that an infectious etiology has been proved.

Diamant and Dahlberg have also been able to estimate the relative risks for the various form of middle ear affections. They show a relative and progressive rise of the risk for the smaller sizes of the air cell system (always within the variation range for each kind of middle ear affection). Diamant has also suggested that the size of the pneumatization may be used for prognostic conclusions concerning the healing possibilities at different forms of operation, especially to be used in cases of myringoplasties. Direct studies of this

kind have not been presented. Attempts to prognosticate surgical intervention relative to the air passage capacity of the eustachian tube are invalid, because such measurements will give only a fleeting idea of a changing functional capability.

III. The cholesteatoma and the size of the air cell system.

It has already been stated that the marginal ear drum perforation has a marked correlation to the small air cell system. Clinically it has been pointed out that the marginal ear drum perforation has a close connection with the presence of cholesteatoma. In reality McKenzie (1931), later supported by Cawthorne (1963), brought forward this correlation. They emphasize that the cholesteatoma is the origin of the marginal perforation by erosion of the bone in this region from the inside and outwards. Diamant has adopted this theory of erosion from the inside, without, however, being able to produce conclusive evidence of his clinical experiments due to technical shortcomings, i.e., he was unable to produce sequential photographs. It should, however, be possible for every otologist to show clinically a slowly growing marginal perforation, which at the start need not include the ear drum at all as it breaks through. M. Diamant disagrees with McKenzie in that this breaking through from the inside does not prove that cholesteatoma is a tumor.

Thus, the magnitude of size of the air cell system is principally heredity-dependent and is an indicator for the frequency of certain forms of otitis media and middle ear disease. This is especially valid for the classification in central and marginal ear drum perforation as in acute otitis media and serous otitis media. The etiology of the cholesteatoma cannot be solved in this manner.

References

1. Alexander, G.: Zur Histologie der Mittelohrschleimhaut. *Monatsschrift fur Ohrenheilkunde*, 61:, 1927.
2. Cawthorne, T.: Congenital cholesteatoma. *Arch. Otolaryng.*, 78:243, 1963.
3. Diamant, M.: Otitis and pneumatization of the mastoid bone. *Acta.* Otolaryng. Suppl., 41:, 1940.
4. Diamant, M.: *Chronic Otitis. A Critical Analysis.* S. Kärger, Basle and New York, 1952.
5. Diamant, M.: The "pathologic size" of the mastoid air cell system. *Acta. Otolaryng.*, 60:, 1964.
6. Diamant, M. and Dahlberg, G.: Inheritance of pneumatization of the mastoid bone. *Hereditas*, 31:441, 1945.
7. Diamant, M. and Lilja, B.: Chronic mastoiditis and its roentgen picture. *Acta. Radiol.*, 29:37, 1948.
8. Flisberg, K. and Zsigmond, M.: The size of the mastoid air cell system. *Acta. Otolaryng.*, 60:, 1965.
9. Friedmann, I.: The comparative pathology of otitis media—experimental and human. *J. Laryngol.*, 69:27, 1955.
10. McKenzie, D.: The pathogeny of aural cholesteatoma. *J. Laryngol.*, 46:163, 1931.
11. Ojala, L.: Contribution to the physiology and pathology of mastoid air cell formation. *Acta. Otolaryng. Suppl.*, 86:, 1950.
12. Opheim, O.: The pneumatic conditions of the human temporal bone in the light of experimental researches on the development of the air space in the chick humerus. *Acta. Otolaryng. Suppl.*, 54:, 1944.
13. Tumarkin, A.: On the nature and vicissitudes of the accessory air space of the middle ear. *J. Laryngol.*, 71:, 1957.
14. Wittmaack, K.: Uber die normale und die pathologoische pneumatisation des sclafenbeines einschliesslich ihrer beziehungen zu den mittelohrerkrankungen. *Jena*, 1918.
15. Wittmaack, K.: Uber die Entstehung der Schleimhautkonstitution des Mittelohres. *Acta. Otolaryng.*, 25:, 1937.

Chapter 7

The Eustachian Tube

FUNCTIONAL EUSTACHIAN TUBE OBSTRUCTION IN ACQUIRED CHOLESTEATOMA AND RELATED CONDITIONS

Charles D. Bluestone, M. D.
Erdem I. Cantekin, Ph. D.
Quinter C. Beery, Ph. D.
Gavin S. Douglas, M. D.
Sylvan E. Stool, M. D.
William J. Doyle, M. A.

Nomenclature

Abbreviations

CHOL	Cholesteatoma
RET-ADOM	Retraction pocket-adhesive otitis media
RET-ATEL	Retraction pocket-atelectasis of the middle ear
TR-PERF	Traumatic perforation
ET	Eustachian tube
ME	Middle ear
TM	Tympanic membrane

Symbols

SWA+	Residual positive pressure remaining in middle ear following open-nose swallowing
SWA-2	Residual negative pressure remaining in middle ear following open-nose swallowing
OP1	First opening pressure
CL1	First closing pressure
CLI+	Residual positive pressure remaining in middle ear after closing pressure and open-nose swallowing
MIN+	Minimum residual positive pressure (SWA+ or CL1+)
TOY+	Residual positive pressure remaining in middle ear following closed-nose swallowing
TOY-2	Residual negative pressure remaining in middle ear following closed-nose swallowing
VALS	Valsalva's test

The presence of keratinizing stratified squamous epithelium with accumulation of desquamating epithelium or keratin within the middle ear (ME) cleft or other pneumatized portions of the temporal bone is called a keratoma or more commonly, a cholesteatoma (CHOL). A congenital CHOL has been defined as an epithelial cyst within the temporal bone that is not in contact with the external auditory canal. An acquired CHOL has been classically associated with a "perforation" of the tympanic membrane (TM) either in the pars flaccida or in the posterosuperior margin or, on occasion, the central portion of the pars tensa. The pathogensis of acquired CHOL has not been resolved. Of the many hypotheses proposed, the following are the most popular: (1) embryonic epidermal rest occurring in the attic (McKenzie, 1931; Teed, 1936; and Diamant, 1952); (2) metaplasia of the ME and attic due to infection (Tumarkin, 1938); (3) invasive hyperplasia of the basal layers of the metal skin adjoining the upper margin of the TM (Nager, 1925; Hellman, 1925; Lange, 1932; Saxen and Ojala, 1952; and Rüedi, 1963) (4) invasive hyperkeratosis of the deep external auditory canal (McGuckin, 1961); and (5) collapse of the TM in the attic or posterosuperior area with invagination, secondary to eustachian tube (ET) obstruction and negative ME pressure (Habermann, 1888).

In an attempt to test the last hypothesis, the ventilatory function of the ET was assessed in older children and adults with acquired CHOL. Since collapse of the TM has been implicated in the pathogenesis, patients with a retraction pocket in the posterosuperior quadrant of the TM were also tested.

Subjects and Methods

Four groups of patients were studied. Group-CHOL, consisted of five patients (five ears) with CHOL who had had tympanostomy tubes inserted prior to reconstructive surgery. The CHOL was in the posterosuperior portion of the TM in three subjects and in the attic in two. Group-RET-ADOM, consisted of three patients (five ears) with a dry deep posterosuperior retraction pocket and otoscopic and tympanometric evidence of high negative ME pressure ($>$-100 mm H_2O), in whom the insertion of tympanostomy tubes failed to alter the position of the retraction pocket. Group-RET-ATEL, consisted of five patients (five ears) who had a deep retraction pocket in the posterosuperior portion of the TM and otoscopic and tympanometric evidence of high negative ME pressure ($>$-150 mm H_2O) or middle ear effusion. Following insertion of a tympanostomy tube, the TM in the posterosuperior quadrant returned to the neutral position. Figure 154 depicts the tympanic membrane—middle ear pathology in the three groups. A comparison group, Group-TR-PERF, consisted of four patients (four ears) who had received traumatic perforation of the TM but who otherwise, had negative otologic histories. Table 50, shows the age distribution of the four groups.

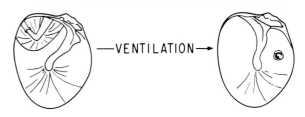

RETRACTION POCKET - ATELECTASIS

—VENTILATION—→

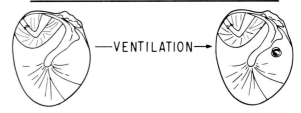

RETRACTION POCKET - ADHESIVE OTITIS

—VENTILATION—→

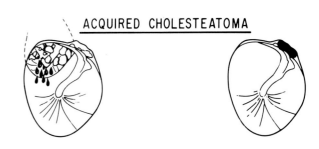

ACQUIRED CHOLESTEATOMA

Fig. 154: Illustration showing the tympanic membrane middle ear pathologic entities studied.

The ventilatory function of the ET was studied by the inflation-deflation technique which is described in detail elsewhere (Cantekin, et al, 1976 and Bluestone, et al, 1976). The experimental arrangement used in the ET function studies described in the present investigation is shown in Figure 155. A closed air pressure system was sealed into the external auditory meatus—ear canal—and into one naris employing a double-lumen balloon catheter (modified Foley). A constant speed syringe pump was used for inflation and deflation of the ME. The pump delivered nominal 6 cc/min air-flow to the external canal.

TABLE 50

Comparison of Ages of Subjects

Age (Yrs)	Traumatic Perforation	Study Group		Cholesteatoma	Total
		Retraction Pocket-Atelectasis	Retraction Pocket Adhesive Otitis		
7-12	1	4	–	3	8
>12	3	1	3	2	9
Total	4	5	3	5	17

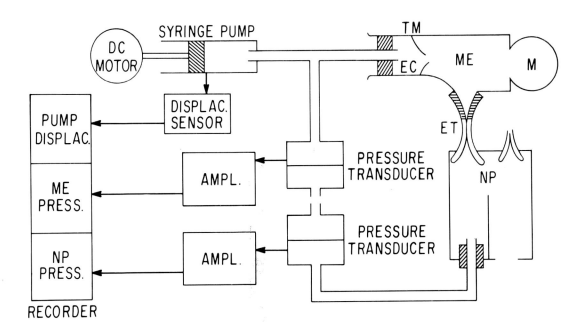

Fig. 155: Schematic representation of the instrumentation. Tympanic membrane (tm); external canal (ec); middle ear (me); mastoid (m); eustachian tube (et); and nasopharynx (np).

The volume of air-flow was monitored by the piston displacement sensor. The rate of applied pressure was 20 to 30 mm H_2O/sec depending upon the subjects' middle ear-mastoid volume and the starting position of the pump piston. ME pressure was measured by a Hewlett-Packard type 1280-C* pressure transducer and simultaneous nasopharyngeal pressure was measured by a Statham type PM-283-TC** pressure transducer. Pressure signals were amplified using Hewlett-Packard 8805-B amplifiers and recorded onto a heat sensitive paper with an MFE model 4-M3-

CAHA*** recorder.

Figure 156 describes the elements of the procedure and the symbols used. All subjects were tested in the sitting position and only wet (water) swallows were employed. Ventilation studies were performed only on subjects whose ears were free of discharge. The results reported here are based on a four part test in the following sequence: (A) active and (B) passive function during open-nose swallowing, (C) active function during closed-nose swallowing (Toynbee's Maneuver), and (D) Valsalva's Test.

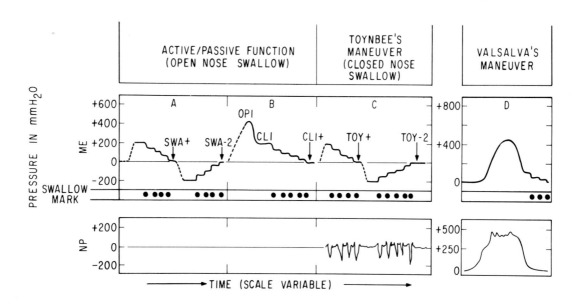

Fig. 156: Sequence of procedures employed in assessing the ventilatory function of the eustachian tube.

*Hewlett-Packard Medical Inst., Waltham, Mass.
**Statham Inst., Inc., Oxnard, Cal.
***MFE Corp., Salem, N.H.

(A) Active Function: After obtaining a hermetic seal in the external canal, 200 mm H_2O of positive pressure+ was applied in the ME (inflation). The subject was then instructed to swallow water to equilibrate. The pressure remaining in the ME following five consecutive swallows without a pressure change is termed the residual positive pressure (SWA+). Then -200 mm H_2O was applied in the ME (deflation) and the patient was instructed to swallow. The pressure remaining in the ME following this test is termed the residual negative pressure (SWA-2).

(B) Passive and Active Function: The ME was inflated with a constant flow of air (flow rate 6 cc/min) until the tube spontaneously opened, at which time the syringe pump was manually stopped. The first passive opening of the ET by ME overpressure is termed the opening pressure (OP1). Following discharge of air through the ET, the tube closed passively without a further decay in ME pressure. This pressure is called the closing pressure (CL1). Then the patient was instructed to swallow water for further equilibration. The residual pressure following passive closing and swallowing is termed CL1+. The minimum residual positive pressure (MIN+) is the lowest recorded pressure remaining in the ME after the active and passive equilibration of ME overpressure (lowest value of CL1+ and SWA+).

(C) Toynbee's Maneuver: Active function of the ET during closed-nose swallowing was assessed by applying a positive pressure of 200 mm H_2O in the ME and manually compressing the unattached naris. The opposite naris was connected to the pressure transducer in order to record the nasal pressure developed during closed-nose swallowing. The residual postive pressure remaining in the ME after closed-nose swallowing (TOY+) was

determined. Next, the ME pressure was reduced to -200 mm H_2O. The residual negative pressure remaining following closed-nose swallowing (TOY-2) was noted.

(D) Valsalva's Test: The passive opening of the ET by nasopharyngeal overpressure (VALS) was determined by instructing the subject to blow against the closed-nose—Valsalva's Maneuver—while the ME pressure was ambient. The nasopharynx pressure corresponding to the first detectable change in ME pressure was taken as the nasopharyngeal opening pressure of the ET.

Results

Figure 157 is a summary of the active function test results for SWA-2, TOY-2, SWA+, TOY+, CL1+, and for Valsalva's test (VALS) for the four groups. "Yes" indicates the change in ME pressure independent of magnitude, and "No" indicates unchanged ME pressure. Active function for the five variables was absent in all ears in Group-CHOL, but was present in all ears in Group-TR-PERF. In addition, CL1+ and TOY-2 were absent in all ears in Group-RET-ADOM and Group-RET-ATEL. Figure 158 shows that as a group, Group-TR-PERF had lower residual negative pressure (SWA-2) than the other three Groups. The minimum residual positive pressure (MIN+) values were greater for Groups-CHOL, RET-ADOM, and RET-ATEL than for Group-TR-PERF, though only the difference between Group-CHOL and Group-TR-PERF was statistically significant at the 5% level of confidence. Although, Figure 159 gives the impression that many of the ears in Groups-CHOL, RET-ADOM and RET-ATEL had opening pressure (OP1) values that were either higher or lower than those in Group-TR-PERF, this was not statistically significant.

+All pressures are in reference to atmospheric (ambient) pressure.

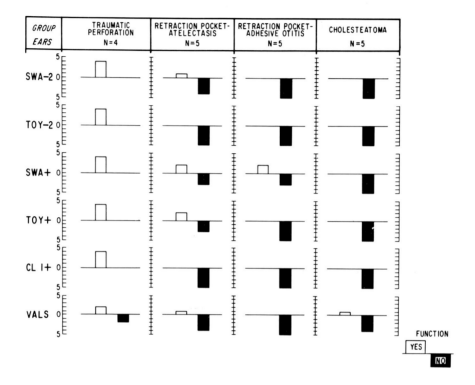

Fig. 157: Active function and Valsalva's test results for the four groups. The variables are defined as: equilibration of applied negative middle ear pressure by open-nose swallowing (SWA−2) and closed-nose swallowing (TOY−2), equilibration of applied positive middle ear pressure by open-nose swallowing (SWA+) and closed-nose swallowing (TOY+), equilibration of middle ear pressure after closing pressure by open-nose swallowing (CL1+), and passive opening of the eustachian tube by nasopharyngeal over-pressure—Valsalva's test—(VALS). Yes indicates change in middle ear pressure independent of magnitude, and no indicates unchanged middle ear pressures.

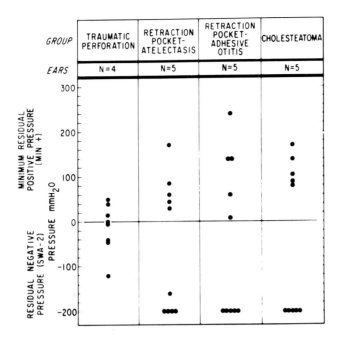

Fig. 158: Minimum residual positive pressure (MIN+) and residual negative pressure (SWA–2) values for the four groups.

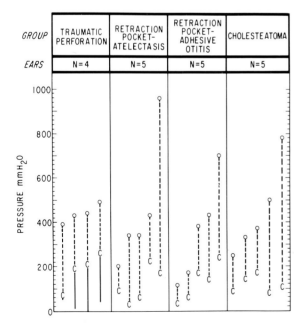

Fig. 159: Active/passive eustachian tube function test findings. Passive function is noted by opening pressure (O=OP1), pressure drop following opening (broken line) and closing pressure (C=CL1). The magnitude of equilibration by active function following passive closing is noted by solid line (CL1+ < CL1). Note that only traumatic perforation group had this function.

There was no difference in closing pressures (CL1) between the four groups. However, only ears in Group-TR-PERF had active function after passive closure of the eustachian tube (CL1+ CL1). (See Table 51 for statistical significance levels.)

Discussion
Interpretation of Function Test Findings

The four patients in Group-TR-PERF who had traumatic perforation of the TM, but who otherwise had negative otologic histories were assumed to have normal ET function as assessed by the inflation-deflation technique. In comparison, the five patients in Group-CHOL, had evidence of functional obstruction of the ET, since all five ears demonstrated the following findings: (1) failure to equilibrate applied positive or negative ME pressure by active function, (2) presence of an opening pressure, (3) closing pressures within normal range, and (4) failure to further equilibrate by active function after passive closing of the ET. If intrinsic or extrinsic mechanical obstruction had

TABLE 51

**Levels of Significance with Respect
To Difference from Group-TR-PERF**

	Variable Name	Group		
		Ret-Atel	Ret-Adom	Chol
DISCRETE VARIABLES*	SWA-2	+	+ +	+ +
	TOY-2	+ +	+ +	+ +
	SWA+	NS	NS	+ +
	TOY+	NS	+ +	+ +
	CL1+	+ +	+ +	+ +
	VALS	NS	NS	NS
CONTINUOUS VARIABLES**	OP1	NS	NS	NS
	CL1	NS	NS	NS
	MIN+	NS	NS	+ +
	SWA-2	+ + +	+ + +	+ + +

NS	NOT SIGNIFICANT
+	SIGNIFICANT $(P < .05)$
+ +	SIGNIFICANT $(P < .01)$
+ + +	SIGNIFICANT $(P < .001)$
*	FISHER'S EXACT PROBABILITY TEST
**	ONE WAY ANALYSIS OF VARIANCE (F-TEST)

Note: SWA-2 is evaluated both as a discrete and as a continuous variable been present, the passive opening and closing pressures would have been either absent or extremely high. However, in other patients with CHOL the finding of mechanical ET obstruction would not be surprising since extension of the disease process into the ME portion of the ET could cause partial or total intrinsic obstruction. The subjects in this study were selected because of the lack of CHOL or mucous membrane disease in that area of the ME. Mechanical ET obstruction might also have been present in their ears, if the disease had been allowed to progress. Anatomic obstruction at the nasopharyngeal end of the ET could be a remote possibility in some patients with acquired CHOL, but this finding was not present in the subjects tested. The patients in this study who were designated as having either adhesive otitis media or atelectasis with a retraction pocket, were also found to have functional ET obstruction, but in a few ears the condition did not appear as severe as in those with CHOL.

Active function following deflation of the ME, when present, usually indicates good ET function, but failure to equilibrate applied negative pressure may not indicate poor function since the tube may have been "locked" (Bluestone and Beery, 1976). Even though all four ears in Group-TR-PERF, in this investigation, could partially or totally equilibrate applied negative pressure, this function has been shown to be absent in previous studies of similar patients (Cantekin, et al, 1976). In the absence of function to applied negative pressure, active function following passive opening and closing of the ET (CL1+ < CL1) may be a better indicator of ET function.

Pathogenetic Implications

Functional obstruction of the ET has been described in children who have had recurrent acute otitis media and chronic middle ear effusions (Cantekin, et al, 1976; Bluestone, et al, 1976; and Bluestone and Beery, 1974), and now documented in patients with an attic or posterosuperior retraction pocket of the TM with either atelectasis or adhesive otitis media, as well

as those with acquired CHOL. This type of obstruction appears to be the result of an inefficient active tubal opening mechanism, or increased tubal compliance, or both (Bluestone, et al, 1972). In this investigation, all of the subjects with retraction pockets had had otoscopic and tympanometric evidence of high ME negative pressure or ME effusion prior to insertion of the ventilation tubes. In some cases the presence of high negative pressure appeared to be persistent. However, the assessment of ME air pressure by tympanometry may not be valid for a severely retracted flaccid TM. Nevertheless in many of these cases, high negative ME pressure was a common finding in the contralateral ear where the TM was not as severely affected. From these preliminary findings, Bezold's (1890) and Wittmaack's (1933) Theory of the pathogenesis of CHOL appears to be supported. In addition, the five patients with CHOL had tympanometric evidence that the TM was intact. What appeared to be a perforation with the operating microscope was actually a deep sac which was not open to the rest of the ME cavity.

Figure 160 describes the proposed chain of

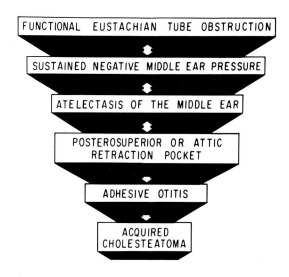

Fig. 160: Schematic representation of chain of events in the development of an acquired cholesteatoma.

events in the pathogenesis of acquired CHOL as derived from the previously proposed hypothesis and from our studies of ET function in children and adults. The basic problem would appear to be functional obstruction of the ET which is severe enough to cause sustained negative ME pressure which, in turn, causes atelectasis of the ME and retraction of the TM. Periodic ME ventilation would occur by either gradient assisted active opening or passive opening of the ET by the gradient alone. This type of ME ventilation would tend to stretch the tympanic membrane thus increasing its compliance. Elner, et al (1971) showed that highly compliant tympanic membranes were associated with reduced ET function. A highly compliant tympanic membrane would tend to collapse even when relatively normal middle ear pressures are present. Khanna and Tonndorf (1972) using time-averaged holography showed the pars flaccida and posterosuperior quadrant are the most compliant portions of the TM. A deep retraction pocket in either of these areas would occur even in the presence of modest amounts of negative ME pressure if the TM was floppy. When the retraction pocket is associated with atelectasis of the ME, the condition may be reversed by a ME ventilation tube. This has previously been reported by Buckingham and Ferrer (1966) who documented, with serial photographs, the return of posterosuperior retraction pockets to the neutral position following the insertion of tympanostomy tubes. However, if adhesive otitis media is present, the retraction pocket may not be reversible and could progress into an acquired CHOL.

Management

Since management of the basic problem, functional ET obstruction, in patients with deep retraction pockets and atelectasis appears to be obscure at present, methods to alleviate the persistent ME negative pressure will be necessary to prevent progression of the disease process. Middle ear inflation techniques, e.g., Polizerization and Valsalva's maneuver, may occasionally be helpful, but in most instances middle ear ventilation tubes will be required. If the retraction pocket is associated with adhesive otitis media in which the TM does not return to normal following the insertion of ventilating tubes, then the patient should be considered "at risk" of developing a CHOL and reconstructive ear surgery may be indicated. When CHOL is present reconstructive surgery including tympanoplasty may be successful, depending upon the ET function. If ET function is poor, recurrence of the atelectasis, retraction pocket and CHOL is a distinct possibility. If a radical mastoidectomy is elected to eradicate the CHOL in a patient with poor ET function then attempts should be made to close the ME end of the ET to prevent reflux of nasopharyngeal secretions.

Conclusions

Functional obstruction of the eustachian tube appears to be the basic abnormality associated with acquired cholesteatoma and with the pathologic tympanic membrane-middle ear conditions related to its development.

Acknowledgements

The authors wish to thank Pamela DeMezza, R.N., and Linda Barto, R.N., who provided technical assistance during the project, and Nancy Gumm and Gayle Tissue, who provided assistance in the preparation of the manuscript.

References

1. Bezold, F.: Cholesteatoma, perforation of Shrapnell's membrane and occlusion of the tubes, an aetiological study (trans. from German) *Arch. Otol.* *N.Y.*, 19:232, 1890, by J. A. Spalding.

2. Bluestone, C. D.; Paradis, J. L.; and Berry, Q. C.: Physiology of the eustachian tube in the

pathogenesis and management of middle ear effusions. *Laryngoscope*, 82: 1654, 1972.

3. Bluestone, C. D.; Berry, Q. C.; and Andrus, W. S.: Mechanics of the eustachian tube as it influences susceptibility to and persistence of middle ear effusions in children. *Ann. Otol., Rhinol., Laryngol., Suppl.* 11, 83:27, 1974.

4. Bluestone, C. D. and Berry, Q. C.: Concepts in the pathogenesis of middle ear effusions. *Ann. Otol., Rhinol. Laryngol., Suppl.* 25, 85: 182, 1976.

5. Bluestone, C. D.; Cantekin, E. I.; and Berry, Q. C.: Effect of inflammation on the ventilatory function of the eustachian tube. Accepted for publication, *Laryngoscope*, 1976.

6. Buckingham, R. A. and Ferrer, J. L.: Reversibility of chronic adhesive otitis media with polyethylene tube, middle ear air-vent, Kodachrome time lapse study. *Laryngoscope*, 76:993-1014, 1966.

7. Cantekin, E. I.; Bluestone, C. D.; and Parkin, L.: Eustachian tube ventilatory function in children. *Ann. Otol., Rhinol., Laryngol., Suppl.* 25, 85:171, 1976.

8. Day, K. M.: Primary pseudocholesteatoma of the ear. *Arch. Otolaryngol.*, 34:1144, 1941.

9. Diamant, M.: *Chronic Otitis. A Critical Analysis.* S. Karger, New York, New York, 1952.

10. Elner, A.; Ingelstedt, S.; and Ivarsson, A.: The elastic properties of the tympanic membrane system. *Acta Otolaryngol.*, 72:397, 1971.

11. Habermann, J.: Zur Entstehung Des Cholesteatoms Des Mittelohrs (Cysten in der Schleimhaut der Paukenhohle, Atrophie der Nerven in der Schnecke). *Arch. f. Ohrenh.* (Leipz), 27:42, 1888.

12. Hellman, K.: Studien Über Das Sekundäre Cholesteatom Des Felsenbeins. *Ztschr. Hals-,*

Nasen-u. Ohrenh., 11:406, 1925.

13. Khanna, S. M. and Tonndorf, J.: Tympanic membrane vibrations in cats studied by time-averaged holography. *J. Acoust. Soc. Am.*, 51:1904, 1972.

14. Lange, W.: Tief Eingezogene Membrana Flaccida Und Cholesteatom. *Ztschr. f. Hals-, Nasen-u. Ohrenh.*, 30:575, 1932.

15. McGuckin, F.: Concerning the pathogenesis of destructive ear disease. *J. Laryngol. Otol.*, 75:949, 1961.

16. McKenzie, D.: The pathogeny of aural cholesteatoma. *J. Laryngol., Otol.*, 46:163, 1931.

17. Nager, F.: The cholesteatoma of the middle ear. *Ann. Otol., Rhinol., Laryngol.*, 34:1249, 1925.

18. Ojala, L. and Saxen, A.: Pathogenesis of middle-ear cholesteatoma arising from Shrappnell's membrane (attic cholesteatoma). *Acta Otolaryngol. (Stockh) Suppl.* 100: 33, 1952.

19. Ruedi, L.: Acquired cholesteatoma. *Arch. Otolaryngol.*, 78:252, 1963.

20. Shambaugh, G.: *Surgery of the Ear.*, W. B. Saunders Co., Philadelphia, Pennsylvania, 1967.

21. Teed, R. W.: Cholesteatoma verum tympani. Its relationship to first epibranchial placode. *Arch. Otolaryngol.*, 24:455, 1936.

22. Tumarkin, A.: A contribution to the study of middle-ear suppuration with special reference to the pathogeny and treatment of cholesteatoma. *J. Laryngol.*, 53:685, 1938.

23. Tumarkin, A.: Attic suppuration, *J. Laryngol., Otol.*, 64:611, 1950.

24. Wittmaack, K.: Wie Ensteht Ein Genuines Cholesteatom? *Arch. f. Ohren-Nasen-u. Kehlkopfh.*, 137:306, 1933.

Chapter 8

Evaluation
of
Surgical Procedures for Cholesteatoma

MASTOIDECTOMY FOR ACQUIRED CHOLESTEATOMA: LONG-TERM RESULTS

D. Thane R. Cody, M.D., Ph.D.
William F. Taylor, Ph.D.

The primary consideration in the treatment of acquired cholesteatoma is the eradication of the disease. Of importance, but less so, is leaving the patient with an ear that provides socially adequate hearing and is easy to care for.

There are three surgical approaches to the management of acquired cholesteatoma in the middle ear cleft. First, there are the classic mastoidectomies, which will be referred to as the "open cavity group." These operations consist of the modified radical mastoidectomy and the radical mastoidectomy. Second, there are the modified radical mastoidectomy and the radical mastoidectomy with obliteration of the mastoid cavity by use of pedicle muscle grafts and other materials. These operations will be referred to as the "obliterated cavity group." Third, there are the mastoidectomies that preserve the posterior and superior bony external auditory canal walls. These operations are the simple mastoidectomy and the simple mastoidectomy with opening of the facial recess. They will be referred to as the "intact canal wall group."

All three surgical approaches have their proponents. Baron and Beales (Derlacki, et al, 1969) have advocated leaving an open mastoid cavity when the cholesteatoma has invaded the epitympanum and mastoid process. They believe that, with the obliterated cavity mastoidectomy or the intact canal wall mastoidectomy, there is a great danger of masking or hiding residual cholesteatoma or of recurrent cholesteatoma developing. These otologists have provided evidence indicating that, with the closed cavity mastoidectomies, residual or recurrent cholesteatoma may not become evident until 10 years or more after opera-

tion. Beales (Derlacki, et al, 1969) has shown that, because the cholesteatoma is often hidden with these types of mastoidectomies, the first indication of residual or recurrent cholesteatoma may be a serious complication, such as facial nerve paralysis or a horizontal semicircular canal fistula. Baron (Derlacki, et al, 1969) has pointed out that most mastoid cavities only require minimal care and that this is a small price to pay for the best chance of eradicating a potentially serious disease.

Rambo (1969) and Palva (1962) are proponents of obliterating mastoid cavities by use of pedicle muscle grafts. Rambo (1969) believes that the posterior and superior bony external auditory canal walls must be removed in order to adequately eradicate disease in the middle ear cleft. However, he found that obliterating the mastoid cavity with muscle grafts reduces postoperative cavity care and the incidence of cavity infection and drainage.

Corgill and Storrs (1967) and Sheehy (Derlacki, et al, 1969) are strong proponents of the intact canal wall mastoidectomy. These otologists believe that, with intact canal wall operations, there is only a small chance of residual or recurrent cholesteatoma. They believe that this risk is offset by little or no postoperative ear care, no problems associated with getting water in the ear, and a better chance of successfully reconstructing the transformer mechanism of the middle ear than with other types of mastoid operations.

To date there has not been a satisfactory comparison of the results that are achieved with these three surgical approaches to the management of acquired cholesteatoma. Most analyses of results obtained with these operations have dealt with chronic suppurative otitis media, in general lumping together inactive disease, chronic infection without cholesteatoma, and cholesteatoma. In addition, when comparisons of the results achieved with these different surgical approaches have been made, usually different operations performed during different eras of otologic surgery are compared. And finally, there are essentially no long-term results reported after these surgical approaches, with the exception of the open cavity group. Sheehy (Derlacki, et al, 1969) drew attention to the latter problem when he stated that only 52% of his patients who had a mastoidectomy for chronic suppurative otitis media had a successful postoperative five-year follow-up.

Many otologists use all three of the surgical approaches under discussion in the management of chronic suppurative otitis media, the method chosen depending on the specific disease. For instance, if there is a pneumatized mastoid process, the surgeon performs an intact canal wall mastoidectomy, whereas if there is a sclerotic mastoid process and an attic defect, an open cavity mastoidectomy or an obliterated cavity mastoidectomy is used (Farrior, 1969). The problem is that no one describes how often a pneumatized mastoid process is encountered with chronic suppurative otitis media and more specifically with acquired cholesteatoma.

The purposes of this analysis of the surgical treatment of acquired cholesteatoma were: first, to define the pathologic changes in the middle ear cleft that are associated with acquired cholesteatoma; second, to compare the results achieved with open cavity, obliterated cavity, and intact canal wall mastoidectomies performed during the same period so that the operative techniques would be relatively uniform; and third, to compare long-term results achieved with these three surgical approaches.

Methods

In order to compare the results of the various types of mastoidectomies used in the treatment of acquired cholesteatoma, the operations performed between January 1, 1963, and December 31, 1969, were studied. This period was chosen because there was the opportunity to follow all patients after surgery for at least four years and the surgical techniques employed were fairly well-standardized. By the latter statement is meant that, in all operations, the operating microscope, electric drill, and continuous suction and irrigation during the drilling were used. Furthermore, during the seven years, the three surgical approaches that were employed in the management of acquired cholesteatoma were: the open cavity mastoidectomy, the obliterated cavity mastoidectomy, and the intact canal wall mastoidectomy. The open cavity mastoidectomies included the classic modified radical and the radical. The obliterated cavity mastoidectomies included the modified radical and the radical. In this group only those patients were included in whom the mastoid cavity was obliterated with pedicle muscle grafts. Occasionally, the pedicle grafts were supplemented by free autogenous muscle grafts. The intact canal wall mastoidectomies included the simple mastoidectomy and the simple mastoidectomy with opening of the facial recess. In most of the intact canal wall mastoidectomies, Silastic sheeting was used to maintain aeration between the middle ear and the mastoid cavity, and thus avoid retraction pockets.

Included in the analysis of results were patients who had been followed up for four years or longer after operation or those whose operation had failed to eradicate disease during the first four postoperative years.

Results

Between January 1, 1963, and December 31, 1969, 473 mastoidectomies that met the outlined criteria were performed for acquired cholesteatoma at the Mayo Clinic.

The Middle Ear Cleft and Acquired Cholesteatoma: The 473 ears with acquired cholesteatoma were studied to determine the pathologic changes in the middle ear cleft that are associated with acquired cholesteatoma. When classified by defect,

389 (82%) of the ears had an attic defect (with or without a tympanic membrane perforation), 65 (14%) had a marginal or total tympanic membrane perforation, and 19 (4%) had a central tympanic membrane perforation. Classification by mastoid process revealed that 323 (68%) were extremely sclerotic, 87 (19%) had a postoperative mastoid cavity, and 63 (13%) were reasonably well pneumatized. Thus, acquired cholesteatoma is usually associated with an attic defect and a sclerotic mastoid process. These pathologic changes in the middle ear cleft are strongly suggestive of inadequate eustachian tube function.

Mastoidectomy: Of the 473 patients, one died of unrelated causes seven months after the operation and 49 have been lost to follow-up. Therefore, 50 (11%) patients are not included in the analysis of results, leaving a total of 423 (89%) patients in the study (Table 52). The near equality of the percentage of patients studied for all surgical groups in-

TABLE 52

Number of Patients Studied, Months Followed
and
Patient Failures by Detailed Type of Surgery*

Characteristics	Type of surgery (both primary and revision)									Total
	Open cavity			Obliterated cavity			Intact canal wall			
	Modified radical	Radical	Total	Modified radical	Radical	Total	Simple	Simple open facial recess	Total	
Patients										
Total	148	42	190	68	22	90	75	118	193	473
Lost to follow-up										
No.	13	5	18	8	2	10	6	16	22	50
%			9			11			11	11
Studied										
No.	135	37	172	60	20	80	69	102	171	423
%	91	88	91	88	91	89	92	86	89	89
Months followed †	10,687	2,942	13,629	4,544	1,772	6,316	3,122	4,699	7,821	27,766
Mean	79.2	79.5	79.2	75.7	88.6	79.0	30.6	68.1	45.7	65.6
Maximum	142	135	142	147	150	150	115	120	120	150
Failures										
No.	25	6	31	17	6	23	46	56	102	156
% failures among pt studied	19	16	18	28	30	29	67	55	60	37
Failure rate/1,000 mo	2.3	2.0	2.3	3.7	3.4	3.6	14.7†	11.9†	13.0†	5.6
% failures within 4 yr	14	14	14	23	20	22	54†	47†	50†	30

dicates that there was no appreciable bias due to these losses. The mean total postoperative follow-up for the 423 patients was seven years, with a range of seven to 150 months (Table 53). (Follow-up shown in Table 52 refers only to "failure-free" intervals.) The follow-up for the intact canal wall group was less, making it necessary to use "failure rates" and "% failures in four years" in comparing various subgroups (Table 52).

Of 423 patients, 348 (82%) underwent primary operations and 75 (18%) had revision mastoidectomies (Table 54).

TABLE 53

Type of Mastoid Operations and Follow-up in 423 Cases of Cholesteatoma

| | | Postop follow-up* (mo) | | Operations | | | |
| | | | | Primary | | Revision | |
Mastoidectomy	No.	Mean	Range	No.	%	No.	%
Open cavity	172	92	34 to 142	141	82	31	18
Obliterated cavity	80	96	26 to 150	55	69	25	31
Intact canal wall	171	70	7 to 139	152	89	19	11
Total	423	84	7 to 150	348	82	75	18

Table 53: *Operations at Mayo Clinic for acquired cholesteatoma, January 1, 1963 to December 31, 1969. †Time from initial observation to failure or to time last known to be free from failure. †Significantly ($P < 0.01$) greater failure among patients with intact canal wall surgery.

TABLE 54

Mastoidectomy Failures and Failure Rates by Type of Mastoidectomy, for Recurrent and Residual Cholesteatomas

| | | Failures due to cholesteatoma | | | | | | | |
| | No. of | Recurrent | | Residual | | Recurrent and residual | | Total | |
Mastoidectomy	patients	No.	Rate*	No.	Rate*	No.	Rate*	No.	Rate*
Open cavity	172	3	0.22	8	0.59	0	0	11	0.81
Obliterated cavity	80	3	0.47	8	1.3	2	0.32	13	2.1
Intact canal wall	171	29	3.7	19	2.4	12	1.5	60	7.7
Total	423	35	1.3	35	1.3	14	0.5	84	3.0

Table 54: Follow-up is total period that patient was under observation. See footnote to Table 53 for a different definition used for purposes of risk measurement.

Mastoidectomy Failures

There were four causes of mastoidectomy failure. The first and most serious cause was recurrent or residual (or both) cholesteatoma. The second cause of failure we refer to as "precholesteatoma." This consists of the development of an attic defect or, when the facial recess has been surgically opened, a facial recess retraction pocket or a retraction pocket in both these regions. The retraction pocket may or may not be associated with tympanic membrane graft failure and infection. The third cause of failure was chronic or frequent recurrent infection, with or without tympanic membrane graft failure, not associated with precholesteatoma or cholesteatoma. The fourth cause of failure was tympanic membrane graft failure without infection, precholesteatoma, or cholesteatoma.

Thirty-one (18%) of the 172 open cavity mastoidectomies were failures, which occurred during 13,629 months at risk. The failure rate* was 2.3 per 1,000 months. Twenty-three (29%) of the 80 obliterated cavity mastoidectomies failed, with a rate of 3.6 per 1,000 months, and 102 (60%) of the 171 intact canal wall mastoidectomies failed with a rate of 13.0 per 1,000 months. The large differences in failure rates between the intact canal wall group (13.0) and the open cavity and obliterated cavity groups (2.3 and 3.6) were statistically significant ($P < 0.01$). The small difference between the open cavity group and the obliterated cavity group was not significant.

The percentage of mastoidectomies that failed by the fourth postoperative year is shown in Table 52. All patients in the analysis had been followed up to this time or their mastoidectomy had failed before the fourth postoperative year. The differences between the open cavity group and intact canal wall group and between the obliterated cavity group and the intact canal wall group were significant ($P < 0.01$).

The percentages of patients still free from failure by years after surgery for the three groups and their subgroups are shown in Figure 161. The failure rates are represented by the slopes of the curves; steeper curves signify greater failure. The obliterated cavity group had significantly greater failure ($P < 0.05$) than the open cavity group only in the first postoperative year; thereafter, the failure rates were nearly equal.

The failure of mastoidectomy for acquired cholesteatoma was lowest among the open cavity operations and highest among the intact canal wall operations. The risk of failure was high for three to five years for the intact canal wall group, and it only leveled off after these times. The other

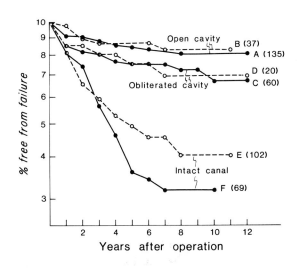

Fig. 161: Percentage of patients free from failure by years after mastoidectomy for acquired cholesteatoma. A = modified radical mastoidectomy. B = radical mastoidectomy. C = modified radical mastoidectomy with obliteration of the cavity with muscle. D = radical mastoidectomy with obliteration of the cavity with muscle. E = simple mastoidectomy with opening of the facial recess. F = simple mastoidectomy.

---

*Failure rate is the ratio of number of failures to number of person-months at risk. It is used here because exposure times differed markedly.

groups' failures occurred steadily but at low rates for 10 years (except the primary obliterated cavity group, which had a high risk during the first year, followed by low risk thereafter).

The differences in results between the modified radical mastoidectomies and the radical mastoidectomies in the open cavity group and in the obliterated cavity group were very small and not significant. For the intact canal wall group, the failure rate was somewhat higher with the simple mastoidectomies than with the simple mastoidectomies and opening of the facial recess, but this difference was not significant.

Failure Due to Cholesteatoma: Recurrent or residual (or both) cholesteatoma was the cause of failure in 11 (6%) of the open cavity mastoidectomies (failure rate 0.81 per 1,000 months at risk), 13 (16%) of the obliterated cavity mastoidectomies (2.1 per 1,000 months), and 60 (35%) of the intact canal wall mastoidectomies (7.7 per 1,000 months) (Table 54). The failure rate due to cholesteatoma in the intact canal wall group was approximately four times that in the obliterated cavity group and nine times that in the open cavity group. Table 54 also shows the failure rates due separately to recurrent and to residual cholesteatoma in these three groups. Sheehy (Derlacki, et al, 1969) and Corgill and Storrs (1967) have stated that the chance of recurrent cholesteatoma is low with the intact canal wall mastoidectomies, which is contrary to our findings. Among the 60 cholesteatoma failures in the intact canal wall group, recurrent cholesteatoma or both recurrent and residual cholesteatoma occurred in 41 (68%) as opposed to five (38%) of the 13 in the obliterated cavity group, and three (27%) of the 11 in the open cavity group. Eight (73%) of the cholesteatoma failures in the open cavity group were due to residual cholesteatoma. This occurred as a result of leaving epithelium in the tympanic cavity or performing inadequate mastoidectomy.

Failure Due to Precholesteatoma: Precholesteatoma in the form of an attic retraction pocket or a facial recess retraction pocket or both, with or without infection and with or without

tympanic membrane graft failure, as would be expected, did not occur in the open cavity group. It occurred in only two (3%) of the obliterated cavity group and in 34 (20%) of the intact canal wall group (Table 55). The postoperative development of attic and facial recess retraction pockets was encountered almost exclusively in the intact canal wall group. These retraction pockets often caused considerable difficulty in the postoperative care. Nineteen of the 34 retraction pockets in the intact canal wall group were associated with chronic or recurrent infection. Occasionally, the pocket became so large that the ear had the appearance of a poorly performed open cavity mastoidectomy and was difficult to clean.

The term "precholesteatoma" for retraction pocket mastoidectomy failure has proved to be appropriate. Many of the cholesteatoma failures in the intact canal wall group originally only had retraction pockets and then later developed cholesteatoma. And since this analysis was completed, at least one intact canal wall mastoidectomy classified as a precholesteatoma failure later developed recurrent cholesteatoma.

Failure Due to Infection: Chronic or frequent actue infections with or without tympanic membrane graft failure but without retraction pockets or cholesteatoma occurred in 14 (8%) of the open cavity group, three (4%) of the obliterated cavity group, and none of the intact canal wall group (Table 55). However, troublesome infection actually was most frequently encountered in the intact canal wall group but always was associated with precholesteatoma or cholesteatoma. Nevertheless, infection by itself was the most common cause of failure in the open cavity group.

Tympanic Membrane Graft Failure: The patients with radical mastoidectomies did not have tympanic membrane perforations repaired so they are not included in this portion of the analysis. Tympanic membrane graft failure without infection, retraction pockets, or cholesteatoma occurred in six (4%) of the patients with modified radical mastoidectomies, five (8%) of those with modified radical mastoidectomies with obliteration of the mastoid cavity, and eight (5%) of those in the intact canal wall group (Table 55). The incidence of tympanic membrane graft failure without other complications was small and similar in the three groups. However, if all mastoidectomy failures are considered, the actual overall incidence of graft failure was the highest in the intact canal wall group. Because this was the most minor cause of mastoidectomy failure and because we (Cody and Taylor, 1973) previously reported long-term results of myringoplasty, we did not analyze

graft failures further.

Primary Versus Revision Operations: The results achieved with primary and revision mastoidectomies were compared. Revision operation involved 18% of the open cavity mastoidectomies, 31% of the obliterated cavity mastoidectomies, and 11% of the intact canal wall mastoidectomies (Table 53). Most revision procedures were second attempts, although some were third procedures.

The failure rates for primary and revision

TABLE 55

Number of Patients by Type of Mastoidectomy and Reason for Failure

Mastoidectomy	No.	Reason for failure							
		Cholesteatoma		Precholesteatoma		Infection		Graft failure	
		No.	%	No.	%	No.	%	No.	%
Open cavity	172								
Modified radical		135	9	7	0	0	10	7	6	4
Radical		37	2	5	0	0	4	11	. . .	. . .
Obliterated cavity	80								
Modified radical		60	8	13	1	2	3	5	5	8
Radical		20	5	25	1	5	0	0	. . .	. . .
Intact canal wall	171								
Simple with opening									
facial recess		102	32	31	18	18	0	0	6	6
Simple		69	28	41	16	23	0	0	2	3

Table 55: *Failure per 1,000 months at risk.

operations in the open cavity group were essentially the same (Table 56, Fig. 162). In the obliterated cavity group, the failure rate was less for the revision operations, and in the intact canal wall group, the failure rate was greater for the revision operations. However, these differences were not statistically significant. The percentage of failures four years after primary operations was significantly greater ($P < 0.01$) in the intact canal group than in the obliterated cavity group and the open cavity group. Results were similar for revision operations.

Pneumatized Versus Sclerotic Mastoid Process: Some otologists (Farrior, 1969) have stated that intact canal wall mastoidectomies should be reserved for patients who have acquired cholesteatomas associated with a pneumatized mastoid process. The assumption is that a pneumatized mastoid process makes the intact canal wall mastoidectomies more feasible and that, when the

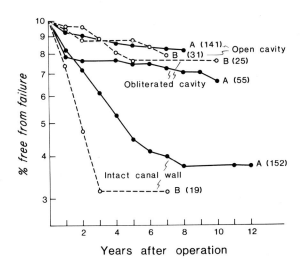

Fig. 162: Percentage of patients free from failure by years after mastoidectomy for acquired cholesteatoma. Primary versus revision operations. A = primary mastoidectomy. B = revision mastoidectomy.

TABLE 56

Number of Patients Studied, Months Followed,
and
Patient Failures by Type of Surgery for Primary and Revision Operations*

| Characteristics | Type of surgery | | | | | | | | | Total |
| | Open cavity | | | Obliterated cavity | | | Intact canal wall | | | |
	Primary	Revision	Total	Primary	Revision	Total	Primary	Revision	Total	
Patients studied	141	31	172	55	25	80	152	19	171	423
Months followed†	11,224	2,405	13,629	4,462	1,854	6,316	7,246	575	7,821	27,766
Mean	80	78	79	81	74	79	48	30	46	65.6
Maximum	142	134	142	150	135	150	120	84	120	150
Failures	25	6	31	17	6	23	89	13	102	156
% of pt studied	18	19	18	31	24	29	59	68	60	37
Rate/1,000 mo	2.2	2.5	2.3	3.8	3.2	3.6	12.3†	22.6†	13.0	5.3
% by 4 yr	14	13	14	24	20	22	47†	68†	50	30

open cavity mastoidectomies are performed on pneumatized mastoids, a large postoperative cavity results, with a greater chance of difficulty during the postoperative period. We have already shown that a well-pneumatized mastoid process is not a common accompaniment of acquired cholesteatoma, being found in only 13% of 473 mastoidectomies. And of the 423 mastoidectomies analyzed, reasonably well pneumatized mastoid processes (Table 57) were noted in only 13 of the open cavity group, 10 of the obliterated cavity group, and 31 of the intact canal wall group. In the remaining group, the mastoids were sclerotic or there was a postoperative mastoid cavity. Since the revision operations (mastoid cavities) already have been analyzed, only the failure rates for the pneumatized and sclerotic mastoid processes were compared (Table 57, Fig. 163). In both the open cavity group and the obliterated cavity group, the

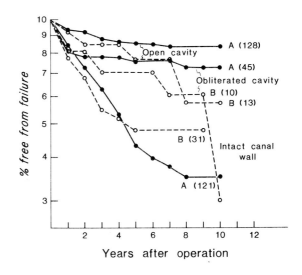

Fig. 163: Percentage of patients free from failure by years after mastoidectomy for acquired cholesteatoma. Pneumatized versus sclerotic mastoid process. A = sclerotic mastoid process. B = pneumatized mastoid process.

TABLE 57

Number of Patients Studied, Months Followed
and
Patient Failures by Type of Surgery for Pneumatized or Sclerotic Cases*

	Type of primary treatment									
	Open cavity			Obliterated cavity			Intact canal wall			
Characteristics	Pneumatized	Sclerotic	Total	Pneumatized	Sclerotic	Total	Pneumatized	Sclerotic	Total	Total
Patients studied	13	128	141	10	45	55	31	121	152	348
Months followed†	895	10,329	11,224	786	3,676	4,462	1,443	5,803	7,246	22,932
Mean	69	81	80	79	82	81	47	48	48	65.9
Maximum	113	142	142	147	150	150	120	120	120	150
Failures	4	21	25	5	12	17	16	73	89	131
% of pt studied	31	16	18	50	26	31	52	60	59	38
Rate/1,000 mo	4.5	2.0	2.2	6.4	3.3	3.8	11.1	12.6†	12.3	5.7
% by 4 yr	15	14	14	30	22	24	48	47†	47	30

Table 57: *Operations at Mayo Clinic for acquired cholesteatoma, January 1, 1963 to December 31, 1969. †Significantly (P < 0.01) greater failure among patients with intact canal wall.

failure rate with a pneumatized mastoid process was almost twice as high (but not significantly so) as with a sclerotic mastoid process. The failure rate was higher (but not significantly) with a pneumatized mastoid process when the cavity was obliterated as compared to when it was left open. In the intact canal wall group, the failure rate with a pneumatized mastoid process was approximately that with a sclerotic mastoid process.

Comment: The most dangerous cause of failure of mastoidectomy for acquired cholesteatoma is either failing to eradicate the cholesteatoma or having the cholesteatoma recur. When postoperative mastoidectomy failures due to cholesteatoma and precholesteatoma were considered together, the incidence rate was 0.81 per 1,000 months at risk for the open cavity group, 2.4 for the obliterated cavity group, and 12.0 for the intact canal wall group. This high incidence of postoperative cholesteatoma and precholesteatoma in the intact canal wall group is disappointing. But, when the basic conditions that are present in the middle ear cleft of these patients are considered, namely, an attic defect or marginal tympanic membrane perforation with a sclerotic mastoid process, it is not surprising that, when the external bony auditory canal walls are left intact, a retraction pocket would develop, with secondary cholesteatoma formation.

Contrary to a commonly held opinion, even in a relatively well pneumatized mastoid process, the chance of failure with the intact canal wall mastoidectomies is only slightly less (and not significantly) than that when the mastoid process is sclerotic. Although with primary intact canal wall mastoidectomies the failure rate is very high, it is even higher with revision intact canal wall operations. Therefore, intact canal wall mastoidectomies should not be used or should be used only under unusual circumstances in the management of acquired cholesteatoma.

In mastoid cavities that were filled with muscle, although the cavities were obliterated immediately after the mastoidectomy, the muscle gradually shrunk with time, and a mastoid cavity developed which was not much smaller than that seen in the open cavity group. There was approximately a threefold increased risk of cholesteatoma or precholesteatoma occurring after obliterated cavity mastoidectomies as compared with the risk after open cavity mastoidectomies. In addition, in the uncommon ear with acquired cholesteatoma that has a relatively well-pneumatized mastoid process, obliterating the cavity with muscle did not decrease the chance of failure as compared with leaving the cavity open. On the contrary, the risk of failure with a pneumatized mastoid process was less in the open cavity group.

Therefore, the open cavity mastoidectomy seems to be the operation of choice in treating acquired cholesteatomas; and mastoid cavity obliteration should be reserved for open cavity mastoidectomy in which mastoid cavity drainage is a significant postoperative problem.

Successful Mastoidectomies

The most frequent criticisms of open cavity mastoidectomies are that they require continuous postoperative care for cleaning of the mastoid cavities of cerumen and epithelial debris and that they are associated with recurrent drainage from the cavities due to superficial infections. Therefore, it was decided to compare the postoperative care required for the open cavity group, the obliterated cavity group, and the intact canal group. The average number of physician-visits per year and the number of acute ear infections or episodes of otorrhea were determined for each group. However, because of the extremely high failure rate in the intact canal wall group, it soon became apparent that this group required far more postoperative care than did the other two groups. Because this did not answer the criticism, the postoperative care required for the successful mastoidectomies in the three groups was compared.

Average Number of Physician-Visits: The average number of physician-visits per year for the successful operations in the three mastoidectomy groups during the postoperative observation period were compared (Table 58). Physician-visits were required once a year or less for 87% of the open cavity group, 93% of the obliterated cavity group, and 97% of the intact canal wall group. These differences were not great and actually show that, as Baron had stressed, successful open cavity mastoidectomies require very little postoperative care. However, the difference in the percentage of mastoidectomies requiring more than one physician-visit per year between the open cavity group (13%) and the intact canal wall group (3%) (Table 58) was statistically significant ($P < 0.02$). However, differences in visits per year between the intact canal wall group and the obliterated cavity group and between the obliterated cavity group and the open cavity group were not statistically significant.

Acute Ear Infections and Otorrhea: The number of acute ear infections and episodes of otorrhea during the postoperative observation period were determined for the successful mastoidectomies in the three groups. The problems did not occur in 66% of the open cavity group, 82% of the obliterated cavity group, and 77% of the intact canal wall group (Table 59). Therefore, fewer mastoidectomy patients in the obliterated cavity group had difficulty with ear infections and otorrhea than did patients in the other two groups, but the differences were not large. However, even a successful intact canal wall mastoidectomy does not assure absence of recurrent acute infections. A comparison of the numbers of ears that had one episode or more of acute infection or otorrhea in each group revealed a statistically significant ($P < 0.02$) difference between the open cavity group and the obliterated cavity group. However, differences between the obliterated cavity group and the intact canal wall group and between the intact canal wall group and the open cavity group were not significant. In ears that had one or more

TABLE 58

Physician-Visits per Year After Successful Mastoidectomies for Cholesteatoma by Type of Mastoidectomy

| Mastoidectomy | No. | Avg visits/yr | | | |
| | | Once or less | | More than once | |
		No.	%	No.	%
Open cavity	141	122	87	19	13*
Obliterated cavity	57	53	93	4	7
Intact canal wall	69	67	97	2	3*

Table 58: *Operations Mayo Clinic for acquired cholesteatoma, January 1, 1963 to December 31, 1969. †Time from initial observation to failure or to time last known to be free from failure. †Significantly (P <0.01) greater failure among patients with intact canal wall (sclerotic cases only).

TABLE 59

Acute Ear Infections and Otorrhea After Successful Mastoidectomies for Cholesteatoma by Type of Mastoidectomy

| Mastoidectomy | No. | Acute ear infections and otorrhea | | | |
| | | None | | One episode or more | |
		No.	%	No.	%
Open cavity	141	93	66	48	34*
Obliterated cavity	57	47	82	10	18*
Intact canal wall	69	53	77	16	23

Table 59: *Significant difference in visits/yr (P<0.02).

acute ear infections or episodes of otorrhea, this occurred during the postoperative observation period only once every two years 11 months in the open cavity group, once every three years in the obliterated cavity group, and once every three years four months in the intact canal wall group. Thus, the frequency of acute infections and otorrhea in those ears that were afflicted with them was similar in the three groups.

Comment: With successful mastoidectomies for acquired cholesteatoma, there is little difference in the postoperative care required for the open cavity group, the obliterated cavity group, and the intact canal wall group. The intact canal group had a statistically significant advantage over the open cavity group regarding the proportion of patients that must visit a physician more than once a year. And the obliterated cavity group had a statistically significant advantage over the open cavity group regarding the number of ears that have one or more episodes of acute infection or otorrhea. However, these small differences in postoperative care are minor considerations compared with the much smaller risk of failure for the open cavity mastoidectomy.

Hearing

Some advocates of intact canal wall mastoidectomies believe that one of its advantages over the open cavity mastoidectomy and the obliterated cavity mastoidectomy is that the hearing results are better. To investigate this assumption, the hearing results of all of the mastoidectomies, with the exception of the radical mastoidectomies, were evaluated. The modified radical mastoidectomies with or without mastoid cavity obliteration were evaluated together and were compared with the intact canal wall group. In analyzing the hearing results, the results of the last preoperative and the last postoperative audiometric tests were compared. The number of ears achieving a mean pure-tone air conduction threshold for the speech frequency range (500, 1,000, and 2,000 Hertz) of 30 decibels (dB) was determined, as were the number

of ears obtaining a closure in the air-bone gap to within 15 dB. A depression in cochlear reserve was considered to have occurred if there was a mean depression in bone-conduction thresholds for the speech frequency range of 10 dB or more, a loss of speech discrimination score of 10% or more, or a combination of these changes.

Only 11% of the modified radical mastoidectomies and 16% of the intact canal wall mastoidectomies resulted in closure of the air-bone gap to within 15 dB (Table 60). This difference was not statistically significant. Seventeen percent of the modified radical mastoidectomies and 26% of the intact canal wall group achieved a 30 dB air conduction level in the speech frequency range; this difference was significant ($P < 0.05$). Therefore, there was small but significant trend for better hearing in the intact canal wall group.

Ten percent of the modified radical mastoidectomies and 15% of the intact canal wall group resulted in depression in cochlear reserve; this difference was not statistically significant. Most depressions in cochlear reserve in these two groups were minor, and a profound sensorineural hearing loss only occurred in 2% of the modified radical mastoidectomies and 1% of the intact canal wall group.

Comment: This analysis revealed that the overall hearing results of mastoidectomy for acquired cholesteatoma were very poor. However, in a large number of the mastoidectomies in each group, no attempt was made to reconstruct a defective ossicular chain, and the operations that failed to eradicate disease or in which there was a recurrence of disease are included. Nevertheless, the analysis shows that the intact canal wall mastoidectomies offer only a slightly better chance of improving hearing and a slightly greater chance of depressing hearing than do the modified radical mastoidectomies. These differences in hearing results indicate that intact canal wall mastoidectomies have no real advantage over the modified radical mastoidectomies in the treatment of acquired cholesteatoma.

TABLE 60

**Hearing Results After Mastoidectomies for Cholesteatoma
by Type of Mastoidectomy**

Mastoidectomy	No.	Air-bone gap closure to within 15 dB		Air-conduction level of 30 dB or better		Sensorineural loss			
						Total with loss		No. with profound loss	
	No.	No.	%	No.	%	No.	%	No.	%
Modified radical with and without cavity obliteration	195	22	11	33	17*	20	10	4	2
Intact canal wall	171	27	16	44	26*	25	15	2	1

Table 60: Significant difference (P < 0.02) in percent episodes of acute ear infections and otorrhea.

Discussion

This study revealed that acquired cholesteatoma is usually associated with an attic defect and a sclerotic mastoid process. Theoretically, these pathologic changes in the middle ear cleft are highly suggestive of underlying eustachian tube dysfunction. Persistent eustachian tube dysfunction would make it impossible for the intact canal wall mastoidectomies to be successful on a long-term basis. Poor eustachian tube function would result in the redevelopment of an attic defect or a facial recess retraction pocket when the recess has been surgically opened and would result in the eventual reformation of a cholesteatoma. Thus, even though an intact canal wall mastoidectomy initially may seem to be successful, because the same factors that gave rise to the acquired cholesteatoma are present, cholesteatoma will recur through a similar mechanism that led to its initial development. This great risk of recurrent cholesteatoma would be added to a significant risk of residual cholesteatoma because of the limitations that the intact canal wall mastoidectomies impose on the surgeon in eradicating disease as compared with the modified radical and radical mastoidectomy.

The present analysis of mastoidectomies for acquired cholesteatoma has substantiated these theoretic considerations. In a series of 171 intact canal wall mastoidectomies, the four year failure rate was 50%. Fifty-five percent of the operations failed because of the development of retraction pockets (precholesteatoma) or cholesteatoma. Even when intact canal wall mastoidectomies were performed on pneumatized mastoid processes, the four year failure rate was 48%, and the failure rate of revision mastoidectomy (68%) was even higher than that of primary operations (47%).

However, the middle ear cleft disease found in the patients in this study theoretically is eminently suited for the modified radical or radical mastoidectomy. The presence of a sclerotic mastoid process should result in a small mastoid cavity requiring minimal postoperative care. Because of good access to the disease in the middle ear cleft and the absence of the opportunity for retraction pockets to develop postoperatively, the risk of failure due to cholesteatoma should be small. If cholesteatoma is the cause of failure, it likely would be due either to residual cholesteatoma left in the middle ear recesses where it is difficult to remove completely or to a less than thorough mastoidectomy.

The present analysis of mastoidectomies for acquired cholesteatoma has borne out these theoretic assumptions. Failure of the open cavity mastoidectomy because of cholesteatoma occurred in 6%, and in 73% of these cases, failure was due to residual cholesteatoma. Precholesteatoma was not a problem. With the open cavity mastoidectomy, the commonest cause of failure was chronic or frequent infection, which occurred in 8%. This confirms the well-known fact that some mastoid cavities give rise to chronic problems. However, the successful open cavity mastoidectomy requires very little more postoperative care than does the successful intact canal wall mastoidectomy or the successful obliterated cavity mastoidectomy. This is a negligible price to pay for an overall chance of failure in four years of 14% compared with 50% for intact canal wall mastoidectomy and 22% for obliterated cavity mastoidectomy (see Table 52).

When a modified radical or radical mastoidectomy is performed on a sclerotic mastoid process, one has to wonder about the necessity or the wisdom of obliterating the resultant small mastoid cavity with muscle. The muscle will gradually degenerate and be replaced by fibrous tissue and thus shrink, and a cavity will eventually result. Theoretically, there would be a smaller chance of chronic cavity drainage with the obliterated cavity mastoidectomies as compared with the open cavity mastoidectomies, but there would also be a greater risk of failure due to cholesteatoma and the development of retraction pockets (precholesteatoma). However, because one has a better operative field with the obliterated cavity mastoidectomies than with the intact canal wall mastoidectomies, the chance of eradicating disease should be better with the former operations than with the latter.

The present analyses of mastoidectomies for acquired cholesteatoma substantiate these theoretic assumptions. There was a three times greater failure rate due to precholesteatoma and cholesteatoma with the obliterated cavity mastoidectomies than with the open cavity mastoidectomies. However, there was almost a three times less chance of failure due to these causes with the obliterated cavity mastoidectomies than with the intact canal wall mastoidectomies. In addition, even when dealing with a pneumatizied mastoid process, the failure rate was less with the open cavity mastoidectomies than with the obliterated cavity mastoidectomies, although these differences were not significant. However, there was a slightly less risk of failure due to cavity infection alone with the obliterated cavity mastoidectomies than with the open cavity mastoidectomies.

The findings in this investigation of the surgical treatment of acquired cholesteatoma have led to certain conclusions. **Because of the underlying middle ear cleft disease associated with acquired cholesteatoma, intact canal wall mastoidectomies will not deal successfully with this disease in a high percentage of cases. Thus, the intact canal wall mastoidectomies ordinarily should not be used in the management of acquired cholesteatoma. Since acquired cholesteatoma is usually associated with a sclerotic mastoid process, and thus there will be a small postoperative mastoid cavity, and since there is a substantial risk of failure of the obliterated cavity mastoidectomies due to precholesteatoma and cholesteatoma, the obliterated cavity mastoidectomies should not be the primary surgical approach in the management of acquired cholesteatoma. However, the open cavity mastoidectomies have an excellent chance of dealing satisfactorily with acquired cholesteatoma and of leaving a small cavity that will require minimal postoperative care. Therefore, the classic open cavity mastoidectomies should be primarily used in the management of acquired cholesteatoma. If postoperative difficulty with the mastoid cavity exists, the cavity can be obliterated with muscle.**

Summary

Long-term results after 423 mastoidectomies for acquired cholesteatoma were analyzed. The mastoidectomies were placed into three groups. The open cavity group consisted of 135 modified radical mastoidectomies and 37 radical mastoidectomies; the obliterated cavity group consisted of 60 modified radical mastoidectomies and 20 radical mastoidectomies in which the mastoid cavities were obliterated with pedicle muscle grafts; and the intact canal wall group consisted of 102 simple mastoidectomies with opening of the facial recess and 69 simple mastoidectomies. The following conclusions were reached:

(1) Acquired cholesteatoma is usually associated with an attic defect and a sclerotic mastoid process.

(2) The overall failure rate was 2.3 per 1,000 months at risk for the open cavity group, 3.6 for the obliterated cavity group, and 13.0 for the intact canal wall group.

(3) Failure rates due to precholesteatoma (retraction pockets) or cholesteatoma were 0.81 per 1,000 months at risk for the open cavity group, 2.4 for the obliterated cavity group, and 12.0 for the intact canal wall group.

(4) When successful mastoidectomies in the three groups were compared, open cavity mastoidectomies required only slightly more postoperative care than did those in the other two groups.

(5) **Open cavity mastoidectomies should be primarily used in the treatment of acquired cholesteatoma.**

References

1. Cody, D. T. R. and Taylor, W. F.: Tympanoplasty: long-term results, *Ann. Otol. Rhinol. Laryngol.*, 82:538, 1973.
2. Corgill, D. A. and Storrs, L. A.: Intact canal wall tympanoplasty: a report of 1000 cases. *Trans. Am. Acad. Ophthal. Otolaryng.*, 71:53, 1967.
3. Derlacki, E. L.; Baron, S. H.; Beales, P. H.; Bellucci, R. J.; Guilford, F. R.; Plester, D.; and Sheehy, J. L.: Round table: selection of closed vs open technique for cholesteatomas. *Arch. Otolaryng.*, 89:211, 1969.
4. Farrior, J. B.: Tympanoplasty (ossicular repositioning in reconstruction): spine of Henle and supporting attic grafts. *Arch. Otolaryng.*, 89:220, 1969.
5. Palva, T.: Reconstruction of ear canal in surgery for chronic ear. *Arch. Otolaryng.*, 75:329, 1962.
6. Rambo, J. H.T.: Musculoplasty for restoration of hearing in chronic suppurative ears. *Arch. Otolaryng.*, 89:184, 1969.

EVALUATION OF SURGERY FOR CHOLESTEATOMA

Claus Jansen, M.D.

The critical evaluation of all techniques for chronic ear surgery raises two essential questions: is complete removal of cholesteatoma possible? Does recurrent cholesteatoma cause complications for the patient?

We have always desired to give the patient a safe ear and with microsurgery, we begin working to restore a functioning ear. The so-called "big and safe" open cavity turned out to be a bad base for reconstructing a functioning sound transforming system. A new era began with all kinds of reanimated, modified, new techniques of reducing the cavity size.

Another alternative was the preservation of the bony wall using a new technique of thinning the posterior bony meatus under microscopical view. There is no doubt that preservation of the meatus is a great advantage, and therefore, it is done in almost all ENT departments of the world. Yet, there is still some doubt whether intact canal technique is sufficient for removal of cholesteatoma. Suspicion is raised by the particularly high rates of recurrences. I would like to have discussed that problem, but unfortunately, the program committee has asked me to "discuss my failures".

The well-known antrostomy or simple or Schwartze mastoidectomy was the canal wall up technique of the last century. Because of the insufficient access to all spaces of the middle ear the posterior bony canal wall was taken down and the open cavity was created. The only way to cut the Gordian knot was to thin the posterior portion of the posterior bony canal wall, which leads automatically to a wide opening into all spaces of the middle ear.

Yet, the thinning caused one of the first and most frequent failures. The technique is sometimes difficult, and in 1958, we perforated the posterior bony wall quite often with the drill. Even a small hole caused a retraction pocket, and it didn't matter in which part of the posterior canal wall the defect was made. The skin retracted into the cavity anyway and the potential risk of a recurrent cholesteatoma was predictable. Covering the defect with any kind of soft tissue usually failed. The retraction pocket occurred somewhat later, but it did occur. Following this, we began partial reconstruction of the posterior bony canal wall with cartilage.

The second failure was trying unsuccessfully to cover a spontaneous attic perforation. Of course, this caused frequent retractions also. Solid cartilage covering still is the best technique in our hands.

Another failure occurred when squamous epithelium grew underneath the posterior bony annulus in the small tympanic cavity of type three tympanoplasty—retracting on top of the mucoperiosteum. From that time on, we preferred to rebuild the new tympanic membrane on the normal level to create a normal-sized tympanic cavity.

A similar failure was the additional enlarging of the meatus close to the posterior bony annulus. Our experience tells us that too large a graft has a tendency to collapse. It gets in firm contact to the promontory and fills the tympanic cavity with squamous epithelium. The bad hearing result is caused by the adherent immobile membrane.

Insufficient thinning particularly in the area of the posterior bony annulus was not a very frequent failure in our hands. It is one of the time-consuming manipulations to open the way to the ossicles. But, especially in cases of an intact ossicular chain, it is an unalterable prerequisite for full eradication of disease. After having had some cases of small pearls of residual cholesteatoma we found the flat angle of view very useful to look underneath the ossicular chain.

Preservation of the ossicular chain at any price is another reason for recurrence. This is not a special problem of the posterior tympanotomy technique but it should be mentioned here. Especially in cases of an epi- and mesotympanal process, cholesteatoma is found on the undersurface of the malleus head. In those ears, the head of the malleus should be removed and of course the remnant part of the incus in most cases.

One of the problems in cholesteatoma surgery is the complete removal of pathological tissue out of the region of the oval window niche, especially if the stapes is intact. Supposing there is additional tympanosclerosis, the potential risk of luxation of the stapes causing a fistula or an inner ear damage is much higher. Unfortunately, no one can prescribe a perfect cure of such a case. In our experience, the second stage operation is advisable. In most of these ears a kind of a pearl was found later which could be removed much more successfully.

Staging is a very important concept for every surgeon who plans to perform intact canal wall operations. In a cholesteatomatous ear, staging can be done to have a "second look" or for later reconstruction of the sound conducting mechanism. For both reasons, a tympanoplasty should be performed at the first stage, for otherwise there is a great risk of squamous epithelium growing in through the perforation. In our experience, we found staging difficult to perform after several years of trying until we introduced posterior tympanotomy in the late fifties. Patients will not return for follow-up if they have no difficulties. We have exerted much effort in the past ten years to follow-up our cases. If there is any suspicion, we perform an endoscopy of the enclosed cavity under local anesthesia. Through the concha, we try at first with a small puncture needle to find the way into the cavity which is very simple following the posterior bony canal wall. Then, with a small trochar, a guiding tube is brought into position. The Ward-Berci pharyngoscope goes with the guiding tube. In the same way, a small ear speculum can be used and the cavity can be inspected by the microscope.

Our first study analyzed our cases followed from 1958 until 1968. In 476 cases, there were 436 with cholesteatoma, 40 with chronically infected ears without cholesteatoma, and five with fistulae in the semicircular system. Of the 476 ears, 455 were moist when they were operated upon, Table 61.

Our 100 patients operated upon from 1969 through 1970, can be followed in Table 62.

In conclusion, the two studies show no significant difference in cholesteatoma recurrence. The rate of recurrent chronic middle ear disease is higher in the second studies than in the first, but there are more dry perforations in the first than in the second. The two facial palsy patients and one partial palsy were the only severe complications. The rate of inner ear damage was higher in the second study.

It is interesting that in the second study, cholesteatoma recurrence took three, four, or five years to recur which gives another reason to follow up patients for at least five years.

TABLE 61

Cases Followed from 1958-1968

Rate of recurrence

Recurrent cholesteatoma	14	(3%)
Recurrent continuous secretion	7	(1.5%)
Recurrent dry perforations	32	(7.5%)

Complications

Brain abscess	0
Inner ear damage	6
Facial palsy	2
(full recovery—1 partial recovery—1)	
Other complications	0

Table 61: *Significant difference between types of surgery (P < 0.05).

TABLE 62

100 Cholesteatoma Cases Operated in 1969-1970

Date of Recurrence	1969	1970	1971	1972	1973	1974	1975
Recurrent Disease							
Cholesteatoma	4				1	1	2
Chronic infection	6	3				3	
Wet and dry	6	5				2	
Dry perforation	2	2					
Complications							
Facial palsy	0						
Brain abscess	0						
Labyrinth trauma (hightone)	9						
Recovering inner 6 months	6						
Persisting	3						

(labyrinth trauma only found in older patients 35-65 years of age)

Location of Recurrence							
Postauricular	2						
Attic	1						
Drumhead	1						

POSTOPERATIVE CHOLESTEATOMA

Gordon D. L. Smyth, M.D.

The concept of avoiding an open mastoidectomy cavity when treating cholesteatomatous middle ear disease is the ultimate goal in chronic ear surgery and much effort and ingenuity have been devoted to the achievement of this concept. Most notably in this effort are the introduction of combined approach tympanoplasty (CAT, or intact canal wall operation) by Jansen (1958) which was subsequently popularized by House and Sheehy (1963) and by Corgill and Storrs (1967) among others in North America and on the other hand, the varieties of obliterative technique proposed originally by Mosher (1911) and Popper (1935) and later modernized by Palva (1963), Schuknecht (1963), Guilford (1961), Austin and Sanabria (1962) and Coyle Shea, et al (1972).

Now after 15 years of endeavor we are looking back to see what has been achieved so that we can decide whether to continue with these "closed" operation, whether we can discover modifications which might contribute to their better success or whether if necessary, we should disband them and start afresh.

The purpose of this is to report the incidence of complications arising so far with one of these "closed" operations in 532 cholesteatomatous ears. These operations were performed between January, 1961 and December, 1974. Over 80% have been followed up regularly until the time of this writing.

Four-hundred and thirty-five operations were intended to be single operations, but 101 of these required at least one revision operation because of complications (Table 63) leaving a total of 334 ears operated upon only once. In a further 97 ears, the operation was carried out in more than one stage as a planned staged procedure (Table 64). In many

TABLE 63

Reason for Revision I	Incidence No.	%
Failure to gain adequate hearing	54	12
Failure TM graft	9	2
Recurrent cholesteatoma	32	7
Residual cholesteatoma		
Epitympanum	2	0.5
Mesotympanum	4	1
Reason for Revision II		
Failure to gain adequate hearing	17	4
Failure TM graft	2	0.5
Recurrent cholesteatoma	1	0.25

TABLE 64

Reasons for staging	Incidence	%
Certainty of leaving mesotympanic cholesteatoma	10	13
Certainty of leaving epitympanic cholesteatoma	6	6
Certainty of leaving mastoid cavity cholesteatoma	1	1
Granulations in oval window	27	28
Tympanosclerotic footplate fixation	4	4
"Second look"	49	50

of the "second look" operations there was difficulty in removing parts of the cholesteatoma because of problems with visualization, usually of the sinus tympani or of the deep aspect of the sulcus tympanicus. Nevertheless, in all, the removal of cholesteatoma was considered to be complete at the end of the operation.

The numbers and types of reoperation are summarized in Table 65. All second and third re-examination of the epitympanum were performed in ears with epitympanic cholesteatoma at the immediate prior operation. Although each second examination of the mesotympanum was carried out in ears with immediate prior mesotympanic cholesteatoma, this was not the case in the group of third mesotympanic operations (58 ears) in whom there had been no immediate prior mesotympanic disease.

TABLE 65

Numbers and Types of Reoperations

Second examination epitympanum	(43 Revised + 42 Staged) =	85
Third examination epitympanum	(5 Revised + 7 Staged) =	12
Total		97
Second examination mesotympanum	(101 Revised + 97 Staged) =	198
Third examination mesotympanum	(20 Revised + 38 Staged) =	58
Total		256

Results

Recurrent Cholesteatoma

This complication (often termed retraction pocket) necessitated a revision operation in 38 (7%) of the 435 intended "only once" ears. In addition, static shallow retraction pockets have been detected in six ears, but are not expected to require further surgical treatment.

Residual Cholesteatoma

If all the operations which were staged because of "certainty of leaving behind cholesteatoma" are excluded and if all those cholesteatomatous ears in which the author was certain of having removed cholesteatoma (both staged and revised groups) when it was present in the immediate prior operation (whether it was a second or third procedure) are considered as a "sample", then some evidence of the ability of CAT to eradicate cholesteatoma for this series is available. Analysis of this sample indicates that in 97 ears where the epitympanum and mastoid were re-explored, residual disease was found unexpectedly in 12 (2%). There were also 198 ears in which only the mesotympanum was re-explored and in these, residual disease was discovered unexpectedly in 31 (11%) (Table 66). In no case was there residual cholesteatoma in the mastoid cavity. If this incidence of unexpected residual disease in the sample is added to that which was detected clinically, the total known incidence of residual cholesteatoma so far in this series of 532 CAT operations becomes 3% in the epitympanum, and 6% in the mesotympanum.

It has been stated that cholesteatoma in children has a different pathogenesis from that

TABLE 66

**Cholesteatomatous Complications in Combined
Children and Adult Groups**

Complication	Known incidence			Sample incidence		
	No. of ears	No.	(%)	No. of ears	No.	(%)
Recurrent cholesteatoma	532	38	(7)	—		
Residual cholesteatoma: Epitympanum	532	14	(3)	97	12	(12)
Mesotympanum	532	33	(6)	198	31	(11)

which occurs in the adult (Baron, 1969 and Derlacki, 1973). Because statistical evidence to decide this issue has so far been lacking, the findings for adults are considered separately from those for children (15 years and below) and within each age group the incidence of recurrent and residual disease has been evaluated independently (Table 67).

TABLE 67

	Residual cholesteatoma				Recurrent cholesteatoma	
	Epitympanum		Mesotympanum			
	Number	%	Number	%	Number	%
Children						
All ears	6/79	8	13/79	16		
					7	9
Re-explored ears (with immediate prior cholesteatoma)	6/33	18	13/54	22		
Adults						
All ears	8/453	2	20/453	4		
					31	7
Re-explored ears (with immediate prior cholesteatoma)	6/64	9	18/144	12		

In children, recurrent cholesteatoma has occurred in seven of 79 CAT operations (9%). Residual cholesteatoma in the epitympanum has been detected so far in six ears (8%), but it should be noted that in only one-half have the epitympanum and mastoid been re-explored. If only the operations in which the epitympanum and mastoid were re-examined are considered separately, then the incidence is much greater. Cholesteatoma was found in the epitympanum unexpectedly in 18%. (In two ears it was found twice.) Re-examination of the mesotympanum was routine in every revised and staged operation and residual cholesteatoma was found here unexpectedly in 22% at the second operation.

In adult patients, recurrent cholesteatoma occurred in 31 of 453 ears (7%). Residual cholesteatoma in the epitympanum has been detected so far in eight (2%). Again, as in the children's group, the incidence becomes much greater if only the ears in which the mastoid and epitympanum were re-explored are considered separately. In these, residual cholesteatoma was present in the epitympanum in 9%. Routine re-examination of the mesotympanum revealed unexpected residual cholesteatoma in 12% at the second operation. The total known incidence of residual cholesteatoma in both the epitympanum and mesotympanum is obviously much larger in children than adults, and these differences are statistically significant (X^2 = 6.79) for the epitympanic (P <0.01) and 9.41 for the mesotympanic rates (P < 0.01). The differences in incidence in the sample are not significant (X^2 = 0.57) for the epitympanum and 3.16 for the mesotympanum).

Time Relationships

Adults

Taking the revised group as a whole, the average time interval between the last operation at which it was believed that cholesteatoma had been removed completely and the most recent examination, was 4.0 years.

In staged operations, the average interval between the first and second operations was six months and when revision was necessary this was carried out between one and two years after the previous staged operation.

In staged operations the average interval between the first operation without cholesteatoma and the most recent follow-up was 2.5 years, except in three operations where this statistic is not available because cholesteatoma was still present and was removed, hopefully in toto, at the most recent operation. In the staged operations which were later revised, the average interval between the first operation without cholesteatoma and the last follow-up was 3.5 years.

Children

Taking the revised group as a whole, the average time interval between the last operation at which it was believed that all cholesteatoma had been removed and the most recent follow-up was 3.5 years.

In once-staged operations, the average interval between the first and second operation was 12 months, whereas revision was carried out on an average two years after the previous staged operation.

In the once-staged operations, the average interval between the first operation at which the ear was seen to be free of cholesteatoma and the most recent follow-up was 2.5 years. In the revised after staged operations, the average interval between the first operation without cholesteatoma and the last follow-up was 3.5 years.

Discussion

(1) Retraction pockets in adults and children. This complication of CAT is the expression of the tendency of cholesteatoma to recur. Initially, cholesteatoma develops because of the combined effects of negative tympanic pressure, lack of rigidity in the tympanic membrane coupled with inward traction from granulation tissue in the tympanum. If the operation fails to correct these factors then it is not surprising that the disease should recur.

A previous analysis for the findings at revision operations had provided evidence that retraction pockets were due to the combined effects of adhesions and lack of support because of loss of part of the sulcus.

This realization led to two important modifications in technique: (1) lining of the tympanum with an inert material such as silastic sheeting, and (2) repair of sulcus defects with cartilage. Consequently, the overall incidence of retraction pockets in this series has shown a marked reduction. The retrospective findings from the 33 ears in which this complication has been noted confirm the basic etiological concept (see table 67). In five other ears the operation notes lack sufficient detail to justify any conclusion as to the cause of the problem. In every instance a defect of the sulcus had been present at the completion of the first operation. In at least one-quarter the notch had resulted from inadvertent damage to the sulcus tympanicus. In 9% this defect had not been repaired at the original operation. In 9% it was found at revision that the repair had been inadequate. In 45.5% silastic sheeting had not been used to control mucosal healing. In at least one-third of cases in which silastic had been used it was obvious at revision that the dimensions of the sheeting had not been adequate to prevent the formation of adhesions deep to the grafted tympanic membrane. In these ears, this deficiency was practically always located in the anterior epitympanum.

Although a statistical analysis of the difference in incidence of recurrent disease in adults and children shows no significance ($X^2 = 1.76$) it must be recognized that this does not entitle the conclusion that there is no difference. Such small percentages are the subject of a large standard error, so it is quite possible that with greater numbers of patients it will be shown that children are significantly more susceptible than adults to recurrent disease after CAT.

On the basis of the evidence of this study, however, it is concluded that retraction pocket formation is usually an unnecessary complication of CAT because it can be prevented by eliminating the factors which were responsible for the development of cholesteatoma in the first instance.

(2) Residual disease in adults and children. The possibility of a high incidence of residual cholesteatoma has figured largely in the controversy over preservation of the osseous canal wall in tympanoplasty. The case against CAT has been that, regardless of the surgeon's skill, maintenance of the most medial part of the canal wall prevents adequate access to cholesteatoma in many cases and will lead to an unacceptable incidence of residual disease.

In the past, it has been stated that the surgical difficulties have been over-emphasized—that in the hands of adequately trained surgeons access to cholesteatoma in CAT is no less than in modified radical mastoidectomy (Smyth, et al, 1971). It has been maintained that the incidence of residual disease is small and far outweighed by the advantages of rapid and secure healing and enhanced chances of functional improvement (Jansen, 1963). At the same time, allowing that difficulties of access may occasionally occur, the advocates of CAT have stipulated that the technique must be abandoned or the operation staged whenever there is doubt about the total removal of cholesteatoma (Smyth, et al, 1969). Both sides in this controversy have agreed that deep extension of cholesteatoma into the sinus tympani creates a problem with any technique (Sheehy and Patterson, 1967).

During the early history of CAT, it was reassuring to find that the predictions of a high incidence of residual cholesteatoma (Baron, 1969) did not appear to be borne out. Nevertheless, it was appreciated that optimism should, of necessity, be guarded because of the expectancy that the growth rate of cholesteatomatous "pearls" might often be slow and that some years development might be required for them to reach proportions sufficient for detection by otoscopy.

However, in this series, as the overall numbers of operations increased and later the numbers of second operations (both staged and revision for failure to gain satisfactory hearing) kept pace, it became increasingly apparent from the findings in ears where the mastoid was opened a second time, that the eventual statistics on residual cholesteatoma would provide little grounds for complacency, and that our earlier predictions would certainly require modification.

The findings in all the second operations on ears where there had been "certainty" of cholesteatoma removal from the epitympanum at the original operation, showed that this opinion had been incorrect 12 out of 97 times (12%), (see Table 66). Admittedly, this group of staged and revised operations does not constitute a random sample and, if anything, there is here a bias towards complications by virtue of the fact that increased difficulty in many of these operations due to bleeding, extensive disease or cramped anatomy, was expressed in the necessity to stage or in their failure to achieve a satisfactory functional outcome.

Not withstanding a bias, the possibility that as many as 54 out of the remaining 449 patients whose mastoids have not been re-examined are still harboring a condition which carries a potential threat to life and will require further surgical treatment is undeniable.

It has been stated that maintenance of the bony meatus should not prejudice the removal of cholesteatoma (Symth, 1972). If this is true, what other explanation can there be for so many instances of a residual cholesteatomy in the epitympanum and mesotympanum as compared to none in the mastoid area? It is the author's belief that the factor which makes the removal of keratinizing squamous epithelium from these areas so much less frequently successful than it is from the mastoid bowl, is the ability of the surgeon, for anatomical reasons, to remove considerable amounts of the bone surrounding cholesteatoma when he is working in the mastoid area. By contrast, in the epi—and mesotympanum, the presence of the facial nerve and the labyrinth prevent any such clearance of bone. As in tumor surgery, success should be greatly enhanced by the removal of a wide margin of uninvolved tissue with the disease.

The criticism of CAT in regard to residual cholesteatoma is not that this occurs more frequently in the epitympanum and mesotympanum because of maintaining the canal wall, but rather, when the disease recurs, its presence in the epitympanum is masked by that canal wall.

This study illustrates the inability of the surgeon to detect the presence of residual cholesteatoma by any means short of an exploratory operation.

(3) Childhood cholesteatoma. It has been stated that cholesteatoma in children is so aggressive, even possessing "malignant" qualities (Derlacki, 1973), that it cannot be treated safely with a closed technique (Baron, 1969). Others have disagreed (Smyth and Law, 1973). The results of this investigation may have helped to resolve this controversy, because the overall known incidence of residual cholesteatoma is much greater in children than adults and this difference is statistically significant for both the epitympanum and the mesotympanum ($X^2 = 6.79$, P <0.01 and 9.41, P < 0.01 respectively). If the "sample" differences had occurred for reasons other than chance, then larger numbers would be necessary to prove significance.

However, just because there is generally more extensive mastoid involvement when cholesteatoma presents in childhood, it does not necessarily follow that this is a fundamentally different disease from that in the adult. It may well be quite simply that cholesteatoma arising as it almost invariably does as a complication of catarrhal otitis media in childhood may have a growth rate which is related inversely to the size of the isthmii anticus and posticus.

Although it can be argued that these separate clinical courses may be as much an expression of anatomical variance as they are of any, as yet unproven, age related differences in the nature of Shrapnell's membrane, it must also be recognized that not all the evidence is necessarily yet available. Most importantly, Palva's (1971) discovery of high cholesteatoma certainly favors the opinion of Baron (1969) in regard to the pervasive nature of the juvenile disease.

Therefore, the argument against CAT in children is twofold: (1) that cholesteatoma in children is a "different" disease—a thesis which gains some support from Palva's biochemical study, and (2) the results of this investigation.

(4) Future developments in the surgery of cholesteatoma. This investigation has provided clear evidence to support the critics of CAT on the grounds of a high complication rate in both adults and children and it is obvious that some of the optimism previously expressed by the author and others about the ability to eradicate cholesteatoma and restore function by means of CAT cannot be sustained.

This is not to say that CAT has no longer any place in the treatment of chronic suppurative otitis media. On the contrary, its use in non-cholesteatomatous ears remains unchallenged where it provides considerable advantages in regard to healing and functional improvement. Nevertheless, it is evident that CAT is not always a satisfactory one and final method of treating cholesteatoma.

Two alternatives are available. Either, (1) CAT must always be carried out as a staged procedure, or (2) an operation in which the canal wall is removed, be used in all cases of extramesotympanic cholesteatoma.

Routine Staging

If it is accepted that staging must be continued until the ear is shown to be free from cholesteatoma, then some patients will certainly require multiple operations. This conclusion is inescapable when one in five of the second operations in this series is known to have failed to eradicate epitympanic cholesteatoma. The concept of once only CAT with its avoidance of an open mastoidectomy cavity has proved extremely attractive to many otologists, but it no longer appears likely that this operation will emerge as the universal solution. Not only will there be patients who cannot or will not accept the necessity for two or more operations, but also there will be surgeons whose

surgical competence, both in training and thereafter, will not be equal to the technical demands of CAT.

Mastoid Obliteration

It may well be that in the future there will be a greater recognition of the merits of an open technique which comprises tympanic reconstruction and obliteration of the mastoid segment with a postaurally based soft tissue graft as originally described by Mosher (1911) and later by Popper (1935). This method has been shown to provide excellent healing (Palva, 1963 and Smyth, et al, 1969) and although the reported functional results have not always been as successful as with CAT, this is not necessarily a problem without a remedy (Smyth, 1976).

In a series of 400 such operations, Palva (1975) has reported residual disease in the epitympanum in 1%. Invariably, this has been managed quite simply by marsupialization usually as an outpatient procedure. In Palva's series residual disease in the mastoid bowl has not been detected and although it can be argued that this awaits discovery, this criticism can be countered by, (1) the evidence from this review in which residual cholesteatoma has not been discovered in any of the mastoid bowls which have been re-explored so far, and (2) the fact that the total removal of squamous epithelium from the mastoid segment is usually facilitated by the possibility of removing uninvolved bone to a depth of several millimeters from the surrounding area.

Conclusion

This long-term survey of the cholesteatomatous complications of CAT has revealed an unexpectedtly high rate of recurrent and residual cholesteatoma. The chief criticism of CAT is not so much that there are cases of residual disease, but rather that they cannot be detected for long periods.

Achievement of the ultimate solution appears to depend initially on a total rejection of the idea that successful tympanoplasty can be achieved only when the osseous canal wall is maintained.

There is evidence that a significantly smaller complication rate can be achieved through a combination of well performed mastoidectomy, cavity obliteration and mesotympanic reconstruction. Obviously, residual cholesteatoma will still occur in the epitympanum, but it is to be hoped that it will be easily managed and pose no threat to the patient. Without doubt, if it is agreed that the prime aim of tympanoplasty is to eradicate irreversible disease and the findings of this investigation are accepted, then it follows that the place of once-only CAT in the routine management of chronic suppurative otitis media with cholesteatoma requires further assessment.

References

1. Austin, D. F. and Sanabria, F.: Mastoidplasty. *Arch. Otolaryngol.* (Chicago), 76: 414, 1962.
2. Baron, S. H.: Management of aural cholesteatoma in children. *Otolaryngol. Clin. N. Amer.*, 71: 88, 1969.
3. Corgill, D. A. and Storrs, L. A.: Intact canal wall tympanoplasty. A report of 1000 cases. *Trans. Amer. Acad. Ophthalmol. Otolaryngol.*, 71: 53, 1967.
4. Derlacki, E. L.: Congenital cholesteatoma of the middle ear and mastoid. A third report. *Arch. Otolaryngol.*, 97: 177, 1973.
5. Guilford, F. R.: Obliteration of the cavity and reconstruction of the auditory canal in temporal bone surgery. *Trans. Amer. Acad. Ophthalmol. Otolaryngol.*, 65: 114, 1961.
6. House, W. F. and Sheehy, J. L.: Functional restoration in tympanoplasty. *Arch. Otolaryngol.* (Chicago), 78: 304, 1963.
7. Jansen, C.: Uber Radikaloperation Und Tympanoplastik. *Sitz Ber. Fortbild. Arztekamm. Ob. v.* 18, February, 1958.
8. Jansen, C.: Cartilage—tympanoplasty. *Laryngoscope*, 73: 1288, 1963.
9. Mosher, H. P.: A method of filling the excavated mastoid with a flap from the back of the auricle. *Laryngoscope*, 21: 1158, 1911.
10. Palva, T.: Surgery of chronic ear without cavity. Results in 130 cases with musculoperiosteal flap and fasciotympanoplasty. *Arch. Otolaryngol.* (Chicago), 77: 570, 1963.
11. Palva, T.: Data presented at Fortbildningskurs Rekonstruktiv mellanörekirurge. Linköping, Sweden, 1975.
12. Popper, O.: Periosteal flap grafts in mastoid operations. *S. African Med. J.*, 9: 77, 1935.
13. Schuknecht, H.; Bocca, E.; Guilford, F. et al: Panel on surgical approach, cavity management and postoperative care in ear surgery. *Arch. Otolaryngol.* (Chicago), 78: 350, 1963.
14. Shea, M. C.; Gardner, G.; and Simpson, M. E.: Mastoid obliteration with bone. *Otol. Clin. N. Amer.*, 5: 161, 1972.
15. Sheehy, J. L. and Patterson, M. E.: Intact canal wall tympanoplasty with mastoidectomy. A review of eight years experience. *Laryngoscope*, 77: 1502, 1967.
16. Smyth, G. D. L.: Outline of surgical management in chronic ear disease. *Otol. Clin. N. Amer.*, 5: 59, 1972.
17. Smyth, G. D. L.: Long-term results in tympanic reconstruction. *J. Laryngol. Otol.*, 1976, in press.
18. Smyth, G. D. L.; Kerr, A. G.; Dowe, A. C. et al: A practical alternative to combined approach tympanoplasty. *J. Laryngol. Otol.*, 83: 1143, 1969.
19. Smyth, G. D. L.; Kerr, A. G.; and Goodey, R. J.: Current thoughts on combined approach tympanoplasty. Part I. Indications and preoperative assessment. *J. Laryngol. Otol.*, 85: 205, 1971.
20. Smyth, G. and Law, K. P.: Surgical management of chronic otitis media in children. *Canad. J. Otolaryngol.*, 2: 296, 1973.

CHOLESTEATOMA SURGERY CANAL WALL DOWN AND MASTOID OBLITERATION

T. Palva, M.D.
P. Karma, M.D.
A. Palva, M.D.

Material

We have analyzed the postoperative state of 100 cholesteatoma ears operated on between January 1, 1967, and May 7, 1969. Every ear with cholesteatoma operated during this period was included in the statistics if there had been no previous ear surgery and the surgical method was basically similar.

The mean age of the patients was 34 years. The average follow-up time was six years, the shortest four years and the longest eight years four months.

Surgical Method

Typical radical mastoid surgery was performed during the period when these ears were operated on. The ear canal was reconstructed using a fascial graft posterior to the canal skin, and the meatally based musculoperiosteal flap was applied to occlude the cavity. In large mastoid bowls, inorganic heterograft bone, and in a few ears, silicone elastomer sponge was employed to fill the remaining cavity. An effort was thus made in all cases to separate the mastoid cavity from the middle ear and to occlude the former.

Extend of Disease

Table 68 gives the recorded data upon the extent of the cholesteatomatous process. In the majority of the ears (92), the epitympanic space was involved, the corresponding figure for the tympanum being 29. Eight ears had cholesteatoma only in the tympanum. In two ears the process extended into the bony portion of the eustachian tube. In addition to the 29 ears of tympanic choles-

TABLE 68

Extent of Cholesteatoma

Tympanum	8
Epitympanum	26
Epitympanum and Tympanum	8
Epitympanum and Antrum	37
Epitympanum, Tympanum and Antrum	11
Epitympanum, Antrum and Mastoid	8
Epitympanum, Tympanum, Antrum and Mastoid	2
TOTAL	**100**

teatoma, squamous epithelium was found in the removed tympanic mucosa in 25 additional ears.

The tympanum was filled with granulation tissue in seven ears and in three the mucosa was granulating in part. Thick mucosa was noted in 11 ears and an adhesive process in 11 ears. In only 14 ears the tympanic mucosa was of normal appearance.

The ossicular chain was found to be intact in 16 ears during surgery. The incus was eroded and the long process necrotic in 42 ears with preserved stapes superstructure. In 42 other ears the footplate only remained.

Preoperatively the majority of the ears were moist or discharging, only seven were dry. The bacterial analysis is given in Table 69 shows that the predominating organism was pseudomonas, followed next by proteus strains. The preoperative treatment had produced 26 culture negative ears

TABLE 69

Preoperative Bacterial Analysis

Aerobic		
	Pseudomonas aeruginosa	23 (ears=%)
	Proteus sp.	16
	St. aureus	15
	St. epidermidis	7
	Diphtheroides	5
	Klebsiella-Aerobacter sp.	5
	E. coli	4
	Alcaligenes faecalis	3
	N. catarrhalis	3
	Providence	1
	B. anitratum	1
Anaerobic		
	Streptococcus	1
Fungi		
	Aspergillus niger	1
	Candida albicans	1

Dry ears	7
Culture negative	26

Monoinfection	53
Di-infection	11
Polyinfection (3 or more strains)	3

and surgery was thus performed on 67 infected ears.

Preoperative Complications Due to Disease Process

Deaf ears. Five ears had become deaf before surgery, two of these dating back over 15 years, and three over two years. At surgery one ear was found to show a horizontal canal fistula, another an extensive oval window cholesteatoma but in three ears there was no obvious cause other than chronic ear disease.

Fistula ears. In this series there were eight fistulae in the horizontal. In four ears the epidermic cover was left in place on top of the fistula and obliteration occurred posterior to this area. Hearing was retained in all. In four ears the squamous epithelium was removed totally with preservation of hearing in three, the fourth being preoperatively deaf.

Facial paralysis. In two ears there was a preoperative facial paralysis of two and five days'

duration. Both these patients were operated on as emergency cases and made a complete recovery. In the third the paresis was of one month's duration and the disease was complicated by a horizontal canal fistula. The facial nerve canal had a granulating surface with a bony defect over an area of only two square mm and this small lesion was probably the cause of a good recovery in three short months.

Surgical Complications

In one ear, inadvertent dislocation of the stapes occurred and in another a footplate fracture. The oval window, and the footplate, respectively, were covered with fascia and hearing was preserved. In a third ear a footplate perforation occurred during cholesteatoma removal. In this ear an initial reconstruction was made using incus transposition and the tympanum was filled with paraffin wax. During a two-month period this ear gradually became totally deaf.

Two more deaf ears resulted after surgery in cases with epitympanic and antral cholesteatoma and squamous epithelium covering the tympanum. Reconstruction after excision of the mucosa was made using two-legged wire from the stapes head and a three-legged wire from the footplate, but there was no known mishap to explain the deaf ears. The preoperative hearing level was 82 and 57 dB, respectively. Thus the total number of deaf ears after surgery is 3% in this series of 100 ears.

Recurrence of Cholesteatoma

Recurring cholesteatoma was found in two ears. One of these, showing pseudomonas infection and extensive mastoid cholesteatoma, was operated in 1968. This ear began to suppurate six months later and the wire columella was removed. In 1972 a revision was made and a hypotympanal cholesteatoma was found. This was removed and cortical bone columellization carried out on top of the stapes. The ear has remained asymptomatic with hearing at the 48 dB level. The other patient was operated in 1968 because of a tympano-antral cholesteatoma but the drum soon perforated and discharge continued intermittently until a revision was performed in 1973. A hypotympanal cholesteatoma was found in this ear also, and after revision the ear has remained stabilized with hearing at the preoperative level of 82 dB.

In both ears the process very probably was residual; in the first ear, islands of squamous epithelium in the tympanum were apparently overlooked and in the second, ear surgery by a resident was not sufficiently well supervised by the senior staff. All in all, recurrence of cholesteatoma was thus noted in 2%.

Marked Postoperative Retraction

Postoperative retraction caused problems in 10 ears in which an adhesive middle ear developed and the musculo-periosteal flap had not been made sufficiently long to fill the antrum and epitympanum. These ears were not self-cleaning and were prone to infection if cleaning was performed at intervals longer than three or four months. In the other ears (Table 70) no treatment problem arose even when the posterior retraction due to large mastoid cavities had made the ear canal wide.

TABLE 70

Postoperative Retraction

Moderate or marked retraction, treatment problems	10
Some retraction, no treatment problems	11
Larger than normal canal	20
Normal canal	54
Cavity left because of fistula	5
Total	100

Recurrence of Suppurative Disease

In ten ears there was postoperative discharge of longer duration, in association with the clinical findings shown in Table 71.

TABLE 71

Recurrence of Suppurative Disease

Silastic sponge in mastoid, infected	3
Heterograft bone in mastoid, infected	1
Recurring cholesteatoma	2
Open cavity fistula ears	2
Closed cavity fistula ears	1
Epidermization of posterior tympanum, open to ear canal	1
Total	10

The first four ears represent those in which retraction caused canal skin perforation due to foreign material. Two of these were revised, the sponge removed after which the ears became dry. In the cases of residual cholesteatoma revision surgery made the ears dry. In six ears there has been no further surgery and the ears have been treated conservatively. Evidently, however, a revision will be required in the two ears in which foreign filling material was used.

In four ears short periods of discharge have occurred. In two, this was associated with the extrusion of the stainless steel wire. When the prosthesis was removed, the ears became dry. A third ear had early postoperative discharge from the open tympanum for five months but has remained dry after epidermization. In the fourth ear there was a period of six months' discharge two years postoperatively but the ear has been dry for the last four years.

Status of Middle Ear Postoperatively

Table 72 shows the methods used for ossicular reconstruction and the outcome of the drumhead repair. In nearly half of the ears (48%) a permanently aerated tympanum was created. In one case a dry perforation developed, in 11 infection resulted in breakage of part of the drumhead. It is worth noticing that an adhesive middle ear developed in 26%; in 14% no attempt was made to

TABLE 72

Ossicular Reconstruction and Outcome of Tympanic Membrane Repair

Ossicular repair	Outcome Aerated Tympanum	Lost Air space	Late Perforation	Discharge	total
Intact chain	7	2	-	-	9
Columellization with bone	13	3	5	2	21
Columellization with wire	27	18	7	6	52
Myringo-stapediopexy	1	3	-	1	4
No ossicular reconstruction	-	9	-	-	9
No drum repair	-	5	-	2	5
Ears = %	48	40	12	11	100

TABLE 73

Reconstruction and Hearing

Reconstruction	No of ears	Socially adequate hearing Preoperatively	Postoperatively
Intact chain	9	6	6
Columellization with bone			
—From stapes head	16	7	7
—From footplate	5	1	2
Columellization with wire			
—From stapes head	26	13	12
—From footplate	26	3	5
Myringo-stapediopexy	4	0	1
No reconstruction	14	1	0
Total	100	30	33

create an air space.

Socially Adequate Hearing

The patients are classified in Table 73 according to the reconstruction method and the socially adequate hearing level (40 dB, average of 500, 1000 & 2000 Hz, ISO-Standard). In 33% of the patients this postoperative level was obtained, the preoperative figure being 30%. In the total material, the average preoperative hearing level was 47 dB and postoperative 48 dB.

Comment

The results in the present series of 100 cholesteatoma ears are thus as follows:

(1) Recurrence of cholesteatoma   2%
(2) Marked post-operative retraction   10%
(3) Recurrence of suppurative disease   10%
(4) Deaf ears   3%
(5) Socially adequate hearing (40 dB
    or better)   33%

In groups 1, 2 and 3 there is overlapping; the four revisions made stabilized the ears reoperated. We ascribe the small figure of 2% for recurring cholesteatoma to the canal down technique, which seems to guarantee the removal of mastoid and epitympanic disease. The window niches and the tympanic sinus are the areas from which the disease cannot always be eradicated.

The 10% postoperative retractions has caused us to modify the surgical technique we now reconstruct the posterior canal wall with homograft dura and cortical bone chips, starting from the epitympanum. When retractions no longer occur, and the use of artificial materials is discarded both in mastoid obliteration and ossicular reconstruction, this seems to lead to nonrecurrence of suppurative disease.

The number of adhesive middle ears (26% unintentional and 14% intentional) suggests that the canal up technique, because of the inevitable formation of an antral retraction pocket under the bridge, would lead to higher percentages of late cholesteatoma than obtained when using mastoid and epitympanic obliteration.

EXPERIENCES WITH SURGERY OF AURAL CHOLESTEATOMA
A CAUSE OF SUDDEN DEAFNESS

Shirley Harold Baron, M.D.

This is a report of the review of the records of 132 patients upon whom I operated for cholesteatoma of the temporal bone. Twenty-nine were excluded because the follow-up has been less than three years, or because of incomplete records. Three were severe cholesterol granulomas, all recovered, but excluded because there was no cholesteatoma matrix.

The one exception to the three or more year follow-up is an unusual case of a woman who suddenly lost her hearing from a cholesteatoma; thus this disease can be added to the list of causes of sudden deafness. In childhood, the left ear became infected, a mastoidectomy was performed, but her left hearing was permanently lost. Her right ear was normal until one year ago when she suddenly became completely deaf in that ear. Examination revealed a right serous otitis media (often an accompaniment of cholesteatoma) and a necrotic posterior canal from which cholesteatomatous debris was removed. A myringotomy was performed, and the hearing returned. There was some concern that there might be some cholesteatomatous destruction of the incus, but at surgery none was found.

Of the 100 cases now reported, the type of surgery performed was a modified radical mastoidectomy in 76, a radical in 21, an intact canal wall procedure in one, a transcanal attico-antrotomy in one, and a combined procedure with a neurosurgeon for a congenital cholesteatoma, which involved the mastoid and occipital bone in one, (Table 74).

There were only 27 attico-antral cholesteatomas with good hearing, ideal for preservation of the matrix. The hearing was maintained or improved in all but two, and one required reopera-

TABLE 74

Cases reported—100

76	Modified radical
21	Radical
1	Intact canal wall procedure
1	Transcanal attico-antrotomy
1	Combined mastoid-neurosurgical operation for congenital cholesteatoma
100	

84% dry   16% wet

tion. Hindsight reveals the reasons for these failures. Had I adhered to my own rules, there would have been no failures in this group. All but the two exceptions remained dry. In seven patients the surgery was performed on the only hearing or better ear.

In 15 other modified radical mastoidectomies bits of matrix covering the stapes footplate or crura, or a possible fistula in the horizontal semicircular canals were left in situ. Of these, three developed intermittent drainage, 12 remained dry. None required further surgery.

The matrix was totally removed in the remaining 34 modified radicals, nine of which were combined with tympanoplasties. Intermittent drainage continued in five, the rest remained dry. Three required further surgery for recurrent cholesteatoma.

Bits of matrix were saved in six of the radicals. Two developed intermittent drainage. One required further surgery.

The matrix was completely removed in the remaining 15 radicals, nine of which were combined with tympanoplasties. Four of these developed intermittent drainage. None required further surgery.

Twenty-three patients had more than one operation upon the same ear. Eleven had their first operation elsewhere, and twelve by me. Four patients had three operations upon the same ear. Two of these had all operations performed by me, and two had their two previous operations performed elsewhere.

It is noteworthy that cholesteatomas developed in the fenestration cavities of four patients.

There were eight revisions for cholesteatoma, an 8% recurrence rate. The revisions of patients first operated upon elsewhere bring the recurrence rate up to 15%. (Cholesteatomas which developed after fenestration surgery are not included because none were present at the initial surgery, (Table 75).

TABLE 75

Recurrent Cholesteatoma Requiring Further Surgery

Modified radicals with matrix saved	2
Modified radicals with matrix removed	3
Radical with bits of matrix saved	1
Transcanal atticotomy	1
Intact canal wall procedure	1
Primary surgery by me (children 4%)	8%
Primary surgery performed elsewhere	7%
	15%

Complications, (Table 76)

Brain abscess was present in two patients. One died and one recovered following brain surgery.

One patient who had had two previous operations with the posterior wall left intact developed a postauricular abscess and a fistula.

In one patient, a horizontal canal fistula was suspected. The matrix was preserved over this fistula, but the remaining matrix was removed.

TABLE 76

Complications

Brain abscess (one died)	2
Epidural abscess, posterior fossa	1
Dead ear	1
Iatrogenic preauricular cholesteatoma	1
Canal atresia with retro-atresia cholesteatoma	1
Facial paralysis with residual cholesteatoma referred the day after surgery	1
Postauricular abscess and fistula	1
Sudden deafness	1

This was unfortunate, for removing the matrix over an unsuspected posterior canal fistula avulsed the membranous labyrinth and resulted in a dead ear. The hearing in her right ear is poor even with a powerful hearing aid.

Another complication was an encapsulated epidural abscess in the left posterior fossa of a 29-year-old woman whose primary operation, a modified radical, was performed two years previously (1956). In this second operation, a radical, the cholesteatoma was under the cochlea. As the dissection progressed medially, pus and spinal fluid suddenly gushed out. It was impossible to remove the posterior fossa matrix which had surrounded the abscess through the small subcochlear opening. It was expected that eventually it would have to be removed by an intracranial approach, but this was never required. The intracranial pocket was aspirated frequently through the subcochlear opening. Finally, in 1966, eight years later, the opening was enlarged, essentially marsupializing the intracranial cholesteatoma. It is now 10 years after her last surgery and 20 years after her first. She has never had any abnormal neurological signs and remains well.

One patient developed an almond-sized mass in front of her left ear which proved to be a cholesteatomatous cyst with a tract from the epitympanum.

There was an extensive recurrent cholesteatoma and evidence of total removal of the tympanic dural plate by the previous surgeon. There was a span of five years between her primary surgery and the appearance of the cyst.

Facial paralysis was a complication in a patient referred to me by the operating surgeon who did a radical for this patient's cholesteatoma. I explored this mastoid about 30 hours after the primary surgery. The facial nerve was bruised but was not severed. There still was cholesteatoma in the sinodural angle. The nerve was decompressed, and its sheath was split. Fortunately, the paralysis completely recovered.

In the one ear upon which I performed a transcanal atticotomy, the patient became violently dizzy four years later. A modified radical was performed for a large recurrent cholesteatoma. The matrix was preserved in this better hearing ear. The patient has been symptom-free for over 16 years.

One patient who had no cholesteatoma at the original tympanoplasty developed an atresia of the meatus and a cholesteatoma behind the atresia.

Referring to the patient with sudden deafness from cholesteatoma, the appearance of her mastoid were similar to that of the first patient in whom I preserved the matrix in 1933. The rule then was, as stated by Day (1934): "The presence of cholesteatoma complicating a chronic suppurative otitis media has been considered a cardinal indication for radical surgery". It seemed reasonable to take advantage of nature's modified radical and preserve the hearing, so, with some trepidation, it was done. It proved to be a good decision, for, as in this patient, the hearing was preserved and the healing was rapid and made me advocate the preservation of the matrix in selective cases (Baron, 1949 and 1967; Baron, 1953), especially in an only hearing ear. The late Theodore Walsh, who opposed the concept, and I debated this controversial modality at the American Academy of Ophthalmology and Otolaryngology in 1952. The year before his death,

Dr. Walsh told me he had come to recognize that this procedure had merit.

The indications and contraindications for preserving the matrix are presented in the following guidelines:

Saving the matrix is recommended for the following reasons:

(1) The layer of matrix that is to be externalized and preserved is squamous epithelium, which serves as a source for complete epidermatization of the mastoid cavity, resulting in a dry ear.

(2) In the attico-antral cholesteatoma, maintenance or improvement of hearing is almost certain, since preserving the matrix leaves the middle structures undisturbed. This is especially desirable if the other ear is deaf.

(3) In sclerotic mastoids, there will be less chance for the formation of recurrent cholesteatomatous cysts. (Reasons for this have been described in a previous paper (Baron, 1953).

(4) In the presence of certain labyrinthine fistulas, the matrix will act as a barrier against infection entering the labyrinth. (Over a fistula its removal could destroy the labyrinth).

(5) In exposed dura mater in any area including the lateral sinus, where there is no clinical evidence of infection, locally or intracranially, the matrix may be firmly adherent. Leaving the matrix will prevent surgical trauma to the dura. The presence of disease in these areas usually will be evidenced by granulations, or a pinkish color of the matrix. In these situations, the matrix may be removed readily.

(6) In facial nerve paralysis caused from the pressure effects of a cholesteatoma, and in which the function may return when the pressure is released, an attempt to remove an adherent matrix from the nerve may produce some injury to the nerve; however, when there is bone necrosis about the nerve,

as evidenced by granulation tissue interspersed with matrix, the matrix should be removed.

When the matrix should be removed

There are certain anatomical and inflammatory factors which make it advisable to remove the matrix:

Anatomical factors:

(1) A pneumatized mastoid. Most cases of chronically discharging ears with cholesteatoma are in sclerotic mastoids, but occasionally the mastoid will be partially pneumatic. Preoperative determination of this by x-ray is important since extensions of the cholesteatoma into pneumatic spaces can occur and will continue to expand if a thorough exenteration is not done. The matrix must be removed to expose the underlying cells.

(2) Perilabyrinthine invaginations of the matrix into the bone should be searched for under magnification and should be removed. Such areas, however, can be dealt with without removing the entire matrix.

(3) In revision mastoid operations, when one has not had a hand in the primary surgery, it may become necessary to remove the matrix to expose important landmarks and to determine the nature of the pathology.

(4) The matrix should be removed whenever there are retrofacial or petrous tip extensions.

(5) If visible invaginations into bone in any area are excessive, the entire matrix in that area should be removed.

(6) With a hearing loss greater than 45 decibels, the matrix should be removed and reconstruction of a conducting mechanism attempted.

(7) In an attico-antral type of cholesteatoma, if the cholesteatoma matrix dips into the middle ear behind the tympanic membrane, this dipped matrix should be removed, and a tympanoplastic procedure to eliminate the perforation caused by this matrix removal should be done.

Inflammatory factors:

(1) Occasionally suppuration occurs between matrix and bone. This will manifest itself by the formation of granulation tissue between the matrix and the bone and by a pinkish color of the matrix. This elevated matrix should be removed and the bone searched for areas of necrosis.

(2) There are cases in which islands of matrix are interspersed with islands of granulation tissue. This indicates bone infection and requires removal of the matrix for complete exposure to search for and remove areas of bone necrosis.

(3) The matrix should be removed when there is clinical or anatomical evidence of a suppurative labyrinthitis, petrositis, meningitis, subdural abscess, epidural abscess or lateral sinus thrombosis.

Discussion

It should be no surprise that I, who have been most vocal against the intact canal wall technique in the presence of a cholesteatoma, have done only one intact canal operation when cholesteatoma was present. I would not have done that had not the hearing been perfect. I had to reoperate upon this patient in two years for recurrent cholesteatoma, and then did a modified radical. It has been three years without a further recurrence, but three years is too short a time to assume that a cholesteatoma has been conquered. To illustrate, in 1964 I performed a radical mastoidectomy upon a 6 year old girl for an advanced, destructive middle ear and epitympanic cholesteatoma and a tympanoplasty with fascia and a bone strut for a columella. This successfully developed a pseudotympanic membrane and a middle ear space, but did not improve the hearing. In three years a cholesteatoma developed in the epitympanum. With the previous open technique this could be seen easily. It could have been opened and externalized as an office procedure, but the patient and her mother were anxious for a hearing improvement, so a second operation was done. The cholesteatoma was eliminated by marsupialization. The middle ear was explored and the bone strut was found adherent to the promontory from bone growth. This was removed and replaced by a cartilage-perichondrial strut made from the tragus—the technique suggested by Brockman (1965). This did result in a hearing improvement. Six years later—nine years—after the first surgery, a new cholesteatoma appeared in the anterioinferior quadrant of the pseudo-tympanic membrane. This was eliminated by a third operation. This is solid evidence that one can never be sure that his surgery has cured a cholesteatoma and is a reason for my wariness of a closed technique.

Conclusion

A surgical technique to guarantee the nonrecurrence of a cholesteatoma has not yet been devised. One can hypothecate the development of a vital stain which will reveal remnants not seen, but it is unlikely that a stained, flaked off epithelial rest that may occur with cholesteatoma removal can be seen with the limited power of the surgical microscope (Begley, 1951). One can hope for the remote possibility of the development of a chemical or other substance which will destroy cholesteatoma without harming adjacent tissues.

Of the techniques available, my favorite is the modified radical with the preservation of the cholesteatoma matrix, a procedure which I have done since 1933 without a serious complication. It is an operation which ends the devastation of a cholesteatoma when the guidelines for its use are followed. Unfortunately, it is ideal only in the attico-antral cholesteatoma which was present in only 27% of my cases. Alternatives for me are the modified radical or radical with removal of all the cholesteatoma with certain exceptions previously mentioned.

Cholesteatoma in children, especially in the middle ear, is a more vicious disease. Four of my 8% recurrences were in children. In them, special care should be taken to choose a procedure which assures their safety.

I agree with Mawson (1975) who, in his presidential address before the Royal Society of Medicine, stated "that in the case of the combined approach tympanoplasties still infected, there is hanging over each patient the threat of further surgery, and over the surgeon the anxiety connected with uncertainty over the safety and extent of residual or recurrent disease".

Special acknowledgment with thanks is due to Doctors Sade, Abramson and McCabe for having organized this meeting. It is hoped that this First International Conference on Cholesteatoma will lead us closer to a solution of the cholesteatoma problem.

References

1. Baron, S. H.: Modified radical mastoidectomy; preservation of the cholesteatoma matrix; a method of making a flap in the endaural technique. *Arch. Otolaryng.*, 49:280, 1949.
2. Baron, S. H.: Why and when I do not remove the matrix. In Symposium: The surgical management of aural cholesteatoma. *Trans. Amer. Acad. Ophthal. Otolaryng.*, 57:694, 1953

3. Baron, S. H.: Preservation of the cholesteatoma matrix in the modified radical mastoidectomy. *Laryngoscope*, 77:905, 1967.
4. Begley, J., Jr. and Williams, H. L.: Cholesteatomatous cysts secondary to incomplete removal of the cholesteatomatous matrix. *Arch. Otolaryng.*, 53:147, 1951.
5. Brockman, S. J.: Cartilage graft tympanoplasty

type III. *Laryngoscope*, 75:1452, 1965.

6. Day, K. M.: The etiological factors in formation of cholesteatoma. *Amer. Otol. Rhinol. Laryng.*, 43:837, 1934.

7. Lindsay, J. R.: The pathogenesis of cholesteatoma and summary of discussion. In: Symposium: The surgical management of aural cholesteatoma. *Trans. Amer. Acad. Ophthal. Otolaryng.*, 57:707, 1953.

8. Mawson, S. R.: Surgery of the mastoid: the first century. *Proceed. Royal Soc. Med.* (Section of Otology), 68:391, 1975.

9. Walsh, T. E.: Why I remove the matrix. In Symposium: The surgical management of aural cholesteatoma. *Trans. Amer. Acad. Ophthal. Otolaryng.*, 57:687, 1953.

A CONCEPT FOR THE MANAGEMENT OF OTITIC CHOLESTEATOMAS

William K. Wright, M.D.

In managing cholesteatomas, all of us ideally prefer to avoid radical and modified radical mastoidectomies because of their known disadvantages. Unfortunately, when any of the conservative operations are used, there is a risk that parts of the cholesteatoma may be incompletely removed and will regrow. Since 1969, I have attempted to neutralize this risk by electively re-exploring every case operated by a conservative technique, and I have devoted my allotted time to analyzing these re-explorations. This study includes only cholesteatomas that were managed by a conservative technique, which enucleates the cholesteatoma while preserving or reconstructing the bony canal wall and tympanic membrane. Between 1969 and 1974, sixty ears in fifty-five patients were studied. I had hoped to re-explore all cases, but eight (or 13.4%) of these patients did not return or refused re-exploration (Table 77). Of the 52 re-explorations, eight (or 15.4%) were positive for a regrowth of cholesteatoma (Table 78). Only one of these regrowths (Table 79) occurred in the mastoid, and since the middle ear was clear of cholesteatoma and the patient was sixty-two years old, I elected to convert her mastoid into a modified radical cavity. All seven of the other cholesteatoma regrowths occurred in the middle ear. They were all small, and I chose to again enucleate them conservatively. Three of these seven cases have been re-explored a second time and have been found to be clear of cholesteatoma. The other four await the end of their two-year interval before a second re-exploration is contemplated. Hopefully, they also will be found clear of cholesteatoma.

Discussion

Regrowth of cholesteatoma after intact bony

TABLE 77

Cholesteatoma Removed with Canal and Drum Preserved or Reconstructed 1969-74

Cholesteatoma Removed with Canal and Drum Preserved or Reconstructed 1969-74	
Re-explored for regrowth or cholesteatoma	52 = 86.7%
Lost to follow-up or refused re-exploration	8 = 13.3%
Total cases	60

(1 or 2 regrowths can be expected among the unoperated cases)

TABLE 78

Surgical Findings at Re-exploration

Negative for cholesteatoma	44 = 84.6%
Positive for regrowth cholesteatoma	8 = 15.4%
Total	52

Judging by size and time interval, these regrowths would not have become manifest for six to twelve years. Therefore, three year follow-up in a cholesteatoma series is meaningless.

TABLE 79

Management of Regrowth Cholesteatomas

Regrowth in mastoid	1	Modified radical mastoidectomy
Regrowth in middle ear	7	Local removal and second re-exploration
Total	8	
Second re-exploration negative	3	
Await second re-exploration	4	
Total	7	

wall and drum technique is an appreciable risk. My series shows a considerably higher incidence (15.4%) than previous studies which have reported about 5%. The obvious explanation would seem to impune my surgical skill, but a more likely explanation is that the percentages in previous studies were based on known clinical returns. My statistics are based on re-exploration, and none of these regrowths were clinically evident. I estimate by the regrowth size and time interval that clinical manifestation would not have occurred for six to twelve years. Therefore, figures based on clinical recurrences with a three-year or more follow-up are meaningless and even misleading.

Case 1: M. O., a four year old male, had a congenital cholesteatoma with erosion of the incus long process and stapes filling the entire middle ear. The cholesteatoma was totally removed with preservation of the ear drum and the malleus. Re-exploration one year later revealed a clear middle ear except for a 3/4 mm cholesteatoma pearl in the posterior one-fourth of the footplate. The drum was opaque, and this regrowth would not have become clinically manifest for many years. The regrowth was enucleated, and the patient now awaits a two-year interval before a second re-exploration.

Case 2: Mrs. A. B., a sixty-seven year old white female, had a right stapedectomy. Thirteen years later she was seen with an anterior perforation and obvious cholesteatoma, although an examination eighteen months earlier had been entirely normal. The cholesteatoma involved the entire undersurface of the drum and malleus. The drum was totally replaced, but an attempt was made to preserve the malleus. Re-exploration eighteen months later showed cholesteatoma piling up beneath the malleus. The malleus and adjacent portions of the drum were resected en bloc, and the resulting defect was patched with a medially placed perichondrial graft. Two years later a second re-exploration showed the ear clear of cholesteatoma. Obviously, active squamous epithelium had been implanted on a raw area of the undersurface of the drum during the original stapedectomy,

but the slow growth of cholesteatoma did not manifest itself for thirteen years. This is one of two known cases of cholesteatoma following stapedectomy in a very large series of stapedectomies done by Guilford and Wright. Other stapedectomy surgeons have acknowledged similar cases, and I also know of a number of cholesteatomas that have followed myringotomy with insertion of indwelling ventilation tubes. I cite these examples because I believe that there is some risk of seeding a cholesteatoma regrowth by spilling active squamous epithelium on raw surgical areas during even the simplest of cholesteatoma enucleation. Therefore, all such ears should be re-explored. On the other hand, even the most extensive and inaccessible cholesteatomas can be successfully enucleated.

Case 3: Mrs. C., a 47 year old white female, had a cholesteatoma of the attic and entire middle ear. The cholesteatoma involved the undersurface of the drum and malleus and grew between the stapes crura into the facial recess and tympanic sinus. It also grew into the round window niche, where it had invaginated the round window membrane at least 2 mm. The cholesteatoma was successfully removed from all of these areas without sacrificing any normal structures except the tympanic membrane, which was entirely replaced, and the incus, which was repositioned onto the stapes head. There was a slight round window perilymph leak which was plugged with gelfoam. It was anticipated that there might be extensive sensory neural loss and a strong possibility of cholesteatoma recurrence, but re-exploration four years later showed no cholesteatoma, and the patient has continued to have a 20 Db hearing level with a 7 Db air bone gap. Re-exploration must be early enough that any cholesteatoma regrowth will be small and can be easily removed, but late enough that any recurrence will have grown sufficiently large to be recognizable.

Case 4: W. A., a four year old male, presented with bilateral posterosuperior cholesteatoma. The right ear was operated first, and the cholesteatoma was entirely removed. The partially eroded incus was repositioned on the stapes under the malleus, and the perforation was closed with a medially placed perichondrial graft. Six months later the left ear had a similar procedure, except that the ossicles were intact. At that time, the right ear was re-explored and thought to be free of cholesteatoma. One year later, the left ear was re-explored and found to be negative for cholesteatoma. As an afterthought and during the same anesthetic, the first ear was re-explored once more. A sausage shaped cholesteatoma regrowth could be seen growing down each stapes crura to within 1 mm of the footplate. The stapes superstructure and incus head were removed. One and one-half years later a third re-exploration showed a middle ear clear of cholesteatoma. The sound conduction was re-established with a prosthesis from the footplate to the malleus, and the hearing is now excellent in both ears. Because of this case, it is felt that re-exploration should not be carried out earlier than one and one-half years.

Eight patients (13.3%) failed to return or refused re-exploration. I would predict that in this group there is at least one patient with a cholesteatoma regrowth, and I am worried over his safety. There are definite advantages of the intact bony canal wall and drum technique over radical mastoidectomy, but creation of a safe ear is not one of these advantages. (That is, unless these patients are re-explored and found to be free of disease.) Incidentally, the modified radical mastoidectomy would not have been adequate for the safety of the patients in this series. Only one regrowth occurred in the mastoid, while the main area for cholesteatoma regrowth was in the middle ear, especially in inaccessible areas such as the undersurface of the malleus, the crotch of the stapes crura, and the tympanic sinus. Only a radical mastoidectomy could have exteriorized these areas. Consequently, it is felt that conservative and reconstructive surgery for removal of cholesteatoma with the re-exploration management plan outlined in this paper provides safety comparable to a radical mastoidectomy with far better functional results. The hearing results on Table 80

TABLE 80

Hearing Reconstruction

Ear drum repair (Ossicles intact)	Air-bone gap 0-10 Db − 81.0%
Repair ear drum and eroded incus	Air-bone gap 0-10 Db = 68.2%
Repair ear drum eroded incus eroded stapes crura	Air-bone gap 0-15 Db = 43.7%

could never have been achieved with radical surgery.

There will be some ears from which I will repeatedly fail to completely remove the cholesteatoma. Two of my failures have occurred in very deep tympanic sinuses. The eustachian tube is another difficult area. However, I can always do a radical mastoidectomy if the patient or I become discouraged. There of course will be some patients who will not return for re-exploration. In my opinion, neither of these reasons justified performing a routine radical mastoidectomy. And, I expect to improve my technique and my follow-up percentage.

Since the answer to the problem is a re-exploration, the key to the problem is an informed patient. In my opinion the doctor should not unilaterally make the decision to try to avoid a radical mastoidectomy. If this conservative surgery is to work, he needs the help of an understanding, cooperative patient who will return for a re-exploration. To strengthen this understanding I have written a small information booklet. Also, in the last 18 months, I have reinforced this whole matter by employing an informed consent questionnaire. Its completion shows that the patient does understand, and it asks the patient to share the responsibility of returning for follow-up at a specific time. He or she signs the questionnaire and receives a copy as a reminder. In paragraph one of the questionnaire, the patient admits that he understands the material and that I will answer any questions. In paragraph two he admits that he understands the seriousness of cholesteatomas. Paragraph number three states the disadvantages of a radical mastoidectomy, which are understood by the patient, and in paragraph four the patient is informed that a radical mastoidectomy cannot always be avoided. However, if conservative surgery is attempted there is a possibility of cholesteatoma recurrence, so an exploratory operation to check for such recurrence must be done approximately two years later. In paragraph five, the patient acknowledges that there are possible risks in both a radical and conservative operations, but that these risks are preferable to continued growth of the cholesteatoma. In paragraph six, the patient states that he prefers conservative treatment if it is possible. Paragraph seven reiterates that a second operation is necessary, and in paragraph eight the patient accepts the responsibility of returning for this operation. I feel very strongly that a questionnaire such as this would be very useful to any surgeon employing the intact canal wall technique.

QUESTIONNAIRE ON CHOLESTEATOMAS OF THE EAR

(1) I have read Dr. Wright's Patient Information booklet on cholesteatoma cysts, and I understand the material. Yes □ No □ Initial   (Dr. Wright is available at this time to answer any questions.)

(2) I understand the possible destructive effects of cholesteatoma and the seriousness of these effects on vital structures deep in the head. Yes □ No □ Initial

(3) I also understand that the radical or modified radical mastoid operation is usually employed to arrest the dangerous progress of a cholesteatoma. In this operation, the mastoid is made part of the ear canal, and the resulting cavity must be cleaned in the doctor's office from one to four times per year on a permanent basis. Furthermore, hearing in the ear sometimes becomes considerably worse, and swimming is prohibited. Yes □ No □ Initial

(4) Sometimes the destructive process and ear structures encountered are such that a radical mastoid operation is unavoidable. However, an effort can be made to avoid this type of radical surgery by microscopically separating and removing the cholesteatoma from the delicate ear structures, thus sparing undamaged structures and hopefully reconstructing what has already been destroyed. To accomplish this, more than one operation may be required. Furthermore, the surgical microscope cannot see single cells, and in spite of meticulous surgical technique, statistics show that there is at least a five per cent chance that the cholesteatoma will recur. Therefore, an exploratory operation to check for early recurrence should be done one and one-half to two years after the cholesteatoma has apparently been removed. Only after such a negative re-exploration is there any assurance that all cholesteatoma cells have been successfully removed. I understand the above. Yes □ No □ Initial

(5) I realize that there are many possible risks involved in any surgical operation and also that the vital and delicate structures deep in the ear might be damaged in performing either a radical or conservative-reconstructive operation. However, since damage to these structures is inevitable by continued growth of the cholesteatoma, I choose to have surgery. Yes □ No □ Initial

(6) I prefer that if possible a radical mastoidectomy be avoided and that a conservative reconstructive operation be done. Yes □ No □ Initial

(7) I realize that this makes necessary another exploratory operation to look for a regrowth of cholesteatoma. Yes □ No □ Initial

(8) This re-exploratory operation should be done one to two years after the first one, and I accept the responsibility of arranging to return at that time. Yes □ No □ Initial

SIGNED WITNESS: William K. Wright, M.D.
DATE

THE SIGNIFICANCE OF THE RETRACTION POCKET IN THE TREATMENT OF CHOLESTEATOMA

David F. Austin, M.D.

The keratinizing epithelial pocket of cholesteatoma has three characteristics important for surgical planning; it's invasive potential, it's progressive destruction of bone and, most important, it's tendency to recur. The similarity of these characteristics to those of neoplasm have resulted in a dichotomy of opinion between surgeons as to the best means of surgical management. Twenty years of experience with conservative surgical approach aimed at preserving the external meatus have allayed some of the dire predictions of those advocating radical surgery for cholesteatoma. Comparative studies of the efficacy of each procedure in obtaining the desired goals of management are still needed. This paper will attempt to supply some data needed for evaluation.

The surgical goals of the treatment of the "pseudoneoplasm" of cholesteatoma are three. First is complete extirpation of the disease process. Second is repair of the damaged middle ear to health and normal function. Third, and largely neglected in surgical reports, is the prevention of recurrence. I have long felt (Austin and Smyth, 1964) that the tendency for recurrence of cholesteatoma is basic to the disease process rather than secondary to the type of surgical approach used for eradication. It is urged that future surgical reports include the recurrence rate of cholesteatoma after a minimum of two years observation in order to evaluate this critical aspect of efficacy of treatment.

Cholesteatoma Recurrence—The Retraction Pocket

The development of conservative canal preserving technics, combined with tympanoplastic reconstruction for the management of cholesteato-

ma allowed the observation of a feature of the disease process not seen with modified radical mastoidectomy—the development of a retraction pocket. The preservation of the attic and antral spaces behind an anatomically placed drumhead allowed the gradual invasion of these spaces by invagination of the posterosuperior portion of the reconstructed membrane. Surgical management of this complication then permits observation of factors responsible for the recurrence of disease.

The natural history of a retraction pocket may be described accurately because the disease appears in the postoperative period when observation is detailed and periodic. The appearance of a retraction pocket is silent and unsuspected. The patient has experienced rapid and uncomplicated recovery from surgery. The drumhead has healed and is functioning. The middle ear is aerated. Canal reconstruction, if necessary, has resulted in an anatomically supportive sulcus. The patient can and does inflate his ear frequently. After the first six months of follow-up, observation is performed at three to six month intervals. A retraction pocket will be seen to develop usually between 18 and 30 months postoperatively. Its appearance is usually unheralded although some patients will note a slight change in hearing. If the pocket is well-developed, some granulation may appear at the posterosuperior margin secondary to erosion and secretion will now be present. In most patients the pocket will acquire all of the characteristics of the original disease; growth, bone destruction and, if operated with the same technic, a second recurrence. If untreated, the growing destructive pocket will cause loss of the thinned posterior canal wall resulting in an unstable mastoid cavity. The best treatment of the retraction pocket is now radical mastoidectomy with mastoid obliteration.

There are many theories concerning the etiology of cholesteatoma. It is instructive to study these to see how they may apply to the development of a retraction pocket. In general, these hypotheses may be divided into three groups; those involving tubal factors or secretory otitis, those involving stimulus by irritation occurring behind the drumhead, and those involving factors present in the deep meatal epithelium and drumhead itself. Detailed exposition of these theories may be found in the writings of Tumarkin (1961), Ruedi (1963), and McGuckin (1961). Other, secondary, mechanisms have been suggested by surgeons concerned with the prevention of retraction pocket formation at the time of the original operation. The most frequently suggested hypotheses have been traction of scar tissue bands in the narrow attic isthmus (to be avoided by the use of sheeting), and/or sagging of the posterosuperior drumhead due to loss of bony support from erosion of the lateral attic wall by disease or surgeon (to be avoided by reconstruction of this portion of the canal). The patient data will be sifted to explore these hypotheses.

Patient Data

The study series consists of all patients operated for cholesteatoma between January, 1969, and January, 1974. No distinction between primary acquired and secondary acquired cholesteatoma was made. For inclusion in the group a minimum two year follow-up was required. Nine patients (12%) were thus lost to follow-up and not included in this series. Table 81 indicates the types and number of operative procedures performed.

The 65 intact canal wall mastoidectomies were all primary procedures as were the 30 modified radical mastoidectomies. The latter operation was done whenever a severely sclerotic mastoid or destruction of the bony canal wall was found. The mastoid obliteration operations were performed on those patients who had had prior radical sur-

TABLE 81

Operations Performed

Procedure	Number
Intact canal operation	65
Modified radical mastoidectomy	30
Mastoid obliteration	29
Total	124

gery for cholesteatoma and required further surgery for reasons of poor hearing or continued disease.

During the same five year period 154 patients were operated for other forms of chronic ear disease via transcanal tympanoplasty. These patients have been recently reported (Austin, 1976). The incidence of retraction pocket formation of this group, together with the cholesteatoma group, is shown in Table 82 categorized by type of disease process.

TABLE 82

Disease	Number	Pockets	Percent
Simple chronic otitis	104	2	2
Atelectatic otitis	50	3	6
Cholesteatoma			
(A) Intact canal	65	15	23
(B) Modified radical	30	1	3
(C) Mastoid obliteration	29	1	3
*(1) Recurrent disease		1	3
*(2) Residual disease		8	22

*These categories are diseases found at secondary surgery following a primary radical operation performed by other surgeons.

The duration of observation for these patients ranges from two to seven years with a mean follow-up of 3.5 years. Retraction pockets were seen to occur over a range of six months (one patient) to five years (three patients). This mean time of initial discovery was at 27 months. For three of the five years (1970 through 1972) silicone sheeting was used to line the middle ear and mastoid. The influence of sheeting upon the incidence of retraction pocket formation is shown in Table 83. The chi-square value indicates that sheeting has no effect upon the incidence of this complication.

TABLE 83

	Pocket	No Pocket	Total
Sheeting	10	34	44
No sheeting	5	16	21
Total	15	50	65

Chi-square: .009 (non-significant)

Tubal function testing was not performed on many patients in this series. Middle ear health was assessed by drumhead mobility on inflation, hearing testing, and presence or absence of fluid in the middle ear as determined by needle myringotomy. Only one patient with a retraction pocket demonstrated inability to inflate the ear and the presence of chronic mucoid secretory otitis. All other patients undergoing revisional surgery had an aerated, healthy middle ear. Findings at revision surgery were limited to a squamous pocket extending from the posterior-superior drumhead margin into the facial recess, attic and antrum. The mastoid and attic bone were covered by healthy mucosa enabling easy dissection of the squamous pocket. In two instances (3% of all patients or 13% of revised patients) residual cholesteatoma in the form of pearls were formed.

Table 84 compares the incidence of complication of patients having intact canal wall surgery with those having modified radical mastoidectomy.

If the incidence of retraction pocket formation is ignored, the problems encountered following modified radical mastoidectomy are double those

TABLE 84

Canal Intact/Modified Radical

	N	N-Comp.	% Comp.
Intact canal wall	60	19 (4)	32 (7)
Modified radical	30	4	13

(The numbers within parentheses represent complications other than retraction pocket formation.)

of the intact canal wall technic. Chi-square analysis does not indicate a significant difference in these numbers, however. Satisfactory results can be expected with modified radical mastoidectomy combined with tympanoplasty.

Discussion of Data

The use of clinical data in arriving at valid conclusions is hazardous. Although the series reported here is small in comparison with some others, it was chosen purposefully to reduce some of the errors otherwise present. The factors influencing this choice were:

(1) The surgical technics employed were constant (other than the use of silicone sheeting) over the period of time studied.

(2) All patients were followed for a minimum of two years.

(3) The operations were sequential over the time of this study to obtain randomness in disease severity.

Surgical conservatism with canal preservation has resulted in persistant disease in 23% of these patients. These recurrences are not manifest in the early post-operative period and, lacking good control of patient follow-up, constitute a definite risk. Early predictions stated that residual disease, hidden behind the intact canal, would lead to severe and life-threatening complications. Such has not been the case. Three percent of this series were found to have residual disease but when compared to the incidence of residual found in those patients having had radical operations (22%), this risk is not a significant factor in determining the type of surgery best suited for extirpation of cholesteatoma.

The retraction pocket, as a novel complication peculiar to intact canal wall technics, was not predictable and has caused recurrent disease in more than 20% of patients. Modification of surgical technic has not resulted in lessening of this incidence of complication. As stated earlier, prevention of recurrent disease must be a goal of surgical therapy. Palva (1975) has stated that he elects modified radical surgery in all cases of cholesteatoma to insure this goal. The advantages of canal preservation for the 75% of patients successfully treated are undeniable. One solution, advocated by many, is surgical staging (Sheehy and Crabtree, 1973). Staging, however, is indicated to eliminate residual disease rather than to treat recurrent disease. My experience has shown that recurrent disease treated by the same surgical technic will have the same result—a second recurrence.

The modern surgical dilemma faced by those advocating canal preservation is not the risk of residual disease but the possibility of recurrent cholesteatoma.

Present Management of Cholesteatoma

For surgeons using canal preservation for the treatment of cholesteatoma, abandonment of their hard-won skills and the attendant advantages to the patient in order to accomplish an unrealizable goal of universal cure is a difficult decision. A 23% failure rate must, however, be a potent factor in this decision. Again we are faced with a dichotomy between conservative and radical surgery for the treatment of the "psuedo-neoplasm" of cholesteatoma.

Compromise in this situation is a possible alternative. For the past five years I have followed the surgical regime outlined below and will continue in the foreseeable future.

(1) Intact canal wall surgery is elected for all patients. In each operation a "Palva" flap is formed and bone paste collected. If anatomic problems or extensive destruction of the canal is encountered, a modified radical with obliteration

is carried out. Such is done in 25% of my patients. They are advised of the likelihood of recurrence and are told that if such appears during the necessary five years postoperative observation, a second operation will be advised.

(2) If residual disease becomes manifest or a retraction pocket appears, a modified radical mastoidectomy with mastoid obliteration is performed.

The above plan eliminates staged surgery for all patients, reserving such for those in whom it is manifestly needed. This plan will result in a single operation for 75% together with anatomic normality. Twenty-five percent of patients will require two procedures culminating in a small cavity requiring minimal care.

Not all surgeons will agree to this compromise. No criticism is made of those who elect modified radical surgery in its various forms as a standard of treatment. Information on the incidence of residual and recurrent disease inherent in this form of therapy is essential for future reevaluation of surgical therapy.

Etiologic Considerations

The conclusions regarding etiology of retraction pocket formation to be drawn from this data are:

(1) Neither negative pressure nor inflammation seem to be factors involved in retraction since neither was observed in this group of patients.

(2) Traction does not seem to be causitive in pocket formation since scarring was not evident at revisional surgery nor did silicone sheeting prevent such recurrence.

(3) Collapse of the drumhead through an eroded portion of the lateral attic wall was not a cause since all eroded areas were repaired.

The hypothesis remaining, unproven but supported by this data, is that retraction pocket formation is caused by a growth-rate error of the drumhead epithelium. Excess growth, meeting a more slowly migrating deep canal epithelium, causes a damming effect and buckling of the drumhead into the attic region posteriorly. This will continue with pocket formation until equilibrium is established or until deepening of the pocket results in relentless progression of the disease. The cause of this proposed hyperactivity is unknown. It is believed, however, that if the cause of the postoperative retraction pocket is established the fundamental nature of cholesteatoma will be nearer solution. Tests of the above hypotheses are possible and are planned for the future.

Summary

The data relative to residual and especially recurrent disease observed in 124 consecutive operations for patients with cholesteatomas are reported. The finding of continuing problems in at least 23% of these patients is noted.

Surgical therapy must be based on the goals of extirpation of the "psuedo-neoplasm" of cholesteatoma, restoration of health and function and prevention of recurrence. Results of "single-barrelled" regimes do not meet these goals. A compromise surgical management regime is offered.

Etiologic implications of the retraction pocket phenomenon are explored and a testable hypothesis offered.

References

1. Austin, D. F. and Smyth, G. D. L. : Cholesteatoma: The vein graft approach. *J. Laryng.*, 78:384, 1964.
2. Austin, D. F. : Transcanal tympanoplasty: A fifteen year report. *Trans. Amer. Acad. Ophthal. Otolaryng.*, 82:30, 1976.
3. McGuckin, F.: Concerning the pathoogenesis of destructive ear disease. *J. Laryng.*, 75:949, 1961.
4. Palva, T.: Mastoid obliteration. *Arch. Otolaryng.*, 101:271, 1975.
5. Ruedi, L.: Acquired cholesteatoma. *Arch. Otolaryng.*, 78:252, 1963.
6. Sheehy, H. P. and Crabtree, J. A.: Tympanoplasty: Staging the operation. *Laryngoscope*, 83:1594, 1973.
7. Tumarkin, A.: Preepidermosis. *J. Laryng.*, 75:487, 1961.

POSTOPERATIVE CHOLESTEATOMA RECURRENCE

J. Sadé, M.D.

In the last two decades conservative surgery for middle ear cholesteatoma has been recommended in various centers (Jansen, 1963; Jako, 1967; Sheehy, 1967; and Sade, 1967) so that it has become routine. The opposite view is that "once a cholesteatoma, always a cholesteatoma" (Baron, 1949), therefore advocating radical surgery. So, the central question is whether cholesteatoma can be eradicated and the ear reconstructed: and, if so, when, how often, and for how long? The present study attempts to answer these questions and assess quantitatively the frequency which ears have been free of cholesteatoma after conservative surgery, i.e., posterior tympanotomies (also called combined approach tympanoplasty, intact canal tympanoplasty, facial recess approach, or canal-up). Only the results of primary surgery have been analyzed; reoperated ears have not been included.

The term "recurrence" of cholesteatoma is used to designate that state in which an ear will show once again a cholesteatoma after surgical removal of this process. Distinction between "residual disease" and "recurrence", though valid (see below), will not be attempted.

Methods and Material

Two groups of patients were analyzed (Table 85):

Group A consisted of 120 patients (124 ears) of which 115 patients (119 ears, i.e. 96%) were available for follow-up. These patients were operated upon in the central Emek Hospital (Afula) during the years 1962-66 (Feiwishewsky, 1967). Of the whole group, 105 (87.5%) had their posterior canal wall preserved, 13 (10.5%) were endaural atticotomies and only two had a radical mastoidectomy. Retrospectively, we asked these questions:

TABLE 85

Number of ears	124 (−4)	68 (−3)
Years	1962-1966	1971-1972
Posterior canal preserved	105 (87.5%)	30 (48%)
Endaural atticotomy	13 (10.5%)	5 (7.5%)
Modified radical	0	6 (9.5%)
Radical mastoidectomy	2 (2%)	12 (18.5%)
Revisions and atypical		12 (18.5%)
Total	120 (96.7%)	65 (97%)

(1) How is the postoperative recurrence rate related to the size of the cholesteatoma found at the operation? Cholesteatomas passing the additus into the mastoid were designated as "large" (59.6%), those which did not (i.e., were confined to the attic) as "small" (40.4%).

(2) How did grafting the tympanic membrane influence postoperative recurrence? When we started, in the early sixties, to preserve the posterior canal wall it was felt (and wrongly so) that in the face of much infection of pus it is preferable to stage the operation leaving even the tympanic graft (and ossiculoplasty) for a second stage—when the ear might be less infected. Most of these patients did not however "dry up." We therefore had a large group of ears, 64 (mostly children), which were not primarily grafted, which we compared with a group (56 ears) which were grafted in the primary operation.

(3) How did the length of time after the operation influence cholesteatoma recurrence?

(4) How did the patient's age relate to cholesteatoma recurrences?

Group A consisted of 68 patients (68 ears) operated upon between the years 1971-72 at the Meir Hospital (Kfar Saba). Thirty ears of these had their posterior wall preserved (posterior tympanotomy) all of which had their tympanic membrane grafted and ossiculoplasty done in the first stage. While after two years 65 patients (i.e., 95.5%) were followed up, at the end of the third year only 21 of the 30 posterior tympanotomies were available for follow-up. Group B (Table 85) contained also five endaural atticotomies, six modified radicals, 12 radicals, and 12 revisions.

Results

Group A: (Fig. 164) Cholesteatoma recurred in 39% of the cases which had their posterior wall preserved when taken as a group over the five years. At the time of follow-up differentiation was not made between recurrence of residual squamous epithelium and the development of deep retraction through missing scutum. However, 7% were noted as presenting shallow retractions of the drum which needed some cleansing but no further surgery. A more complete picture emerged when the patients were divided into different groups. Then cholesteatoma recurrence showed the following pattern:

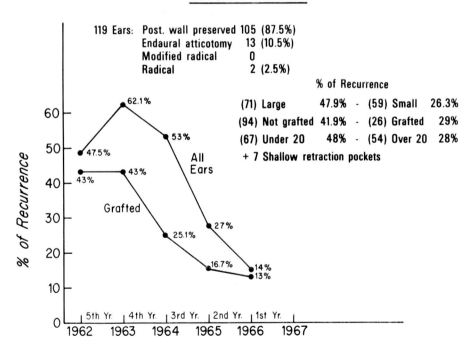

Fig. 164: Group A 105 posterior tympanotomies followed up for five years.

(1) Grafted versus non-grafted.

Recurrences occurred in 41.9% of the ears which were not grafted and in 29% of the grafted ears.

(2) Size of the cholesteatoma at operation when the group was taken as a whole.

Recurrences occurred in 47.9% of the large cholesteatomas and in 26.3% of the small cholesteatomas.

(3) Length of time after the operation when the group was taken as a whole.

Non-grafted ears: Cholesteatoma occurred in 27% after a follow-up of two years as compared with 54% after three-five years.

Grafted ears: In 16% after two years as compared with 43% after four-five years.

(4) Age of patients when group was taken as a whole.

Patients under 20 years had recurrences in 48%. Patients older than 20 years showed recurrences in 28%.

Group B: Cholesteatomas were found to have recurred after:

(1) One year in two ears (7%), after two years in four ears (14%) of 30 ears with posterior tympanotomies. However, after three years, out of 21 ears which were available for follow-up, seven ears (33%) showed the presence of cholesteatoma—once again. In four of these seven, atrophy of part of the posterior wall of skin into the mastoid which was however, self-cleansing in two.

(2) After two years in one ear of the five endaural atticotomies.

Discussion

Several problems may arise after conservative surgery for chronic ears—only some of which are specifically associated with cholesteatomatous ears. Thus, hearing gained might deteriorate, or a grafted tympanic membrane might sink toward the promontorium (atelectasis formation), (Sadé and Berco, 1976). Granulation tissue and reperforation of the new tympanic membrane may also occur. Spontaneous breakdown of the posterior wall (Weinberg and Sadé, 1971) in intact canal technique is seen in cholesteatoma surgery mainly because most intact canal techniques are done when cholesteatoma is present—but this breakdown is probably not seen only in cholesteatomatous ears and is probably secondary to thinning the canal wall. However, this present study deals only with specific features belonging to cholesteatomatous ears and are, as stressed by Sheehy (1967), essentially of two types: (A) recurrence of epidermoid cyst-line structure (i.e., cholesteatomas) in the middle ear cleft which might be due either to stratified squamous epithelium left behind or new formation of the same through a metaplastic process (Sadé, 1974 and Sadé and Weissman, 1976): these will often present themselves as small epidermoid cysts or "pearls". (B) In ears where portions of the scutum or posterior canal wall are missing the canal skin may collapse at this point into the attic and mastoid creating a deep-seated keratin-producing pocket which does not cleanse itself and will often become secondarily infected. This phenomenon is well-recognized but its mechanism is not completely understood. Invagination of external canal skin through a secondary breakthrough of the posterior canal (Weinberg and Sadé, 1971) wall also belongs to this group. The importance of these retraction pockets is in their frequent inability of self-cleansing and secondary infection ensuing thereafter.

The conclusions derived from our follow-up of Group A are: (a) recurrences are about 13% less when the ear is grafted than when it is not, (b) recurrence of "young" cases, i.e., two years postoperative are about half (27%) of those found after a longer follow-up (54%), (c) when the cholesteatoma is confined to the attic (small cholesteatomas) recurrence rate is about half (26.3%) when compared with those ears where extension is to the mastoid (47.9%) (large cholesteatomas), (d) there is about half as much a chance (24%) for recurrence after the age of 20 as for the younger patients (48%). When looking at Group B we see that the recurrence rate within the first three years is not very significantly different from the corresponding grafted patients in Group A. Altogether it seems that at least during the first five years after conservative surgery for cholesteatoma, recurrence of the basic disease is considerable but not inevitable. One facet of the problem is to recognize the higher risk group and treat it accordingly.

This analysis furnishes us with some valuable information, but it does not answer all of our questions. Thus we do not have crossed information on the various parameters (size of cholesteatoma, age of patient, grafted T.M., length of follow-up). So we don't know how an adult ear which had a small cholesteatoma, and had its tympanic membrane grafted will fare in the long run. We have assessed each parameter by itself but not with each other. It is possible, for example, that the poorer prognosis for large cholesteatomas in the young is in effect, one parameter. Yet it stands to reason from this study that older people with small cholesteatomas who had a posterior tympanotomy (and therefore had their tympanic membrane grafted) and have a minimal scutum erosion have less chance of a recurrence. Whether the satisfactory results are maintained for longer periods such as five-ten years is unknown. Unfortunately this study does not give the prognostic distinction between retraction pockets through a missing scutum and residual cholesteatoma.

The relatively higher incidence of cholesteatoma recurrence in the ungrafted group may be due to the special conditions existing here, i.e.: perforation concomitant with absence of middle ear epithelium—the latter having been removed at surgery. Under such conditions the epithelium will probably find its ways unopposed into the middle ear cleft.

Radical surgery should not be generally advocated for cholesteatomatous ears. Yet total reconstruction of such ears is not always possible. We should tailor the operation for each specific ear, according to the pathology of that particular ear.

A posterior tympanotomy which often leaves the patient with a relatively normal ear with no open mastoid bowl is a very desirable and reasonable procedure. Yet, these patients should be followed as there is always the possibility of recurrence. Perhaps the routine second look, often advocated, should be practiced mandatorily after the closed technique is used (Crabtree, 1976). And, one way to enforce this policy would be to defer the oc-

ciculoplasty for a second procedure.

When we choose a specific operation for a given ear other factors besides the presence of cholesteatoma should be taken into account. Some ears might just not be suitable for "total reconstruction" as the posterior tympanotomy attempts to be. Thus, irreversible chronic changes of the middle ear mucosa (Fig. 165) or the rare case of real mechanical obstruction of the eustachian tube are not inducive for reconstruction of the tympanic cavity. We have found the attempts to overcome some of these difficulties with silastic disappointing. Also, the greater the destruction of the ossicular chain the lesser are the chances of closing the air bone gap. This is particularly true when the stapes is missing or fixed. Therefore, total or subtotal ossicles destruction, extensive footplate tymanosclerosis, and important mucosal destruction or irreversible mucosal hyperthropy (often covered with stratified squamous epithelium, see Fig. 165) and especially in the presence of extensive cholesteatoma penetrating deep into the cellular crevices of the temporal bone, are usually not suitable candidates for conservative surgery.

These difficulties are not always present simultaneously and therefore some operations which are of compromising nature are at times in place. Thus, destruction of important areas of the scutum or posterior wall by disease (or by previous surgery) or important involvement of the mastoid region, such as cholesteatoma penetrating into the apex of the pyramid in the presence of relative intactness of the tympanic cavity may be suitable for endaural atticotomies or modified radical operations.

At present, postoperative cholesteatoma recurrences are viewed with greater trepidation than they deserve. In over 20 years of practice, I have not seen a serious complication arising from postoperative cholesteatoma recurrences. We have been taught to dread the intracranial complications which may occur in recurrent postoperative cholesteatomas, but very very rarely. Most complications are due to relatively rapid progressive infection and concommitant

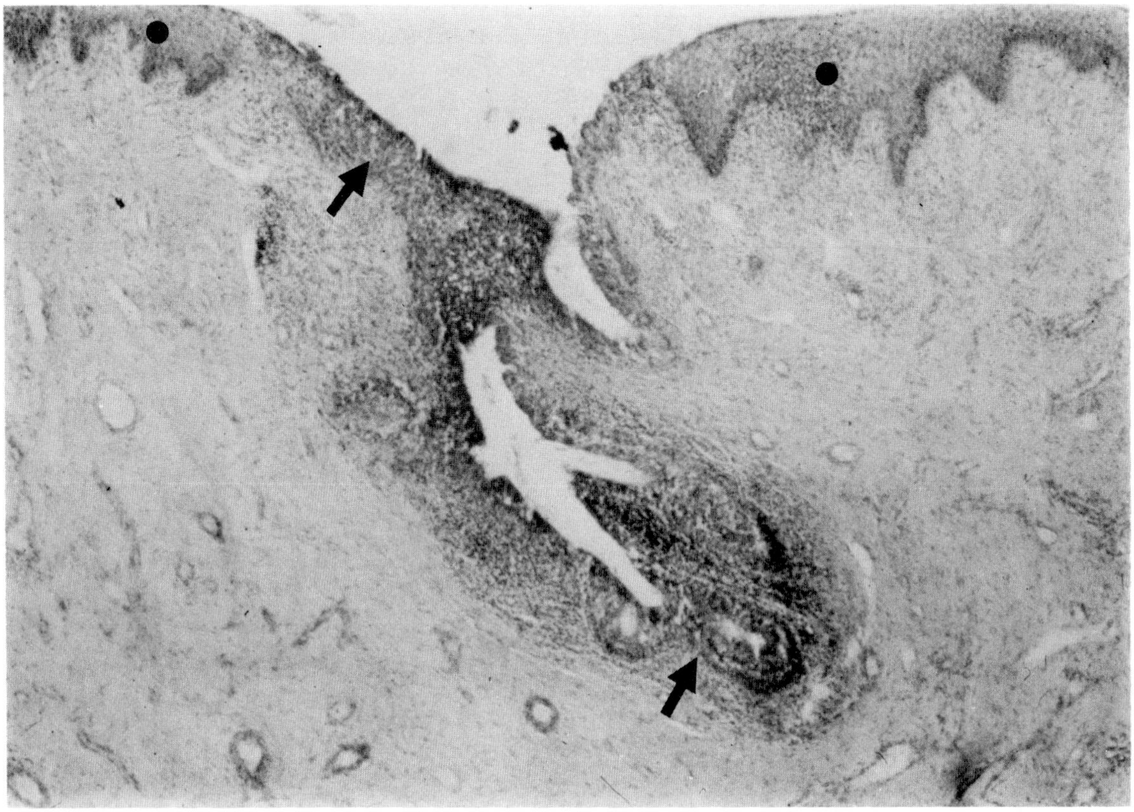

Fig. 165: Biopsy of hypertrophic mucosa from a promontorium showing metaplastic squamous epithelium (black dot) passing into inflammed respiratory mucosa forming glands (arrows).

bone resorption in ears which have not been previously operated upon—and their path of least resistance is medial. This changes once the ear is operated upon. Thus of 124 cholesteatomatous ears we have seen, 14 presented themselves as acute mastoiditis and showed eight labyrinthine fistulas, seven perisinusal abcesses, and four sinus thrombophlebitis. The other 110 ears showed one fistula, one perisinus abscess, and one facial paralysis. None of these complications was observed in a previously operated ear.

Today we do have a better way to manage cholesteatomatous ears than we did in the past, but further progress will be made less on technical considerations and more on the understanding of the major questions:

(1) When and why does the grafted drum retract through a missing scutum into the middle ear cleft? And, why does it not always occur?

(2) Why do we have neo-pearl formation in closed cavities and what is their actual fate? It seems that not all stratified squamous epithelium which is left behind will form an epidermoid cyst once again! The advocacy of closed technique takes it for granted that the surgeon is able to remove all cholesteatoma which can be seen with the microscope. It should be noted however that more and more attempts are made to reconstruct the destroyed scutum—the result of such endeavors are as yet unknown. Gordon Smyth, Blair Simmons, Brian McCabe, Arnold Schuring and Michael Glasscock have told me that they have all seen one or more cases where S.S.E. was left behind over a fistula—or the footplate—or over

the promontory—only to disappear on the second look. This could only be due to a metaplasia in reverse which theoretically could certainly occur (Sadé, 1974 and Sadé and Weissman, 1976).

(3) What is the fate of a small epidermoid formed behind an intact canal and grafted drum? From the various "second looks" such small epidermoid cysts are not rare, yet we don't know their growth rate, or whether they all progress, or some might regress, depending upon their blood supply.

Summary

Recurrence rates of cholesteatoma after conservative middle ear surgery (i.e., posterior tympanotomies) were studied. Two groups of operated ears were analyzed after having been followed from two to five years—one of which was a retrospective study (105) ears), the other was a prospective one (30 ears).

Conclusion

(A) Cholesteatomatous ears can be operated upon conservatively. A significant number of these will not show recurrence of the disease within the first five years after the operation. However, recurrence rate of cholesteatoma in posterior tympanotomies present themselves in increasing number the longer the time since the initial operation. Accurate assessment of what really happens is critically related to a longer follow-up and to the percentage of patients seen after their operation.

(B) The prognosis of these operations is in direct relation to (1) the age of the patient, (2) grafting the tympanic membrane, and (3) size of the cholesteatoma.

(C) Once the scutum is eroded the chances of retraction pockets are considerable and thought should be given to an atticotomy or modified radical if the tympanic cavity itself is relatively intact. Altogether one should refrain from having a dogmatic approach to chronic ear surgery—instead, armed with the various operations at hand, one should tailor a particular operation to a particular ear or pathology.

(D) In view of the apparent inevitability of some recurrence rate making itself apparent with time after conservative surgery—all such ears having had a closed technique operation should be followed routinely with a "second look" within the second year postoperatively.

(E) While progress in ear surgery has been done through the last 20 years the future depends probably more on understanding the pathobiology of cholesteatoma than on new techniques.

References

1. Baron, S. H.: Modified radical mastoidectomy. *Arch. Otolaryng.*, 49:280, 1949.
2. Crabtree, J.: Shambaugh workshop on microsurgery. Chicago, Mar., 1976.
3. Feiwishewsky, A.: Postoperative recurrences of aural cholesteatoma. *M. D. Thesis, Hebrew University*, Jerusalem, Oct. 1967.
4. Jako, G. J.: Posterior route to the middle ear. Posterior tympanotomy. *Laryngoscope*, 77:306, 1967.
5. Jansen, C.: Cartilage—tympanoplasty. *Laryngoscope*, 73:1288, 1963.
6. Sadé, J.: Present concepts of reconstructive middle ear surgery. *EENT Monthly*, 46:1121, 1967.
7. Sadé, J.: Biopathological aspects of s.o.m. *Ann. Otol. Rhinol. Laryng. Suppl.*, 83:59, 1974.
8. Sadé, J. and Berco, E.: Atelectasis and secretory otitis media. *Ann. Otol. Rhinol. Laryng. Suppl.*, April 1976.
9. Sadé, J. and Weissman, Z.: The phenotypic expression of middle ear mucosa. *First International Conference on Cholesteatoma*. Aesculapius Publishing Company, Birmingham, Alabama, 1977.
10. Sheehy, J. L. and Patterson, M. D.: Tympanoplasty with mast. *Laryngoscope*, 77:1502, 1967.
11. Weinberg, J. and Sadé, J.: Postoperative cholesteatoma recurrence through the posterior wall. *J. Laryng. Otol.*, 85:1189, 1971.

PROBLEMS IN SURGICAL CONTROL OF CHOLESTEATOMA

Richard J. Bellucci, M.D.

The origin and pathogenesis of cholesteatoma as well as the unusual energy of growth which it demonstrates remain unsolved problems. When the cholesteatoma becomes established, however, the cure may be obtained by complete surgical excision. The efficiency of this surgery and the problems associated with this method of control are the objectives of this investigation.

Origin and Pathogenesis

Three theories (Lindsay, 1953) have been proposed for the origin of middle ear cholesteatoma. The congenital or primary cholesteatoma originates as epidermal inclusions which develop into the mature cholesteatoma. A tympanic membrane perforation is not found usually in these cases and the epidermal rests tend to occupy a position deep in the petrous region of the temporal bone. These cases fortunately are rarely seen and definite proof of congenital origin has not been established.

The metaplasia theory proposes the conversion of the middle ear mucosa to squamous epithelium resembling skin as a result of chronic inflammation or trauma. This theory, however, lacks support of convincing histopathologic evidence. The existence of cholesterol granulomas possibly can be explained by this theory. A middle ear exudate may exist behind an intact tympanic membrane for an extended period of time. At surgery small yellowish cholesterol granulomas may be found which are composed of granulation tissue, giant cells, blood pigment and cholesterol crystals. The negative pressure as a result of eustachian tube dysfunction causes engorgement of blood vessels releasing blood pigments and exudate which ultimately will cause granulation tissue to develop. Tumarkin explains the blue tympanic membrane on the basis of this theory (Tumarkin, 1958).

The mass of evidence, both clinical and histopathological, indicates the cholesteatoma originates from the epidermis of the canal and tympanic membrane. The migration theory stipulates that a retraction pocket or perforation develops in the tympanic membrane through which epithelium of the edge of the external auditory canal or tympanic membrane invaginates into the middle ear. The driving force for development of a retraction pocket in Shrapnell's membrane is believed to be the negative middle ear pressure caused by eustachian tube dysfunction as postulated in the Bezold-Habermann theory. Epithelial migration through the perforation forms the cholesteatoma sac which ultimately collects desquamated epithelial debris. Reduced pneumatization of the mastoid is usually found when the disease starts early in life. A hypocellular mastoid is always abnormal and results from inhibition of pneumatization due to middle ear vacuum or condensing osteitis (Tumarkin, 1958).

Most otologists agree that the origin of cholesteatoma is due to eustachian tube dysfunction which creates a middle ear vacuum. The vacuum in turn causes a retraction pocket which then may develop into the cholesteatoma (Jordan, 1963). Periodic middle ear infection usually occurs in ears having negative middle ear pressure. Perforation of the tympanic membrane follows permitting the epithelial edge to proliferate and invade the middle ear. In other cases the retraction pocket may slowly collect debris, enlarge and extend into the middle ear.

The matrix or wall of the cholesteatoma sac is composed of keratinizing stratified squamous epithelium (epithelium layer) which lies over 1-2 mm of connective tissue (sub-epithelial layer). The epithelial layer closely resembles skin but is thinner. There are no pilosebaceous units but all characteristics of the stratum germinativum are present (Schechter, 1968). The subepithelial layer is in intimate contact with the underlying bone. Just beneath the basal cells are found reticulin fibrils and elastic fibers which make up a loose tissue network. The defects of the underlying bone as well as the vascular channels are invaded by this tissue. Layers of collagen are also intimately connected with the adventitial layers of the blood vessels of the bone. The most common cells of the subepithelial layer are the fibroblasts which appear to be the elements, along with the osteoclasts and osteoblasts, actively engaged in the invasion and destruction of the underlying bone (Harris, 1962).

Considerable controversy exists concerning the influence of the subepithelial layer on the underlying bone. Bone erosion under this layer is seen in almost all cases of long standing. Clinically, the bone is flattened and absorbed. Prominent middle ear structures such as the ossicles, facial nerve and lateral semicircular canal are involved in the destructive process. Large cholesteatoma which erode the tegmen are frequently responsible for intracranial complications.

The exact modus operandi of the subepithelial layer in absorbing bone remains in doubt. Many otologists believe that pressure alone exerted on the bone by the impacted epithelial debris produced by desquamation is responsible for the erosion of underlying bone and extension of the cholesteatoma (Harris, 1962 and Baron, 1953). These otologists believe that exteriorization and marsupialization of the cholesteatoma sac relieves the pressure on the bone and the cholesteatoma will be inactivated. Since the matrix, however, so closely resembles skin its removal will not be required. Following this mode of treatment, complications will be reduced and the tissues conserved will permit better hearing (Baron, 1953 and McGuckin, 1963). Frequent postoperative care will be required in order to ensure stability in mastoid

cavities with this type of epidermal tissue.

Other otologists consider the exteriorization of the cholesteatoma for the relief of pressure on the underlying bone insufficient treatment (Walsh, 1953). They cite the invasion of the vascular spaces by the subepithelial layer and believe enzymes are produced in this layer which cause erosion of the underlying bone (Walsh, 1953 and Abramson, 1967). Others have indicated a special invasive property of the subepithelial layer especially near the periosteum which has a close resemblance to the invasiveness which is characteristic of neoplastic tumors (Maeda, et al and Abramson, 1967). The clinical and laboratory evidence on which these theories are based has not been clearly described. Bone erosion is peculiar to cholesteatoma. Increased vascularity associated with certain tumors (angiomas and glomus tumors) are known to be responsible for bone absorption. Highest levels of enzyme activity have been demonstrated in the presence of highly vascularized granulation tissue. In turn, granulation tissue usually is associated with active infectious processes.

Since the erosion of the underlying bone by the subepithelial layer of the matrix has not been definitely excluded by experimental evidence, all cholesteatoma should be considered potentially invasive. The subepithelial layer of the cholesteatoma, therefore, should be removed in all cases.

Preoperative Study and Treatment

The treatment of cholesteatoma to date remains surgical. It has been generally agreed that cholesteatoma in most cases is a complication of otitis media. Measures to control frequent attacks of otitis media, therefore, will ultimately reduce the incidence of cholesteatoma.

Recurrent attacks of middle ear infection can be reduced but not eliminated entirely by preventive measures. Eustachian tube dysfunction is becoming better accepted as the basic cause of middle ear infection (Bellucci, 1976). All factors which are responsible for eustachian tube dysfunction, however, have not been precisely defined.

Malformation of the nasopharynx in varying degrees may change the action of the eustachian tube musculature which ultimately accounts for eustachian tube malfunction. Added factors such as nasal obstruction due to hypertrophic adenoid, deviated septum, allergic rhinitis and hypertrophic inferior turbinates play a significant and complementary role. General nutrition, resistance to infection, poor personal habits of nose-blowing and frequent exposure to other people with upper respiratory infections are also important in the frequency of attacks of otitis media (Bellucci, 1976).

It must be stressed, however, that surgery of the ear cannot be uniformly successful if the basic cause for middle ear infection rests in the eustachian tube and remains untreated. Although the surgery may be skillfully performed, the ultimate stability of the ear will depend on whether the postoperative ear becomes reinfected. Selection of cases for tympanoplasty with a good possibility of stability after surgery is possible in ears without cholesteatoma. When cholesteatoma is present, however, surgical removal is required regardless of the coexistant eustachian tube dysfunction. The middle ear infection should be brought to the most quiescent state by local debridement and by medicating the patient before the operation. In this manner, it is possible to determine the degree of eustachian tube malfunction which may coexist with the cholesteatoma. If the ear becomes quiescent under treatment, saprophitic organisms may be found in cultures of middle ear secretion and few organisms due to eustachian tube contamination such as pneumococcus, hemophilus influenzae, B-hemolytic streptoccus and Neisseria catarrhalis will be present (Bellucci, 1976).

Surgery of Cholesteatoma

Following careful preoperative debridement, the inflammation of the middle ear mucosa subsides. Consequently, at the time of surgery it is possible to identify easily the metaplastic from normal tissues permitting conservation of tissues for tympanoplasty. Regardless of prognosis for stability in any case, cholesteatoma demands surgery as it follows a course of progressive invasion and destruction.

Today, conservation of hearing has become a primary consideration, and the surgical management of aural cholesteatoma has become a challenge to the otologist. Complete removal of the cholesteatoma in most cases would not be too difficult if conservation of tissues for the tympanoplasty were not a major consideration. In most cases, therefore, a line of demarcation between normal and diseased tissues based on general appearance under inadequate magnification must be established at the time of surgery. The final decision between what is normal and what is diseased tissue is usually a compromised judgement. Furthermore, in order to obtain a good postoperative level of hearing, the normal anatomical structure of the middle ear should be maintained as close to normal as permitted by the disease process. At the same time, adequate exposure is required for removal of all the cholesteatoma. Again, two opposing decisions are possible, and a compromise is made usually between the preservation of the anatomy and providing enough latitude in exposure for control of the disease. When making these decisions in aural cholesteatoma, the experience and surgical judgement of the otologist are of paramount importance.

After all the visible squamous elements have been removed, often there is doubt in the minds of most otologists whether cholesteatoma still remains in the ear. The uncertainty regarding the total removal of all cholesteatoma in every case has been expressed frequently. Some otologists have recommended a second operation at a later date to be sure the cholesteatoma has been controlled (Bellucci, 1973). It is very probable that some few fragments of squamous or metaplastic tissue remain in all cases. During healing and in the absence of infection, these elements are most likely absorbed. It can be theorized that in the postoperative ear, under favorable conditions and in the absence of infection, the few cells which have undergone metaplasia may revert to normal. When unfavorable middle ear conditions and infection persist, metaplastic cells can continue to proliferate and may develop into a clinical cholesteatoma. This opinion regarding the behavior of middle ear cholesteatoma is not based on any known experimental work. It is inconceivable that all the metaplastic cells and shreds of squamous debris have been removed in every case under the magnification and with the instruments currently in use. Cholesteatoma is a cellular diagnosis and present surgical techniques to ensure positive identification and thorough elimination of cells are grossly inadequate. It is possible that the remaining small metaplastic areas may revert to normal. Squamous debris may be absorbed when they exist in small quantities. It is doubtful, however, that larger masses of squamous tissue can be absorbed. Instead, these remain to proliferate if not completely removed.

Surgical Technique

The control of cholesteatoma requires complete exposure and meticulous exenteration. The middle ear anatomy must be maintained close to normal and, whenever possible, the posterior canal wall should be preserved. The technique currently in use conforms to these prerequisites and details of this surgery have been reported (Bellucci, 1973). A brief description will be included here. The surgery is started by widening the osseous portion of the external auditory canal in all directions. In the superoposterior quadrant, a control window is made into the attic which at the same time preserves the rim of annulus (the bridge). This window permits the inspection of the antrum to determine the limits of cholesteatoma and, if necessary, the window can be extended anteriorly over the head of the malleus to expose the attic recess anterior to this ossicle. The annulus over the ossicles is preserved whenever possible as this assures the correct lateral dimensions of the middle ear. In most cases, cholesteatoma is limited to the attic and middle ear and by following this technique, mastoidectomy has been found unnecessary

in 60% of the cases. Should the cholesteatoma extend beyond reach into the antrum when observed through the control window, a trans-cortical mastoidectomy is performed. The posterior canal wall is preserved, however, in a more posterior position than normal because it has already been widened posteriorly during the initial steps of the operation when exposing the middle ear. This combined exposure provides very adequate access to the mastoid and middle ear and the cholesteatoma can be approached through the mastoid area as well as through the middle ear. The mastoid cavity is drained posteriorly. The ossicles and tympanic membrane are reconstructed using the commonly employed methods. The tympanic membrane perforation is grafted usually with fascia and the external auditory canal is reconstructed using canal skin or a very thin Thiersch graft taken from the abdomen (Bellucci, 1973).

In this technique, the middle ear which is the critical area to evaluate, is exposed first. The extent of the cholesteatoma is determined and the degree of middle ear damage is evaluated permitting early modification of the surgical procedure in accordance with the pathology encountered. This early appraisal of the middle ear has an important influence on the remainder of the operation. Surgery can be extended step by step from the middle ear into the epitympanic area and finally into the mastoid if this is required. This wide external auditory canal technique offers the best opportunity for maximum conservation of healthy tissues in their normal anatomical relationship for use in the tympanoplasty. Extensive mastoid surgery is very often unnecessary as the cholesteatoma involves only the middle ear and the epitympanic space.

Results

Essentially three types of middle ear operations were performed. The radical mastoidectomy was required when middle ear mucosal changes and ossicular destruction were so extensive that a tympanoplasty could offer only a very poor opportunity for improvement in hearing. In most cases of very chronic infection, the mastoid pneumatization was reduced by chronic osteitis. Consequently, preservation of the posterior canal wall often was not considered necessary. Routinely, in performing a radical mastoidectomy, all soft tissues of the middle ear and the mastoid, and all ossicles except the stapes were removed. The mastoid bowl was polished and the posterior canal wall was lowered to a level close to the Fallopian canal. The entire cavity was grafted with a very thin Thiersch graft taken from the abdomen.

Recurrence rate of cholesteatoma was low in this group, 3% after at least two years of observation. This is a low percentage considering 90% of cases in this group had extensive cholesteatoma involving the middle ear, attic and mastoid, Table 86. In some cases the middle ear orifice of the eustachian tube was plugged firmly with fascia. This procedure was considered necessary when severe eustachian tube dysfunction existed and contamination of the middle ear through the eustachian tube could not be controlled.

TABLE 86

Tympanoplasty Residual or Recurrence of Cholesteatoma

Type of tympanoplasty	Total number	Cholesteatoma		Residual or Recurrence	
		number	percent	number	percent
Type I Ossicles intact	120	16	13	1	6
Type II Mal-stapes wire	140	63	45	13	21
Type III Ossicular-trans Cortical incus	135	59	44	15	25
Radical Mastoidectomy	90	81	90	4	3
Total	485	219	45	33	15
Total of Type II and III	275	122	44	28	23

Although a large number of radical mastoidectomies are included in this study, this type of surgery is being done less frequently today. Better exposure of the middle ear and epitympanic space using the wide external canal approach accounts for this change. The recurrence rate of cholesteatoma, however, remains high (23%) in Types II and III tympanoplasty, indicating that the present surgical techniques used are inadequate for identification and surgical control of squamous and metaplastic tissues. In these cases, further surgical procedures are required. When all soft tissues of the middle ear and mastoid are removed, as in

the radical mastoidectomy, the recurrence rate of cholesteatoma is low (3%). The difference in these figures demonstrates that in attempting to preserve hearing by doing a tympanoplasty some risk of incomplete surgical removal of the cholesteatoma must be accepted. A radical mastoidectomy in selected cases has a place in modern otology. This operation is given further importance when considering that the postoperative grafted ear has a hearing level ranging from 30-50 dB and the ear has a high degree of stability.

When the ossicles were found to be intact, a tympanoplasty Type I was performed (Wullstein,

1956). Usually an epitympanic retraction pocket filled with cholesteatoma was the typical pathology. The body of the incus and head of the malleus may have shown evidence of erosion but the cholesteatoma was limited and accessible. In a group of 16 cases, only 6% had recurrence of cholesteatoma. This low percentage was expected since the cholesteatoma, because of its location, could be removed as an intact sac.

The majority of cases required a Type II or III reconstruction. The position of the cholesteatoma in the posterosuperior quadrant of the tympanic membrane caused erosion of the lenticular process or stapedial crura. In other ears the epitympanic cholesteatoma extended medial to the body of incus or head of malleus requiring disarticulation and repositioning of the ossicles. When the body of the incus was found to be extensively eroded by cholesteatoma making it unsuitable for transposition and the stapes crura were intact, the malleus-stapes wire was used. The wire was also used when the distance between the handle of the malleus and head of stapes measured more than 3 mm. This extreme anatomical variation makes ossicular transposition technically difficult. The wire prosthesis is classified as a Type II tympanoplasty because it functions in a manner similar to the normal incus. When the crura of the stapes were absent, a cortical bone prosthesis was used to bridge the gap between the handle of the malleus and the mobile footplate of the stapes. In most cases cholesteatoma was found to be extensive with involvement of the epitympanic space, the medial side of the ossicles and the middle ear surface of the tympanic membrane. Occasionally, extension of cholesteatoma was found anterior to the head of malleus and to the processus cochleariformus. These areas are always difficult to visualize and some question always arises concerning completeness of removal of every shred of squamous epithelium.

Statistical analysis of results in cases with advanced cholesteatoma reflects the difficulties anticipated in complete removal. In Type II and III reconstruction of 122 cases of cholesteatoma, 28 patients or 23% had recurrence of cholesteatoma. This finding seems acceptable but it must be realized that many cases in this study had a radical mastoidectomy. Therefore, many of the ears with very advanced cholesteatoma, were not classed as a tympanoplasty. Only suitable ears without widespread tissue destruction and with cholesteatoma which appeared to be surgically controllable, had a tympanoplasty. In spite of observing these strict prerequisites for tympanoplasty, a recurrence developed in 23%. This figure would be higher if a tympanoplasty was attempted in every ear, including those with far advanced soft tissue destruction.

Conclusions

Based on experimental evidence and clinical experience, the migration theory of cholesteatoma appears to be most valid explanation for cholesteatoma.

Whether the subepithelial layer exerts its energy for the absorption of underlying bone by chemical effect or by pressure necrosis is unknown. Until scientifically determined, it is best to remove the subepithelial layer and thus terminate the destructive action of the cholesteatoma.

Cholesteatoma must be considered as a complication of middle ear infection or trauma. The control of middle ear infection by improvement in general health and early treatment of nasal pathology may reduce the incidence of cholesteatoma. Eustachian tube dysfunction is becoming better accepted as a strong etiological factor in middle ear infection. If this theory is correct, the course of middle ear infection in some cases cannot be permanently altered by any means of treatment because the factors causing eustachian tube dysfunction are difficult to correct. Consequently, middle ear stability in certain cases is difficult to achieve and permanently cure.

Complete surgical removal of cholesteatoma may be impossible using the methods and magnification available. Some vestige of cholesteatoma or a metaplastic cell must remain in every case until some method is developed for better identification of these tissues at the time of surgery. Recurrence of cholesteatoma remains a possibility in all cases and is the problem to be solved in future investigation.

Although carefully selected cases were used in this study, of 219 ears with cholesteatoma, 15% showed evidence of recurrent cholesteatoma. Included in the 219 cases are 81 ears on which a radical mastoidectomy was performed. Excluding these ears from the statistics, the rate of recurrence increases to 23%. A tympanoplasty performed for ears with widespread cholesteatoma and for advanced mucosal squamous metaplasia may be a more radical approach to the management of this disease. A radical mastoidectomy has a definite place in aural surgery as it may eliminate a second operation. Routine control of cholesteatoma of the middle ear and mastoid is never a foregone conclusion. Patients should be informed of this fact and urged to follow a routine of regular inspection and treatment of the postoperative ear for evidence of recurrence of cholesteatoma and early correction if it is necessary.

References

1. Abramson, M.: Collagenolytic activity in middle ear cholesteatoma. *Ann. Otol. Rhinol. Laryngol:* 78:112, 1969.
2. Baron, S. H.: Why and when I do not remove the matrix. *Trans. Amer. Acad. Ophthalmol. Otolaryngol.,* 57:694, 1953.
3. Bellucci, R. J.: Selection of cases for tympanoplasty. Presented at the Shambaugh Fifth International Workshop on Middle Ear Microsurgery and Fluctuant Hearing Loss, February 29-March 5, 1976, Chicago, Illinois, 1976.
4. Bellucci, R. J.: Preservation of the posterior canal wall. *Arch. Otolaryngol.,* 97: 198, 1973.
5. Harris, A. J.: Cholesteatosis and chronic otitis media: The histopathology of osseous and soft tissues. *Laryngoscope,* 72: 954, 1962.
6. Jordan, R. E.: Secretory otitis media in etiology of cholesteatoma. *Arch. Otolaryngol.,* 78: 261, 1963.
7. Lindsay, J. R.: The pathogenesis of cholesteatoma and summary of discussions on the removal of the matrix. *Trans. Amer. Acad. Ophthalmol. Otolaryngol.,* 57:707, 1953.
8. McGuckin, F.: A critical analysis of certain cases of destructive ear disease. *J. Laryngol. Otol.,* 77: 115, 1963.
9. Maeda, M., Tabata, T., Shimada, T. et al: Histological and histochemical studies on cholesteatoma epidermis. *Ann. Otol. Rhinol. Laryngol.,* 76: 1043, 1967.
10. Schechter, G.: A review of cholesteatoma pathology. *Laryngoscope,* 79: 1907, 1969.
11. Sheehy, J. L. and Patterson, M. E.: Intact canal wall tympanoplasty with mastoidectomy. A review of eight years experience. *Laryngoscope,* 77: 1502, 1967.
12. Tumarkin, A.: Attic cholesteatosis. *J. Laryng. Otol.,* 72: 610, 1958.
13. Walsh, T. E.: Why I remove the matrix. *Trans. Amer. Acad. Ophthal. Otolaryng.,* 57:687, 1953.
14. Wullstein, H.: Theory and practice of tympanoplasty. *Laryngoscope,* 66:1076, 1956.

CHOLESTEATOMA RECURRENCES IN TYPE IV TYMPANOPLASTY

Harold F. Schuknecht, M.D.

At the Mass Eye and Ear Infirmary we remove all of the cholesteatomatous matrix (squamous epithelium) whenever possible, even when fistulae of the bony labyrinth develop. For ears with extensive involvement of the epitympanum or mastoid, the "canal-down" technique, in association with Type III or IV tympanoplasty and facial-muscle obliteration of the epitympanum and mastoid, is preferred. In 1971, Dr. Keatjin Lee and I reported the findings in 936 major surgical procedures performed at the Mass Eye and Ear Infirmary (Table 87). The incidence of preoperative cholesteatoma was 37%, and the incidence of postoperative recurrence (mean observation time: five years) was 2.7%. In 1976, Dr. Victor Gotay-Rodriguez and I reviewed the results of 70 Type IV tympanomastoidectomies performed by me over an 11 year period. The criteria for performing this operation is total destruction of the tympanic membrane and all ossicles except the footplate of the stapes. Cholesteatoma was present preoperatively in 83% and postoperative recur-

TABLE 87

Incidence of Cholesteatoma

	Number	Preoperative Cholesteatoma	Postoperative Cholesteatoma			
			Graft	Middle Ear	Mastoid	Total
Tympanoplasty	331	18 (5.4%)	2	3	1	6
Tympanoplasty and mastoidectomy	409	213 (52%)	4	9	2	15
Tympanoplasty and atticoantrostomy	29	14 (48%)	0	0	0	0
Mastoidectomy only	158	101 (64%)	0	1	3	4
Rambo	9	1 (11%)	0	0	0	0
	936	347 (37%)	6	13	6	25 (2.7%)

rences were noted in 4.28% (mean observation time: 4.17 years), (Fig. 166).

For non-clinicians who may not realize its possible morbid implications, the following brief report is of interest:

Mr. S. D., a 23-year-old man with a history of recurring bilateral otorrhea for many years. He now complained of right ear pain and tinnitus, as well as vertigo. An antibiotic drug was prescribed by a hospital emergency care physician. Twelve

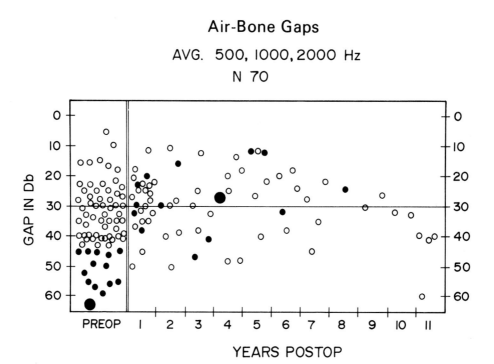

Air-Bone Gaps
AVG. 500, 1000, 2000 Hz
N 70

Fig. 166: Tympanomastoidectomy type IV. Bone-air gaps from the preoperative and the last available postoperative audiometric test for each of 70 ears. The solid circles represent data on the 14 ears with the largest preoperative bone-air gaps.

days later, he was brought to the hospital because of headaches, drowsiness, vertigo, and vomiting. It was reported that there were no meningeal signs or nystagmus (which in retrospect is difficult to believe). Radiologic studies were compatible with right epitympanic cholesteatoma. Despite intensive antibiotic therapy, his condition gradually deteriorated, and he died on the eighth day of hospitalization. Autopsy revealed meningitis and right temporal lobe abscess. Both temporal bones were removed for histological study (Figs. 167 & 168).

The right temporal bone shows advanced acute and chronic inflammatory changes in the middle ear, mastoid, and inner ear. Only remnants of the tympanic membrane, embedded in granulation tissue remain. The middle ear contains fibrous tissue, cystic spaces with acidophilic fluid, granulation tissue, and lakes of pus. The antrum is lined with squamous epithelium and contains a central plug of keratin debris. There is a 3 mm defect in the tegmen of the mastoid. The fistulous tract contains granulation tissue and extends into the middle cranial fossa. There is pus in the internal

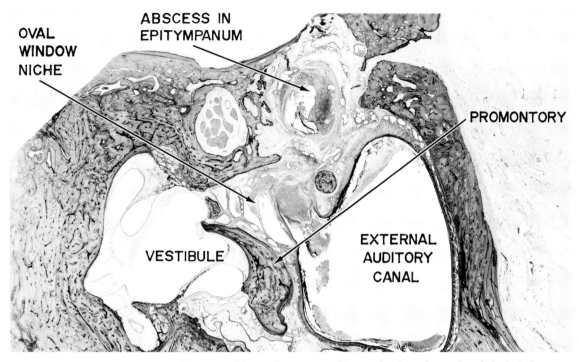

Fig. 167: Vertical section of the right temporal bone of a 23 year old man showing advanced pathological changes resulting from chronic suppurative otitis media. *(Courtesy of Dr. C. Morales-Garcia, Santiago, Chile.)*

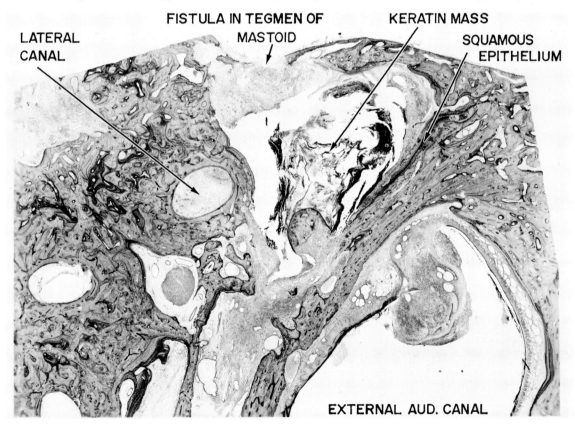

Fig. 168: Vertical section of the same ear showing cholesteatoma of the mastoid and a fistulous tract in the tegmen of the mastoid communicating with the middle cranial fossa. *(Courtesy of Dr. C. Morales-Garcia, Santiago, Chile.)*

auditory canal.

The superior and lateral semicircular canals contain granulation tissue and pus, and the cristi show a severe subepithelial edema. The stroma of the cristae and the maculae are infiltrated with acute and chronic inflammatory cells. There is an acidophilic precipitate in both the endolymphatic and perilymphatic spaces of the canals, vestibule, and scalae of the cochlea. Hair cells are seen thoughout the vestibular sense organs. The organ of Corti shows compression artefact; however, hair cells can be seen throughout. The cochlear, vestibular, and facial nerve trunks appear normal.

Diagnoses

(1) Chronic suppurative otitis media and mastoiditis, right.

(2) Cholesteatoma, mastoid, right.

(3) Mastoid—middle fossa fistula, right.

(4) Otitic meningitis.

(5) Temporal lobe abscess, right.

References

1. Gotay-Rodriquez, V. and Schuknecht, H.: Experiences with Type IV tympanomastoidectomy. *Laryngoscope*, 1976, in press.

2. Lee, K. and Schuknecht, H.: Results of tympanoplasty and mastoidectomy at the Massachusetts Eye and Ear Infirmary. *Laryngoscope*, 81:529, 1971.

RESULTS IN CHOLESTEATOMA SURGERY

Michael E. Glasscock, III, M.D., F.A.C.S.

Surgery of cholesteatoma remains a controversial subject after many years of debate. Should the ear be routinely marsupialized to the outside, as in the radical and modified procedures, or should a more conservative approach be taken in an attempt to preserve the anatomical function of the ear? The purpose of this writing is to review the complications and results in a series of patients who were managed with an intact canal wall procedure. The follow-up period is a minimum of one year and a maximum of five years. The surgical technique in all of these patients has been a facial recess type approach leaving the posterior canal wall intact. The grafting procedure employed fascia as an underlay graft.

Postoperative Complications

Complications of cholesteatoma surgery can be divided into two groups: (1) those iatrogenic injuries to the contents of the temporal bone resulting from a mishap in surgery, and (2) those arising from a lack of control of the primary disease.

(1) Iatrogenic injuries: The unskilled or careless surgeon can produce severe injury to the contents of the temporal bone. Operating upon a diseased ear which has lost its normal antomy, it is possible to dislocate ossicles and injure the labyrinth with resulting sensorineural hearing loss. Certainly the uncovered facial nerve is easily damaged if special precautions are not taken to protect it.

(2) Control of disease: If the cholesteatoma is not removed completely, residual disease will cause problems. Residual disease should be differentiated from recurrent disease, in which the original disease process starts over again. Recurrent disease refers to retraction pockets in the attic and posterosuperior quadrant that go on to produce cholesteatoma.

Case Material

The patients in this series were operated on between January 1, 1970, and December 31, 1974, allowing for at least one year to as much as five years of follow-up. Five hundred ninety (590) primary chronic ear operations were performed during this period and of this number, 179 or 30% involved removal of cholesteatoma. The 179 operations were performed in 153 patients, 26 of whom had bilateral disease. Consequently, the basis of this report is 130 patients who underwent 154 operative procedures. The overall follow-up rate in this group was 85% and the five year rate was 75%. Twenty percent (20%) of these individuals had undergone unsuccessful previous surgery. Eighty-five percent (85%) of the patients presented with secondary acquired cholesteatomas while 15% had primary acquired disease. One patient had both a primary and secondary acquired lesion. Twenty-two percent (22%) of the patients had cholesteatomas limited to the tympanic cavity. One hundred and four (104) procedures were performed as planned two stage operations with an average interval of six months. All patients were treated medically prior to surgery with daily irrigations of 1.5% acetic acid followed by an antibiotic-cortisone otic drop. The majority of the ears were dry at the time of surgery, but 35 had purulent drainage at the time of their operations. Two individuals had large horizontal canal fistulae and two had fistulae on the superior canal. There were three oval window fistulae. In all of these cases except one, the matrix of the cholesteatoma was left intact over the opening at the first stage and removed at the second. Four individuals presented with large aural polyps. In seven cases, there were exposure of the facial nerve, but there were no preoperative or postoperative facial palsies. Two patients had dural exposure due to disease at the time of surgery. No patient complained of vertigo prior to surgery and none had a positive fistula test. When the cholesteatoma was limited to the middle ear, the mastoid was not opened. One patient had a 2 cm acoustic tumor removed from the involved ear after the cholesteatoma had been removed.

Results

In reviewing the results in these 154 cases, the author was primarily interested in residual or recurrent disease and postoperative complications. Hearing results have not been considered here as they have been reported elsewhere (Glasscock, 1976).

In this series of patients using underlay technique, the graft take was 96%, which coincides with my previous results (Glasscock, 1973). There was a 6% incidence of frank wound infections in the postoperative period. There was no particular correlation between preoperative and postoperative infections. However, all of the postoperative perforations were associated with infections with the exception of one, and in this particular case the silastic sheeting had been made too large for the middle ear and had rolled up so that it touched the new eardrum, causing a pressure necrosis. There were no dead ears and only one ear demonstrated any loss of bone conduction of 15 dB or more (0.6%). Only one patient had severe vertigo after surgery and this was an individual who had a very large superior canal fistula that was uncovered inadvertently at the first procedure.

Recurrent cholesteatoma has certainly been the greatest problem in this series of patients, in that there was return of the original disease process in 21 cases (14%). It is interesting to note that if the primary disease was an attic cholesteatoma the recurrence would be in the attic, and if it was a posterosuperior quadrant retraction, the same type of lesion would recur.

There were 19 patients in which residual disease was found at their planned second stage. Eight of these (5%) had cholesteatoma left on purpose at the first operation either over a fistula, over an oval window, or wrapped around the crus of the stapes. Eleven (7%), however, were completely unsuspected. When residual pearls were found, 8% were in the middle ear, 3% in the attic, and 1% were in the antrum. Of the 12 middle ear pearls, eight had purposely been allowed to remain. Two antrum pearls had also purposely been allowed to remain on the canal fistulae at the first procedure. There were no residual pearls found in the mastoid of any of these cases. Cholesteatoma had been allowed to remain in seven patients, and at their second stage procedure, the disease had disappeared. I have no explanation for this and certainly feel that one should not find any false security in the fact that the skin does occasionally disappear. A total of 40 ears (26%) had either residual or recurrent disease. This would seem to be rather high; however, I feel that residual disease can be removed by a planned second stage procedure, leaving as our main problem the 14% who develop recurrent disease.

Discussion

Only by carefully reviewing our cases will we be able to determine the success of our operative procedures. It behooves every otologic surgeon, whether or not he publishes his results, to periodically review his cases to determine what his actual results are. Whether one decides to exteriorize the ear or to use a more conservative approach will depend a great deal on his training, philosophy, and ability as a surgeon. Certainly, one must be honest with himself and never leave cholesteatoma unless he is convinced that a second procedure is feasible. If it is impossible at a second or third stage to remove the disease, the ear must be marsupialized. While there is a rather high incidence of recurrent disease in this series, it would appear that 86% of the individuals maintained a dry ear, normally functioning tympanic membrane, and normal posterior canal wall. These individuals do not require cleansing of their cavities, they do not have recurrent infections, and can actively participate in water sports.

Many of these individuals obtained satisfactory hearing levels.

Residual disease is a problem but it can be managed simply by performing the procedures as planned two stage operations. This allows the surgeon to thoroughly inspect the mastoid, antrum, attic, and middle ear for any disease that was inadvertently allowed to remain at the initial procedure. The low incidence of sensorineural hearing loss (6%) would indicate that staging in fistula cases is a very worthwhile approach.

The intact canal wall tympanoplasty has many advantages, but if one is going to use this technique, there are certain prerequisites that must be met. First, the surgeon must become familiar with the technique itself and the surgical anatomy of the temporal bone. This knowledge can, of course, be acquired by attending a temporal bone surgical dissection course. Modern instrumentation has made intact canal wall tympanoplasty possible and the surgeon must train himself in the use of the operating microscope, irrigation-suction, and high speed dental-type drills.

Summary

A series of 154 cases of cholesteatoma managed by an intact canal wall tympanoplasty was reviewed, with 85% overall follow-up. The complications and results of this procedure were discussed, the worst complication in this series being recurrent disease (14%). Residual disease was managed by planned two stage procedures.

References

1. Glasscock, M. E.: Tympanic membrane grafting: Overlay vs. undersurface technique. *Laryngoscope*, 83:754, 1973.
2. Glasscock, M. E.: Ossicular chain reconstruction. *Laryngoscope*, 86:211, 1976.

VITAMIN "A" THERAPY OF AURAL CHOLESTEATOMA

R. Bruce Duncan, F.R.C.S.

Preface by Dr. Brian F. McCabe

When lecturing in New Zealand recently, Dr. Duncan, an otolaryngologist, showed me his material on the vitamin A therapy of cholesteatoma. For many years, we have searched for a medical treatment for this condition, and his results indicate that there may be something quite important in using vitamin A therapy for the treatment of aural cholesteatoma. As the manuscript reached me only three days before the conference, I will read it to you, though there are some points which are obscure to me. Recent contacts by the Roche Company to my department promise that a multinational approach to this modality of treatment will commence.

Although Dr. Duncan's results sound incredible, I've had reasonably good contact with him and would qualify him as a good observer with solid credentials.

The Effect of Vitamin A* Acetate Therapy

(1) Improvement is evident in three-five weeks.

(2) The mucous membrane of the middle ear becomes vascular and thicker. It begins to extend, pushing back the cholesteatomatous membrane.

(3) Cholesteatoma desquamation is less adherent and can be peeled off the underlying membrane without bleeding.

(4) Cholesteatoma membrane retracts and may disappear from the middle ear. The last sites are roof of attic and lower lip of oval window and promontory, suggesting a metaplasia etiology.

(5) The unpleasant smell of moist or wet mastoid cavities and drum perforations disappears.

(6) Mucus production increases and appears to possess immune properties. The daily production of mucus is controlled by frequency of therapy, and vitamin A concentration.

(7) Mastoid cavities and drum perforations are less painful to clean and dress.

(8) The affected ear or cavity feels more comfortable and sensations or pains over the temple disappear.

(9) Hearing may improve.

(10) Labyrinthine symptoms may abate.

Introduction and methods

Vitamin A acetate (100,000 I.U. per ml parenteral) was used for uncomplicated anosmia (Duncan, 1962) and one patient with bilateral modified mastoidectomy cavities reported improvement in smell and ear disease (1958). The cholesteatoma spontaneously disappeared and later bilateral tympanoplasty operations, 1960 and 1964, using pinna cartilage columella, improved hearing. No recurrence has occurred up to 1974. I used the injectable form of vitamin A (300,000 I.U. per ml) topically on a patient from 1973 with noticeable improvement when supplies were available. A regular supply was obtained in May, 1975, for this series of 80 patients.

The vitamin A concentrate (1 ml equals 1,000,-000 I.U. units) is in peanut oil. It is diluted

---

*Vitamin A: Hoffman La Roche, 16 The Terrace, Wellington, New Zealand.

(150,000 I.U. per ml) with olive, corn, or mineral oil. At first 50,000 I.U. then 100,000 I.U. per ml were tried. Concentrations higher than 150,000 I.U. per mil do not give enhanced effects. The patient instills drops in the ear at night for at least 20 minutes and should go to sleep with the treated ear uppermost. It is best to treat alternative ears daily when bilateral disease is present. No serious effects have occurred, but comments on an oily taste in the nose on waking, itching, and excess mucus were reported. Allergy to peanut oil which is in the concentrate has affected six patients to date, but a less allergic concentrate vehicle will soon be available. Because treatment is long-term, atopic patients should be asked about allergy to vegetable oils, as five patients reacted to olive and two to corn oil. If the ear is heavily infected an antibiotic topically or orally is used when vitamin A therapy begins. It takes three-five weeks for its effect to occur and thereafter antibiotics are seldom used, perhaps only during a heavy nasal infection. After three-five weeks, perhaps earlier, mucus production will be excessive and perhaps pour from the ear. The drops are then instilled every second or third day to decrease the mucus flow. Eventually most patients will instill vitamin A drops once every four days to keep the ear or cavity free from smell and infection and inhibit cholesteatoma regeneration.

At first the disappearance of smell and pus from cavities caused me to assume high vitamin A dosage had an antibiotic action. Eight untreated mastoid cavities were swabbed and cultures made for bacteria and fungi. The bacteria were the usual skin commensals, and a number of non-pathogenic fungi were identified. Vitamin A discs of various concentrations and media with vitamin A were overgrown by the commensals. There was no inhibiting effect after three weeks culture. Vitamin A in vivo must stimulate immune substances, possibly immunoglobulin A in the rejuvenated mucosa and increased mucus.

Biopsies of middle ear tissue before and after therapy have been difficult to interpret due to lack of facilities in Wellington.

Results of survey, May, 1975 to April, 1976

One hundred-thirteen patients were treated, but 33 were excluded (21 treated less than three months, and no reply from 12). The 30-60 age group included 42 of the 80 assessed. The type of disease was predominantly acquired cholesteatoma (Table 88).

TABLE 88

Clinical Disease Types	Patients
Acquired cholesteatoma	55
Childhood cholesteatoma	18
Congenital cholesteatoma	1
Hyperkeratosis attic	3
Tympanosclerosis	1
Adhesive middle ear	1
Infected chronic otitis	1

Table 89 lists the types of drum perforations and the numbers and conditions of open mastoid

TABLE 89

Clinical Conditions of Ears	Patients
Perforations marginal (1 bilateral)	15
Perforations attic (6 bilateral)	36
Perforations central (2 bilateral)	12
Mastoid cavity single	37
Mastoid cavities bilateral	12
Cholesteatoma	98
Epithelitis cavity	26
Dry ears or cavities	11

cavities. Table 90, the numbers of patients with surgery. The high number of open cavities was necessary because good access is essential for therapy. The effect of vitamin A therapy is shown in Table 91.

TABLE 90

Surgery	Patients
Single open cavity	37
Bilateral cavities	12
No operation	31
Total	80

TABLE 91

Effect of Vitamin A Therapy	Patients
Disappearance of cholesteatoma (9 bilateral)	50
Decrease of cholesteatoma (8 bilateral)	43
Disappearance of smell (26 bilateral)	91
Change to mucus secreting lining (3 bilateral)	32
Change to thin red skin (18 bilateral)	71
Both effects present	7
Increased mucus production (2 bilateral)	28
Infection remains	7
No effect from therapy	5

Increased mucus production persisted in 10 ears, but all other ears were controlled by frequency or alteration in dosage. Smell disappeared from all ears except four. The response to treatment was unpredictable as was the stimulation of mucus. Forty patients commented on reduction of pain during ear dressings and 29 of lack of sensations around the ear and face they had associated with ear disease. Improvement of hearing occurred in 42 patients of the 50 who commented on this and 16 noticed less vertigo. Three patients had surgery because it was considered there was no access of vitamin A through the aditus. Treatment has been continuous for 6-12 months in 49 of the patients. Allergic reactions may occur with itching and increased mucus production, and requires a change of the main oil vehicle. As a precaution in all patients I have changed the vehicle after three-four months therapy and used mineral oil for a few.

Case report: E. S., female, white, age 52. Bilateral discharging ears as a child in Britain. Ear dry since 1956. Deafness increasing and slight vertigo. Right ear large central perforation yielding a little desquamation when cleaned. Left ear a wide central and marginal perforation with stapes surrounded by adherent cholesteatoma. Vitamin A treatment began September, 1975. Within three weeks, moistness, no smell and no masses of desquamations. Frequent suctioning, every four days as patient became alarmed. The quantity of desquamation began to reduce by December, 1975 and in March, 1976, ears were still moist with no smell, and hearing and vertigo were much improved. A throbbing sensation in the right temple area disappeared after 15 years. This patient had two large cholesteatoma sacs which are now probably empty of desquamations.

Case report: S. P., male, white, age 19. Left childhood cholesteatoma and open mastoid cavity at age 9. Cytotoxic food testing at age 17 resulted in a "dry" cavity. Right attic perforation and cholesteatoma became active at age 18 and vitamin A therapy began May, 1975. The cholesteatoma decreased in size but the deafness increased.

February, 1975, atticotomy and simple mastoidectomy. Glue mucus in mastoid cells and cholesteatoma in the aditus. The cholesteatomatous membrane could be sucked out easily leaving a red moist surface. It has not involved the mesotympanum. Hearing much improved two months after operation.

Case report: V. D. C., female, white, age 45. Bilateral discharging ears as a child in Holland. In 1966, age 35, her ears were discharging and there was foul smell and cholesteatoma. Surgery was performed in 1967 and 1973, with bilateral open cavities. Cholesteatoma recurred around the remaining ossicles, but hearing was of moderate degree. Instillations of vitamin A was started in May, 1975, and the foul smell disappeared. Instillations of vitamin A were continued and only a trace of cholesteatoma remained by February, 1976. Over a year later, April, 1976, the disease was cured and the ear was improved. Peanut allergy occurred and may interfere with therapy. This was a dramatic result as antibiotics would not control the smell.

Surgical technic

Cholesteatoma may persist in the roof or posterior limits of a cavity because head positioning is difficult. This highlights the inadequacy of ear drops. Small marginal and attic perforations may impede vitamin A penetration especially when an increase in desquamation is evoked. Debris is suctioned frequently and some vitamin A solution placed in the perforation with a canula. Progress may not occur because of obstruction in the aditus, or cholesteatoma disease in the mastoid. A combined approach using a wide atticotomy with removal of the scutum and simple mastoidectomy permits removal of cholesteatoma in the mastoid and opening of the attic to vitamin A solution. The aditus is enlarged laterally, superiorly, and if necessary inferiorly to give a 3 or 4 mm space, but there is no need to open the facial recess. An exploratory tympanotomy allows middle ear webs around the incus and stapes to be broken, occasionally releasing pockets of glue mucus. The

effect of vitamin A on cholesteatoma may render unnecessary surgical removal from the facial recess and posterior tympanic sulcus.

A mastoidotomy and tympanotomy with simple mastoidectomy and enlargement of aditus has allowed access of vitamin A to the middle ear cleft with apparent disappearance of mucus effusion, pounding and deafness. Vitamin A access had eliminated the disease from the middle ear in one patient, but a blocked aditus allowed the disease to persist in the antrum and some facial cells. Another patient had oily globules in the mucus of the mastoid cells and antrum, but no cholesteatoma except a small area in webs on the lower lip of the oval window.

The atticotomy did not depress the hearing in the diseased ears. The opening may tend to close, but can be curetted using local anesthesia. Debris needs to be suctioned frequently at first, but after six weeks of post-operative vitamin A therapy, there is little to be removed. Hearing may improve at this stage, but I suspect hearing improvement can be caused by other factors. Vitamin A therapy should be started at least six weeks before surgery as it may loosen the cholesteatoma membrane allowing gentle suction removal. Some contraction of the cholesteatoma areas does occur and the increased vascularity aids healing. As yet I do not know if vitamin A therapy increases middle ear adhesions, but I suspect it decreased the tendency. I am using vitamin A for two months before middle ear reconstructive surgery and for two months after a fascial graft viability appears to be enhanced.

Discussion

A search of literature failed to locate any study on topical vitamin A therapy of aural cholesteatoma. Fell and Mellanby (1953 and 1957) demonstrated that vitamin A acted on the germinal layer of chicken embryo skin coverting it to a mucous membrane with cilia. This effect probably occurs to the cholesteatomatous membrane as the desquamations strip off after three-six weeks of treatment. There could be another effect, a stimulation of pockets of the original mucous membrane which lifts off an overlying cholesteatoma membrane and then advances, displacing the cholesteatoma from the periosteum. The last remaining areas of cholesteatoma are the attic roof and the promontory near the lower lip of the oval window. More frequently it retreats to the drum margin. This could indicate the origin of the disease, a metaplasia (Sadé, 1966) or 'in vacuo' invasion (Tos, Pederson, 1975). Surgery and bone disease could have distorted this observation! The effect is so profound that I believe vitamin A therapy will greatly reduce surgery if its access is adequate. Eventually it will be known if the disease recurs inspite of continuing therapy. It has persisted in small pockets (surgically removable) in four patients who have had therapy for 9-12 months. Another problem is when to close the atticotomy or mastoidectomy after the combined approach.

Vitamin A has long been known to stimulate mucus production and the first mucus appearing after two or three weeks therapy in a dry ear is similar to the glue mucus seen in children.

During the next one-three weeks, it changes to a more fluid odorless mucus. A wet smelling ear begins to form clear mucus after three-six weeks treatment. This clear mucus must have normal or increased immune activity (Jurin and Tannock, 1971 and Cohen and Cohen, 1973). It appears to displace viscous mucus in the middle ear cleft and may be more suitable for ciliary activity. Vitamin A may, however, stimulate ciliary activity because mucus appears to be quickly cleared from the middle ear and patients report returning eustachian tube patency. Although urea (Bauer, 1970) may temporarily clear a middle ear of mucus, it does not stimulate the normal middle ear mucosal processes. A venting tube may fail for the same reason. The vascular, ciliary, mucosal and mucus effects of vitamin A have been reported in the post nasal space (Stanbygard, 1954; Duncan, 1956; Alk, 1974). Four patients of this series reported such improvement, probably from drainage of vitamin A via the eustachian tube. I have not been able to make any i.g.A. or immune assays of this provoked mucus.

Forty-two patients reported varying degrees of hearing improvement, some confirmed by audiogram. This improvement results from elimination of cholesteatoma membrane and desquamation and possibly the disappearance of viscid mucus pockets. The increased vascularity of the mucus membrane over the ossicles may increase flexibility of the joint capsules, annular ligament and round window membrane. Vitamin A may pass through the round window membrane and stimulate the membranous labyrinth (Ruedi, 1954) in a similar manner to its affect on the olfactory mucosa (Duncan, 1962).

Vitamin A therapy requires patient cooperation; therapy may increase the mucus and desquamation discharge after two-three weeks and require frequent attendances. A large cholesteatoma sac may take up to eight weeks to empty. The frequency of dosage must be regulated to avoid excess mucus production which may frighten the patient, but in time a twice-weekly treatment is enough to keep most ears clean and free from cholesteatoma disease. Open cavities and wide perforations were selected because good access of vitamin A without surgery was considered necessary for the first clinical trial. If vitamin A proves to be useful in the therapy of cholesteatoma, the future lies with surgery designed to give access, because the parenteral route is unpredictable*.

---

*Editor's note: This manuscript was received from the author in New Zealand shortly before the conference. Its importance is obvious. We hope the reader will accept its principal point, that vitamin A may have a profound curative effect upon cholesteatoma.

B. F. M.

Summary

Vitamin A acetate (150,000 I.U. per ml) therapy was used for 3-12 months on 74 patients with aural cholesteatoma, three with hyperkeratosis of the drum and one each with tympanosclerosis, chronic discharging otitis media and adhesive middle ear disease. A profound stimulating effect was noticed on the middle ear cleft mucosa causing it to produce mucus and the rejection or retraction of cholesteatomatous membrane. Infection and smell were greatly reduced without using topical antibiotics. To permit access of vitamin A to the mastoid, a combined approach of mastoidotomy or atticotomy and simple mastoidectomy with enlargement of the aditus is occasionally necessary.

Discussion by Dr. Sheehy and Dr. McCabe

Dr. Sheehy: May I ask if it was your impression, Dr. McCabe, that Dr. Duncan still considers cholesteatoma a surgical condition?

Dr. McCabe: The role of surgery is to provide access to wherever the cholesteatoma exists. If it is tympanomastoid, then an access must be created so that the vitamin A can get into the mastoid.

References

1. Alk, G. P.: Clinical study of nasal oil containing vitamin A. *Wein Med. Wochenshr.*, 124:473, 1974.

2. Bauer, F.: The use of urea in exudative otitis media. *Otol. Clin. N. Amer.*, 3:57, 1970.

3. Cohen, B. E. and Cohen, I. K.: Vitamin A enhancement of normal and steroid-suppressed immune reactivity. *Surgical Forum*, 24:276, 1973.

4. Duncan, R. B. and Briggs, M.: Treatment of uncomplicated anosmia by vitamin A. *Arch. Otolaryng.*, 75:116, 1962.

5. Duncan, R. B.: Vitamin A therapy in atrophic nasopharyngitis and rhinitis. *New Zealand Med. J.*, 55:322, 1956.

6. Fell, H.: The effect of excess vitamin A on cultures of embryonic chicken skin explanted at different stages of differentiation. *Proc. Roy. Soc. B.*, 146:242, 1957.

7. Fell, H. and Mellanby, E.: Metaplasia produced in cultures of chicken ectoderm by high vitamin A. *J. Physiol.*, 119:470, 1953.

8. Jurin, M. and Tannock, I.F.: Influence of vitamin A on immunological response. *Immunology*, 23:283, 1971.

9. Ruedi, L.: Actions of vitamin A on human and animal ear. *Acta Otolaryng.*, 44:502, 1954.

10. Sadé, J.: Pathology and pathogenesis of serous otitis media. *Arch. Otolaryng.*, 84:79, 1966.

11. Standbygard, E.: Treatment of Ozena and rhinopharyngitis sicca with vitamin A. *Arch. Otolaryng.*, 59:485, 1964.

12. Tos, M. and Pederson, K.: The onset of chronic secretory otitis media. *Arch. Otolaryng.*, 101:123, 1975.

QUESTIONS AND ANSWERS
RESULTS OF THERAPY "TELL ME ABOUT YOUR FAILURES!"

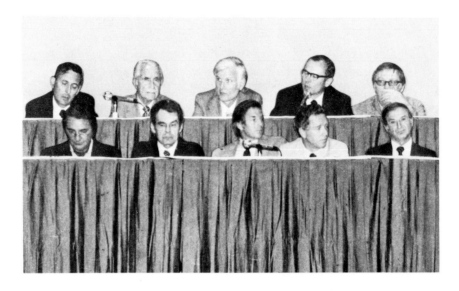

Panel: Evaluation of Surgical Procedures for Cholesteatoma, "Tell Me About Your Failures!" Left to right, front row: B.F. McCabe, M.D.; W. Wright, M.D.; G. Smyth, M.D.; C. Jansen, M.D.; R. Bellucci, M.D. Back row: J. Sadé, M.D.; S. Baron, M.D.; T. Palva, M.D.; T. Cody, M.D.; and D. Austin, M.D.

Dr. McCabe: All of our speakers have done a splendid job of carrying out their assignment. Each was asked to report their failures, and avoid descriptions of techniques. We are not interested in techniques, except to know what techniques they are reporting.

Now, to the task. It seems that in upper midwestern USA, the recurrence rate of cholesteatoma is 35%. In Germany it is 3%. In Texas it is 15%. In the Great Lakes area it is 23%. In northern Ireland, it is 16%. In Israel, it is 33%. In Finland, it is 2%. In California, it is 8%. Are we talking about the same disease? The disease can't vary that much around the world, and so there must be another variable that we don't have a handle on. I hope that might come out. I would like to ask Thane: Your recurrence was among the highest.

Why do you think this is? How many of these were done by residents and how many by senior staff?

Dr. Cody: First of all, of the overall 35% cholesteatoma failure rate, 24% were recurrences and 11% were residual. Secondly, in most of the operations, a portion, if not all, was done by a resident, but in all operations a staff man was there and often interceded. That is not a principal factor to my mind because our biggest cause of failure was recurrent cholesteatoma, or attic retraction pockets which haven't as yet developed into cholesteatoma. That is our biggest cause of failure. A lot of those ears are excellent for six months, a year, a year and a half, two years, and at various times developed retraction pockets, which went on to form cholesteatomas. I find it hard to relate that to the original surgery. Now, many people here apparently have not had this problem, but I know at least Dr. Austin and Dr. Sadé have. They reported a rather high recurrence rate with retraction pockets.

Dr. McCabe: Let's talk about that retraction pocket business. David Austin said in only one instance did he ever see a retraction pocket fail to go on to a cholesteatoma. Is that right, David?

Dr. Austin: Yes.

Dr. McCabe: What is the experience of the panel?

Dr. Bellucci: Well, I think the original disease probably came from eustachian tube dysfunction. Now, if that is the case, and we have done nothing to the eustachian tube, it will persist. We take out the cholesteatoma, and the ground rules are the same for this ear, and therefore we expect that there is a negative pressure again, and a retraction pocket would develop, and ultimately there is a good chance of getting a cholesteatoma in it.

Dr. McCabe: Dr. Palva, I noted, unless I am wrong, that, although your frank recurrence rate was 2%, using Cody's pre-cholesteatoma terminology, would that add an additional 10% to yours?

Dr. Palva: That is to say, do retraction pockets go on to develop cholesteatoma? I wholeheartedly second David here when he says that if you have an intact canal wall and you have a retraction pocket, that is going to develop into a cholesteatoma. But when you have removed the bony posterior canal wall as I do, it is an entirely different matter because your whole posterior canal wall is yielding. There is no such space as you have with the canal wall up and the retraction pocket creeps behind the wall.

Dr. McCabe: Dr. Palva, your membranous posterior canal slowly fades back. Is that right?

Dr. Palva: Right.

Dr. McCabe: So that the canal is several times normal size?

Dr. Palva: It doesn't yield so much. It may well be sometimes double the size, but that is I consider an extreme than in a very rare case. Maybe 1.3 or 1.5 times larger than normally.

Dr. McCabe: Do any of the panelists have an opposite opinion? That is, retraction pockets develop and then remain stationary, and then do not go into a keratotic phase and then cholesteatoma?

Dr. Sadé: I don't have a contrary view, but how do we know? Have we counted? Unless we take a certain number of cases which started to retract, and follow them up several years and see what percentage develop a deep retraction pocket, which we call cholesteatoma, our conclusions would be based on our impressions, and this cannot be accepted as solid evidence. It is true that those retraction pockets are secondary to eustachian tube malfunction, but it is possible that some people get over this eustachian tube malfunction. We don't know what percentage.

Dr. McCabe: Dr. Cody did have some evidence of the rate of retraction pockets going into cholesteatoma. He had some figures.

Dr. Cody: No, I just said that because these retraction pockets develop at different periods of time, I assume that there were varying degrees of underlying eustachian tube dysfunction.

Dr. McCabe: Well, we don't really know whether it is eustachian tube dysfunction or not, or a combination of factors that produces the slow retraction pocket. We are not talking about the cause of the retraction pocket, but the state.

Dr. Cody: We watched many of them go right through the sequence of events. We have observed that in front of our eyes. At the same time we are watching other retraction pockets that haven't gone into cholesteatoma.

Dr. Baron: May I ask Dr. Cody what he means by pre-cholesteatoma? Does that refer to a retraction pocket?

Dr. Cody: Yes, most commonly in the attic or through the surgically opened facial recess.

Dr. McCabe: Bill Wright reported a 12% rate of significant retraction pocket. Is that right?

Dr. Wright: Yes.

Dr. McCabe: What do you do with these?

Dr. Wright: I surgically remove them. I don't wait for them to form cholesteatomas.

Dr. McCabe: So, you surgically remove pre-cholesteatomas without waiting to see if they become keratotic. What comes after that?

Dr. Wright: Well, some of these have been due to poor eustachian tube function, and I put a button ventilating tube through the eardrum, and I have not had them recur.

Dr. McCabe: Has anyone else had the same experience? I have had an opposite experience. It makes a difference in some, but not in many.

Dr. Wright: I also put some thick silastic in the bone gap to try to fill this up, so that I won't get a recurrence. I think that the eustachian tube is a big part of the problem with the ones that have the recurrence. They definitely suck back into the mastoid, and I think that if they don't have cholesteatoma in them, they certainly have the potential. All the patient has to do is go swimming about once, and he will have some cholesteatoma start forming.

Dr. Austin: Well, to be a little disputative, I had no luck whatsoever with buttons or silastic in prevention of these pockets, and I have tried both systems. Frankly I think I have tried just about everything that anybody has ever suggested, and I feel they are out of my control. You are questioning why there are differing reports of incidence figures. In my paper I state that this disease is a "pseudo-neoplasm," and I think it would benefit all of us in terms of our learning to do what Dr. Cody did today. You called it by a different name, but it is essentially "at risk" reporting, just as our head and neck colleagues do. When we are talking about cholesteatoma we will learn a lot more about the occurrence of this complication in relation to the time that elapses if we do adopt these time scales. I suspect that this has something to do with the variation of incidence of recurrence of which we have heard.

Dr. Wright: That is a good point. With any type of surgery, the longer the follow-up, the worse the statistics become.

Dr. McCabe: Claus appears to probably do the highest rate of "canal-up" mastoidectomies of the whole panel. Claus, do you have any contraindications to "canal-up" mastoidectomies?

Dr. Jansen: I would say at the moment, maybe cancer.

Dr. McCabe: You can take on all comers.

Dr. Jansen: I normally keep the "canal-up".

Dr. McCabe: How about malignant external otitis?

Dr. Jansen: Yes, of course, that too.

Dr. McCabe: There must be some others.

Dr. Jansen: Normally in clinical surgery, we don't take the posterior bony canal wall down. May I make another remark on retraction pockets? I do not believe that all these retraction pockets are caused by dysfunction of the tube. I don't believe in that, because I would like to put the question back to those people, and ask them what kind of proof do you have?

Dr. Bellucci: I had one patient, and that is enough to prove it. She had ear disease all her life. She came to me with two operations on each ear. We controlled her nasal allergies, and the ears dried up. We performed a tympanoplasty on one ear, had a beautiful result, and she heard very well. She had a very thin control window membrane. She got a severe cold, and that pulled right in, and she has a cholesteatoma pocket again. Now both ears periodically discharge after they have been completely stabilized for a length of time. When she gets a bad nasal problem which compromises eustachian tube function, then it affects the ear again. I am sure that no matter what we do it is always going to follow the same course.

Dr. Jansen: Richard, I didn't say always. I just said that I think it is seldom that we have dysfunction of the tube. I have retraction pockets, too, when we have no dysfunction of the tube. That is my experience.

Dr. Bellucci: Well, what does it do then?

Dr. Jansen: That is another question, but we do have retraction pockets without having a malfunction of the tube.

Dr. Sadé: I think that what Dick said really sums up how much we know about the eustachian tube, and I think that Claus' question is totally legitimate. What are the proofs? We don't have proofs. We have some gut feeling, but we don't have proofs. I would tell you that, contrary to David and not totally contrary to you, I agree about the ventilating tubes but I can't agree about the silastic. I have in several instances been able to abolish a retraction pocket with a ventilating tube. I know very little about it, but I take this rightly or wrongly as evidence that we are dealing with a ventilating deficiency of the middle ear, and therefore that we are dealing with a eustachian tube which is malfunctioning.

Dr. McCabe: Dr. Palva?

Dr. Palva: It is true that we don't know very much about the function of the eustachian tube but we do have some data. I think that Claus Jansen a little bit overemphasized the concept that a retraction pocket comes from some other cause than eustachian tube malfunction. We have methods of testing eustachian tube function preoperatively. We have various methods of testing, and quite accurate methods, and I am wondering how he can have such a low recurrence rate if he operates upon hundreds of ears. There must be at least 15 to 20% with poor tubal function. These cases over the years must develop retraction pockets if he has the canal wall up. There simply must be retraction pockets. I don't think the German people are that good with their eustachian tubes that they would function in every case, when we know that in every other country there are people with tubes that don't function.

Dr. Wright: We really have only three possibilities for these retraction pockets. One is a vacuum which you can correct by a ventilating tube. The other is traction, like a traction diverticulum in the esophagus, which is due to scar tissue attached to the under surface, pulling the retraction pocket back in, which you can correct, hopefully with silastic, and the last one is an innate tendency for retraction, like my golf swing, which produces a slice invariably.

Dr. Smyth: It seems to me a pity that if at this stage we forget everything we learned in the first two days. I don't think there is too much evidence yet, one way or the other, about the eustachian

tube, but Dr. Lim referred in his paper earlier to the effect of the basement membrane in terms of wound healing. He published a paper last year referring to his experimental work on wound healing which indicated that the direction in which the epithelium would grow during the wound healing phase was related to the direction of the fibers which underlaid the squamous epithelium. It seems to me that it might be worth considering whether or not the fibers which are formed in the connective tissue during the healing phase don't have something to do with the direction in which the squamous epithelium will grow. If the squamous epithelium support is pointing inwards to the facial recess of the epitympanum, it will grow in that direction, and it doesn't matter what the eustachian tube function is like. Now, eustachian tube function is probably very relevant in the younger patients, and may well be the cause of the increased incidences of problems in the child not only because of eustachian tube function which is producing negative pressure, but also because it is creating an environment in the middle ear space which affects the possibility of metaplasia or some other predisposing factor. Perhaps we should look a little more past the eustachian tube problems.

Dr. McCabe: Gordon, you are to be congratulated in being one of the few clinicians to do what we tried to design this conference to foster: bring basic information to bear on the understanding of this disease process. Richard?

Dr. Bellucci: I agree that we have this problem more frequently in childhood, and we have been studying this problem for about ten years, and of course our scientist friends here want figures. Now, it is very difficult to measure this eustachian tube and its angles. Ratnesar today showed differences but to get down to a figure that this angle is different from that angle, therefore this one will have eustachian tube malfunction and this is most difficult. I am sure you will find it, too, very difficult as you begin to study this. However, circumstantial evidence does show that there is a problem.

Dr. Baron: I wanted to ask Dr. Jansen why he

feels that eustachian tube dysfunction is not the main cause of retraction. You must have a reason.

Dr. McCabe: Dr. Jansen?

Dr. Jansen: We did a lot of tube function testing before, and that gave me the nice opportunity to invite Tauno Palva to come to Germany maybe to perform his techniques of tube function. So we did it before tympanoplasty or a radical, and we did it afterwards, and we found in about the 50 cases where we did this, that we had bad function when we saw a kind of ingrowing epithelium. We did this about 20 years prior, because we had the same problem, and took down the posterior bony canal wall. We had the problem, too, because we sometimes left the so-called red skin. Now we take it out, and have no significant difference between the tube function before and afterward.

Dr. McCabe: Dr. Cody?

Dr. Cody: Brian, unless I interpreted Dr. Bluestone's work incorrectly, I thought he showed very nicely in five consecutive cases of very small cholesteatomas confined to the posterior tympanum or the attic with not a great deal of inflammation and no encroachment on the eustachian tube orifice area, all had eustachian tube dysfunction. So, if I am interpreting his presentation correctly, then this is in contradistinction to Dr. Jansen's concept. This is a hundred percent.

Dr. McCabe: Dr. Cody, there is no question in my mind that Bluestone's work and this panel's impression, with the exception of Claus Jansen, strongly indicates the eustachian tube as the culprit in canal-up failure. A couple more questions. David Austin and Jacob Sadé have come to be greatly selective in their mastoid operations. Would each of them tell us what is the best kind of an ear, in their opinion, for "canal-up" mastoidectomy, and what is the worst kind of an ear for a "canal-up" mastoidectomy? David, would you start?

Dr. Austin: The answer is simple. The best kind of ear for a "canal-up" operation is one in which I can do it easily and quickly, and if I can't do it easy and quickly, I will take down the canal. It is a technical selection. The other kind of ear in which it is easy to choose is that in which disease has recurred, and then I think once this potential has been proven, there is no sense in keeping the space back there to get new disease in and so I eliminate that space. So, the two instances are when I can't easily maintain the canal, and these are the cases which are operated exactly as Dr. Palva does, with certain non-essential modifications; the other is that in which the disease reappears, and in those again I tend to find myself doing Dr. Palva's operation.

Dr. McCabe: That makes sense to me. Dr. Sadé?

Dr. Sadé: My reasoning takes into account the other ear. Is there a lot of destruction? If there is total ossicular destruction, I know that my chances of restoring the hearing is less good. What is the state of the mucosa? If it is a very hyperplastic mucosa, I doubt that I can create an air cavity. Then there is the extent of the cholesteatoma. There is also the extent of the scutum destruction. If there is a lot of scutum destruction, I would hesitate to do it. A lot of scutum destruction is tantamount to me to an invitation for a retraction pocket. Then there is the size of the air system. If there is an extremely small mastoid, it is much easier for me to do an atticotomy and if there is a big air system, it is much more conducive to do a "canal-up" technique. Then there is, of course, the age of the patient. The younger he is, the less enthusiastic I am about a closed cavity technique.

Dr. McCabe: Panel members, we are ready for our second phase. What questions do you want to ask of your fellow panelists? Richard, and then Claus.

Dr. Bellucci: Dr. Jansen, you rarely perform an open cavity technique except in cancer. Now, when you have a sclerotic mastoid, can you do this canal wall technique via facial recess?

Dr. Jansen: Yes, I can.

Dr. McCabe: Dr. Jansen, you had a question.

Dr. Jansen: Dr. Cody, in your statistics, you told us that when you do a "canal-up" technique, you do a simple mastoidectomy. Would you please define what that is?

Dr. Cody: Complete mastoidectomy. We use the words synonymously.

Dr. Jansen: Would you please tell me what kind of operation your canal-up technique is, for as you know we have several kinds of these techniques.

Dr. Cody: Would you prefer the term, "complete mastoidectomy"?

Dr. Jansen: Yes, "complete mastoidectomy".

Dr. Cody: Well, as on the slide, the number of intact canal wall procedures is 170.

Dr. McCabe: Dr. Palva.

Dr. Palva: Well, while we're talking about eustachian tube function, we might elaborate this question a bit more. I would like to ask Dr. Jansen now—let's suppose that he had a group of patients where the patient cannot do a positive Valsalva maneuver. Let's say he had a perforation in the pars tensa. You put plus 200 mm positive pressure, and it doesn't go through. You put minus 200 mm negative pressure, and he cannot equalize with swallowing. Do you believe in this whole group of patients with the intact canal wall technique you are improving the eustachian tube function? And you will get no retraction pockets?

Dr. Jansen: Well, I think at first I have to ask you, do you have a perforated drum or not?

Dr. Palva: Yes, I said you have a perforation.

Dr. Jansen: Fine, Is pressure equalization not possible from the tympanic side or from the other side?

Dr. Palva: From neither.

Dr. Jansen: You find the tube obstructed from both sides, is that so?

Dr. Palva: Well, I said that a patient couldn't do the Valsalva maneuver.

Dr. Jansen: Well, we have a lot of patients that cannot do the Valsalva maneuver.

Dr. Palva: I said that we couldn't put 200 mm. Hg. positive pressure through, and he couldn't equalize minus 200 mm. Hg. negative pressure. These are the prerequisites.

Dr. Jansen: All right, let's follow that question. I would say that first I would try to get down to the disease, to find out what is going on, because we sometimes have a one way obstruction of the tube, as you probably know by polyps, cells, etc. So, then I would push something through, like a very small

tube. I wouldn't perform a posterior tympanotomy. If I find a complete obstruction, I would do a posterior tympanotomy, too, but I would try to get a grommet into my new tympanic membrane. That's it. Have you another question?

Dr. Palva: I just wonder when you are probing your tube, are you making a great insult to the mucosa there? I would think you would be afraid of a complete stricture or stenosis if you are probing.

Dr. Jansen: No, not in my experience.

Dr. Palva: It is contrary to any physiologic experience.

Dr. Jansen: Maybe it is against your experience, but not of the mucosa of the tube. This is undesirable, and we shouldn't force it through. But even if there is complete obstruction, I would perform posterior tympanotomy because I would like to have the canal intact. Why should I take down the canal in such a case? I would put a grommet in the tympanic membrane, and that's it. May I ask you what you would do in such a case?

Dr. Palva: I never preserve the canal wall in such a case.

Dr. Jansen: Why?

Dr. Palva: Because I don't want to get the retraction pocket that would inevitably, in my thinking, go into the mastoid cavity. It will if you have a lowered pressure in the middle ear, or if you have a eustachian tube that doesn't return air when you swallow.

Dr. Jansen: If you have a grommet in your tympanic membrane?

Dr. Palva: In my experience, that does not solve the problem in these ears.

Dr. McCabe: Dr. Austin?

Dr. Austin: I have been involved in some of these discussions in the past, and rather than let Claus take all the raff, I personally think that one of the subjects that really must be discussed at the next international conference is just this, because I have heard so many people throw out this idea that the eustachian tube is at fault. Of course, it is bound to be. It must be at fault. This has got to be where the disease comes from, but I submit that there is absolutely no objective evidence of this in any literature any place. I haven't read your 30-page paper yet, Dick, but if you have objective evidence, how did you get it? The tympanometry machine does not measure eustachian tube function. It does not reflect middle ear pressure. It gives fallacious information. First of all, nobody has ever defined what function it is they are talking about. Dr. Inglestedt is over here. His group has told us that the only air the middle ear needs in a 24-hour period is less than one ml. They don't consider ventilation to be a function of the eustachian tube, merely equalization of pressure. So, already, there seems to be some basic conceptual defect here, and I don't think that there is anything to be gained about sitting here and theorizing that the eustachian tube is at fault, or it isn't, until some objective evidence is presented on one side or the other. This patient got over her cold, what happened to the disease?

Dr. Bellucci: She got a cholesteatoma.

Dr. Austin: It should have regressed as the tube got well, shouldn't it?

Dr. McCabe: Gentlemen, now we will open the panel to questions from the floor.

Dr. Ratnesar: I did mention this morning that I did assess the function of the eustachian tube using a catheter. May I answer Dr. Palva that if a surgeon can use a catheter through the ureters and not cause any damage to the mucosal epithelium, I feel that is quite justifiable for me to insert a catheter through the eustachian tube to assess the patency, and also assess the size of the tube in relation to the catheter by using different sized catheters.

Dr. Palva: You can assess the patency, but you cannot assess function.

Dr. McCabe: It should also be mentioned that in the case of the ureter, there is no rigid passage, there is no bony or cartilaginous framework. The two then are not comparable.

Dr. Bellucci: That's right.

Dr. Palva: Function is another subject and I agree with Dr. Austin that what they do in tympanometry is not always physiologic.

Voice: Still it is about the best we have, isn't it?

Dr. McCabe: Panel? No response? I guess then that what we have available is the best of a bad lot.

Dr. Friedberg: A retraction pocket is in fact a result of a ventilatory problem, but not necessarily of the eustachian tube. A local ventilatory problem is all you have to postulate, and that can be in the posterior recess, in the attic area, due to adhesions, redundant mucosa, or granulation tissue. So, the eustachian tube may or may not be involved. The other thing is we started out talking about pockets versus cholesteatoma two days ago, and we have not solved the problem of what a pocket is yet. I think a pocket is an area that is supported by a rigid rim and has a collapsible center to it, somewhere in the middle ear. If it is self-cleansing, it is not a problem, it is just a pocket. If it is not self-cleansing, it has to be dealt with. There are two ways you can deal with a pocket. You can either support the collapsible center by a myringostomy tube, fascia, whatever, or you can reduce the rim. I prefer to reduce the rim, but that is my personal attitude.

The things that concern me are two major opinions that I have heard today. One is Dr. Smyth's, that there are factors responsible for a recurrence which he believes, and I believe, you can prevent. On the other hand, Dr. Austin, on several occasions, has stated that he believes there is something inherent about cholesteatoma, which causes its recurrence, which cannot be prevented. I hope he is wrong. I wonder if other members of the panel can tell me whether they think it is preventable or not preventable.

Dr. McCabe: Anyone care to respond to that?

Dr. Jansen: I think that retraction pockets become a danger when they become wet. If the pocket produces a draining ear, I think then that the self-cleaning system is stopped, and that produces the problem of recurrent cholesteatoma. Does that answer your question?

Dr. Jansen: What kind of procedure is that? Would you please let me know?

Dr. Cody: The posterior bony wall canal was left, and all of the superior canal wall that was there. If there was an attic defect, there was a defect in the superior bony canal wall. In a majority of those cases, and I can't tell you exactly the figures but we could put on the slide and see it, the facial recess was opened as well, to give access into the facial recess and oval window area.

Dr. Jansen: May I have another question? How many of those ears did you do yourself?

Dr. Cody: Very few.

Dr. Jansen: Thank you very much.

Dr. Cody: May I say one more thing in regard to that? It is very interesting that, although I mentioned that our residents had performed a portion or the entire operation of many of the cases, in cases that I showed with the intact canal wall procedures, a large number were done almost in entirety by a nationally known otologic surgeon, not me.

Dr. McCabe: Dr. Wali, may we have your question?

Dr. Wali: We have heard Dr. Wright and Dr. Sadé say that they close the perforation by doing tympanoplasties, and yet they put ventilation tubes in them. How long do they leave them in? Do they get retraction after they take the tube out?

Dr. Sadé: I don't take this tube out. Unfortunately, the tube falls out, and then sometimes the tympanic membrane collapses and sometimes it doesn't, and I don't have numbers. The difference between a perforation and a ventilating tube is probably due to its size. A secondary infection can occur through a ventilating tube, but this is a rare occurrence. As to its permanence, I think Dr. Ingelstedt is right, a perforation is a God-sent ventilating tube.

Dr. McCabe: Any other response?

Dr. Palva: If I could make one comment about the question that was asked from the back microphone, about Dr. Smyth's and Dr. David Austin's comments seeming to be contrary. We have been reviewing a series of cases that are something like 20 years old, all radical mastoids. We have seen that if a good operation has been performed and the disease has not been in the middle ear primarily, but in the epitympanic space and has gone into the mastoid, you have had

a perfectly good result for all this 20-year period.

Dr. Baron: When I showed that little girl who first had a cholesteatoma recurrence in three years, and then in nine years, I wanted to make an important point, which is that I believe that the reason why one can't remove all of the cholesteatoma is that microscopic flakes of epithelium drop off as seeds. These little seeds occur wherever you are working. In this case it was the epitympanum, and nine years later it was in the middle ear. I think that is one of the reasons for our failures.

Dr. McCabe: Dr. Wright?

Dr. Wright: I certainly agree with that, Shirley. I think these are microscopic seeds, and they take years to manifest themselves. That is why you either have to go in early and find them, or you have to sit around until they become big boys, and then they are a mess to clean up. As far as the ventilating tube is concerned, I think that indications are exactly the same as in an ordinary serous otitis media. In fact, if I am doing one of these cases, and I don't trust the eustachian tube, I would place a tube. Claus was talking about passing a dilator. If I was worried enough to pass that tube in the first place, I would put a ventilating tube in that ear, and then after healing had taken place and the tissues were a little stronger, I would very gingerly take out the tube - it might be three months—and I would watch that very carefully over the next three weeks. If it started to retract or had any problem, I would put the tube back in and probably try to get a permanent perforation.

Dr. McCabe: Dr. Sheehy?

Dr. Sheehy: There is a comment which is appropriate to make now. We found in reviewing between 850 and 875 intact canal wall procedures that had one year or more follow-up, a 4% incidence of serous otitis. We don't do eustachian tube function tests preoperatively so that is not a selective factor. It happened to be 6% in the four to six year age group, a small group of about 30, and only 2% in the older age group. So, it is rather small.

Dr. McCabe: Dr. Dequine is at the first microphone.

Dr. Dequine: Just a few words to try to bring you an experience about contradictions noted by the Chairman about an important point concerning residual cholesteatoma. When I started the intact canal wall technique, I was, like everyone, afraid of the possibility of recurrence of cholesteatoma without any means of control. So, I decided to do a routine one year revision, and I found, interestingly enough, 54% residual cholesteatoma. This is very high compared to figures presented by the members of the panel. I may find one, two, or even three recurrences one to three millimeters in size. That does not mean, I hope, the failure of the technique but the failure of the surgeon. It may take many years for the recurrence in the mastoid to become evident and give clinical complications. So, in my opinion it is a good thing to make a systematic revision. There is no problem with the patient if you properly prepare him before the first stage.

Dr. Abramson: Two days ago Dr. Roth summarized the disease as a problem of growth control. I wonder if any of the panel members would care to comment as to whether they accept this as a significant part of the disease, and if they do, how does their particular operation influence this problem?

Dr. McCabe: Dr. Sadé?

Dr. Sadé: I have some comments on what Dr. Abramson has said and on what Dr. Dequine has said to show us how things are more complicated than we imagine. If you made a wound, and it heals, there is always a cholesteatoma which is forming invariably—a cholesteatoma, according to what we know histologically, and it disappears. Then, there are several experiments, among them some by Dr. Abramson, in which skin has been implanted under skin or in muscle or mucosa, and the small epidermoid cyst formed but did not grow. It stayed small. There are other experiments which show us that tumors are really growing in relationship to their vascularization. There are various factors which are involved here, but the point that I wanted really to raise is that it is also possible that of those 50% of recurrences which you found in your ears, some of them might have stayed small all their life. Some of them might have even regressed. We don't know.

Dr. McCabe: We are at the end of our panel discussion, but Dr. Sheehy has some comments before we adjourn. Dr. Sheehy?

Dr. Sheehy: My comments are to emphasize a few points that were well made, and to try to answer a question or two that I have been asked. One thing you noticed was that in many of the papers the incidence of residual disease was highest in the middle ear. Now, I want to point this out to you because when you are doing tympanoplasties, you are closing the area where you are most likely to have residual disease.

Secondly, in reference to Bill Wright's comments about timing the second stage, we have had the experience of seeing a one and a half millimeter cyst in the mastoid in a planned second stage operation after three years. I have also had the experience in a case in which I used a Palva flap in an ear that had three previous radicals. We got a nice healed, dry ear, and then years later I went back to help the hearing, and there was a one and a half centimeter cyst with no clinical evidence of it. The timing is important, and if you are looking for residual disease, don't go back in too quickly.

Finally, there is serious question as to whether you should relegate everyone to an open cavity knowing that if you use some type of closed procedure, you may still end up with 20% eventually with an open cavity, but you have to think of the 80% that didn't end up that way.

Chapter 9
Complications

COMPLICATIONS OF CHOLESTEATOMA:
A Report on 1024 Cases

James L. Sheehy, M.D.
Derald E. Brackmann, M.D.
Malcolm D. Graham, M.D.

Complications resulting from chronic otitis media with cholesteatoma were common, often serious, and at times fatal, prior to the modern era of antibiotics. Complications are still commonplace in many of the developing areas of the world.

We were asked to review the complications seen at the Otologic Medical Group and to determine what if any correlation there might be between these complications and various factors in the patient's history and findings at surgery.

Selection of Cases

We selected for study the charts of patients operated upon during the ten years, 1965 through 1974, who met the following criteria:

1. The patient had not had prior middle ear or mastoid surgery, other than simple mastoidectomy or myringotomy.
2. Mastoidectomy was performed.
3. Cholesteatoma involved the epitympanum or mastoid, or both.

There were 1024 operations (in 949 patients), which met these criteria. This number represents 14% of all operations for chronic otitis media during the ten years and 23% of the primary operations.

Chart Identification

The study charts were identified by referring to our chronic ear surgical data sheet, a section of which is reproduced for your information (Table 92).

We have been using the same data sheet, with minor modifications and periodic updating, since

TABLE 92

Chronic Ear Surgical Data Sheet: Procedure	
Myringoplasty	16-1
Radical mastoidectomy	16-2
Modified radical mastoidectomy	16-3
Mastoid obliteration operation	16-4
Tympanoplasty without mastoidectomy	16-5
Tympanoplasty with mastoidectomy	
Intact canal wall	
Routine	16-6
Reconstruction—partial	16-12
total	16-11
(Cartilage 17-1)	
(Bone 17-2)	
Obliteration technique	
Soft tissue	18-7
Bone	18-10
Plastic	18-11
Cavity remains	18-8
Other procedure	18-9

mid-1963. The surgical data sheet is an integral part of the patient's chart and serves as a quick reference for the surgeon as he sees the patient in the office. The surgical data, with short-term follow-up information, is stored on a computer tape. This information is used for yearly short-term statistical reports. The stored data may be used for chart identification in long-term studies and detailed reviews as in this report.

Method of Study

Using information stored on computer tapes, we obtained a printout of chart numbers of all cases which met the criteria for this study. Each chart was reviewed in detail by one of the three authors to extract the information for analysis.

This report will be limited to a discussion of

complications of cholesteatoma as related to age of patient, duration of disease and other items which we felt would be of interest in relationship to the patient population. Additional information obtained in the chart review in regard to surgical management and postoperative results will be presented at the American Otological Society Meeting in 1977.

General Information

The patient population at the Otologic Medical Group may not be typical of an otologic practice, and this must be kept in mind in reviewing the statistical information.

Twenty-five percent of our new patients are referred by otolaryngologists, and the percentage of these cases which are surgical is higher than the twelve percent of our overall new patient load which eventually have surgery. Ten percent of the new patients come from outside California and the percentage of these that are surgical candidates is also higher.

During the ten year period covered in this report the average number of patients operated upon for correction of chronic ear disease was 717 per year, one-third of which were revision operations. One-third of these revisions were operations on patients originally operated elsewhere, a third were planned second stage procedures and one-third were unplanned revisions of our own graft failures or hearing failures or reconstructive operations on old radical mastoidectomies.

Duration of Disease

Table 93 shows the distribution of cases in this study in regard to duration of disease. A third stated that their problem had existed five years or less and a third indicated greater than twenty years.

Type of Hearing Impairment

In reviewing the cases we recorded the type of hearing impairment as none, conductive, mixed or total loss.

An individual was considered to have no hear-

TABLE 93

Chronic Otitis Media with Cholesteatoma
Duration of disease (N-1024)

Duration of Disease	Incidence
year or less	16%
5 years or less	37%
6 to 20 years	29%
21 years or more	34%
51 years or more	4%

ing impairment if the pure tone air conduction average (500-2000 Hz.) was 25 dB or less, and the hearing level was within five to ten dB of the opposite ear.

If the bone conduction level was worse than 25 dB at any single speech hearing frequency the hearing impairment was recorded as a mixed loss, regardless of the status of the opposite ear.

Total loss of hearing indicates no measurable air or bone conduction.

The type of impairment was recorded as conductive if it did not meet any of the above-mentioned criteria.

Two-thirds of the cases had a pure conductive impairment and 5% had no hearing impairment (Table 94). Eleven cases (1%) had a dead ear preoperatively.

TABLE 94

Chronic Otitis Media with Cholesteatoma
Type of hearing impairment (N-1024)

Type of Hearing Impairment	Incidence
Conductive	68%
Mixed	26%
None	5%
Total Loss	1%

Type of Perforation

Table 95 lists the type of perforation noted at the initial examination. Three percent of the cases had an intact tympanic membrane at the time of surgery.

TABLE 95

Chronic Otitis Media with Cholesteatoma
Type of perforation (N-1024)

Perforation	Incidence
Attic	42%
Posterior Superior	31%
Total	18%
Central	6%
None	3%

Aural Discharge

The extent and type of discharge by history and the status of the ear at the time of surgery are shown in Table 96.

TABLE 96

Chronic Otitis Media with Cholesteatoma
Aural discharge (N-1024)

Aural Discharge	Incidence
By History	
None or rarely	26%
Intermittent	53%
Continuous	21%
At Time of Surgery	
Dry	47%
Mucoid	10%
Purulent*	43%

*Refer to text for description of purulent discharge.

You will note that one-fourth of the patients had had little or no discharge in recent years; some of these had had considerable otorrhea in years past, however.

A comment is indicated in regard to the 43% of cases that are listed as having a purulent discharge at the time of surgery. It is our custom to record "purulent" on the surgical data sheet if the ear has any purulent discharge, regardless of the extent. We estimate that less than 10% of these cases had a profuse purulent discharge.

Age at Time of Surgery

Three percent of the patients were under the age of seven at the time of surgery (Table 97). The youngest was four.

TABLE 97

Chronic Otitis Media with Cholesteatoma
Age of patient at time of surgery (N-1024)

Age at Time of Surgery	Incidence
4 to 6 years	3.2%
7 to 15 years	14.5%
16 to 65 years	78.3%
66 years or older	4.0%

Two-thirds of the patients were between 20 and 59 years of age and 2% were in their 70's.

Surgical Procedure

Table 98 shows the surgical procedures performed on these 1024 cases. Eighty-eight percent were managed by the intact canal wall technique (Sheehy, 1972).

TABLE 98

Chronic Otitis Media with Cholesteatoma
Operative procedure performed (N-1024)

Procedure		Incidence
Tympanoplasty		97.6%
Intact canal wall	88.1%	
Obliteration	6.9%	
Cavity remains	2.6%	
Modified Radical or Radical		2.4%

There were some minor age-at-surgery related differences. In the 33 cases between the age of four and six, there was not a single radical or modified radical mastoidectomy performed. Both the intact canal wall technique and cavity remaining technique were used more frequently, and obliterative techniques less frequent in patients under the age of 16.

The frequency with which various surgical procedures were performed varied in different years. In 1965 only 74% of the cases were managed with the intact canal wall technique and 22% had a soft tissue obliteration of the mastoid at the time of tympanoplasty. In 1971 and 1972 96% of the cases were managed with the intact canal wall procedure and only 2% had mastoid obliteration.

The incidence of radical or modified radical mastoidectomy varied from less than 1% in 1966 to 6% in 1970.

Complications of the Disease

This study was initiated to analyze the complications of cholesteatoma and to attempt to relate the incidence of these complications to age, duration of disease and any other factors in the patient's history or the findings at surgery.

We looked at seven problems: Labyrinthine fistula, facial nerve paralysis, acute exacerbation of the disease (including preoperative pain), dizziness, meningeal or intracranial complication and total loss of hearing.

Each complication was initially analyzed in age-related groups in regard to duration of disease, the extent of otorrhea, type of perforation, presence of diabetes and extent of disease. Upon looking at the data we found that the number of cases in two of the age groups, and the number of major complications in three of the four age groups, were too small to give us meaningful information.

The complications which will be considered in some detail are labyrinthine fistula, facial nerve paralysis, meningeal involvement and total hearing loss. The incidence for each of these is shown in Table 99.

TABLE 99

Chronic Otitis Media with Cholesteatoma
Complications of the disease (N-1024)

Complications of the Disease	Incidence
Labyrinthine fistula	10.0%
Facial nerve weakness	1.1%
Meningeal involvement	0.3%
Epidural abscess (2 cases) Meningitis (later brain abscess) (1 case) Total hearing loss	1.1%

Labyrinthine Fistula

Cholesteatoma had involved the labyrinth, usually limited to the lateral semicircular canal, in 104 patients (10%).

The incidence of labyrinthine fistula was much higher in those whose disease had existed 20 years or more and lower in those whose disease was of less than 10 years' duration (Table 100).

The fistula incidence at various ages was approximately the same with the exception of the seven to 15 year age group: 3%. All complications were less common in this group (Table 101).

Meningeal Complications

A meningeal complication was recognized once preoperatively (meningitis) and twice at the time of surgery (chronic epidural abscess). All three were in adults.

Total Hearing Loss

Eleven patients (1%) had a total loss of hearing preoperatively. Less than half had labyrinthine fistulae.

All of the dead ears occurred in the 16 to 65 year age group. Although only one-third of the 1024 patients had been aware of their disease 20 years or more, three-fourths of the dead ears occurred in this group.

Miscellaneous Age Related Information

In the process of obtaining age-group related

TABLE 100

Complications of Cholesteatoma re Duration of Disease

Distribution of Complications re Duration of Disease

Duration of Disease	% of 1024 In Cases Each Group	All Complications N-114	Fistula N-104	Facial N-11	Meningeal N-3	Dead Ear N-11
1 year or less	17%	11%	11%	17%	33%	9%
2-5 years	21%	12%	12%	8%	33%	-
6-9 years	13%	7%	7%	-	-	9%
10-19 years	15%	13%	14%	-	-	9%
20 years or more	34%	57%	56%	75%	34%	73%
	100%	100%	100%	100%	100%	100%

Table 100: Percentages refer to distribution of complications in each duration of disease group. A higher complication percentage figure compared with the percentage distribution of cases figure in the lefthand column indicates a greater than expected incidence of complications in that duration group.

TABLE 101

Complications of Cholesteatoma re Age of Patient

Complications	N	All Cases N-1024	Incidence re Age of Patient 1-6 N-33	7-15 N-148	16-65 N-802	66+ N-41
Labyrinthine fistula	104	10.0%	9.1%	3.4%	11.6%	7.3%
Facial nerve weakness	11	1.1%	3.0%	—	1.2%	—
Meningeal involvement	3	0.3%	—	—	0.4%	—
Total hearing loss	11	1.1%	—	—	1.4%	—
Total cases with above complications	114	11.0%	12.0%	3.5%	13.0%	7.0%

Table 101: Percentages refer to incidence of complications in various age groups. Compare percentages in each age group column with overall incidence.

information relative to complications we explored other areas in which we felt there might be significant differences in various age groups: Staging the operation and reasons therefore, graft take and postoperative serous otitis media.

Staging the Operation

We perform tympanoplasty in two stages for one of two reasons: To obtain a better hearing result or to obtain an ear free of both residual cholesteatoma and recurrent cholesteatoma (Sheehy and Crabtree, 1973). Considered in making this decision are the status of the ossicular chain, the mucosal status and the possibility of residual cho-

lesteatoma.

There were 996 tympanoplasties in this series, 39% of which were staged. The reasons for staging, and the age related differences, are shown in Table 102.

Staging was more commonly performed in the younger patients, and the reason for this was the possibility of residual disease. This possibility of residual disease was a significant factor, however, in all age groups, but with decreasing frequency with age.

A mucosal or ossicular problem, or both, was the most common reason for staging in those 16 years of age or older.

TABLE 102

Tympanoplasty with Mastoidectomy for Cholesteatoma

	All Cases N-996	Age of Patient			
		1-6 N-32	7-15 N-145	16-65 N-780	66+ N-39
Operation staged	39%	68%	46%	36%	36%
Reason					
Mucosal and/or ossicular problems only	44%	27%	27%	49%	63%
Mucosal and ossicular problem, and concern re residual cholesteatoma	18%	50%	23%	16%	6%
Residual disease only reason	12%	9%	14%	11%	—
Residual disease involved in decision for staging	50%	68%	71%	45%	38%

Table 102: Reason for staging the operation related to age of the patient at time of surgery.

Graft Take

There were 887 tympanoplasties in which a fascia graft was used and in which we had six months or more follow-up information. The graft take rate at 6 months was 97% with a 2% late failure rate. There were no significant differences in the various age groups (Table 103).

Postoperative Serous Otitis Media

We were very interested in comparing the incidence of postoperative serous otitis media in the different age groups. The overall incidence of persistent serous otitis media (requiring a ventilation tube) was 4%. The incidence was slightly higher in those six years old and younger and lower in those over 65 years (see Table 103).

Facial Nerve Paralysis

Facial nerve paralysis was apparent in eleven cases (1%).

In four cases this was a total paralysis. Facial function returned to normal in two weeks in two cases, three months in one and six months in the fourth.

In seven cases the paralysis was partial. Facial function returned to normal within a month in five cases, within a year in one and has not returned to normal in the seventh case.

The number of patients with preoperative facial nerve paralysis was small (11 cases), but we thought it would be of interest to note some correlations. Three-fourths of the paralyses occurred in those who had had their disease 20 years or more, although only one-third of the 1024 patients fell into this group.

One-fourth of the patients had had little or no otorrhea and yet 40% of the facial paralyses occurred in this group. One-third of the 1024 patients had a posterior superior marginal perforation and yet half of the facial paralyses occurred in this group.

Acute Exacerbation of the Disease

Six percent of the patients had an acute exacerbation of their disease immediately prior to surgery. This was manifested by pain (usually a subacute mastoiditis or empyema in the cholesteatoma) and may have been associated with a sudden

TABLE 103

Tympanoplasty with Mastoidectomy for Cholesteatoma

| Age of Patient | Fascia Graft Cases | | P.O. Serous Otitis Media | |
	Graft Take	Late Failure	Temporary	Persistent
All ages	96.7%	2.3%	2.9%	4.0%
1-6 years	97.0%	0	0	6.3%
7-15 years	97.7%	1.6%	2.2%	0.7%
16-65 years	96.5%	2.5%	3.1%	4.6%
66 years or older	97.2%	0	5.3%	2.6%

Table 103: Age of patient re graft take and re postoperative serous otitis media. Refer to text for definitions and discussions.

onset of facial paralysis or labyrinthine fistula or both of these. In one case there was a subperiosteal abscess.

The incidence of acute exacerbation varied from 3% in the four to six year age group to 7% in the 16 to 65 year age group. We suspect that this difference may not be significant due to both the small number of cases in the younger age group and the difference in incidence in regard to duration of disease in the older age group.

Dizziness

Twenty percent of the patients are recorded as having some type of dizziness in the year prior to their surgery. This symptom was much more frequent in those with a labyrinthine fistula (although not present in some), but was otherwise primarily related to the age of the patient and probably represented inner ear changes not related to the mastoid disease.

Discussion

Most of the data presented was in agreement with the information we had obtained on yearly evaluations and with our clinical impressions. We had not, however, previously evaluated in detail many of these complications.

Labyrinthine Fistulae

Some of the younger men in our Group were surprised at the 10% incidence of labyrinthine fistulae, but many of us remembered that there were fistulae in 13% of the 555 mastoidectomy cases reported in a 1967 article (Sheehy and Patterson, 1967). The fistula incidence has decreased in recent years, and ranged from a high of 17% in the 1966 cases to a low of 3% in the 1970 cases.

The cases reported here are a selected group: They are the 75% of primary mastoid surgery cases with more advanced disease, and there is a selective element in the fact that the patient was referred to us for surgery in the first place.

We do not know what if any effect this selective factor had on the statistics. Fistulae were certainly much more common in those with long-standing disease. This fact presumably explains the decreased incidence in recent years: patients are being referred sooner for surgery.

It is of interest that 12 of the 104 fistula cases developed a total loss of hearing postoperatively. This 12% incidence should be compared with the 1% incidence of postoperative dead ear in the remaining 1000 cases.

Details of the management and outcome of fistula cases will be the subject of a subsequent report.

Facial Nerve Complications

The incidence of preoperative facial nerve paralysis was low (1%). As such it is questionable if the statistics are significant.

The majority of facials occurred in those who had had their disease 20 years or more. Six of the 11 patients with preoperative facial nerve paralysis also had recently developed pain in the mastoid, although these 6 represent only 10% of those with an acute exacerbation of their disease. Four of the 11 patients with facial nerve paralysis had a concomitant labyrinthine fistula.

Surgically Related Complications

Surgical and postoperative complications are not the subject of this report, but we thought it would be of interest to comment on these in regard to the facial nerve.

We reported one operative facial nerve damage requiring a nerve graft in 555 cases in 1967. There was one additional case in this series of 1024 operations. This case and five mild, temporary, (immediate) facial nerve weaknesses occurred in 902 cases managed by the intact canal wall technique.

Delayed postoperative facial nerve paralysis occurred in three cases, all managed by the intact canal wall technique. In one of these the paralysis was total and has persisted; this ear had extensive labyrinthine destruction and exposure of the internal auditory canal; radical mastoidectomy was necessary later for control of the disease.

Miscellaneous Findings

There was one case with a congenital cerebral spinal fluid leak identified at surgery and one case of a congenital herniation of a portion of the temporal lobe into the mastoid.

Three cases were identified in which there were one or more cholesteatoma cysts in the mastoid isolated from the main cholesteatoma mass. In none of these was there any clear indication (that is, new bone growth) as to the cause of the finding.

Sensori-Neural Hearing Impairment

It is surprising that only a fourth of the patients presented with a mixed impairment in light of the extent of the disease and the commonly discussed influence of chronic otitis media on inner ear function. We plan to look at all the unilateral cases and further evaluate this finding.

Tympanoplasty on Draining Ears

We try to obtain a dry ear prior to surgery, but do not postpone surgery on cholesteatoma cases if the ear continues to drain. As a result, 43% of the operations in this series still had some purulent discharge.

Twenty percent of the patients had had continuous aural discharge when first seen and few of these were we able to dry up prior to surgery. Half of those with intermittent discharge by history were still discharging some at the time of surgery. Only 5% of the total group were in an acute exacerbation.

Our surgical management of the ear that continues to drain is the same as for the dry ear with cholesteatoma, with one exception: In the profusely draining ear we will usually place a catheter drain into the antrum at the conclusion of surgery.

The fascia graft take rate was slightly lower in the draining ears: 95% versus 98% in the dry ears. We were not aware of this difference, based on our yearly short-term evaluation, and suspect that the difference is a manifestation of the case selection for this study.

Tympanoplasty on Children

One frequently hears the statement that tympanoplasty should not be performed under the age of six or seven, or even ten.

We believe that if there is an indication for mastoid surgery the patient's age, per se, is not a relevant factor. The youngest patient in this series was four and no radical or modified radical mastoidectomies were performed on any of the 33 patients under six years of age. The fascia graft take rate was the same as for the entire group (97%). The frequency of staging the operation was almost twice that of adults due primarily to our concern in regard to possible residual disease.

Conclusions

(1) A labyrinthine fistula was found in 10% of 1024 primary operations for mastoid cholesteatoma during a 10 year period. Twelve of these 104 fistula cases developed a total hearing loss postoperatively.

(2) Facial nerve paralysis was present preoperatively in 1% of 1024 cases. The paralysis was total in four and partial in seven.

(3) Eleven patients (1%) had a total loss of hearing prior to surgery.

(4) Meningeal complications were rare (0.3%) in this series.

(5) The above complications were more common in those patients whose disease was known to have existed 20 years or more and less common in those existing in nine years or less.

References

1. Sheehy, J. L. and Patterson, M. D.: Intact canal wall tympanoplasty and mastoidectomy: A review of eight years experience. *The Laryngoscope,* 77:1502, 1967.
2. Sheehy, J. L.: *Surgery of Chronic Otitis Media in Otolaryngology.* Harper and Row Publishers, Inc., Hagerstown, Maryland, 1972.
3. Sheehy, J. L. and Crabtree, J. A.: Tympanoplasty: Staging the operation. *The Laryngoscope,* 83:1594, 1973.

COMPLICATIONS OF CHOLESTEATOMA

Frank N. Ritter, M.D.

A quantitative assessment related to the length of the patient's history of disease. Are complications less or different in type now as compared to the pre-antibiotic era?

Epidemiological studies demonstrate that over a given period of time, almost all infections change in their virulence and behavior. Today, infections are modified, not only by chemotherapeutic agents, antitoxins and vaccines, but by a host who lives in an era where socio-economic conditions permit a high level of nutrition, which in turn generates a strong internal resistance to infection. Accountably, in the last three decades, suppurative otitis media has also changed, undergoing a dramatic conversion from a dangerous illness, with sometimes fatal complications, to one which still occurs frequently in the acute phase, but seems relatively rare as a chronic illness and not prone to complications. It is naturally legitimate to ask what has happened during this same time to one of the pathologies of otitis media, specifically cholesteatoma. Has it changed in its presentation, behavior, destructive ability and tendency to produce complications?

This question, which is most concisely posed by the title of this portion of the symposium, seeks the answer by comparing clinically two groups of patients: one from the pre-antibiotic era, the other from the more recent times. Because the University of Michigan maintains on file, like other institutions, large numbers of patient records, it would seem that this comparison would not be difficult to make.

Pre-Antibiotic Era

The pre-antibiotic era is generally recognized to be that time in medical history prior to World War II. The initial portion of this study began by selecting records of patients who had undergone mastoidectomy during 1937-1942. However, the master code sheets for this period of time and those prior to it, were so worn from use as to be unreadable. When records were obtained, they too were in the same condition with torn or missing pages, badly worn and too indistinct for proper study. Of those records able to be obtained and studied, the operative notes usually mentioned cholesteatoma as being present, but rarely described its extension. Consequently, the only recourse to understanding the behavior of cholesteatoma in the pre-antibiotic era was to search the literature.

The literature search proved to be almost as barren. While cholesteatoma was the subject of quite a few papers in the pre-antibiotic era, the discussions were usually philosophical ones debating the origin of this disease as to whether it was congenital or acquired. Infrequent papers did report one or several case histories of patients having cholesteatoma, but these reports were about the clinical course of patients who were critically ill from the extensiveness of the cholesteatoma and its subsequent infection in its spread to vital structures. One paper did analyze statistically a group of cholesteatomas and this one is most germane for comparison and use in this symposium.

In 1938, Holmes reported a study of the records of 303 patients from the Massachusetts Eye & Ear Infirmary who had cholesteatomas (Holmes, 1938). The time interval was an eleven year period from 1925-1936, and in each of his cases, cholesteatoma was found at operation and sometimes verified by pathological examination (Fig. 169).

CHOLESTEATOMA INCIDENCE

Massachusetts.......303 cases
1925 - 1936

Michigan................152 cases
1965 - 1970

Fig. 169: A comparison of the incidence of cholesteatomas in the time span for each of these series.

Massachusetts Eye and Ear Series

Age of Patient At the Time of Surgery

Figure 170 is a reproduction of the plot of the age of these patients at the time of their surgical operation. Eleven percent of the patients were op-

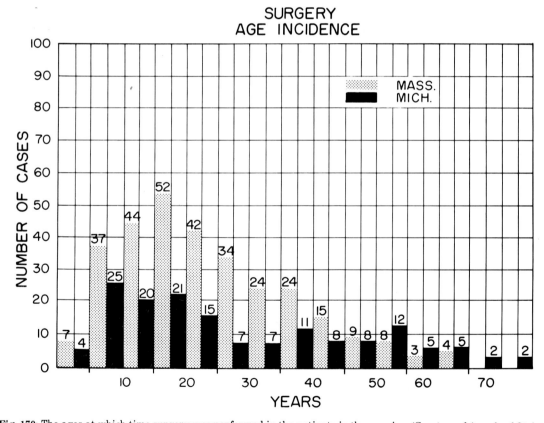

Fig. 170: The ages at which time surgery was performed in the patients in these series. *(Courtesy of Annals of Otology, Rhinology and Laryngology.)*

erated upon under 10 years of age, 43% under 20 years of age, and 56% under 26 years of age. Most patients (87%) had undergone surgery by 40 years of age, so cholesteatoma was then an illness occurring in young people, even the youngster (Fig. 171).

Aural Discharge

The Massachusetts series demonstrated that 35% of the ears started to discharge under six years of age and 63% began their symptoms under 11 years of age. As to length of time of the aural discharge, 20% of the patients noted it less than one year in duration and about 70% noticed it less than six years. Thus, cholesteatoma was associated with discharge developing early in life (Figs. 172 & 173).

CHOLESTEATOMA
AGE AT SURGERY

	<10 yrs	<20 yrs	<26 yrs
Mass.	11%	43%	57%
Mich.	19%	46%	56%

Fig. 171: The age at which surgery was carried out in the patients in these series.

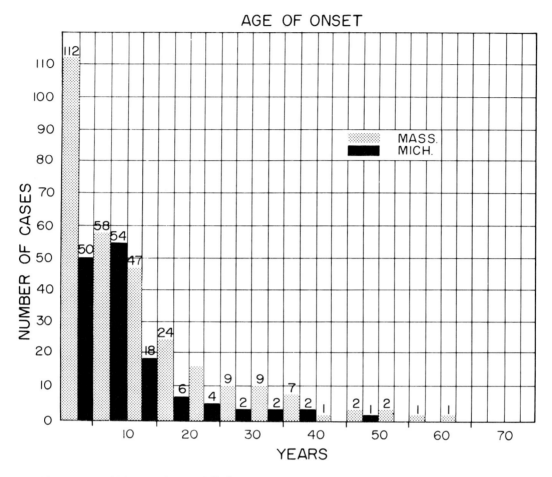

Fig. 172: The ages at which time the aural discharge began by comparison in these series. *(Courtesy of Annals of Otology, Rhinology and Laryngology.)*

CHOLESTEATOMA
ONSET AURAL DISCHARGE

	5 yrs	11 yrs
Mass.	35%	63%
Mich.	33%	68%

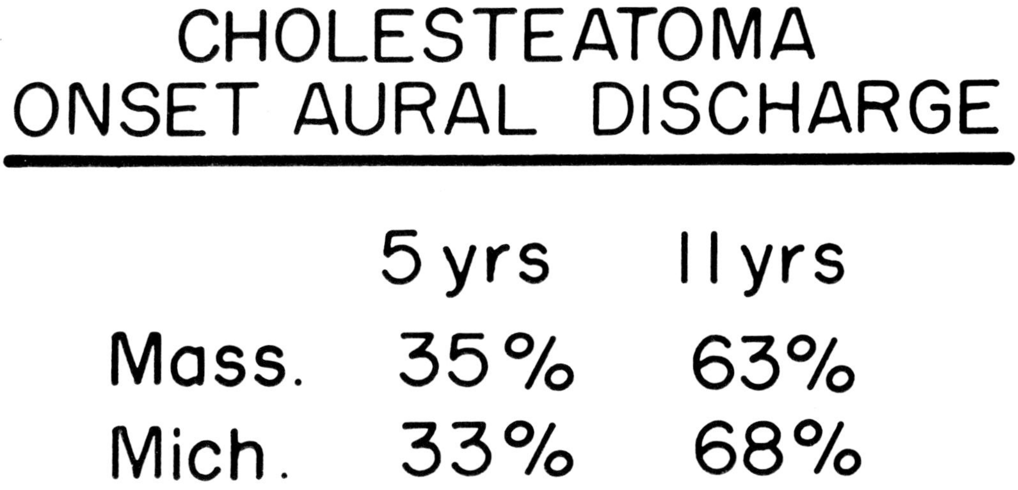

Fig. 173: A comparison of the onset of the aural discharge in each of these series. *(Courtesy of Annals of Otology, Rhinology and Laryngology.)*

Perforation Of The Tympanic Membrane

Holmes found in most cases, the perforation was hidden by exhuberant polypoid granulation tissue in the ear canal, but when detected, it was noted to occur in Shrapnell's membrane in 25% of the cases; the posterior superior quadrant of the pars tensa in 25%, centrally located in 14%, and the whole drum head was absent in 36% (Fig. 174).

In summary, the Massachusetts series contained 303 surgical operative cases for cholesteatoma over 11 years. The aural discharge was of short duration and issued from an attic or posteromarginal perforation of the tympanic membrane. Most of the patients were young individuals. Complications were not tabulated in these patients.

Post-Antibiotic Era University of Michigan Series

The present search of the Michigan Medical Center records was done over a six year period from January 1965 to December 1970, in which 315 mastoidectomy-tympanoplasty procedures were performed. Of these 315 patients, a cholesteatoma was found at surgery and frequently verified by pathological examination in 152 ears. In an effort to provide as an exact comparison with the Massachusetts study, the format Holmes chose to use is also used in this paper.

Age Of Patient At The Time Of Surgery

Nineteen percent of the patients were under 10 years of age at the time of their surgical procedure, 46% were under 20 years of age and 56% were under 26 years of age. Most cases, 72%, were under 40 years of age. These statistics are very close and almost identical to those of the Massachusetts series.

Aural Discharge

In the Michigan series, 50 ears (33%) began to discharge under five years of age and 104 (68%) of the patients noted the symptoms beginning under 11 years of age. As to length of time of the discharge, 1% noted it less than one year in duration and 36 (24%) of the patients noted it less than six years. The Michigan statistics vary from the Massachusetts series only in the duration of the

CHOLESTEATOMA PERFORATION

	Mass.	Mich.
Shrapnels	25%	25%
Post. Sup.	25%	40%
Central	14%	21%
Whole	36%	14%

Fig. 174: A comparison of a location of perforations in the Massachusetts and Michigan series.

discharge. The time of onset by age is almost identical. (By 11 years of age: 63% Massachusetts, 68% Michigan.)

Perforation Of The Tympanic Membrane

Perforations were usually visible otoscopically at initial examination. In the Michigan series, Shrapnell's area contained the perforation in 39 (25%) of the ears; the posterior superior part of the pars tensa in 61 (40%); centrally located in 32 (21%); and the whole drum head was missing in 20 (14%). The Michigan study contains more posterior superior located perforations and less whole tympanic membrane destructions, but is otherwise very close statistically to the Massachusetts study.

Ossicular Destruction

The Massachusetts series did not study ossicular destruction, but in the present series, the malleus head was at least partially destroyed in 58 (30%) of the patients; the incus, especially the long arm in 133 (87%), and the superstructure of the stapes in 51 patients (33%).

Location Of The Cholesteatoma

In all patients in the Michigan series, the cholesteatoma was found in at least the middle ear or epitympanum. It invaded the antrum in 70 cases (46%) and the mastoid in 21 cases (14%).

Hearing

There was a loss of hearing of these patients in whom 137 of 152 had hearing tests. In six of these 137 patients, a non-functioning ear for hearing was noted. In addition to these six, there were 11 ears that had discrimination scores below 80% in which the loss ranged from 28% to 76%. For all the rest, the S.R.T. averaged 42.2 db.

Complications

Figure 175 tabulates the complications and cites their percentage. This compares favorably with a previous study on the present day complications from chronic suppurative otitis media (Ritter, 1970).

Comment

The Massachusetts study had 303 cholesteatomas in 11 years and this study reports 152 in just half that time. Identically, in both series, 56% were operated on under 26 years of age. Thirty-five percent of the ears from the Massachusetts series had begun to discharge by 6 years of age and 63% by 11 years. In the Michigan study for these same periods, 33% and 68% of the ears began

COMPLICATIONS

	CASES	
Lateral Semicircular Canal Fistula	16	10%
Facial Nerve Exposure (paralysis in 2)	12	7%
Dural Exposure, Pathological	12	7%
Sigmoid Sinus Thrombosis	2	
Cerebellar Extra-Dural Abscess	1	
Temporal Lobe Abscess	1	

Fig. 175: A compilation of the complications and type of each in the Michigan series.

to discharge—again, also almost identical.

In the Massachusetts series, 25% of the perforations were in Shrapnell's membrane, 24% were in the posterior superior quadrant of the pars tensa; 14% were central and in 36%, the whole drum head was missing. In the Michigan series, 25% of the perforations were also Shrapnell's, but 40% were in the posterior superior quadrant; 21% centrally located and in 13% the whole drum head was destroyed. Likely, the reason for the discrepancy is that infections are nowadays treated with antibiotics, so are not apt to be as severe and provide so abundant an infection which would destroy the whole drum head.

Thus, the size of each of these series, the age at which time the aural discharge began and was later surgically treated, its duration, the site of perforation in the tympanic membrane, are so similar or are almost identical. However, there were still differences in the series.

In the Massachusetts series, the antrum was almost always invaded and enlarged by the cholesteatoma. Often, it was accompanied with radiographic evidence of destruction. When added to the fact that one-third of the Massachusetts patients had exuberant granulation tissue polyps in the ear canal, so that the drum head was hidden otoscopically, an impression is gained of severe and extensive disease in the pre-antibiotic era. Likely, the complications were also more frequent and sometimes, life threatening, but the series fails to quote them. In the Michigan series, the tympanic membrane was never difficult to examine, even on initial patient presentation as large aural polyps were not noted in any ear. Further, the antrum was invaded by the cholesteatoma in only 46% of the ears and the mastoid segment in 14%. These statistics point to a less extensive illness and allude to the fact that a complete mastoid air cell exenteration does not often need to be presently done at surgery. With less extensive infections, present day surgeons can legitimately concentrate on more conservative aural surgery for hearing reconstruction. Yet, the surgeon should not be trapped because 21% of the central perforations in the Michigan series, were associated with cholesteatoma, a few of which even invaded the mastoid.

As a spillover, might these statistics, in comparison, permit any clue as to the etiology of cholesteatoma? It is interesting that despite better diagnostic methods, improved medical facilities, antibiotics and better socioeconomic times, with a more robust and healthy population that lives longer, that cholesteatomas appear to have changed little in presentation, behavior and their effects upon tissue destruction. Confronted with this lack of change in the illness, and the fact that cholesteatoma is predominately a disease of early life, causes the authors of both of these series to conclude that it is an illness more often of congenital cause than one gains from reading the literature.

Present day otologists always "wonder where all the operative ear cases are", and that chronic ear disease seems less frequent because of the antibiotics. While this is true of acute mastoiditis, now very rare, the chronic ears in both of these series are almost identical in number per time span studied. Thus, no change in frequency over the years with as many ears on which to do surgery as ever before, but more capable surgeons available to perform surgery.

Conclusion

Two series of patients were compared to answer the question: what effect have antibiotics had on the behavior of cholesteatoma. The series used to provide the statistics for the comparison study were not from the same institution, but this would seem to be only a slight criticism. The comparison reveals nearly identical behavior of onset, duration of discharge, site of tympanic membrane perforation from the cholesteatoma despite the patient cases being separated by an interval of 40 years. Further, because the comparison still shows the illness to be mainly one of the first three decades of life and has not changed over the years, the congenital theory of the causation of cholesteatoma seems particularly strong.

References

1. Holmes, E. M.: A review of three hundred and three cases of cholesteatoma. *Ann. Oto. Rhino. Laryngol.*, 47: 135, 1938.

2. Ritter, F. N.: Chronic suppurative otitis media and the pathologic labyrinthine fistula. *The Laryngoscope*, 80:1025, 1970.

SENSORINEURAL HEARING LOSS RESULTING FROM CHRONIC OTITIS MEDIA

Michael M. Paparella, M.D.

Introduction

In previous studies we described sensorineural hearing loss as a common and significant concomitant in chronic otitis media (Paparella, 1970 and 1972). Prior to our initial report there were few articles in the literature documenting the presence of sensorineural hearing loss with otitis media (Bluvshtein, 1963; Gardenghi, 1955; Hulka, 1941; Thorburn, 1965; and Verhoeven 1961). Since our initial reports we continue to observe the presence of sensorineural hearing loss, especially high frequency loss, in our patients.

Clinical Studies

As was partially described earlier, the charts and audiograms of 500 patients with chronic otitis media who ultimately went to surgery, were reviewed. Of these, only 279 ears, representing 232 patients, were considered eligible for this study. The remaining patients were rejected for this study because of any other causes which might have resulted in a sensorineural hearing loss, such as systemic or local exposure to ototoxic drugs, fistula confirmed at operation, exposure to loud noises, etc. Thorough audiometric data was available for all patients included in this study. Both ears of 47 patients were included. The median age of the group was 30 years. There were 197 male ears and 82 female ears.

Most of the patients in this group had conductive hearing losses, many with a sensorineural component. In this report only cochlear losses will be considered. Thirty percent of this group were found to have otalgia, 13% a history of vertigo, while 25% had tinnitus.

Of the 279 ears included in this study group, 245 were draining actively at the time audiograms were taken. The remaining 34 ears had a history of intermittent drainage in the past, but they did not have active otorrhea at the time of examination. Mean bone conduction thresholds for those ears with no drainage and for those with active drainage are compared in Figure 176.

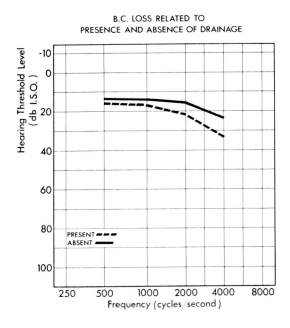

B.C. LOSS RELATED TO PRESENCE AND ABSENCE OF DRAINAGE

Fig. 176: Self-explanatory.

The length of time that inflammation of the middle ear was present and how this variable affected cochlear function were considered next. Initially it was believed that the longer the period of active suppuration, the greater the sensorineural involvement. The subjects, therefore, were divided into subgroups according to the duration of the ear drainage; mean bone conduction audiograms for each group are presented in Figure 177. The results, in general, seem to corroborate our empirical observations.

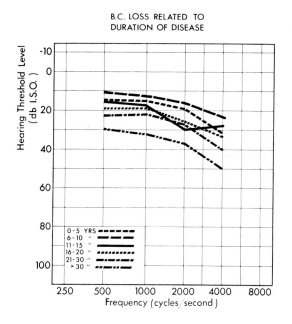

Fig. 177: Self-explanatory.

All but 21 ears were noted to have a drumhead perforation; most of the remaining ears, however, showed evidence of old healed perforations. The pathology described at the time of surgery was documented and assessed. Cholesteatomas were found in 115 ears and granulation tissue in 125 ears.

An arbitrary definition of the extent of the pathology was determined by involvement of (1) the attic region, (2) the mesotympanum and hypotympanum, and (3) the antrum and mastoid air cells. With cholesteatoma or granulation tissue in just one of the three regions, the involvement was called mild, while those with two or three areas involved were classified as moderate or severe, respectively. The mean bone conduction thresholds for each of these groups are seen in Figure 178.

The effect of middle ear pathology (granulations, cholesteatoma, and pus), manifesting as apparent bone conduction loss in partially obstructing both windows or tamponading the round window in such manner as to alter the phase differential, was considered. In general, bone conduction

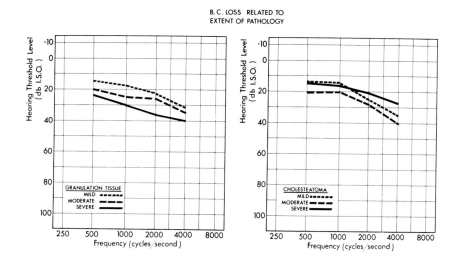

Fig. 178: Self-explanatory.

losses, persisting after surgery in which there was removal of middle ear pathologic tissues, suggest that mechanical window occlusion is not the cause of the cochlear involvement.

In all the audiograms mentioned above, the effects of presbycusis are still present and are probably responsible for some of the deficit seen, especially in the high frequency losses of older patients. Patients with severe cochlear involvement greatly affect the average audiometric results.

Audiograms by decades were established for the entire study group (Fig. 179). The younger age groups demonstrate a significant degree of bone conduction loss.

B.C. LOSS BY DECADES

Age (Yrs.)	No. of Cases	CPS			
		500	1000	2000	4000
0-9	20	6.8	8.0	6.8	11.1
10-19	80	7.3	9.6	10.8	16.2
20-29	27	15.4	14.8	19.8	30.8
30-39	41	19.8	19.8	31.2	32.0
40-49	46	23.3	22.7	29.7	40.2
50-59	39	25.9	26.7	32.8	48.1
60+	26	33.5	39.0	48.7	69.8
TOTAL	279	19.5	19.1	24.0	32.8

(Decibel Loss)

Fig. 179: Self-explanatory.

Presbycusis must be taken into consideration. In an attempt to determine the proportion of perceptive loss due to presbycusis, the average bone conduction thresholds by decade for the three groups over 40 years of age were then compared with data from a study by Glorig and Nixon (Fig. 180).

A built-in control in this study is the normal ear in patients with unilateral disease. A comparison between the diseased and normal ears serves to substantiate the existence of sensorineural involvement and also helps to exclude the consideration of presbycusis for older patients (Fig. 181). Comparison of the differences between the bone conduction thresholds in the diseased and the non-diseased ears, yields significant ratios ($P < 0.01$) at 1,000, 2,000 and 4,000 Hz, but not at 500 Hz.

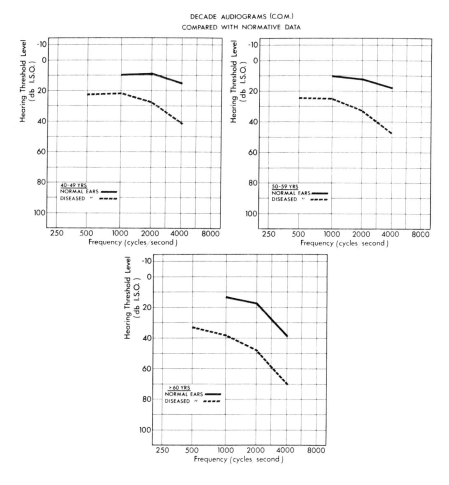

Fig. 180: Self-explanatory.

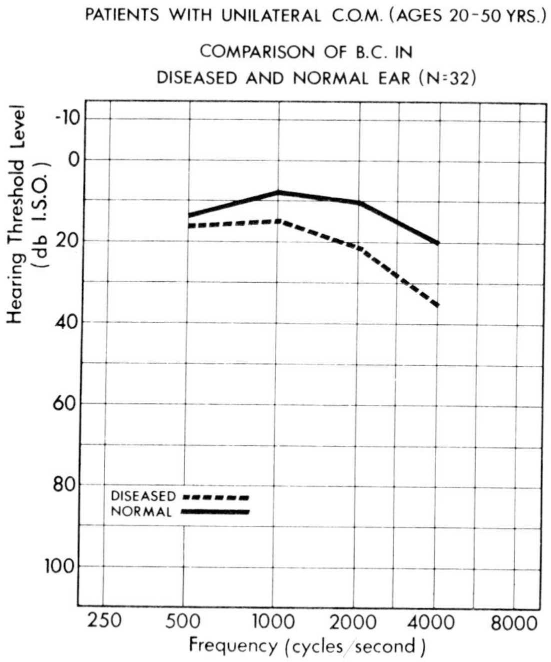

Fig. 181: Self-explanatory.

The Round Window

The fine structure of the round window membrane in primates has been described by Kawabata and Paparella (1971). The membrane has three layers: (1) the epithelial layer, consisting of nonciliated flat cells contiguous with the middle ear lining; (2) the middle layer (immediately beneath the basement membrane of the epithelial layer), in which fibrocytes with extensions form a network of continuous cells with large intercellular spaces filled with collagen and elastic fibers; and (3) the inner layer (facing the scala tympani) consisting of elongated thin cells with thin cytoplasmic extensions (Fig. 182). The membrane

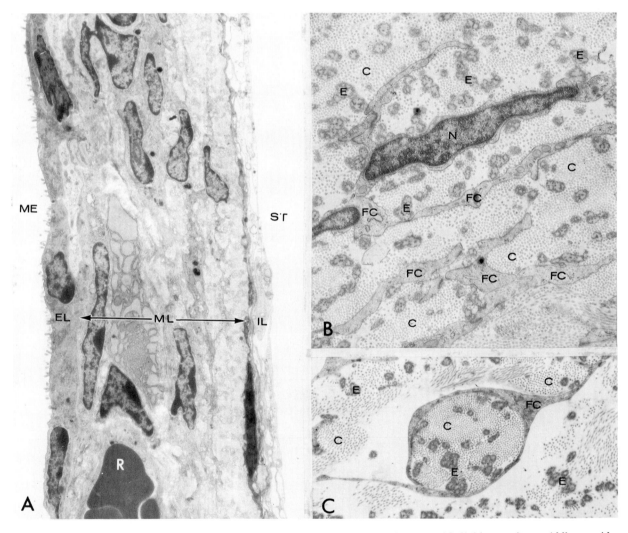

Fig. 182: (**A**) Round window membrane of squirrel monkey demonstrating three layers: epithelial layer (el) on middle ear side (me); large middle layer; inner layer lining scala tympani (st); red blood cell (r). (**B and C**) Higher power view of middle layer showing fibrocytes (fc); collagen fibers (c); elastic fibers (e); and nucleus (n).

measures approximately .065 mm in thickness.

According to Dean and Wolff (1934) the round window niche is approximately 1 mm in depth and 2 mms in diameter. Detailed anatomical dimensions of the niche were described by Donaldson (1968). There are essentially no ciliated cells in the region of the round window under normal circumstances. Pus can be pooled in the adjacent sinus tympani space especially when the patient is in an upright position. Remnants of mesenchyme in the niche and sinus tympani are slow to be resorbed and can become infected in infants. These factors encourage pus or infected tissue to be concentrated at the round window thereby encouraging absorption through it.

Pathology

We previously described temporal bones of patients with tympanogenic suppurative labyrinthitis resulting from otitis media with extensive cochlear loss but preservation of vestibular function. We have also seen patients in whom vestibular function is lost by invasion of cholesteatoma with preservation of cochlear function. These represented gross examples of destruction of pars superior or pars inferior with preservation of its counterpart (Fig. 183).

Studies of the pathological influence of chronic

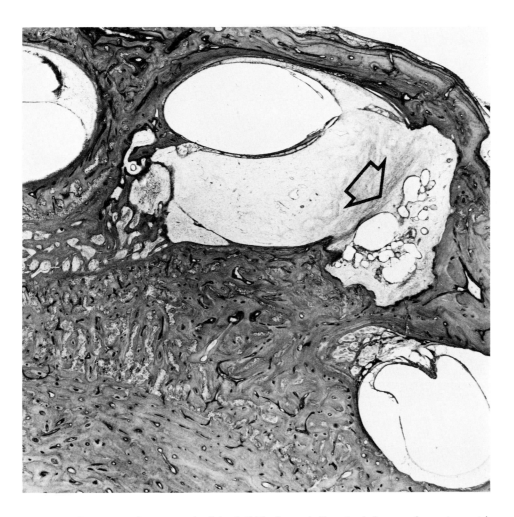

Fig. 183: Tympanogenic suppurative labyrinthitis (human). Round window membrane (arrow) is difficult to see and is surrounded by a fibrous tissue response in the round window niche to the right and in the scala to the left.

otitis media on the inner ear was assessed in animals. Eleven animals (six guinea pigs, one squirrel monkey, one dog and three cats) with spontaneously occurring otitis media were studied. Similar changes were seen in the middle ears of all the animals. Cystic dilatation, infiltration of inflammatory cells and formation of granular tissue were found. Some specimens showed new bone formation. Varying degrees of involvement of the round window membrane and the scala tympani of the basal turn adjacent to the round window membrane were noted in all specimens. The round window membrane was thickened and invasion of inflammatory cells through the membrane was seen in some cases. Numerous inflammatory cells and serofibrinous precipitates were present in the perilymphatic space, particularly in the scala tympani (Fig. 184).

We also studied 334 human temporal bones, of which 75 were found to have middle ear inflammation with effusion, 35 serous and 40 purulent. Of the 40 ears with purulent effusion, 10 were

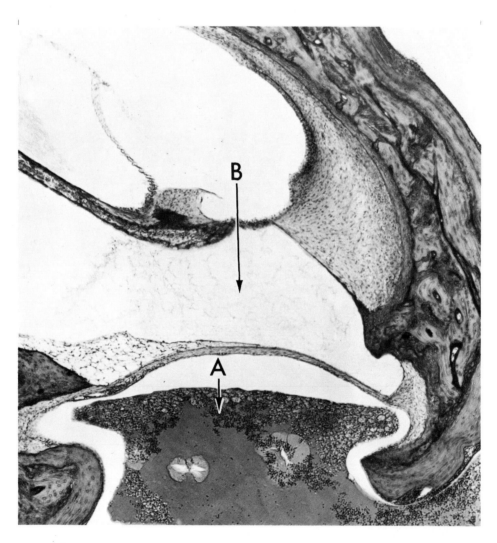

Fig. 184: Round window and perilymph pathology. Pus cells are seen in the region of the round window (**A**) and serofibrinous precipitates are seen in the perilymph of the scala tympani (**B**).

classified as chronic and 30 as acute. Cells were seen in the middle ear space and infiltrating the subepithelial layer of the middle ear mucosa. There was also edema of the mucosa and dilatation of capillaries.

In the group of 75 ears with inflammation, slight hyperplasia and metaplasia of the outer layer were found in all specimens. Gross changes consisted of dilatation of the vessels within the fibrous layer, thickening of the membrane, infiltration of inflammatory cells, marked metaplasia or hyperplasia, or cystic changes. Such changes were more prevalent in the purulent group than in the serous or control groups.

Basal turn pathology: The inner ears were studied and the most significant findings were changes in the perilymph of the scala tympani near the round window membrane, although perilymph changes in other areas were occasionally seen. These alterations consisted of either serofibrinous precipitates or inflammatory cells in the perilymph or both. Of the 75 ears with middle ear effusion, a total of 50 demonstrated pathological changes in the scala tympani. In the acute purulent group both cells and precipitates were seen in 13 ears, cells alone in five and precipitates alone in five. In the chronic purulent group, both findings were seen in two ears, cells alone in four and precipitates alone in four ears. In the serous group, both cells and precipitates were seen in five ears, cells only in nine and precipitates only in three.

Table 104 categorizes the results of the pathology in the normal and abnormal groups.

TABLE 104

Pathological Changes in the Scala Tympani

	Cases with Middle Ear Inflammation and Effusion (Total cases—75)			Controls (Total cases—269)	
	Acute Purulent	Chronic Purulent	Serous	Blood in Middle Ear	Normal
Number of Specimens	28	13	34	31	238
Number with Scala Tympani Pathology	23	10	17	12	8

Figure 185 demonstrates examples of round window pathology in humans with inflammatory cells on the inner ear side of the round window membranes.

Examples of serifibrinous precipitates localized to the perilymph of the scala tympani are seen in Figure 186.

Quantitative hair cell analysis using the method of cochlear graphic reconstruction was done whenever possible. In the acute purulent group (mostly children) 17 cases were not considered suitable for study because of autolytic or hypotonic degenerative changes. Of the remaining 11 cases eight appeared normal while three showed distinct lower basal turn lesions of the organ of Corti, manifested mainly by missing outer hair cells.

Of the chronic purulent group (mostly adults) 10 demonstrated hypotonic degeneration and two

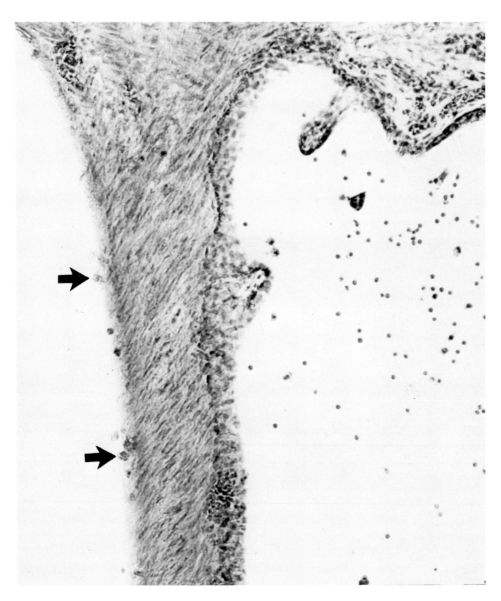

Fig. 185: Round window pathology as seen in one human temporal bone case. Inflammatory cells are seen in the perilymph on the scala tympani side of the round window membrane (arrows).

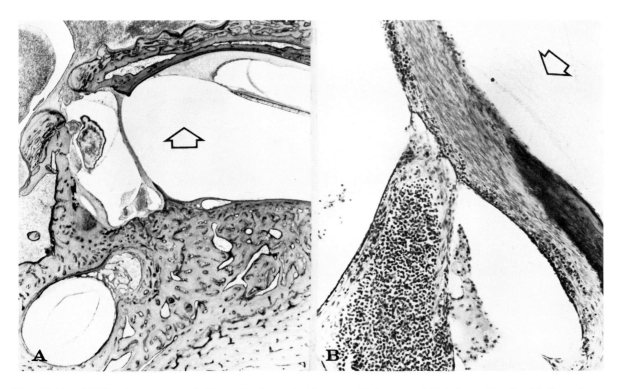

Fig. 186: (A and B) Two human cases of otitis media demonstrating a serofibrinous precipitate (arrow) localized to the scala tympani of the basal turn.

autolysis rendering interpretation difficult. Five with hypotonic degeneration seemed to have lower basal turn lesions, but this was uncertain, and in any case presbycusis could not be ruled out. In one case, a child with good hair cell preservation, scattered outer hair losses were seen in the lower basal turn.

In the control groups the findings were essentially normal.

At the present time we are studying the biochemical effects of perilymph in the presence of acute and chronic otitis media. Distinct changes, indeed, occur in perilymph including elevated levels of the enzymes lactic acid dehydrogenase (LDH), malic acid dehydrogenase (MDH), as well as other biochemical alterations. These will be described subsequently by Dr. Juhn of our laboratories.

Very High Frequency Studies in Otitis Media

At the present time, using both animal and human subjects with acute and chronic otitis media, we are concentrating our attention upon auditory changes which occur in the basal turn. Since chronic otitis media with, and/or without cholesteatoma, may follow earlier bouts of acute otitis media, we are interested in studying acute otitis media, using behavioral methods in chinchillas and using very high frequency audiometry in humans. We are also assessing very high frequency losses in patients with chronic otitis media. The following examples relate to acute otitis media in human subjects. There are 8 patients with 14 ears to date studied by this method.

In addition to obtaining the standard audiogram, thresholds are obtained at 4,000, 6,000, 8,000, 10,000, 12,000, 14,000, 16,000 and 18,000 Hz, in these patients. To date, our data substantiates our preliminary findings. Without fail, in these patients, thus far, we have observed a dramatic loss in the frequency range of 4,000 to 18,000 Hz in patients with acute otitis media. There is remission of the loss after treatment, however, it appears that there may be some residual damage at the extreme high frequencies. We hope to be able to show the course of the hearing loss during infection and the recovery functions over time. It may be that recovery functions will be different for chronic cases in comparison with acute cases (Figs. 187, 188, & 189).

Summary

Audiometric studies in patients have shown sensorineural hearing loss, especially of a high tone type, to be a frequent and sometimes serious complication of chronic otitis media. Presence or absence of cholesteatoma does not appear to relate significantly to the development of sensorineural hearing loss, whereas duration and activity of disease does.

Patients and temporal bones are described with gross suppurative tympanogenic labyrinthitis resulting from invasion of otitis media through the round window. Cochlear function is lost, vestibular function is preserved, thus illustrating the existence of localized labyrinthitis.

Preliminary very high frequency audiometric data in patients with acute otitis media indicates temporary as well as permanent threshold shifts occurring at the extreme end of the basal turn.

Based upon pathological studies of human and animal temporal bones, the following sequence of events (pathogenesis) leading to the development of sensorineural hearing loss (pathology) can be described. Acute or chronic otitis media appears to commonly result in the passage of toxins (enzymes) and infective elements (diapedesis of leukocytes) through the round window membrane leading to perilymphatic serous labyrinthitis localized to the basal turn (high frequency TTS) with the ultimate possibility of damage of sensory elements and spread apical-ward (high and eventually lower frequency PTS).

Clinicians dealing with patients with otitis media should keep this common complication in mind. The presence and growth of sensorineural hearing loss in patients with otitis media becomes an additional consideration for surgical intervention.

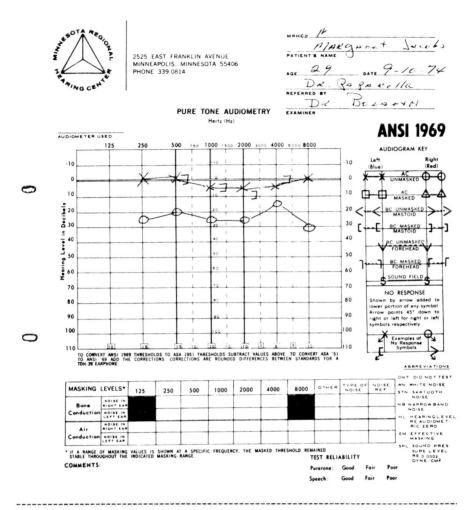

Fig. 187: Standard audiogram for patient M.S.

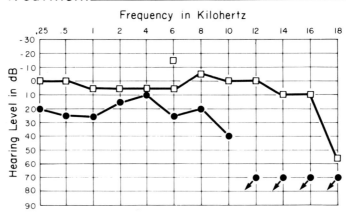

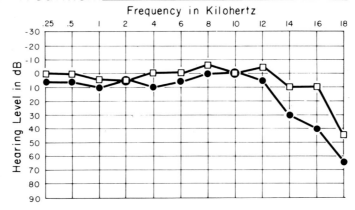

Fig. 188: Pretreatment (above) and post-treatment (below) high frequency audiogram showing loss and recovery.

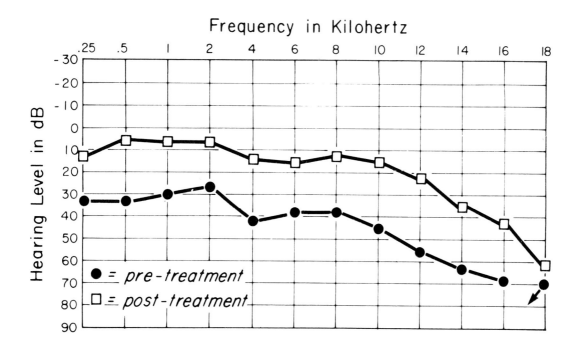

Fig. 189: Self-explanatory.

References

1. Bluvshtein, G. M.: Audiologicheskaia kharakteristika khronicheskikh gnoinykh srednikh otitov. *Vestn. Otorinolaring*, 25:64, 1963.
2. Dean, L. W. and Wolff, D.: Pathology and routes of infection in labyrinthitis secondary to middle ear otitis. *Ann. Otol.*, 43: 702, 1934.
3. Donaldson, J. A.: Fossula of the cochlear fenestra. *Arch. Otolaryng.*, 88:124, 1968.
4. Gardenghi, G.: Contributo allo studio della funzione cocleare nell'otite media purulenta cronica. *Bull. Mal. Orecch.*, 73:587, 1955.
5. Hulka, J. H.: Bone conduction changes in acute otitis media. *Arch. Otolaryng.*, 33:333, 1941.
6. Kawabata, I. and Paparella, M. M.: Fine structure of the round window membrane. *Ann. Otol.*, 80:13, 1971.
7. Paparella, M. M.; Brady, D. R.; and Hoel, R.: Sensori-neural hearing loss in chronic otitis media and mastoiditis. *Trans. Amer. Acad. Ophthal. Otolaryng.*, 74:108, 1970.
8. Paparella, M. M.; Oda, M.; Hiraide, F.; and Brady, D.: Pathology of sensorineural hearing loss in otitis media. *Ann. Otol.*, 81:632, 1972.
9. Thorburn, I. B.: Chronic disease of the middle ear cleft. In Scott-Brown, W. B.; Ballantyne, J.; and Groves, J.: *Diseases of the Ear, Nose and Throat.* (Ed. 2) Butterworths, Inc., Washington, D.C., 1965.
10. Verhoeven, L.: The examination of the ear in chronic otitis media. *J. Laryng.*, 75:962, 1961.

NERVE DEAFNESS RELATED TO CHOLESTEATOMA

John R. Lindsay, M.D.

This presentation is concerned only with nerve deafness associated with cholesteatoma in the middle ear spaces and connected with the external canal. Primary cholesteatoma which has not invaded middle ear spaces may produce sensorineural or nerve deafness by direct erosion of the labyrinthine capsule and invasion of the inner ear or by compression of nerves in the inner meatus.

Cholesteatoma in middle ear spaces may erode the bony capsule of the inner ear. This may occur in situations where desquamation is active and desquamated cells and debris are retained in the cholesteatoma cavity. The vestibular area is usually the site where erosion of the capsule occurs. A fistula symptom may develop with or without evidence of sensorineural impairment. Adequate surgical exenteration of the cholesteatoma cavity and exteriorization of the area may prevent further neural impairment due to the presence of the fistula.

Most instances of sensorineural impairment of hearing or of profound deafness associated with middle ear cholesteatoma can be attributed to the inflammatory, infectious, granulomatous or suppurative processes with which it is associated.

The possible role that viral disease may play in the development of attic cholesteatoma or of nerve deafness of tympanogenic origin usually is not clear.

Inflammation or bacterial infection associated with middle ear cholesteatoma may invade the inner ear by several routes.

The common routes have been: (1) by erosion of the labyrinthine capsule by cholesteatoma, usually the vestibular part, creating a potential pathway for invasion by infection, or (2) by extension of the inflammatory process through the oval window or round window membrane.

Invasion of the inner ear through the oval window by infection has occurred in our experience only under certain predisposing conditions. These have included: (1) lowered resistance to infection due for example, to uncontrolled diabetes, (2) a congenital bony dehiscence in the stapidial footplate, sealed off only by mucosa and endosteal membrane, and (3) a late complication following stapes surgery.

An acute temporary labyrinthine irritation has been indicated in a few instances in the course of severe acute middle ear suppuration, also occasionally following stapedectomy, by the temporary complaint of severe hypersenitivity to loud high-pitched sounds.

Extension of an inflammatory process to the inner ear through the round window membrane has been demonstrated in several instances in our histopathological collection.

Case 1: A 79 year old female gave a history of scarlet fever in childhood followed by chronic bilateral discharge from the ears.

Many years later an operative procedure was done on the right ear through the external canal. The histopathological findings on the right ear include a completely fibrosed and ossified mastoid area, a dry cavity consisting of posterior epitympanum and part of the antrum, lined by squamous epithelium and communicating widely with the external canal (Fig. 190).

The middle ear space is sealed off from the attic and antrum region. With the retracted drum adherent to the remnant of the lenticular process and head of the stapes.

The partially eroded head of the malleus is still present in the scar tissue in the anterior part of the epitympanum.

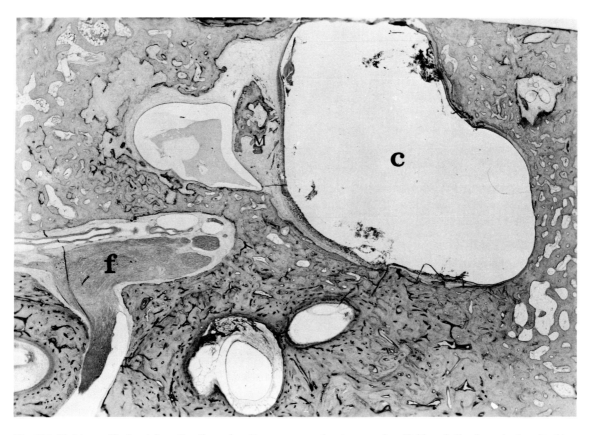

Fig. 190: Right ear. Horizontal section through epitympanum and antrum region. Epidermis lined surgical cavity (c). Remnant of head of malleus (m). Facial nerve (f). Sclerosed mastoid at right margin.

The hearing for low tones was at the 40 dB level by air conduction at age 75, falling off at the higher frequencies.

The left ear shows bony and fibrous sclerosis in the mastoid and epitympanic areas, particle absorption of both ossicles in the epitympanum, retracted and distorted tympanic membrane, with a dense fibrous adhesion to the promontory. The round window niche contains thickened fibrous mucosa which is continuous with a thickened round window membrane. Fibrosis and new bone are also present in the adjoining lower end of the scala tympani. Degeneration of sensory and neural components is marked in the lower end of the lower basal coil (Fig. 191).

The "labyrinthitis ossificans" is confined to the

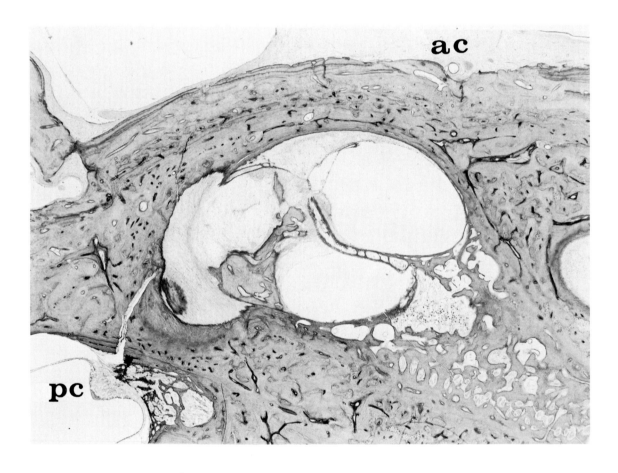

Fig. 191: Left ear. Horizontal section through round window and posterior canal regions. Localized fibrosis and new bone in the scala tympani at the round window. Fibrosis in the round window niche extends through the membrane into the scala tympani. Posterior canal (pc). Fibrous middle ear adhesion (ad).

area of the scala tympani adjoining the round window.

The audiogram showed the threshold for low tones to be depressed more than on the right, but to be similar in the 2000 to 4000 Hz. region (Fig. 192).

The operative procedure on the right ear apparently consisted of an "incudectomy", along with adequate exteriorization, a procedure sometimes used at that time. A localized extension of epidermis lining the cavity represents the final healing process.

The labyrinthitis ossificans in the left scala tympani represents an inflammatory reaction

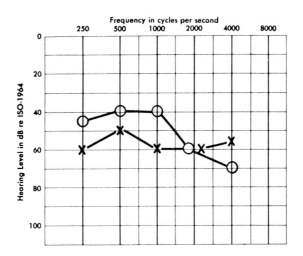

Fig. 192: Audiogram. Right ear (o). Left ear (x).

transmitted through the round window membrane probably without bacterial invasion.

Case 2: The bilateral chronic middle ear suppuration was of many years duration in this case. The middle ears are lined partly by stratified squamous or "cholesteatomatous" membrane and partly by polypoid infected mucosa. The round window membrane on one side is thickened by fibrosis which extends to almost fill the round window niche (Suga and Lindsay, 1975). Localized labyrinthitis ossificans fills the adjoining lower end of the scala tympani (Fig. 193).

In both of the above cases it appears that the localized labyrinthitis occurred during an active

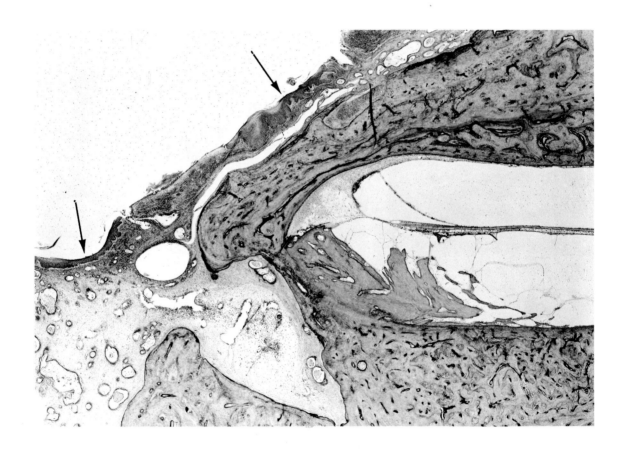

Fig. 193: Horizontal section through the round window niche. New bone and fibrous tissue occupy the scala tympani in the round window region. Fibrosis fills the round window niche. Epidermis (arrows) interspersed with polypoid mucosa lines the middle ear space.

stage of a suppurative process in the middle ear.

The pathway of extension of acute suppurative infection from middle ear spaces to the labyrinth has usually not been found to be through the windows. In the absence of antibiotic therapy the pattern of pneumatization in the deeper parts of the pyramid was frequently the key to extension of an undrained focus of suppuration to the meninges and the labyrinth.

Direct extension of an inflammatory process into the labyrinth through the round window has also been observed in disorders in which there has been a generalized depression of immunity.

Case 3: A case of Wegener's granulomatosis first recognized in early 1965, developed bilateral serous otitis media in June, 1965. Nerve deafness developed in left ear despite general improvement under therapy followed by gradual nerve deafness in right ear. Radical mastoidectomy on the left was performed after appearance of 7th nerve palsy (Hanotia, et al, 1969). In February, 1967, total deafness on both sides had developed. Death occurred two years later.

Examination of the temporal bones* shows a direct extension of fibrosis in the round window niche through a less dense but broadened round window membrane in the scala tympani. Labyrinthitis ossificans and fibrosis are scattered throughout the labyrinthine spaces on both sides (Figs. 194 and 195).

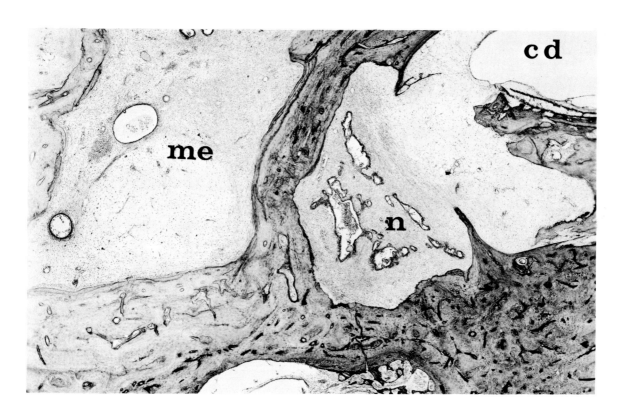

Fig. 194: Left ear. Section through the round window region. Diffuse fibrosis in middle ear (me), fills the round window niche (n), and extends through the membrane into the scala tympani. Fibrosis and new bone occupy the perilymphatic space. Dilated cochlear duct (cd).

---

*Temporal bones received from Dr. Maxine Bennett

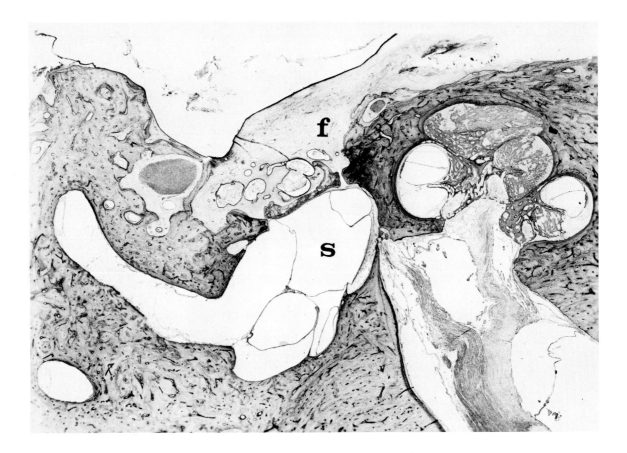

Fig. 195: Left ear. Horizontal section through stapes footplate and cochlea showing ossification in cochlea, dilated saccule (s), and cochlear duct. Fibrosis of middle ear mucosa (f).

In this instance the bilateral ear disease complicating the nasopharyngeal inflammation progressed despite apparent general improvement of the granulomatous process to invade both inner ears, through the round window membranes.

Case 4: A 48 year old female complained of trouble in her right ear and pains in various joints in July, 1971 (Suga and Lindsay, in press). Thick fluid drained from right ear after myringotomy. Joint symptoms and impaired hearing continued. In April 1972, bilateral myringotomy and insertion of tubes again allowed drainage of fluid. Conduction impairment of hearing was found on the left but on the right there was also moderate sensorineural high tone hearing impairment. Six months later the right ear was totally deaf. Her

rheumatoid arthritis increased and affected many joints. Rheumatoid lung disease, and several cranial nerve palsies developed. Despite general medical therapy, including an immuno-depressive agent, progression of her general disease resulted in death approximately two years after initial symptom had appeared.

The microscopic examination of the deafened ear showed diffuse fibrotic changes in the round window niche and the scala tympani, continuous with the round window membrane. There was new bone in the semicircular canals and basal coil of the cochlea, with diffuse fibrinoid changes in the perilymphatic system and marked endolymphatic hydrops (Figs. 196-200). There was no evidence of meningitis.

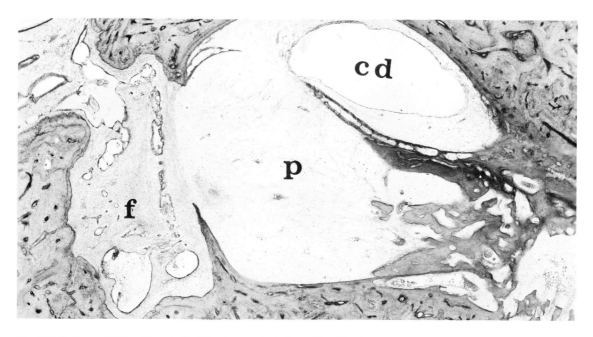

Fig. 196: Left ear. Diffuse fibrosis (f), fills the round window niche, blends with the round window membrane and fills the adjoining perilymphatic spaces (p). New bone has formed in scala tympani. Cochlear duct (cd) is dilated.

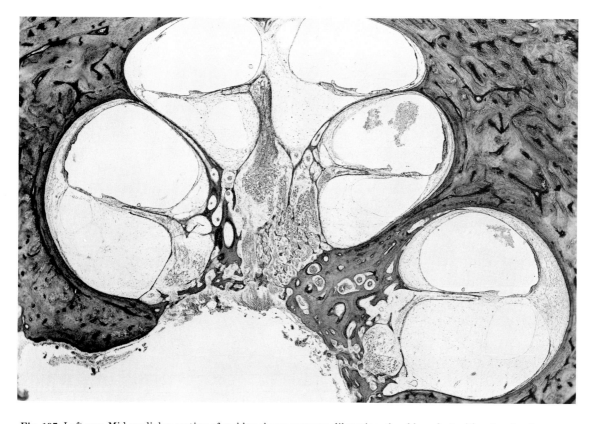

Fig. 197: Left ear. Mid-modiolar section of cochlea shows extreme dilatation of cochlear duct with extensive degeneration of tectorial membrane and organ of Corti. Loose fibrosis has extended to the apex in perilymphatic spaces. Ganglion cell degeneration is evident in upper basal and lower middle coils.

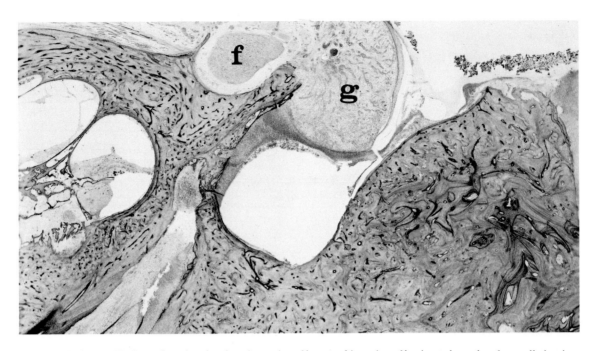

Fig. 198: Right ear. Horizontal section showing absorption of bone and invasion of horizontal canal and ampulla by cholesteatoma. Facial nerve (f). Granuloma (g). Covered by squamous epithelium lining the cholesteatoma cavity. Purulent exudate in cochlea and internal meatus.

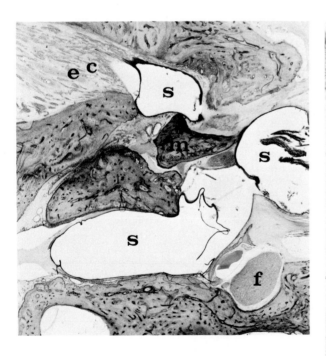

Fig. 199: Left ear. Horizontal section through the attic and upper edge of external canal wall (ec). An epidermis—lined dry sac (s) occupies most of epitympanic space, with a broad opening into external canal through pars flaccida and upper part of pars tensa. Malleus (m). Incus (i). Facial nerve (f). Vestibule (v).

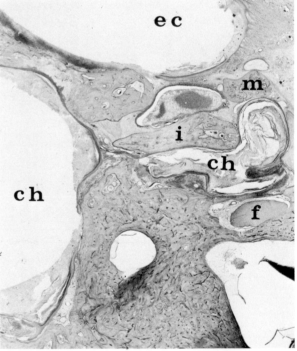

Fig. 200: Horizontal section through the upper part of external canal (ec). Cholesteatoma occupies the epitympanum and mastoid areas (ch). Incus (i). Malleus (m). Facial nerve (f).

The case illustrates the extension of a mild type of inflammatory process through the round window, causing a diffuse labyrinthitis in the presence of a progressive systemic fatal disease and immuno-depression.

Case 5: A 24 year old man developed a common complication of untreated cholesteatoma in his right middle ear. The illustration shows extensive erosion of bone and invasion of the horizontal canal. The extent of absorption of bone and the large granuloma indicates that diffuse labyrinthitis had been present for some time before the fatal diffuse meningitis occurred.

The left ear shows a dry epidermis-lined sac in the epitympanic space, an extension from the external canal through the pars flaccida and the upper margin of the pars tensa. The presence of a large opening to the external canal had apparently permitted extrusion of any moisture of desquamated debris. The middle ear was sealed off from the epitympanum and filled with fluid, stained pink with eosin, due to tubal blockage, possibly terminal.

Case 6: The cholesteatoma in this patient invaded the horizontal canal and destroyed the inner ear. At a later stage the cholesteatoma invaded the cerebellum with a fatal result (Suga and Lindsay, in press).

Case 7: A 26 year old male developed an attic cholesteatoma which has replaced the mastoid cell system and invaded the middle cranial fossa from the attic and mastoid without destroying the labyrinthine capsule or the membrana propria.

Pulmonary abscesses were the main fatal complication.

Discussion

Nerve deafness associated with middle ear cholesteatoma has usually been a complication of the associated inflammatory reaction, due to bacterial infection.

The formation of a cholesteatomatous fistula in the labyrinthine capsule is usually accompanied by some degree of inflammatory reaction.

The reaction apparently induces changes in the perilymph which tend to become diffuse and to affect sensory and neural components. The process may occur without actual invasion of the labyrinthine spaces by the bacterial agent.

Evidence that a somewhat similar process of transmission by the perilymph is involved in the production of nerve deafness in advanced Paget's disease and in osteitis fibrosa has recently been reported (Lindsay and Suga, 1976 and Lindsay and Suga, in press).

The normal stapes footplate and annular ligament appear to be highly resistant to invasion of the labyrinth by infection or inflammation. Invasion has been observed in the presence of lowered general resistance due to untreated diabetes, also in cases of congenital defect of the bony footplate and also as a late complication following stapes surgery.

The round window membrane has shown decreased resistance to extension of infection, resulting in diffuse labyrinthitis in the presence of general immuno-depression.

A localized labyrinthitis ossificans has been presented in two instances, in the round window region. This was found in cases with a history of chronic suppuration since childhood, but apparently has been an unusual complication.

The fatal complications of middle ear cholesteatoma have in our experience occurred more frequently by direct invasion of either the meninges, the temporal lobe, the cerebellum or the blood stream, than by an extension by way of the labyrinthine spaces to the meninges.

References

1. Hanotia, P.; Peters, H.; Bennett, M.; and Brown, R.: Chelation therapy in Wegener's granulomatosis treated with EDTA. *Ann. Otol. Rhin. Otol.*, 78:388, 1969.

2. Lindsay, J. R. and Suga, F.: Sensorineural deafness due to osteitis fibrosa. *Arch. Otol.*, 102:37, 1976.

3. Lindsay, J. R. and Suga, F.: Paget's disease and sensorineural deafness. *Laryngoscope*, (in press).

4. Suga, F. and Lindsay, J. R.: Labyrinthitis ossificans due to chronic otitis media. *Ann. Otol.*, 84:37,1975.

5. Suga, F. and Lindsay, J. R.: Labyrinthitis ossificans. *Ann. Otol. Rhin. Laryng.*, (in press).

ANALYSIS OF ONE HUNDRED CASES OF FISTULAS OF THE EXTERNAL SEMI-CIRCULAR CANAL

M. R. Wayoff, M.D.
J. M. Friot, M.D.

From the years 1966 to 1975, we observed 100 cases of fistulas of the horizontal semi-circular canal due to cholesteatomatous mastoiditis. There was no significant sexual or right-or-left incidence. The opposite ear was abnormal in 70%.

The otoscopic findings (Table 105) show chiefly pars flaccida perforation (32%) or total eardrum defects (40%). It is significant that a postoperative mastoid cavity was present in 12%.

TABLE 105

Otoscopic Findings

Intact eardrum	1%
Pars flaccida defect	32%
Pars flaccida plus post-sup. defect	9%
Post-sup. defect only	6%
Total eardrum defect	40%
Postoperative cavity	12%

During the operation, size and location of the fistulas were noted. The fistula was 2 mm or greater in length in 65%. There were seven ears with "prefistulas" manifested as a blue line. The fistula was located on the dome of the canal in 50, posteriorly placed in 26, and anteriorly placed in eight. The full length of the canal was open in 16 ears. The ossicular chain was always interrupted, and the other associated lesions are seen in Table 106.

The clinical history of these patients extended over a long period of time, even ten to twenty years.

TABLE 106

Associated Lesion

Fallopian canal open	25
Canal open with facial palsy	8
Dura denuded	22
Lateral sinus exposed	3
Carotid artery exposed	1

A positive fistula test was present in only 40%, associated with a history of dizziness. The vertigo can be present without nystagmus (40%). Often the fistula is an intraoperative discovery and X-ray studies and tomographs can be misleading.

The auditory function is surveyed in Figure 201. The shift to the left of the air conduction envelopes demonstrate an average improvement of 14 dB in the group as a whole.

Figure 202 shows the postoperative results in 63 cases supervised over a period of more than two years. The matrix was always removed even in the radical technique. We consider that preservation of the matrix provides only short-term safety, ultimately indicated only on an only-hearing ear. It is incorrect to compare the fistula ear with a fenestrated ear as their futures will be different. In 12 ears, the fistula appeared in old mastoid cavities, most of them being quiescent. Undoubtedly, the removal of the matrix represents a risk to the cochlea, but it is a calculated risk. Statistically, the values of the bone conduction do sustain our opinion.

In this paper, we have not considered the details of the surgical procedure. Usually, the extent of the cholesteatoma and associated disease

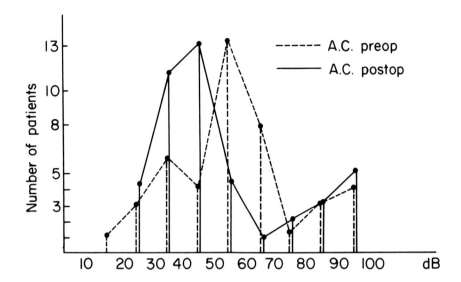

Fig. 201: Fistulae of the external S.C. canal preop and postop audiograms.

		Radical Technique	Open Cavity with Fascia ± Type III	Closed Technique	Total
A.C.	↑	3	20	0	23
	=	7	12	1	20
	↓	12	7	1	20
B.C.	↑	1	2	0	3
	=	9	31	2	42
	↓	12	6	0	18
Total		22	39	2	63

Fig. 202: Comparing results and techniques.

necessitated an open cavity technique with fascia graft and Type III columellar reconstruction. In some ears, the closed technique was possible, but was always done as a two-staged procedure.

At the present time, the labryinthine fistula is the more frequent complication of cholesteatoma (11% incidence in our total series 1966-1975). Nearly all were located on the external semicircular canal. The surgical treatment has been discussed by many authors. It is our opinion that the matrix must be removed routinely with subsequent covering with a fascial graft to control this condition.

QUESTIONS AND ANSWERS

Dr. Harker: Well, you've heard very lucid, clear presentations on the complications of cholesteatoma and we do have some time for questions.

Voice: I asked Dr. Ritter if there is a percentage figure on the number of his cases which were reoperations or were these all primary cases?

Dr. Ritter: These were all primary cases in the Michigan series, but this was not stipulated in the Massachusetts series. However, I would suspect that 98% of these were primary also. No revisions.

Dr. Bellucci: Dr. Ritter, you said the condition is ultimately congenital. Now, congenital what? Congenital cholesteatoma?

Dr. Ritter: The question as to the origin of cholesteatoma is certainly one that's been kicked around for centuries, and I don't claim to have the answer here. The literature contains little reference to the etiology frequently being a congenital one. The stress is primarily on other causes. Our statistics show that the disease does not vary. Furthermore, it occurs in the very young. With the knowledge that youngsters' ears are difficult to evaluate, I strongly submit the proposition that many or most cholesteatomas are congenital embryonic rests and they start their discharge early in life and they begin at that time.

Dr. Harker: Dr. Sheehy, have you further comments?

Dr. Sheehy: I would point out that preoperative facial paralysis (1.1%) occurred more commonly in dry ears and more commonly in posterosuperior marginal perforations.

It is of interest that the intra-operative paralysis case and all postoperative paralyses occurred in intact canal wall cases. There were 902 intact canal wall cases. There was one operative facial paralysis, and one facial nerve cut in 902 patients. The five temporary mild ones were indeed so mild that if you hadn't looked carefully you wouldn't have noticed it.

The postoperative paralyses, all delayed, were small in number but they likewise occurred in the 902 intact canal walls. Whether that's significant or not I don't know because there weren't that many cases.

Dr. Katz: Dr. Sheehy, concerning your conductive hearing loss complications, how do you handle a dry myringostapediopexy that appears to be eroding the incus?

Dr. Sheehy: There is active disease?

Dr. Katz: There is no drainage. The tympanic membrane is just lying on the incus.

Dr. Sheehy: And the hearing is good?

Dr. Katz: Perfect.

Dr. Sheehy: I don't do a thing to it. Despite what one might think, most of us in the Otologic Medical Group are conservative, and do not operate on ears unless there is a reasonably clear cut indication that surgery either is indicated now or is certainly going to be and that you'd better operate in order to prevent a problem which you're certain is going to develop.

Dr. Baron: May I take issue with Dr. Ritter on his assumption that the cholesteatomas in children are congenital. With no proof to the contrary, I refer to a patient in whom I inserted tubes for a bilateral serous otitis media. One became purulent and the other did not. The purulent ear developed a cholesteatoma. I think cholesteatoma develops in children rather rapidly. It doesn't have to be congenital and I think that one must assume that the purulent otitis media in children is a much more vicious disease and can lead to cholesteatoma.

Dr. Ritter: Before the thought on congenital cholesteatoma becomes much larger than it is, let me say both Dr. Holmes and I merely thought from our series that more stress should be placed on the concept that it may be a congenital disease and more often appreciated as such than the literature would lead us to believe. Neither of us offer it as the sole cause of a cholesteatoma. As far as the congenital theory having some merit in fact, it was in 1928 when Dr. Teed from the University of Iowa described histopathologically in an iced temporal bone section a congenital cholesteatoma from an infant. That was almost fifty years ago.

Dr. Ruben: Dr. Ritter, you made a most interesting analysis; however, there are some pitfalls in that you really don't know the population area that was being drained and whether or not the cases were being referred to Dr. Holmes.

Secondly, and Dr. Hinchcliffe can help me out here, there was a paper published from the Northern Health District in Glasgow in which they looked at the incidence before and after the use of the ventilating tube. My memory is a little bit hazy but I think there was a decided decrease in the number of mastoidectomies that were done in the same kinetic and same socioeconomic class population. Whether or not this article specified a decrease in cholesteatoma, I do not know.

A third point is that in our experience, which is essentially in urban ghetto situations, the incidence of complications from cholesteatoma is much higher. Again we're working with really the lowest of the lowest class and the least tended medically.

Dr. Harker: Dr. Hinchcliffe, have you any comments?

Dr. Hinchcliffe: No, I don't remember that paper. Certainly there are great problems in trying to assess how things were in the preantibiotic era compared with the antibiotic era. Clearly Dr. Ritter is limited by the data available to him, and he's performed an excellent service. Epidemiologists can become very critical and say well you should perhaps try to find some population in the world which antibiotics have not reached, do your survey and see what happens after the introduction of antibiotics, especially if you do something like an incidence study.

Dr. Sheehy: I would like to comment on one thing Dr. Ruben mentioned. Our lack of preoperative CNS complications is not I suspect due to the socioeconomic aspect. It is due to the fact that in

Los Angeles County all patients who develop a meningitis that is not clear-cut as to the exact cause have to go to one specific hospital. Therefore, if you look in our residency training program, you find a much higher incidence than you would expect. The only one we recognized preoperatively was a patient who walked into the office with a low grade meningitis. He later got a brain abscess after I'd done a modified radical. The other two were diagnosed only at surgery as chronic epidural abscesses. They were essentially asymptomatic.

Dr. Harker: We have one more comment. Dr. Sadé?

Dr. Sadé: Dr. Ritter is to be complimented on his study. It is valuable and it supplies us with data and we will have to look at it in print to get its entire value. But, the surprising thing is that the occurrence of cholesteatoma seems to be the same today as in the pre-antibiotic era. This striking finding may lead us to some conclusion.

One paramater which has not been mentioned is the difference between chronic ears and acute ears with cholesteatoma. In the analysis of the 124 cases which I presented yesterday, there is a tremendous difference between those which presented with acute mastoiditis and those with chronic mastoiditis.

Dr. Sheehy: Could I make a comment? In 6% of our series we recorded acute exacerbation of chronic disease if they had a primary complaint of pain or if they had an acute complication. Pain meant either an empyema in the mastoid or a subacute mastoiditis in a cellular mastoid filled with cholesterol granuloma that had been blocked by cholesteatoma. Six percent of our patients fell into that category. Some had a facial paralysis, some had a fistula, but the majority did not.

Dr. Harker: Are there any questions for Dr. Lindsay or Dr. Paparella?

Voice: Very briefly, it would be difficult to do justice to these wonderful demonstrations of Dr. Lindsay, from whom we have so much to learn, even today. Do you think that the newborn formation in the labyrinth is a sort of localized process? I have been struck by the point Dr. Paparella has made about the localized labyrinth hiatus, which I have also referred to in our animal experiment. In other words, is the new bone formation just limited in your cases to the labyrinth or have you found any osteogenesis also in other parts of those tempral bones?

Dr. Lindsay: I will try to answer your question, but I'm not sure I can. In the chronic cases in whom we found a labyrinthitis it was a localized process. In those ears the effects of the chronic otitis were very evident.

Dr. Webster: In the light of the very interesting study of the effects of chronic inflammation causing hearing loss, I would like to ask Dr. Paparella if he has any evidence of the potentially ototoxic topical medications that we put into the middle ear having any curative effect? It would appear in your studies with high frequency audiometry that might be an ideal situation where you could treat some patients with antibiotics topically and other patients with only systemic antibiotics and see if there is any difference in the hearing in the two groups.

Dr. Paparella: Mainly the acute otitis media study provides us a model wherein there is no possibility of ototoxic drug effect, because the patients just didn't have it. There is a high frequency cochlear loss which is sometimes temporary and sometimes permanent. As I mentioned briefly, we didn't dwell on it, but we did try very diligently—in looking at the original 500 patients studied audiometrically—to exclude all with any suspicion of ototoxic drug effect, local or systemic. Those are the only two things we've done. But still there's a question as to whether drugs indeed do cause a cochlear loss and I think in some instances they might well have. That needs to be studied.

Dr. Austin: If one measures bone conduction preoperatively and then compares these scores postoperatively after reconstruction of the ossicular chain when broken you will find a consistent average 11.5 dB pseudohypacusis for bone conduction over the speech range. I've read Dr. Paparella's papers and this value is very close to

the values that he first reported, but ascribed to inflammatory depression of hearing. I wondered if he has measured the change in bone conduction with loss of ossicular continuity?

Dr. Paparella: We do, of course, try carefully to get postoperative audiograms and we have not seen that the pre-versus the postoperative bone conduction thresholds vary. I might say that we have better luck with our audiologists in getting consistency with our bone conduction measurements pre- and postoperative much more so than we do in our otosclerotic patients. So, I think we're looking at, at least from an audiometric point of view, a valid result. Also, when we look at those graphs, we're looking at average data. Now this means that many patients of course have no observable bone conduction threshold shifts with routine audiometry. What I think we're indicating here is that they probably have a great deal going on in the basal turn. As you know, if you look at the basal turn this represents a substantial part of the entire cochlear partition. So there is an awful lot that can go on there before it reaches a place where it might be measured audiometrically. But those that show cochlear losses are genuine losses.

Dr. Smyth: Dr. Glasscock, I was reassured to find that your experience was the same as mine in terms of epithelial pearls in the mastoidectomy cavity having virtually not been a problem. I hope that this will be encouraging for those that feel that maybe the Palva operation has something to offer for them. You drew attention to one matter that has really escaped attention so far, rather surprisingly, and that is what happens to the cochlea in these operations for cholesteatoma. I was I'll say envious of your very small incidence of cochlear problems in this intact canal wall tympanoplasty. You also referred to your treatment of fistula, which brings us to this most difficult management problem: what do we do with the fistula in the cholesteatomatous ear? I gather that you do not advocate a one stage removal of matrix from the lateral semicircular canal fistula. Is that correct?

Dr. Glasscock: I'm afraid to exteriorize an ear

like that and leave the cholesteatoma matrix because I think that the chances of chronic infection over the fistula would make the fistula larger and the hearing may, over a period of time, deteriorate. I would prefer to leave the cholesteatoma, stage it, and go back and remove the matrix off the fistula. I personally don't like to take cholesteatoma off a fistula at the primary stage because to me it would be very similar to removing the stapes and opening the perilymphatic space. We'd never take out a stapes in an ear that has a perforation so it just seems logical not to open up the perilymph in a chronic ear.

Chapter 10

Applications

IS CHOLESTEATOMA TO BE REGARDED AS A PROBLEM REQUIRING RELATIVELY URGENT SURGERY?

Panel One: Moderator: Charles J. Krause, M.D.
Panelists: S. Baron, M.D.; J. V. D. Hough, M.D.; C. M. Kos, M.D.; G. Nager, M.D.; and D. Plester, M.D.

Dr. Krause: It's with a great deal of pleasure that I chair this distinguished panel. The general format will be one of discussing some general questions first that have been circulated and then we'll take questions from the floor, directed to our panel members. First of all, panel, do you operate on every ear that you see in which you identify a cholesteatoma? Dr. Kos?

Dr. Kos: When I first read this question, I almost reverted to my younger days as a student in suspecting that there was a trap in it somewhere. But, after giving it further thought, I've come to the conclusion that the answer should be no.

Dr. Krause: How about the other panel members? Do you operate on every ear that you see in which there is a cholesteatoma? Dr. Baron?

Dr. Baron: No.

Dr. Krause: Any others with the same opinion?

Dr. Hough: I will say no, also. Do you want us to?

Dr. Krause: We'll get a little more specific in a moment.

Dr. Plester: My experience also leads me to say no.

Dr. Krause: Everyone says no. So there are some ears in which a cholesteatoma is identified in which surgery is not indicated. Now, I am interested in knowing the panelists' opinion as to what size indicates that the ear is safe and does not require surgery and conversely what size indicates danger and requires surgery. Dr. Hough?

Dr. Hough: There are a number of factors to consider. You look at the patient in general.

Their age makes some difference in your decision as to whether to operate and indeed whether or not this is a safe procedure. In the older age group, you would be less anxious to proceed rapidly with a big operation—depending upon the physical condition of the patient. Systemic diseases may accompany the cholesteatoma. I think the attitude of the patient toward you and toward the operation makes a great deal of difference.

If the ear has a cholesteatoma with a wide mouth that is dry and has a history of very little recurrent infection, that cleanses itself well and without history compatible with impending complications, all of these factors lead one to consider leaving the ear alone. Another factor is the x-ray appearance. If it is a pneumatized temporal bone, as Dr. Lindsay has pointed out, the danger is greater. All of these things should be taken into consideration.

Dr. Krause: Dr. Plester?

Dr. Plester: There is hardly anything to add to what Dr. Hough has said, and we have to consider hearing as well. If a patient's only hearing ear would have a cholesteatoma, I would certainly be much more conservative. Also, if one ear has normal hearing and the other ear has cholesteatoma in a dry ear and a profound hearing loss and I don't believe I can improve hearing in this ear to near normal, I would also be conservative. Another consideration is a fistula in the only hearing ear. If the ear is dry and doesn't give much trouble, I would leave it alone, carefully observing the patient regularly.

Dr. Krause: Dr. Baron?

Dr. Baron: I agree with Dr. Hough. You have to consider the age of the patient. I would not include children in this group. I would operate on a child virtually every time. I would like to call your attention to a paper that was written by Kenneth Day. I referred to it yesterday because in those days when you had a cholesteatoma, the rule was that you were going to do a radical. He was concerned about destroying the hearing, as I was. He wrote an article describing 50 successive patients. On 37 he was able to, by irrigating the attic with alcohol or ether a couple of times a week, render 31 dry. There were six failures, three of which were in children. For the other seven cases, read the article. So it is possible in a cholesteatoma with a large attic opening to safely treat them without surgery.

Dr. Krause: From what we've heard here this week, maybe vitamin A needs to be added to that regimen. Dr. Kos?

Dr. Kos: It would seem facetious to say that the absence of signs and symptoms constitued a safe ear when we're talking about cholesteatoma. Often the definition of a safe ear with cholesteatoma is dependent on retrospection. There are some conditions, while it may not be considered a dangerous ear such as a retraction pocket into the sinus tympani with granulation tissue, that I believe should require early surgery in order to have any reasonable chance of stopping progression of the disease. At the same time, in those instances one should be much aware of the possibility of a mastoid cholesteatoma peeking through the retrofacial tracts to the sinus tympani. Attic perforations, as has been stated, are treacherous and have a potential for much more threat than one usually observes. But, if attic erosion has created a natural atticotomy where the sac or the retraction pocket is adequately visualized and instrumentally accessible, it could be considered a safe ear. There are varying degrees, of course.

Dr. Krause: Dr. Nager, do you have any comments?

Dr. Nager: I certainly agree with all the panelists. I think the important information falls perhaps in four or five categories. First, the patient's history. The absence of drainage over a long period of time is something to consider. Second, the absence of sudden cessation of secretion which may be an alarming symptom indicating retention. Third, the presence of symptoms suggesting involvement of the membranous labyrinth. Fourth, the otoscopic examination. A lot depends on the size and location of the perforation. Last, the roentgenology evaluation may give one fairly good information on the extent of the cholesteatoma within the temporal bone and its relationship to nearby structures.

Dr. Hough: In case we leave the impression that cholesteatoma is not a surgical disease, it certainly is in my mind a definite surgical disease. We are talking about the rare instance when there is no surgical indication.

Dr. Krause: Can you give any sort of indication of the percentage of patients that you see with cholesteatoma that you treat conservatively?

Dr. Hough: I'd say in the neighborhood of 10%.

Dr. Plester: I think about 5%.

Dr. Baron: I'd say that currently I have three patients under observation. One is a man now 83 whom I've been treating for 15 years. He had a wide mouth attic perforation but he is also physically unfit. He had pulmonary tuberculosis. He has progressed to blindness, but is very faithful in coming in once every six to eight weeks to have this cleaned. I think this is important. If you are going to treat a patient without surgery, he must be a reliable patient for follow-up; if he is not going to be a good patient for follow-up, then you should consider surgery.

Dr. Krause: Excellent point. Now, we hear otologists talk about an impending complication. What indicators do you gentlemen use to view that an impending complication is present? Dr. Baron?

Dr. Baron: Well, we have the usual physical signs of intracranial disease such as meningeal signs or high fever or pain or dizziness or excess discharge, very odorous.

Dr. Hough: An acute or sudden change in the picture of the course of a disease is the most important indicator. This patient was doing well yesterday and today "this" symptom has been added.

Dr. Plester: I think also that these sudden changes are most important. In addition, beginning facial palsy might be very important.

Dr. Kos: I regard impending complications referred to here as insiduous symptoms which announce that a complication has already begun to develop. False alarms such as thermal stimulation from ear drops or irrigation must be excluded. Other false alarms are referred otalgia and disease processes in other parts of the body, such as cervical arthritis, sinusitis, occipital tension, whether occupational or stress, and temporomandibular joint syndromes. I don't think that everyone should jump into a surgical procedure because he's made up his mind from some of these false alarms that this is an impending complication.

There are other considerations such as facial numbness which can point to a facial paresis. Episodes of mental confusion may be precursors to meningitis, as can retro-orbital pain and rapidly increasing sepsis. As a resident many years ago with wards holding 50 to 60 otologic patients with varying stages of complications I was taught and soon realized that walking up and down the ward and speaking to each of the patients gave me some of the earliest hints of potential complications. If there was an uncharacteristic euphoria I watched that patient very carefully, and many times they went on to develop meningitis. Similarly, if there was a change in personality and drowsiness, that often meant to me the possibility of a complication, and many of them did develop them. So, my concept of an impending complication are these precursor symptoms which may or may not be indicative of a complication developing.

Dr. Krause: Dr. Nager?

Dr. Nager: Again I'm in agreement with all the panelists. If we look at the patient's history and he presents the first time to your office with a history of continuous rather profuse, purulent, malodorous discharge indicating osteitis and he mentions that there has been a sudden arrest of discharge, I would become very concerned about retention and possibly break-through in an undesirable direction. Finally, the otologic examination reveals the site, location and size of the perforation. A large perforation is generally less likely to produce serious complications.

Dr. Baron: May I mention the obvious fact that if the patient under observation shows by x-ray that there has been ·ı increase in the size of the cholesteatoma, surgery is indicated.

Dr. Krause: In this morning's discussion, we've assumed that our surgery improves these patients, but would the panel state what evidence we really have that the patients are improved. Are there certain patients we made worse by doing a surgical procedure? Dr. Plester?

Dr. Plester: In the so-called closed technique the ear is only safe if we had a second look after three to four years. Otherwise, a relatively safe ear is an ear with an open cavity which can be looked over easily.

Dr. Kos: This depends on the thoroughness of the initial surgery and the anatomical variations encountered. Generally, an adequately exteriorized ear properly cared for postoperatively might include taking a second or even a third look. More specifically, the patient should be followed frequently to control granulations or subsequently to re-operate a cavity that is ulcerating and draining. I find this most distracting in pneumatized mastoids where the cells of the petrous apex have been invaded, especially those contiguous with the solid angle. As long as there is exteriorization where pressures are not likely to build up, and invasion is curtailed or inhibited by keeping the cavity clean, I regard that as making the patient a lot safer than not operating on him.

Dr. Krause: Dr. Hough?

Dr. Hough: There are several factors here other than just making the operation safe for Life. We put a capital "L" on life and we're talking about abundant life as well. We're trying to save the patient's life and we're also trying to save function, so that life will be better. So, to achieve both of these is our goal. I don't believe that we can honestly say that there is any hard scientific epidemiological data that proves that an operated ear is more safe than a non-operated ear. We in this room have not debated about whether or not this is a surgical disease. That point we haven't really discussed much in this whole conference. I believe the real proof would be that if I had or you had a cholesteatoma and it was one of the types that we discussed, if we had a proper surgeon to do the operation, it would be carried out. I think we have here a group of scientists who have studied this problem more than any other in the world. This group would say our experience tells us very strongly that this is a surgical disease. We make these ears more safe by doing surgery and we have repeatedly seen patients who have not had surgery who had these terrible complications, such as intracranial complications, loss of hearing, etc., even death. The evidence is that there isn't any question as we speak to the world that this is a surgical disease.

Dr. Krause: Dr. Baron?

Dr. Baron: The "proof of the pudding" is in personal experience. Not a patient upon whom I've done surgery for cholesteatoma has ever developed a serious complication early or late. I think that in itself proves that the ear is then a safe ear as far as the patient's life is concerned.

Dr. Krause: How about the patient who has had canal-up mastoidectomy and subsequently develops acute otitis media? Is there a greater chance of that patient developing CNS infections than the one who's had the canal wall taken down?

Dr. Hough: I don't think there would be any question but that they'd have a greater chance because they have a closed cavity. If they have an open cavity there's no problem with drainage. But this would be true in a normal mastoid as well. I think they are probably a little more susceptible than a normal mastoid, but they were predisposed and more susceptible originally. So I don't know that you've made them any worse, but you may have carried a little of a burden following the surgery of a little more risk.

Dr. Plester: I think doing the canal wall technique we rather frequently might hurt the tegmen and expose the dura mainly if the antrum is rather small and therefore the danger might be increased, at least in relatively inexperienced hands.

Dr. Krause: One other question I have for the panel before we open it up to questions on the floor. There's been a tremendous amount of information presented here in the past few days, much of it very sophisticated experimental information and a great deal clinically oriented. Are there any concepts that you as individuals have found particularly interesting and that you might utilize in your own practice?

Dr. Kos: Yes. There have been many concepts described during this meeting and in much more detail than was available in past years. I couldn't help but be reminded of my own career and thinking that of the variations of concepts that were presented here by scientists of different durations of experience, wonder if they wouldn't after thirty years remember how many times they changed their mind during that interval. In general, I learned a great deal but the central theme has been a concept that I have not had to change my mind about over the years, although certainly applications and various satellite considerations have caused me to change a great deal.

Dr. Hough: We sometimes wonder. We realize of course that the disease is an enemy and the enemy is far from being conquered. We still really have not done anything about preparing this patient so that they do not have the disease. We've done nothing preventative. We have a few things that help to still the complications, but we have nothing to treat the disease itself to stop it. So, we control it in confines. It was interesting to me this morning to realize that we are fighting the same enemy and the enemy is just as strong as it ever was. When I heard Dr. Ritter's paper—the same disease was there four decades ago and it was there 400 years ago. The power of the enemy has not been stilled at all. We have some more tools to fight with, but that's it. It seems to me as I have heard the papers that we have accumulated a vast amount of knowledge that has stimulated all of us and will make us more observant in the future, but we've also come to many blind ends that indicate our total ignorance. There are many, many things that we need to have another conference on.

Dr. Baron: I was very impressed with Dr. Paparella's presentation this morning to show that there is actually involvement of the round window. Actually, I personally haven't thought much about it. I think the suggestion that was made that we pursue the studies further to see if topical application of medications are toxic to the inner ear would be very important to our knowledge.

Dr. Kos: One thing occurred to me. I wasn't able to attend all the meetings, though I was here for about 98% of them. I didn't hear any reference to the role of genetics in this condition of cholesteatoma except from Dr. Plester and I wonder if some of the questions we're asking might have solutions in the field of genetics.

Dr. Krause: Dr. Nager?

Dr. Nager: I certainly leave greatly impressed and again with great respect for the many several contributing factors that lead to the origin of cholesteatoma, genetics being certainly one factor that was very beautifully discussed by Dr. Plester. There is just no doubt about the genetic factor and its role in pneumatization in the architectural structure and pathophysiology of the eustachian tube. Also, in the remnants of embryonic collective tissue it was brought out that all are well known factors that play a part in the genesis of cholesteatoma.

Dr. Plester: I think one of the main results of this conference is certainly an enormous stimulus for further research. Not too many questions have been answered but very many new questions came out during this conference and I'm looking forward very much to the next one. I hope to get at least some answers.

Dr. Krause: Now, are there questions from the floor?

Dr. Sheehy: There were a couple of remarks made and generally agreed with by the panelists. Let me call attention to the fact that we have looked at all our complications in terms of aural discharge and type of perforation. Interestingly enough there was essentially no difference in the ears that had drained and that had not drained, with one exception. That was in the case of the facial nerve paralysis and admittedly there were only 11 cases out of a thousand. But they were twice as common in the posterior superior

marginal perforations as opposed to the attic perforation. They were also more common by about double in the ears that had not been draining. But as regards the fistula cases we could see absolutely no correlation, looking at it the way we did. We all draw conclusions from our clinical experiences which sometimes we cannot substantiate.

Dr. Delvillar: I was surprised that very few references are made in this conference to the x-ray findings, principally by polytomography. I don't know why, because we usually judge the behavior of cholesteatoma by polytomographic study. We deal with only small cholesteatoma in the attic, but not with the very big cholesteatomas that are usually not so termed because they are not real cysts. However, cholesteatosis can destroy all the bone which is well evidenced by polytomography. It is a surprise that a radiologist is not participating in this conference.

Dr. Krause: I'd be interested in knowing from the panel how important to you are x-ray findings relative to your assessment of the patient?

Dr. Kos: It's so routine and so much a part of the complete examination that I personally took it for granted that these studies were being made, both initially and even serially, if necessary. That is taken for granted and that is the reason I ignored it.

Dr. Plester: We certainly do the same in every patient with cholesteatoma, but mainly to get the anatomical structure of the ear and of course for medicolegal reasons. I think that radiography is not too reliable in determining the extent of the disease, at least not in the usual projections. I think polytomography might be done, but it is rare that we do it.

Dr. Hough: I would agree that I cannot evaluate extent of the disease particularly with x-ray but I too would have liked to have seen a little more emphasis on radiologic findings because this is how I determine my philosophy of what I'm going to do surgically to the ear. If I see a cholesteatoma that clinically appears to me to be essentially confined to the attic and has a sclerotid mastoid with a small antrum, I have no hesitation to go ahead and take down whatever canal wall I need to and remove the cholesteatoma, because we'll have a small bowl and this is a self-cleansing, easily handled bowl that's safe. It's academic whether or not we take down the canal wall. This constitutes a fairly large percentage of ears, incidentally. However, in a patient with a large pneumatized mastoid, I'm more reluctant to take that canal wall down because of the large cavity which will be present postoperatively. So, x-ray findings help us to decide upon our approach to the problem.

Dr. Krause: We have time for two more quick questions.

Dr. Abramson: I was struck by the fact that the panel in discussing this problem felt comfortable in waiting on cholesteatomas when the mouth of the sac was wide as compared to narrow. I think that we've heard enough about the nature of bone resorption in this conference to seriously question the fact that bone resorption occurs just by pressure and we know that bone resorption can occur in the absence of active suppuration that is seen from the outside. Now, I'd like to relate a detail in my own experience on the problem of wideness of the sac. The ultimate in wide sac is nature's modified radical and nature's atticotomy. During my residency I was following all the cholesteatomas that came for surgery at the Massachusetts Eye and Ear Infirmary. One of the senior otologists in Boston was a man with a very large practice who routinely treated these patients by aspiration of debris. In one year three patients who had dry ears and nature's modified radicals were admitted to that hospital for inner ear fistulas. The process that had destroyed the canal wall and the attic wall had eventually gone on to destroy the bone over the labyrinth.

Dr. Baron: I'd like to comment on that. The patients to whom I refer and whom I treat conservatively are carefully x-rayed. The cholesteatoma has not extended to perform nature's modified radical and that type of case I would not treat con-

servatively. It's the patient with a large attic opening and by x-ray a relatively small cholesteatoma—either by conventional or polytome x-rays—and I also mentioned once before this patient is to be followed very carefully. In no case where the cholesteatoma is large, as you've stated in the modified radical, would I hesitate to operate.

Dr. Hough: I think this demonstrates how easily it is to be misunderstood and how we can leave wrong impressions. We were talking about a host of factors, including age groups, etc., but you take a patient who is 75 years old and has a small retraction in the attic that you can see the edges of with a wide mouth that you can cleanse easily, this is what we were speaking of.

Dr. Plester: Yes, I think I also would like to mention that in 100% of children or young people I would certainly go on to do surgery but at least 5% in the age group over 60 I was speaking of were going to be treated conservatively.

Dr. Benda: Dr. Day's successor told me that for the first few years after he inherited Dr. Day's practice, it was necessary for him to operate on many of the patients that had been managed medically.

Dr. Bellucci: We have concluded more or less that congenital cholesteatoma is fairly rare. Therefore, what we're dealing with is acquired cholesteatoma. Now how do we acquire this cholesteatoma? Seems to me it is the complication of a middle ear infection. Something has perforated the drum and then it begins to develop a cholesteatoma. I think what we have to do is concentrate a little bit more on now how to get this out of the ear once it's started but concentrate our research and our efforts on what causes middle ear infection in the first place and how to control the problem to eliminate the process. I feel that the eustachian tube function is the problem here. I feel we have to concentrate every effort to solve it.

PROBLEM: WHAT ARE THE PRINCIPLES GOVERNING CHOLESTEATOMA SURGERY

Panel Two: Moderator: George E. Shambaugh, Jr., M.D.
Panelists: V. Goodhill, M.D.; H. Schuknecht, M.D.; D. Austin, M.D.; G. Smyth, M.D.; and T. Palva, M.D.

Dr. Shambaugh: The task before me is formidable—to condense into fifteen minutes the meat of this conference. Fortunately, Dr. McCabe asked me to moderate this last panel and that gives me a chance to spend more time and at the same time to get a playback from these authorities on the comments that I will make. If they disagree with me, so much the better.

First of all, terminology. The name cholesteatoma is still, I think, the best for this non-neoplastic tumor of desquamating epithelium that destroys hearing and can destroy life. During this meeting bone necrosis was rather loosely confused with bone destruction or resorption. There is a great and crystal-clear difference. Necrotic bone is dead bone, a sequestrum. Cholesteatoma does not kill bone, it causes bone resorption by enzyme action, osteoclasts, and histiocytes, induced by various factors, the most important being infection with inflammation and granulation tissue. I think that this was brought out very beautifully the first two days of this conference. The bone is resorbed by cellular action as a result of an infected cholesteatoma, but it is not bone necrosis. The infection is in the desquamated debris of the cholesteatoma, where organisms can thrive free from the antibodies and leukocytes brought by the blood circulation. In other words, infection elsewhere in the middle ear without cholesteatoma can be combated by the normal process of the immune reaction brought by the blood. But cholesteatoma is different. Remove the debris and granulation tissue and the infection and inflammation subside. The bone resorption ceases and bone deposition takes its place. Now, we all must remember that bone remodeling is a constant process that goes on from the time we're born until we die and that in

the presence of infection bone resorption outpaces bone deposition. As infection subsides the process changes and bone deposition takes its place and this is why we see sclerosis in these chronic ears eventually rather than bone destruction.

I would like a comment from the panel on what I've just said about bone necrosis and bone resorption in cholesteatomas. Do you agree that we ought not to use the term bone necrosis in these cases?

Dr. Jansen: Dr. Shambaugh, I'm not quite sure what I should say. I'm not quite sure which expression, bone necrosis or bone resorption.

Dr. Palva: I think that necrotic bone is entirely different than resorbed bone. The point you made is right. In the cholesteatoma we have living bone that is being absorbed or in the process of being absorbed.

Dr. Smyth: I really don't think, Dr. Shambaugh, that I have anything to add to what Dr. Palva has said.

Dr. Austin: I'm afraid I'll have to plead ignorance of the ultimate process. I know we have many processes involved. Infection causes osteitis and resorption and I'm sure we've seen that there is an active osteolytic enzymatic process involved as well.

Dr. Baron: The words "osteomyelitis of the temporal bone" is bandied about. Yet, osteomyelitis is infection of the bone marrow and the only marrow in the mastoid bone is probably in the tip; I'm not sure about the ossicles. We should use the term "osteitis" rather than "osteomyelitis".

Dr. Shambaugh: I would certainly agree with that. Marrow bone is not involved in most of these ear infections. In the old days when infection got into the petrous apex where there was marrow, we could have osteomyelitis, but that is unusual. We don't see this in these cholesteatoma cases.

Now, my next point is that we must differentiate the three stages of cholesteatoma. The first is the skin-lined cavity or pocket, so situated that it cannot clean itself. This we have heard called a pre-cholesteatoma or we might say an inactive cholesteatoma pocket. Second, is the pocket filled with desquamated debris that is not yet infected? This is an active cholesteatoma, but not very active. Bone resorption is not yet a big factor because there is not the inflammation in the subepithelial connective tissue which is required for active bone resorption. Such an ear is dry. The third state is when the debris is infected, the ear discharges, and we have inflammation of the subepithelial connective tissue and the cholesteatoma actively and rapidly enlarges. This is the stage which of course we must try to control. Any comments on this differentiation of the three stages of cholesteatoma?

Dr. Jansen: No comments. I agree.

Dr. Palva: You left out the cholesteatoma that grows out of the basal cells from the Shrapnell's membrane. For instance, when you have just the inflammatory reaction in the middle ear and the basal cell starts to migrate, that certainly leads to cholesteatomas. I think this should be included.

Dr. Shambaugh: Thank you. I also did not mention the congenital cholesteatoma.

Dr. Smyth: I would agree in every way except maybe with your second stage in which you say that there is not much bone absorption. But it's been my experience that in patients who have a natural myringostapediopexy that very often you can see the long process slowly eroded and not in an ear whose anatomy is normal. This to me implies there has been resorption of bone in these cases but they're still dry and not infected.

Dr. Austin: It's very difficult to reconstruct the natural history of the disease when we see the end point only. In other words we try to look back and guess about it, but it is a disease which seems to me to be a continuum without interruption and I fail to see how you can divide it into parts. It's one

whole continuous dynamic process. I don't know about three "stages."

Dr. Shambaugh: Well, this is my concept, and I would like some more comments from the panel on this—that a cholesteatoma which is dry is relatively inactive. It may have a little debris in it. If it's perfectly clean it's completely inactive and harmless. I think you can divide it into three stages. The stage of inactivity which is what you strive to attain by treatment either through local treatment which was mentioned in the previous panel, by local cleaning of the ear or by surgery. Do you want to comment on that, Dave?

Dr. Austin: Well, you know it becomes inactive when the patient dies. When we're dealing with living, growing, abnormal tissue, I really don't quite accede to the thought that there is an inactive stage to this disease.

Dr. Shambaugh: I would like to take issue with that. I think during this conference it was stated rather repeatedly that the skin lining a cholesteatoma is skin. There is nothing mysterious or different about it than skin elsewhere. The only difference is its location. If the skin is not inflamed, if there is no infected debris upon it, why is it a progressive disease?

Dr. Palva: May I have here one word? The statement that we are dealing with skin is not correct. It was pointed out earlier that we are not dealing with skin because we don't have glands there, so that stratified squamous epithelium is different from skin, even from ear canal skin. I would venture the opinion that once you have a 1 cm cholesteatoma, even if it is totally dry, it is an advancing disease. Even though there is a promoter of this absorption which may be collagenase or other enzymes, we still have this factor that biologists call pressure characterization that is effective and which may cause slight advancement of the disease all the time the debris or cholesteatoma is there.

Dr. Shambaugh: Supposing there is no debris?

Dr. Palva: I think you are much safer if there is no debris, but if you have a sac, I wouldn't be happy with it. I would be watching this ear even if the sac would not be in contact with any bone.

Dr. Baron: May I say a word? I would like to agree with you, George. I disagree with the concept that once you have a cholesteatoma you go to your grave with it. We have seen many years of marsupialization of a cholesteatoma and the moisture and infection has gone. It may stay clean and healthy, not get larger.

Dr. Shambaugh: I'd like the first slide, please. We have heard Dr. Derlacki talk about his type of congenital cholesteatoma. This is the Cawthorne type of congenital cholesteatoma. This woman came to me with a history of a draining ear for many years, a facial paralysis of many years' duration which preceded the draining ear by three years, a dead ear on that side, no cochlear response and no caloric response. (Fig. 203). Next

slide. On your left hand side looking at the x-ray there you see the contrast medium introduced into the operative defect after I'd evacuated the cholesteatoma which reached to the petrous apex. (Fig. 204). The entire cochlea has been destroyed, the carotic artery lay exposed, the dura was widely exposed, and this cavity was filled with foul cho-

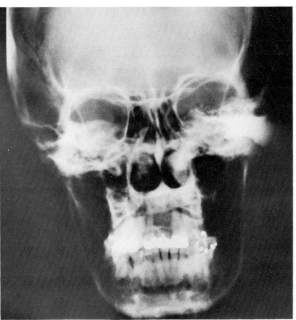

Fig. 204: X-ray of patient in Figure 203.

lesteatoma debris. All I did was to clean out the debris, open it widely to the outside so that I could gain access to it and keep it clean. I have kept it clean now for six years. She returns to see me about once every six months. I have her use Johnson's Baby Oil in the ear for four or five nights before she comes in. This is something I would recommend for a dry cholesteatoma pocket that you want to keep clean. This preparation is very effective in softening up the debris so that it comes out very easily. We use it also in our fenestration cavities. This was essentially a marsupialization. Now, why didn't we remove the matrix? It was unsafe to remove the matrix. We would possibly have gotten meningitis, injured the

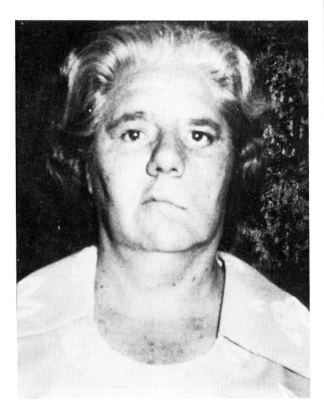

Fig. 203: Female with history of draining ear for many years, facial paralysis of many years' duration which preceded the draining ear by three years. Also the ear on that side was dead, had no cochlear response and no caloric response.

carotid artery or caused other problems even if we had been able to, and I doubt if we could have, removed the matrix down to the apex. So marsupialization made this a safe ear. It is a dry ear. I would agree with Shirley Baron that such an ear is effectively treated, maybe not ideally, but effectively. We otologists, and I include Shirley Baron with me in this, did many fenestrations in the old days, and we still follow these patients, many hundreds of them who must come back to have their ear cleaned. They have a large cavity lined by skin, by stratified squamous epithelium, and if you don't clean it out this cavity tends to fill with cholesteatoma debris. They essentially have an active cholesteatoma if they neglect it and don't come back for cleaning. Under this debris they develop granulation tissue, bone resorption, deep pockets in the tip of the mastoid, and may become a great problem. On the other hand, if you clean it out regularly, keep the ear cleaned of any debris, it remains inactive and harmless. Would you agree, Shirley, that these are essentially large cholesteatoma cavities?

Dr. Baron: Yes, I have four fenestration patients upon whom I've had to do surgery for cholesteatoma. They certainly can develop it, and there are a few that can develop it whether you keep them clean or not. I hate to say this but one of your own cases, George, had some cells up above the horizontal semicircular canal from which the debris was hard to clean and a cholesteatoma developed which required surgery.

Dr. Shambaugh: I saw the same, usually in the mastoid tip, where the epithelium grew in and I wasn't able to keep it clean and had to do surgery. Fortunately, these cases are unusual.

Dr. Palva: Dr. Shambaugh, may I have a word here? I don't think that you used the right expression if you were referring to the fenestration cavity as cholesteatoma cavities. I count myself in that generation also. I do see quite a number of these cases and I think it an entirely different situation. You have a healthy epidermis in these cavities and you have very little debris to remove. Some, in fact, are self-cleansing. On occasion

there are some cells that get infected, they break down and you may get a cholesteatoma-like situation where you have keratin accumulating. Well, we remove just the surface and it heals. Nothing more needs to be done. So I think there is a total difference between cholesteatoma epithelium and this stratified skin type that covers the fenestration cavity. I do not agree at all.

Dr. Shambaugh: How about a Bondy operation where you leave the matrix? I have had a number of these that I have followed through the years and they act exactly like the fenestration cavity. No difference.

Dr. Palva: I take your word that they behave in the same way. If they behave in that way, that means they don't form keratin in the amount that they are forming in the cholesteatoma situation. I still think there are some biochemical things that we don't understand that tells the basal cells and then the maturing cells in the granular cell layer to form much, much more keratin than ordinarily would be the case. We are far from knowing really what are the messages to the granular cell layer that regulate the amount of keratin.

Dr. Baron: When you talk about the Bondy operation, when you are doing a modified radical, whether or not you preserve the matrix, if you do not lower the bone over the facial ridge to the level of the ear canal, you will develop a pocket which will be very troublesome. This is a word of warning. When you do this surgery, please remember this point in technique.

Dr. Palva: I agree.

Dr. Shambaugh: The topic of this panel is on the principles governing cholesteatoma surgery. So far we've talked just about general principles. First of all I think I should mention something about the terminology of cholesteatoma, primary acquired versus secondary acquired. I started otology in an era before antibiotics when I was on the staff of the Municipal Contagious Disease Hospital in Chicago and would do five or six mastoidectomies a week on children with scarlet fever. Some of these children had the necrotizing type of otitis media which led to a large or total perforation and eventually cholesteatoma. The mucosa of the middle ear in these cases sloughed and in the healing process, skin grew in from the canal. These are secondary acquired cholesteatomas because they are secondary to an acute infection. The primary acquired is the type which develops in the perfectly normal ear as a result of an attic retraction. I think perhaps we should also include as a sub type that which occurs in a chronic secretory otitis, where the posterior superior quadrant is sharply retracted and we get a pocket and eventual cholesteatoma. The congenital cholesteatoma is the type which is from an epidermal rest. Facial paralysis may be the first symptom.

We see cases of extensive cholesteatoma in small children. These may be congenital, I don't know. They can occur in cellular mastoids and they may be congenital. Do the panel members have any ideas on this? Cholesteatosis in children?

Dr. Baron: I don't think that most of them are congenital. Most of them are due to the development of a purulent otitis media. There is some property of bone in children that makes it possible for a cholesteatoma to develop very rapidly. For instance, in the patient I spoke of in which I put tubes in both ears and one developed a purulent otitis media, a cholesteatoma developed within ten months. Perhaps it is the property of the softness of the bone which may be basically due to stimulation by infection.

Dr. Shambaugh: Any other comments on childhood cholesteatosis?

Dr. Smyth: One of the difficulties we have is with the ones which one sees developing in the posterior pocket of the tympanic membrane. Frequently enough, if you are observing the child over a period of time you can watch the development of the disease and I wouldn't suspect that these have a congenital basis. I think the matter is rather different with those that occur behind Shrapnell's membrane. I don't think I ever see these in very young children before they have actually developed a perforation or a retraction. I think it would be impossible for me to say in those cases whether they originated in the middle ear space or occurred because of an ingrowing of the epithelium from the outside in.

Dr. Palva: Well, I have the impression that these are not really congenital and I think that they do not develop from these retraction pockets in the posterior inferior area either. I think in these cases we have, again, the same pathogenesis starting from the basal cells. Once you have inflammatory reaction in the middle ear you get the mucosal lining from the inner side of the tympanic membrane away and you get a break in the basement membrane. Then basal cells start to proliferate into that inflammatory connective tissue and there is cholesteatoma developing behind them in that drum. Many people say this is then congenital disease, but it is acquired.

Dr. Shambaugh: That would be the metaplasia theory that Sadé proposed?

Dr. Palva: No, this would be the Ruedi theory.

Dr. Austin: You made a very important point just before that which was a source of confusion for many of us younger otologists. That is the first time I ever heard exactly the definition of secondary acquired cholesteatoma from you and I must say that I believe and I know for a fact that many of us refer to the atelectatic posterior superior pocketing as a secondary acquired cholesteatoma. Perhaps we need three terms or a subset as you suggest.

Dr. Shambaugh: The true secondary acquired cholesteatoma is almost unknown now in our country. I think that perhaps in undeveloped parts of the world where they have no antibiotics nor good nutrition, etc, you might see it, but not in our country.

We come to the principles governing cholesteatoma surgery. I have been very impressed at this and other conferences at the increasing number of canal-up operations which are found to have cholesteatoma residue or recurrence as years go by. Now, in this conference the difference between a recurrence and a residue is not too clear. As a matter of fact, a number of authors said they couldn't be sure whether it was a recurrence or a residue. The fact is that these patients after canal-up operations were found later on to have cholesteatoma, so they still had their disease. Cody's statistics were very fine: on the basis of four years or longer follow-up, 35% had cholesteatomas that either recurred or were residual. When he used the open cavity technique, the old-fashioned radical mastoid which I still think is an excellent operation, or the Bondy operation, open cavity technique, there were only 6% recurrent cholesteatomas. There is a very great difference in the incidence of persistent disease if you do a closed cavity technique. Gordon Smyth reports 16% failures to eradicate disease by the canal-up technique. Palva uses the canal wall down open cavity which he then obliterates with a pedicle facial muscle graft, with only 2% failure to eradicate disease. Now, is this correct, Dr. Palva?

Dr. Palva: Yes.

Dr. Shambaugh: So he has the best statistics of all as far as getting rid of disease is concerned. He takes the wall down. His hearing results were not bad but not spectacular. I compare his hearing results in my notes with those of Dr. Wright. Wright recognized the frequency of cholesteatoma disease either continuing or recurring with the canal-up technique and reexplores every case two years later. He finds residual cholesteatoma. He calls it residual; now, whether it's residual or recurrence, I'm not certain. He reported 15%. In every one of these cases Dr. Wright reported the ear was clinically free from disease and the patient was without symptoms. He estimates that most of these would not have developed symptoms for another six to 12 years because of the slow growth of this cholesteatoma. I was greatly impressed by Dr. Wright's questionnaire that he has his patients complete before they are operated upon. The patient understands exactly what's going on, why it is being done, they have a choice between a radical or a canal-up technique, and with the clear understanding that they must return in two years to have the ear reoperated and that it is their responsibility to do so. I think this is excellent. As a matter of fact, I'm going to ask him

to send me a copy of this. Dr. Austin, I was glad to see that you use a Bondy operation in a third of your patients with cholesteatoma. Now I say I was glad because I think the Bondy operation is still one of our best tympanoplasties. These are cases where the tympanic membrane is intact, the cholesteatoma is confined to the attic, you can evacuate the cholesteatoma, and leave the matrix if it's smooth and healthy looking. I take the matrix out nowadays, but it can be left. Do not touch the tympanic membrane where it is attached to the stapes, and these patients can have normal hearing after this operation.

Bellucci had a high incidence of residual or recurrent cholesteatoma with the canal-up technique, and a low incidence with an open cavity. So in summary it seems to me quite clear that if your primary aim is to get rid of disease, the open cavity radical or Bondy modified radical should be done. If you want to improve upon cavity size, use Palva's method of obliteration. If your primary aid is to improve hearing, the canal-up technique can be used but the second look is mandatory one or two years later. Now, I would like some comments.

Dr. Jansen: We did many Bondy operations, Dr. Shambaugh, but I think to cover the attic perforation with cartilage and to cover the cartilage with fascia and put the skin on top to close the perforation in our experience worked out better than the Bondy operation. So I think there is a potential risk of getting another retraction pocket which is going into the tip of the mastoid. It could be a nice change to do a Bondy and cover the attic perforation with cartilage.

Dr. Shambaugh: That's getting a smaller ear canal. Dr. Palva?

Dr. Palva: Well, Dr. Shambaugh, I think your conclusions were quite right and I agree with all you said. I am primarily concerned with the safety of the ear, that's what I always explain to the patient before I operate. That's why I do the radical mastoid surgery first. Then I reconstruct, but before I reconstruct I have the old-fashioned radical mastoid surgery done. I have sometimes intended to do the canal-up technique which I of course do in a way, if there is no cholesteatoma, but I have not been able to convince myself that this has been sufficient surgery to free the patient of disease. Of course, when you talk about hearing results, the anatomy of the radical mastoidectomy is not as good for hearing reconstruction, and not as easy if you have the canal wall in place, I quite agree. Then you have to take many other factors into account, too. One thing that is often not considered is that we are operating for the most part on patients who have one normal ear. It does not matter too much if your hearing result is 30 dB or 40 dB or even 20 dB because that ear is inferior anyway. That patient, at least in my country, appreciates much more a safe ear than an ear that we must have a second look at. If I tell every patient that now we will operate and in two years we will operate again, he will go to seek another doctor.

Dr. Shambaugh: This second look idea has never appealed to me in the first place. We have a very mobile population in the Chicago area. Our patients are always moving to California or to Florida and if we tell a patient he must come back in two years and be reoperated the chances are fifty-fifty they will be many miles away and won't come back. Secondly, consider human frailty. How many of your patients go to their dentists regularly twice a year, simply because the dentist says they must have their teeth checked? They don't. They go when they have a toothache. As to their ears, if they are having no symptoms one could never be certain the patient would return, submit to an anesthetic, be in the hospital, be cut into for the nebulous possibility that there may be some trouble there. It doesn't appeal to me. Possibly when we have the lawyers after us for unnecessary surgery we'll find ourselves being sued for operating some of these cases that have nothing wrong with their ears. There are many aspects of this that I don't like personally. Now, I'd like some comments from Dr. Smyth on this because he does the second look technique.

Dr. Smyth: I would like to say a number of things about this, Dr. Shambaugh, very very briefly.

First, yesterday I was only reporting what you might term an experiment. It was an evaluation of a number of those types of operations. The purpose of the report was to invite information. Maybe I should also have reported my experience with Professor Palva's operation, as I have had a great deal of experience with this also. I was very disappointed when I found I had such a high incidence in my sample—it was 23%. I only knew about 9% overall, but I suspect in due course there is quite a chance that the incidence of residual disease in all my patients would go to that high figure. It's all right for me to carry out this operation in my own closed community where there are no other ear doctors and there is nowhere else they can go, and under the present political and social conditions. I wouldn't like it to be thought that my paper yesterday suggested that I necessarily would advise everyone to do a two-stage combined approach—far from it. Under certain situations, the second operation would be highly inadvisable for the reasons you have mentioned.

Professor Palva has indicated that he sacrifices something in terms of functional improvement and certainly this is a very important consideration for me because 63% of my children have bilateral cholesteatoma. In this last survey in which I went back over the 15 years' experience I discovered to my pleasure that the majority of patients with the Palva operation in whom the stapes were missing, my reconstructed chain with a cartilage stuck between the footplate and the deep surface of the tympanic membrane produced results which were better in terms of closing the gap to 10 dB or less. These differences were strongly significant. So I think that if you can be prepared to find another method of ossicular reconstruction, you may find the hearing results are better.

Dr. Palva: May I comment here? Those slides I showed were from a period in my life that I regret. The reconstruction was done with a stainless steel wire prosthesis in the middle ear. I don't do that anymore. I quite agree with Gordon that hearing results are no worse with this operation, but I was experimenting with the stainless steel wire reconstruction. That wasn't a good method and I have said it several times.

Dr. Shambaugh: Now, I'd like to ask Dr. Baron to comment on what I've said because I think he agrees with me.

Dr. Baron: I do and I'd like to say that the reports in this meeting have vindicated my prediction at the time of your first Chicago meeting that someday all those doing the intact canal wall technique would come up with higher recurrences. That's exactly what's happened at this meeting, and I think if there is another meeting the percentages of recurrences will be even higher.

Dr. Shambaugh: Do you want to say anything, Dr. Austin?

Dr. Austin: Yes, because I have a little different point of view. If I could remind Shirley, he predicted a high percentage of residual disease, not recurrent disease, because we didn't know that pocketing was such a factor in those days. We discovered that later. Lest we go away thinking that we should all do modified radical operations, I find that their criteria are seldom encountered in cholesteatoma surgery. Those modified radicals were modified radicals with tympanoplastic reconstruction which is a little different thing. I look at the statistics reported here a little differently. It seems that every author reporting recurrence or residual disease reported the high incidence and in the tympanum, either epitympanum or mesotympanum. I fail to see how the modified radical changes this incidence of recurrence. As a matter of fact, in my written report I found 22% residual disease in these people who had had modified radical surgery done. So I don't think the modified radical is any safer a procedure than is the intact canal wall. I have never seen a life-threatening complication following an intact canal wall procedure because fortunately this disease has the ability to erode bone and erode the canal wall and thus exteriorize itself naturally. I don't advocate or tell others to do primarily a

modified radical, nor do I like to do it. The modified radical is my second stage procedure. I think that first attempts should be to preserve the canal wall, and upon seeing recurrence, then a modified radical can be done with more safety because then you not only prevent recurrence but you do get a second look at the middle ear to control the residual disease. I think perhaps my statistics were misinterpreted on presentation because my 30% at that time was a happenstance and it's not what I'm doing at the present time.

Dr. Shambaugh: There are two more topics which deserve brief mention. The tubal problem was emphasized several times during this week, especially by Bellucci. I think that Sade' also emphasized it. Certainly the incompetent eustachian tube is a tremendously important factor in the retraction cholesteatomas which we're seeing more of nowadays than we used to. I believe that the allergic factor in these children is extremely important and unless the otolaryngologist or the otologist learns how to manage these cases himself, he won't get anywhere by sending them to the general allergist. Now, in allergy, there are two opposing schools of thought—one the Rinkle School, which was developed from Hansel, the otolaryngologic allergist, whose concept is quite different from those of the general allergists in our big universities. Rinkle's methods work on these children most effectively. Dr. Derlacki rarely tubes his children patients with secretory otitis because he is able to cure them with allergic management. Interesting to me was the incidence of tubal problems and cholesteatoma in cleft palate children. These children get milk into their middle ear when they try to drink milk because of their problem, and then they develop an allergy. Milk allergy is extremely important to recognize in children with ear problems. Unless you are alert to allergic problems and know how to diagnose and treat them, you'll miss them entirely. I would urge the younger men here who are interested in ear disease to learn the Rinkle method of treatment. They'll be very pleased with the results obtainable.

I want to ask one final question of the panel. What type of operation do you do in a small child with extensive cholesteatosis? Do you do a canal-up technique or do you do something different? Dr. Jansen?

Dr. Jansen: I would do the technique of posterior tympanotomy to get out the disease and follow the child. I think it's much better to do it this way; otherwise, we have maybe later to reconstruct the posterior bony canal wall. We have very good results doing this.

Dr. Shambaugh: Dr. Palva.

Dr. Palva: May I first make a short comment upon allergy, because I do second you very strongly and I urge the ENT people to get more into these allergic problems. We are doing at the present time a large scale study of secretory otitis media. As Dr. Shambaugh pointed out, milk is the chief offender. When you really study some hundreds of children, you come up with figures that show milk, weed, tomatoes are really the factors that take a toll of these patients. Once you correct this, then you have a healthy child.

Now back to the question of how to handle big cholesteatoma in a child. Without hesitation, I would perform a classic radical mastoidectomy and put down my graft to cover the posterior sigmoid sinus area and the antrum and have the skin grow on top of that. That healed canal would not be much wider than the ordinary ear canal in a child.

Dr. Smyth: My personal method with children is to do a staged intact canal wall tympanoplasty—for a number of reasons. I refer to the hearing in the Palva operation and although it's better when the crura are missing, it's significantly worse with other reconstructive methods. As I said earlier, 63% of my children patients have bilateral cholesteatoma so the hearing aspects are very important in this group. I think that intact canal wall tympanoplasty is getting a bit of a battering this morning. I think we must not ignore the fact that it's a very useful operation. In my experience, over a third of the patients do not have cholesteatoma, but generalized granulation tissue disease, which is very effectively treated by this method. I hope we won't go away thinking that it's an operation with no future. I can't believe that.

Dr. Baron: In the presence of a cholesteatoma I use the open technique. I try to do a modified radical; if not, I do a radical with a tympanoplasty.

Dr. Austin: After telling the parents the dire prognosis in this kind of condition—which I think is very dire—I will probably embark on a series of multiple operations, the first of which will be an intact canal wall procedure.

Dr. Shambaugh: This completes our panel and I thank all of our panelists and all of our participants in the audience for their superb cooperation in one of the best meetings ever held.

SUMMARY AND CONCLUSIONS

Brian F. McCabe, M.D.
Jacob Sadé, M.D.
Maxwell Abramson, M.D.

At the beginning, a definition of cholesteatoma was attempted in biological as well as clinical terms. Cholesteatoma is not simply skin in the wrong place, but a three dimensional epidermoid structure exhibiting independent growth, displacing or replacing middle ear mucosa, resorbing underlying bone, and tending to recur after removal. This biological definition of cholesteatoma permits a more abstract discussion so biological models may be used by scientists in the application of a new understanding of the disease. Important are growth control as related to control of mitosis in skin, differentiation of cells under various influences as related to metaplasia, competition in the interphase between different epithelia in terms of cell surface properties, wound healing as a model for cell movement, epithelial mesenchymal interactions, and other factors influencing patterns of cell migration, to name some.

There appears to be a definite relationship between the inability for self-cleansing in a cholesteatoma as compared to canal skin, with the promotion of a subepithelial inflammatory reaction. The inflammatory connective tissue promotes bone resorption through decalcification followed by sequential enzymatic breakdown of bone matrix. While osteoclasts are capable of resorbing bone under normal conditions, the evidence is that localized bone resorption can occur from inflammatory connective tissue, the action of cells "turned on" by inflammation. This inflammatory connective tissue while always present under the epithelium of cholesteatoma is also present in chronic otitis media without cholesteatoma. No evidence was evinced that stratified squamous epithelium of itself had any destructive or noxious properties.

Ten experienced otologic surgeons presented their longest term results available on different operative techniques, especially including "closed cavity" techniques. This series of presentations entitled "Tell Me About Your Failures!" was followed by a panel discussion among them which engendered a considerable difference of opinion indicating that we are far from the final word. Indeed, there is evidence we may be in some state of regression from the enthusiastic acceptance of the "canal up" mastoidectomy of the past decade. At the same time, in presentations on rates of complication, it is evident that not only have complications from cholesteatomatous disease in itself dropped dramatically from earlier years, but "canal up" procedures do not seem to have been attendant with any reversal of this trend. Circumscribed mastoiditis (positive fistula test) is by far the most common complication today, excluding progressive conductive deafness. The two most noteworthy features of this part of the conference were, (a) there is a definite need for longer followup in these newer operations for adequate evaluation, and (b) at least a few surgeons voiced willingness to give them up.

Epidemiologic studies point out that ethnic groups with a high rate of central perforations (Eskimos, Indians) do not have a disproportionately high cholesteatoma rate, whereas groups with a high rate of eustachian tube "insufficiency" (cleft palate patients) do. Moreover, cholesteatoma patients have a higher rate of eustachian tube "insufficiency" than noncholesteatoma patients, it appears from existing work, admitting the comparatively primitive state of the art. Other studies seem to establish at least a frequently genetically established mastoid hypocellularity, a feature of this disease chronically underestimated in terms of middle ear aerodynamics.

The three theories of genesis of cholesteatoma, viz., migration, congenital, and metaplastic, were presented and discussed in detail. The concensus is that most are due to epithelial migration, some are certainly congenital, and some may be due to metaplasia.

While it was evident that most otologists today view cholesteatoma as a purely surgical disease, it is evident that selected patients are best served by office management. Further, there may be a new form of medical management (without to date suitable controls or long term followup) which could be revolutionary in cholesteatoma management: topical vitamin A therapy (New Zealand). Plans were laid for the evaluation of this modality multinationally.

We have made an auspicious new beginning in understanding the pathophysiology and treatment of this disease. At the same time it is evident that we have raised many more questions than we have answered. Perhaps the greatest yield of the conference was in bringing the expertise and interest of our colleagues in basic science to bear on our problem. Future such conferences we hope will extend this, and through mutual effort result in the eradication of this disease.

INDEX OF CONTRIBUTORS

INDEX